Clinical Decision-Making Study Guide for

Medical-Surgical Nursing
Patient-Centered Collaborative Care

Seventh Edition
Revised Reprint

Donna D. Ignatavicius, MS, RN, ANEF

Speaker and Curriculum Consultant for
Academic Nursing Programs
Founder, Boot Camp for Nurse
Educators®
President, DI Associates, Inc.
Placitas, New Mexico

M. Linda Workman, PhD, RN, FAAN

Senior Volunteer Faculty
College of Nursing
University of Cincinnati
Cincinnati, Ohio;
Formerly Gertrude Perkins Oliva
Professor of Oncology
Frances Payne Bolton School of Nursing
Case Western Reserve University
Cleveland, Ohio

Clinical Decision-Making Study Guide prepared by

Patricia Conley, MSN, RN

Staff Nurse
Cardio-Pulmonary Telemetry/PCU
Research Medical Center
Kansas City, Missouri

Donna Rose, MSN, RN

Senior Lecturer
School of Nursing
Old Dominion University
Norfolk, Virginia

Amy H. Lee, MSN, RN

Senior Lecturer
School of Nursing
Old Dominion University
Norfolk, Virginia

ELSEVIER
SAUNDERS

ELSEVIER
SAUNDERS

3251 Riverport Lane
Maryland Heights, Missouri 63043

CLINICAL DECISION-MAKING STUDY GUIDE FOR
MEDICAL-SURGICAL NURSING:
Patient-Centered Collaborative Care, Seventh Edition
Revised Reprint   ISBN: 978-1-4557-7565-1

Notice

Knowledge and best practice in this field are constantly changing. As new research and experience broaden our knowledge, changes in practice, treatment and drug therapy may become necessary or appropriate. Readers are advised to check the most current information provided (i) on procedures featured or (ii) by the manufacturer of each product to be administered, to verify the recommended dose or formula, the method and duration of administration, and contraindications. It is the responsibility of the practitioner, relying on their own experience and knowledge of the patient, to make diagnoses, to determine dosages and the best treatment for each individual patient, and to take all appropriate safety precautions. To the fullest extent of the law, neither the Publisher nor the Authors assume any liability for any injury and/or damage to persons or property arising out of or related to any use of the material contained in this book.

The Publisher

Nursing Diagnoses—Definitions and Classification 2012-2014. Copyright © 2011, 2009, 2007, 2005, 2003, 2001, 1998, 1996, 1994 by NANDA International. Used by arrangement with Wiley-Blackwell Publishing, a company of John Wiley and Sons, Inc. In order to make safe and effective judgments using NANDA-I nursing diagnoses it is essential that nurses refer to the definitions and defining characteristics of the diagnoses listed in the work.

Executive Content Strategist: Lee Henderson
Senior Content Development Specialist: Rae L. Robertson
Senior Project Manager: Jodi Willard
Publishing Services Manager: Debbie Vogel

Printed in the United States of America

Last digit is the print number: 9 8 7 6 5 4 3 2 1

Preface

The *Clinical Decision-Making Study Guide* is a companion publication for Ignatavicius & Workman's *Medical-Surgical Nursing: Patient-Centered Collaborative Care, 7*th Edition. This Study Guide, written by experts in the fields of adult medical-surgical nursing and nursing education, will help to ensure mastery of the textbook content and help you learn about collaborative practice in the care of the adult medical-surgical patient.

The 7th edition has been carefully revised and updated for an increased emphasis on clinical decision-making, and the use of Case Studies has been expanded.

The overall organization of the *Clinical Decision-Making Study Guide* directly corresponds to the unit/chapter name and number in the textbook so that you or your instructor can readily select the corresponding learning exercises in the Study Guide. Chapters are organized by the following sections:

- **Study/Review Questions** are designed to encourage prioritizing, clinical decision-making, and application of the steps of the nursing process. Questions have been updated to focus on the question formats of the NCLEX Examination, and emphasize the NCLEX priorities of delegation, management of care, and pharmacology.
- Additional "real-world" **Case Studies** are included in this edition, along with the addition of documentation-focused questions, allowing you to further develop your decision-making and charting abilities in a variety of clinical situations.

Answers to the Study/Review Questions are provided in the back of the Study Guide. Answer guidelines for the Case Studies are available on your Evolve website at http://evolve.elsevier.com/Iggy/ in the "Prepare for Class" folder. Each chapter's Case Studies can also be downloaded and completed as a word processing file, if preferred.

The Evolve website also features an introductory "pre-chapter" that includes concrete study tips to help you make the most of your individual learning style.

The *Clinical Decision-Making Study Guide* is a practical tool to help you prepare for classroom examinations and standardized tests, as well as a review for clinical practice. This improved format will help you review and apply medical-surgical content and help you prepare for the NCLEX Examination.

Contents

1 CHAPTER

Introduction to Medical-Surgical Nursing

STUDY/REVIEW QUESTIONS

1. The Institute of Medicine report *To Err Is Human* highlighted the need to improve patient safety. Which national organization requires its accredited agencies to meet specific national patient safety goals?
   a. National Hospital Council
   b. *Healthy People 2020*
   c. National Patient Safety Foundation
   d. The Joint Commission

2. What is the purpose of the Rapid Response Team (RRT)?
   a. Provide Code Blue teams in case of simultaneous emergencies
   b. Enable the nurse to recognize changes in patient status before an acute emergency
   c. Replace immediate consultation with the physician or medical resident
   d. Comprise teams of staff already familiar with the patient's medical diagnosis

3. In addition to being able to provide care with skill in techniques and procedures, what must the medical-surgical nurse also be prepared to utilize when caring for the patient? *(Select all that apply.)*
   a. Teaching
   b. Patient advocacy
   c. Spiritual counseling and support
   d. Rehabilitation strategies and methods
   e. Administrative scheduling and budgeting
   f. Coordination of care

4. Which factors are likely to be causes of medical errors? *(Select all that apply.)*
   a. Lack of technical experience
   b. Overload of information
   c. Poor communication
   d. Maliciousness and criminal intent
   e. Failure to follow accepted facility practices

5. Which is the best way for the nurse to assess the patient's learning after teaching?
   a. Have the patient write a summary of the points covered.
   b. Ask the patient to repeat the information back.
   c. Quiz the patient on relevant points in the instruction.
   d. Repeat the important points to the patient.

6. Which type of evidence is rated highest on a Level of Evidence scale?
   a. Well-designed case control with cohort studies
   b. Randomized trials of small descriptive studies
   c. Well-designed controlled trials without randomization
   d. Systematic review or meta-analysis of all randomized controlled trials

7. Which is the best use of information from electronic sources, such as websites or e-mail, in retrieving data for the evidence-based practice process?
   a. Being sure to include links to articles so the reader can follow up on subsequent results
   b. Evaluating the information for credibility and reliability before putting it into use
   c. Using only university-related sources to ensure the most current results
   d. Assessing the number of hits the sources have on a search engine to determine popularity

8. Which action exemplifies the goal of case management in an acute care setting?
   a. Making sure the patient's dietary choices meet prescribed nutritional needs
   b. Scheduling home visits after discharge and monitoring patient progress
   c. Monitoring the patient's vital signs and noting trends of elevations
   d. Reviewing the patient's hospital bill for accuracy and any excessive charges

9. Which actions best demonstrate a collaborative nursing function? *(Select all that apply.)*
   a. Requesting the assistance of another staff member to turn a patient
   b. Administering medications as prescribed by the health care provider
   c. Maintaining patient confidentiality by not notifying the family members of a change in the patient's condition
   d. Making a referral to the case manager to assist with discharge planning
   e. Ensuring clear communication with other health care providers

10. Which occurrence does the Joint Commission's National Patient Safety Goals designate as a high-risk issue?
   a. Health care workers' exposure to infectious diseases in the workplace
   b. Violating privacy considerations of patients' confidential information
   c. Administering medication that is not familiar to the nurse
   d. Failure to review patients' food allergies before serving meals

2

CHAPTER

Introduction to Complementary and Alternative Therapies

STUDY/REVIEW QUESTIONS

1. Which are ways that the National Center for Complementary and Alternative Medicine advances scientific research? *(Select all that apply.)*
   a. Provides funding for research examining the effectiveness of complementary therapies
   b. Makes complementary therapies available to certain patients
   c. Provides patient handouts on the benefits of complementary medicine
   d. Investigates and evaluates efficacy of complementary therapies, and ensures that this information is available to health care professionals
   e. Acts as a clearinghouse for information about complementary therapies

2. Which therapies have been identified as complementary and alternative domains by the National Center for Complementary and Alternative Medicine? *(Select all that apply.)*
   a. Cognitive behavioral therapies
   b. Mind-body therapies
   c. Manipulative and body-based therapies
   d. Biologically based therapies
   e. Energy therapies

Matching. *Match the education that the nurse should provide to the patient with the herbal preparations listed below.*

Herbal Preparation
a. Ginkgo biloba
b. Saw palmetto
c. Garlic
d. Glucosamine sulfate
e. Ginseng

Education

_____ 3. May potentiate antidiabetic drugs; may cause bleeding when used with antiplatelet drugs

_____ 4. Discontinue use 2 weeks before surgery; may inhibit platelet aggregation

_____ 5. May take several weeks of use before effectiveness noted; may cause GI upset, so take with meals

_____ 6. Use carefully with anticoagulant therapy because bleeding may occur

_____ 7. Monitor INR if used when taking warfarin

8. For what purposes might imagery be used? *(Select all that apply.)*
   a. Decrease pain
   b. Lessen fatigue
   c. Reduce nausea
   d. Promote arousal
   e. Decrease anxiety

9. What are the benefits of massage therapy? *(Select all that apply.)*
   a. Produces patient relaxation
   b. Eliminates bruising with injury
   c. Lessens aggressive behaviors in patients with dementia
   d. Reduces pain
   e. Eliminates the need for drug therapy

10. The nurse prepares to give a massage to an older adult who has been bedridden for 3 days. When the patient's back is exposed, the nurse notes an area of redness on the sacrum that is about 6 cm in diameter. What is the best action for the nurse to take?
    a. Massage the area vigorously using long, flowing strokes.
    b. Massage the area with rhythmic stroking using light touch.
    c. Avoid massaging over an area of skin that is reddened or bruised.
    d. Use rapid, continuous strokes while massaging.

11. Which statements about aromatherapy are true? *(Select all that apply.)*
    a. Aromatherapy involves the use of essential oils to stimulate the sense of smell.
    b. Essential oils may be applied in compresses, used in baths, or applied to the skin.
    c. Because essential oils are natural, they do not need to be diluted before being applied topically.
    d. Lavender has been used for stimulation and to promote concentration.
    e. Rose oil has been used to promote relaxation and sleep.
    f. Allergies should be assessed before using essential oils.

12. A patient is using herbal preparations in their health care regimen. What safety education information should the nurse relay to the patient? *(Select all that apply.)*
    a. "Make sure you discuss your use of herbal preparations with your health care provider."
    b. "You should use reliable sources of information regarding herbal preparations."
    c. "Continue to visit your health care provider as recommended to ensure that your use of herbal preparations do not make you overlook a problem with your health."
    d. "Herbal preparations are wonderful; you may take them as the need arises."
    e. "All herbal preparations are manufactured at the same strength."

13. The patient has been diagnosed with chronic pain. Before suggesting that the patient try meditation as a pain management method, what must the nurse consider?
    a. The patient's personal preference and medical condition
    b. The patient's ability to ambulate
    c. Possible negative outcomes such as grief
    d. The patient's willingness to commit to meditation three times per day

14. The nurse is teaching the patient about massage therapy. Which statement by the patient demonstrates a correct understanding of the nurse's instruction?
    a. "Firm finger pressure is applied to certain points on the body."
    b. "After 5 minutes, a gentle tingling sensation is felt."
    c. "Massage is sometimes painful."
    d. "Using various stroke techniques will produce relaxation."

15. The patient is taking garlic to lower cholesterol levels. What information does the nurse provide to the patient about this herbal supplement?
    a. Blood glucose levels should be monitored when taking garlic.
    b. Look for unusual bleeding or bruising.
    c. Garlic is not effective in the capsule form.
    d. Avoid taking garlic with coffee, tea, or cola.

16. The nurse is caring for a patient who has antibiotic-associated diarrhea. The patient would like to begin probiotic therapy for this condition. What are the best responses about this therapy by the nurse? *(Select all that apply.)*
    a. "Probiotics may be found in yogurt."
    b. "This therapy may cause an increase in gas and abdominal bloating."
    c. "This therapy should be taken with meals."
    d. "It is not necessary to check with your health care provider before beginning therapy."
    e. "Probiotics are live microorganisms that may stabilize the GI mucosal barrier."

3 CHAPTER

Common Health Problems of Older Adults

STUDY/REVIEW QUESTIONS

1. Which statements about the health of older adults in the United States are true? *(Select all that apply.)*
   a. The fastest growing group is between 85 and 95 years of age.
   b. Only 5% of older adults are in nursing homes.
   c. Older adults are at risk for poor nutrition.
   d. Older adults 85-95 years old are often wrongly referred to as the "frail elderly."
   e. Men live longer than women.

2. The nurse is caring for an older adult patient. What are the best interventions to help reduce relocation stress in this patient? *(Select all that apply.)*
   a. Explain all procedures to the patient before they occur.
   b. Reorient the patient frequently to location.
   c. Allow for the patient to have adequate time for rest, and encourage family and friends to keep their visits to a minimum.
   d. Provide ample opportunity and time for the patient to participate in decision making.
   e. Arrange for familiar keepsakes to be at the patient's bedside.

3. Which statements would be included in an educational program on wellness behaviors for the older adult? *(Select all that apply.)*
   a. Allow at least 10 to 15 minutes of sun exposure 2 to 3 times weekly.
   b. Take one aspirin twice a day.
   c. Obtain a yearly influenza vaccination.
   d. Create a hazard-free environment to prevent falls.
   e. Increased dietary needs include calcium and vitamins A, D, and C.
   f. Reduce dietary intake of complex carbohydrates and fiber.
   g. Drink 6-8 glasses of water per day to prevent dehydration.

4. Which statement about how nutrition is affected in older adults is true?
   a. Changes in smell and taste can result in decreased use of sugar.
   b. Older adults need increased calorie intake to maintain ideal body weight.
   c. Loneliness and boredom may impact the older adult's incentive to eat.
   d. Obesity is the most common nutritional problem in nursing homes.

5. What are the direct benefits of exercise? *(Select all that apply.)*
   a. Decreases depression symptoms
   b. Reduces muscle strength
   c. Improves sleep apnea
   d. Increases mobility
   e. Decreases risk of heart disease
   f. Reduces or maintains body weight

6. Which assessment findings in the older adult indicate an increased risk for falls? *(Select all that apply.)*
   a. Increased mobility
   b. Macular degeneration
   c. Balance instability
   d. Full joint range of motion (ROM)
   e. Peripheral neuropathy

7. The nurse is caring for the confused older patient who is at risk for falls. Which interventions should the nurse implement to ensure patient safety? *(Select all that apply.)*
   a. Remind the patient to use ambulatory devices as needed.
   b. Instruct the patient to limit activity as much as possible.
   c. Provide appropriate lighting in the patient's environment.
   d. Make sure the patient's eyeglasses are functional, and routine eye examinations have been performed.
   e. Implement facility-specific fall protocols.

8. The patient requires physical restraints. Which interventions must the nurse perform for this patient? *(Select all that apply.)*
   a. Check the patient every 30 to 60 minutes.
   b. Release the restraints at least every 4 hours.
   c. Turn on the television to provide distraction.
   d. Place the patient in an area for careful observation.
   e. Decrease communication with the patient.

9. Which type of psychoactive drug requires the most careful monitoring by the nurse because of the drug's potential for causing confusion and incontinence?
   a. Tricyclic antidepressants
   b. Antipsychotics
   c. Antianxiety agents
   d. Sedative-hypnotics

10. Which factors must the nurse acknowledge and include in discharge education for the older adult about medication administration? *(Select all that apply.)*
    a. Suggest a simple type of reminder to take daily medications.
    b Ensure that medication labels have large print to assist patients with identification.
    c. Request easy-open caps for medication bottles and ensure that they remain out of reach for visiting children.
    d. Provide a complete list of the patient's regularly taken over-the-counter medications to health care providers.
    e. Alert health care providers if medication side effects are affecting the patient's ability to take his or her medications.

11. Which physiologic changes must the nurse teach the older adult who is taking medication to be aware of? *(Select all that apply.)*
    a. Oral drugs will be ineffective because of an age-related increase in GI motility.
    b. There may be an alteration in the ratio of adipose tissue to lean body mass which may affect the distribution of a drug.
    c. Decreased function of the liver may alter the metabolism of certain drugs.
    d. Altered kidney function may affect excretion of drugs causing increased plasma concentrations of drugs.
    e. Most older adults will not have any significant physiologic alterations.

12. Which interventions are effective in helping to reorient the older adult who is suffering from delirium? *(Select all that apply.)*
    a. Talk to the patient using a calm voice.
    b. Restrict visitors during periods of agitation.
    c. Remove personal items and store them safely.
    d. Apply wrist restraints to keep the patient from endangering himself or herself.
    e. Provide calming music.

13. Which symptoms of depression in older adults should be carefully evaluated by the health care provider? *(Select all that apply.)*
    a. Early morning insomnia
    b. Reluctance to participate in social activities
    c. Reminiscing about the past
    d. Normalization of appetite and intake
    e. Excessive daytime sleeping

14. In planning care for the older adult with dementia, the nurse identifies which intervention as the first priority goal of care?
    a. Prevent cognitive decline.
    b. Reorient on a regular basis.
    c. Prevent injury.
    d. Assist with ambulation.

15. Which statements regarding elder abuse are true? *(Select all that apply.)*
    a. The abuser is often a close family member or caregiver.
    b. Only physically dependent older adults are vulnerable to elder abuse.
    c. Elder neglect is categorized as a type of elder abuse.
    d. 700,000 to 1.2 million older adults suffer from elder abuse each year.
    e. There is a need for mandatory reporting laws for suspected elder abuse.

Matching. *Match the type of elder abuse with its definition.*

Types of Abuse
a. Neglect
b. Physical abuse
c. Financial abuse
d. Emotional abuse

Definitions
_____ 16. Mismanagement or misuse of an older patient's property or resources
_____ 17. Intentional use of threats, humiliation, intimidation, and isolation
_____ 18. Examples include hitting, burning, pushing, and molesting the patient
_____ 19. Failure to provide for basic needs, such as food and clothing

20. What are signs indicating that the older adult is experiencing dementia or delirium? *(Select all that apply.)*
    a. Temporary, acute confusion
    b Progressive loss of cognitive function
    c. Agitation, combative behavior
    d. Extreme violence
    e. Sudden onset of apathy, withdrawn behavior

Matching. *Match the terms with their definitions.*

Term
a. Fallophobia
b. Presbyopia
c. Polypharmacy
d. Nocturia

Descriptions
_____ 21. Urination at night
_____ 22. The use of multiple drugs
_____ 23. Psychological fear of falling in older adults
_____ 24. Farsightedness that worsens with aging

CASE STUDY: MEDICATION USE IN OLDER ADULTS

Use a separate sheet of paper to answer the questions in this Case Study, or go to the "Prepare for Class" folder on your Evolve website at http://evolve.elsevier.com/Iggy/ to download and complete as a word processing file. Answer guidelines for this Case Study are also available on your Evolve website.

An 80-year-old patient is brought to the emergency department (ED) after fainting at home. His serum digoxin level is 2.3 ng/mL. He is transferred to a medical-telemetry nursing unit. The next day the nurse asks the patient to tell her about his routine for taking his daily digoxin tablets. He states that he was told to check his pulse every morning before taking a pill. He does this in his kitchen because the clock on the wall has big numbers and he can see the second hand go around. The nurse asks him how long he measures his pulse. He replies "I keep counting the beats until I get to 60. Sometimes it takes a long time. Then I take my heart pill." Later he tells you that he hates "having so many pills to take" and admits having trouble remembering to take his pills. He states that he sometimes can't remember which pills to take with breakfast and which to take at night.

1. Identify two statements made by this patient that are a safety concern.
2. What specific pharmacokinetic factor should be considered when giving digoxin to an older adult?
3. What can the nurse suggest to assist this patient to take his multiple medications correctly?
4. Devise a teaching-learning plan to reteach this patient about taking digoxin at home.
5. Who should be included in the teaching session with this patient?
6. Discuss how the nurse can validate whether the teaching plan has been effective.

4 CHAPTER

Cultural Aspects of Health and Illness

STUDY/REVIEW QUESTIONS

Matching. Match the terms with the appropriate definitions.

Terms
a. Culture
b. Subculture
c. Cultural diversity
d. Cultural competence
e. Culture care accommodation
f. Cultural assessment
g. Cultural sensitivity
h. Transcultural nursing
i. Ethnocentrism

Definitions

_____ 1. Differences among people which may or may not be visible

_____ 2. The process of examining one's own feelings and experiences about diversity, and learning about specific cultural differences so that appreciation for the values and beliefs of others may be respected

_____ 3. An integrated pattern of human behavior which is learned and transmitted to succeeding generations that includes thought, speech, action, and artifacts

_____ 4. The judging of others through the exclusive lens of one's own cultural beliefs

_____ 5. An area of study and practice that focuses on the care, health, and illness patterns of people with similarities and differences in their cultural beliefs, values, and practices

_____ 6. Data collected or research conducted to learn about the culture of patients

_____ 7. The process through which one becomes respectful, appreciative, and sensitive to the values, beliefs, lifeways, practices, and problem-solving strategies of a patient's culture

_____ 8. Part of a larger culture of the patient

_____ 9. Professional actions and decisions that help people of a designated culture adapt to or negotiate with others for a beneficial or satisfying health outcome with professional care providers

10. What is the most important aspect of culture that the nurse must consider when caring for a patient?
    a. Language and dialect
    b. Religious practices
    c. Dietary needs
    d. Cultural shock

True or False? *Read each statement and write T for true or F for false in the blanks provided. If the statement is false, correct the statement to make it true.*

_____ 11. Cultural practices that should be included as part of a cultural assessment include nutrition, family roles, pregnancy and childbirth, death rituals, and spirituality.

_____ 12. Transcultural nursing focuses on the care, health, and illness patterns of people with various cultural beliefs, values, and practices.

_____ 13. In the 2008 census, minorities accounted for 31% of the total population in the United States.

_____ 14. All people within the same country have the same health care needs.

_____ 15. Garlic worn around the neck is thought to protect against cold and flu viruses in some cultures.

_____ 16. Pain is displayed the same way in all cultures.

17. How is "hypertension" referred to in some cultures?
    a. "High blood"
    b. "Low blood"
    c. "Hot blood"
    d. "Sour blood"

18. Which question or statement reflects the best way to consider a patient's religious or spiritual practice?
    a. "Do you have any dietary restrictions?"
    b. "Are you a Christian?"
    c. "Please tell me whether your religion allows you to accept blood products."
    d. "How can I help you in meeting any religious or spiritual needs you may have?"

19. Which are the most appropriate choices in selecting an interpreter for a patient who does not speak the same language as the nurse? *(Select all that apply.)*
    a. Using a friend or family member of the patient
    b. Using a health care team member
    c. Using a person from the community or a local university
    d. Using the mechanical interpretation method approved by the facility
    e. Accepting the patient's decision that he or she does not need an interpreter

20. The nurse is admitting an older adult who has cellulitis of her lower leg. The patient has been applying a homemade poultice to the leg for a week and refuses to remove it during the admission assessment. Which actions demonstrate that the nurse is sensitive to the patient's cultural beliefs? *(Select all that apply.)*
    a. Express understanding that the patient may feel the poultice will help the leg heal, and ask permission to remove it temporarily so that the leg may be assessed.
    b. Inform the health care provider that the patient will not remove the poultice.
    c. Ask the patient about the poultice and how it has worked for her.
    d. Tell the patient that the leg will not heal until the doctor's orders are followed.
    e. Discuss with the patient her past experiences using this type of poultice.

21. Which factors must the nurse be aware of when providing care to patients who are categorized as homeless? *(Select all that apply.)*
    a. They are a rapidly growing population.
    b. They may have mistrust of health care providers.
    c. There may be a language barrier.
    d. They all suffer from mental illness.
    e. They may have an inability to adhere to treatment due to their lack of permanent living space.

CASE STUDY: ASSESSMENT OF A CULTURE

Use a separate sheet of paper to answer the questions in this Case Study, or go to the "Prepare for Class" folder on your Evolve website at http://evolve.elsevier.com/Iggy/ to download and complete as a word processing file. Answer guidelines for this Case Study are also available on your Evolve website.

The hospital is opening an outreach clinic and has asked the nurse manager to help set it up. The clinic is located in a community with many recent immigrants from Guatemala.

1. What does the nurse need to know to be prepared to provide culturally appropriate care for the patients of this new clinic?

2. How will the nurse find that information?

3. How would the nurse address and work through issues related to spiritual beliefs that may be affecting a patient's condition?

4. What are some ways to ensure proper communication when working with the Guatemalan patients in this clinic?

5 CHAPTER

Pain: The Fifth Vital Sign

STUDY/REVIEW QUESTIONS

1. Which statements are true about the assessment of a patient's pain? *(Select all that apply.)*
   a. "Pain is a universal experience" means that it is experienced by all patients in the same way.
   b. Pain alters the quality of life more than any other single health-related problem.
   c. Over the years, there have been major advances in how pain is managed.
   d. Unrelieved and untreated pain is a major public health problem in the United States.
   e. The nurse's primary role in managing pain is to administer analgesics as ordered.

2. Which factors may affect a patient's perception of and response to pain? *(Select all that apply.)*
   a. Age
   b. Disease process
   c. Gender
   d. Sociocultural background
   e. Genetics

3. Which statement best describes the gate control theory?
   a. It is a complex phenomenon composed of sensory mechanisms located in the brain.
   b. Pain transmission is regulated by specialized cells located in the spinal column.
   c. Pain occurs because of increased sensitivity to painful stimuli.
   d. Perception of pain occurs by way of the stimulus transmitted directly to the brain.

4. Pain is a response caused by stimuli to the free nerve endings or receptors. What are these receptors called?
   a. Axons
   b. Fibers
   c. Nociceptors
   d. Endorphins

5. Which are body responses of acute pain? *(Select all that apply.)*
   a. Dilated pupils
   b. Diaphoresis
   c. Increased respirations
   d. Increased heart rate
   e. Decreased heart rate

6. The nurse is taking a health history of a patient who reports lower back pain for 10 months. How does the nurse categorize this pain?
   a. Acute pain
   b. Chronic cancer pain
   c. Non-cancer pain
   d. Somatic pain

7. Which characteristics pertain to somatic pain? *(Select all that apply.)*
   a. Sharp, burning or dull, aching, or cramping
   b. Diffuse, deep, and stabbing
   c. Painful numbness or shooting, burning, or fiery
   d. Poorly localized
   e. Skeletal muscle spasms
   f. Nerve compression
   g. Insertion site of wound drain
   h. Bladder spasms
   i. Pancreatitis
   j. Bony metastasis

8. Which characteristics pertain to neuropathic pain? *(Select all that apply.)*
   a. Sharp, burning or dull, aching, or cramping
   b. Diffuse, deep, and stabbing
   c. Painful numbness or shooting, burning, or fiery
   d. Poorly localized
   e. Skeletal muscle spasms
   f. Nerve compression
   g. Insertion site of wound drain
   h. Bladder spasms
   i. Pancreatitis
   j. Bony metastasis

9. Which characteristics pertain to visceral pain? *(Select all that apply.)*
   a. Sharp, burning or dull, aching, or cramping
   b. Diffuse, deep, and stabbing
   c. Painful numbness or shooting, burning, or fiery
   d. Poorly localized
   e. Skeletal muscle spasms
   f. Nerve compression
   g. Insertion site of wound drain
   h. Bladder spasms
   i. Pancreatitis
   j. Bony metastasis

10. Which statements are true about pain control barriers in an older adult patient? *(Select all that apply.)*
    a. Older adults tend to underreport pain.
    b. Pain perception increases with age.
    c. The pain assessment scales are inaccurate.
    d. Cognitive impairment limits reliable pain assessment.
    e. Barriers are caused by lack of participation from professional health care staff.
    f. Communication issues between the patient and caregivers do not cause barriers.

Matching. Match the type of pain with its source.

Source
a. Nerve fibers, spinal cord, and central nervous system
b. Skin, subcutaneous tissues, and musculoskeletal structures
c. Organs and the linings of the body cavities

Pain Type
_____ 11. Somatic pain
_____ 12. Visceral pain
_____ 13. Neuropathic pain

14. A patient reports a deep, poorly localized, cramping type of pain. These assessment findings indicate which type of pain?
    a. Somatic
    b. Psychosomatic
    c. Neuropathic
    d. Visceral

15. A patient reports a constant "achy" type of pain after abdominal surgery. This is an indication of which type of pain?
    a. Somatic
    b. Visceral
    c. Neuropathic
    d. Psychosomatic

Matching. For each of the characteristics listed, mark "AP" for acute pain, "CP" for chronic pain, or "B" for both.

Characteristics

AP = Acute pain

CP = Chronic pain

B = Both

Pain Description

_____ 16. Duration greater than 3 months

_____ 17. Intensity ranges from mild to severe

_____ 18. May be accompanied by anxiety and restlessness

_____ 19. May be accompanied by depression, fatigue, and decreased functional ability

_____ 20. Begins gradually and persists

_____ 21. Cause may be well-defined

_____ 22. Reversible

23. Which are physiologic responses that indicate a patient is experiencing pain? *(Select all that apply.)*
    a. Diaphoresis
    b. Restlessness
    c. Bradycardia
    d. Hypotension
    e. Bradypnea

24. What is the best type of pain scale to use for patients who have language barriers or reading problems, or for children?
    a. 0 to 10 numeric rating scale
    b. FACES (smile to frown)
    c. Verbal description scales
    d. No type of scale

25. Which therapies might be used for the relief of chronic pain? *(Select all that apply.)*
    a. Opioids
    b. NSAIDs
    c. Adjuvants
    d. Cutaneous stimulation
    e. Cognitive behavioral measures

26. The nurse monitors for gastric irritation, signs of bleeding, and bruising as side effects of which pain medications? *(Select all that apply.)*
    a. Aspirin (non-opioid analgesic, NSAID)
    b. Acetaminophen (non-opioid analgesic)
    c. Ibuprofen (non-opioid analgesic, NSAID)
    d. Morphine (opioid analgesic)
    e. Demerol (opioid analgesic)

27. A patient with chronic bone pain as a result of osteoarthritis or rheumatoid arthritis may be prescribed which agents? *(Select all that apply.)*
    a. Aspirin
    b. COX-2 inhibitor such as celecoxib (Celebrex)
    c. Opioid such as morphine
    d. Acetaminophen (Tylenol)
    e. NSAID such as ibuprofen (Motrin, Advil)

28. Which are advantages of the patient-controlled analgesia (PCA) method of medication administration? *(Select all that apply.)*
    a. It allows for a predetermined bolus.
    b. It maintains a constant level of pain relief.
    c. It diminishes patient anxiety by allowing patient control over administration.
    d. It eliminates the need for repeated injections.
    e. The patient needs no education for effectiveness.

29. Which drugs can cause life-threatening seizures, particularly in an older adult, because of an accumulation of toxic metabolites? *(Select all that apply.)*
    a. Ibuprofen (Advil, Motrin)
    b. Morphine
    c. Meperidine (Demerol)
    d. Acetaminophen (Tylenol)
    e. Codeine

30. A patient is prescribed morphine sulfate, an opioid analgesic, for pain. Which nursing interventions decrease the risk of constipation? *(Select all that apply.)*
    a. Give foods low in bulk and roughage.
    b. Instruct the patient to increase water consumption.
    c. Administer a stool softener every morning.
    d. Change the dose of the opioid.
    e. Encourage activity.

31. Which statements are true regarding the side effects of respiratory depression as a result of administering an opioid analgesic? *(Select all that apply.)*
    a. Respiratory depression develops when opioid tolerance occurs.
    b. Monitor for respiratory depression in patients receiving opioids by IV administration, especially monitor opioid-naive adults.
    c. The pain, stress, and anxiety experienced by the patient are potent respiratory stimulants that may override or negate the respiratory depression resulting from the drugs.
    d. Respiratory depression is less of a problem in the older adult.
    e. The drug used to reverse respiratory depression is known as naloxone (Narcan).
    f. A one-time dose of naloxone (Narcan) is all that is needed to reverse the effects of the opioid.
    g. Sedation will occur before opioid-induced respiratory depression.

32. Which statement about the adverse side effects of opioids is true?
    a. Bolus administration is less likely to produce central nervous system changes.
    b. Stimulants such as caffeine may counteract opioid-induced sedation.
    c. Opioid antagonists produce more respiratory depression than opioid agonists.
    d. Peripheral effects include vasoconstriction and elevated blood pressure.

Matching. *Match the definitions of physiologic sequelae associated with opioid use with their correct terms. Answers may be used more than once, and more than one term may apply to each sequela.*

Terms

a.   Physical dependency
b.   Tolerance
c.   Addiction

Physiologic Sequelae

_____ 33.   Persistent drug craving

_____ 34.   Withdrawal symptoms upon abrupt cessation

_____ 35.   Occurs in everyone who takes opioids over a period of time

_____ 36.   Gradual resistance to effect of the opioid

_____ 37.   Abuse for recreational purposes

_____ 38.   Higher doses needed to achieve pain relief

_____ 39.   A common fear in patients and health professionals

_____ 40.   Genetic, psychosocial, and environmental factors influence development

_____ 41.   Problem with amount of medication given to a patient with substance abuse

42.   The nurse may find the mnemonic PQRST a helpful guide for a thorough assessment of a patient's pain. Briefly identify what each of the letters in the mnemonic stands for.

P   _____

Q   _____

R   _____

S   _____

T   _____

43.   Which statements are true about the use of an epidural catheter for pain management? *(Select all that apply.)*

a.   It is an external catheter placed in the lumbar or thoracic region near the spinal cord.
b.   It is used for hospitalized patients with any type of postoperative pain.
c.   Morphine and hydromorphone (Dilaudid) may be used, along with a local anesthetic such as bupivacaine.
d.   The nurse monitors for nausea and vomiting, pruritus, and infection at the insertion site.
e.   Catheters are in place for a maximum of 12 to 24 hours.
f.   Urinary retention and weakness in the legs can occur.
g.   Pain assessments can be performed less frequently while receiving pain medications through epidural catheters.

44. Which nonpharmacologic therapies stimulate the skin and subcutaneous tissues to produce pain relief? *(Select all that apply.)*
    a. Massage
    b. Imagery
    c. Vibration
    d. Heat application
    e. Therapeutic touch

45. A patient using a transcutaneous electrical nerve stimulation (TENS) unit asks the nurse how it works to decrease pain. What is the best response?
    a. "It delivers an electric shock to relieve muscle tension."
    b. "Low voltage electrical currents are delivered to the painful area."
    c. "Endorphins are blocked, which inhibits pain transmission."
    d. "The nerves causing pain will swell, raising the pain threshold."

46. Which statement about the strategy of distraction is true?
    a. Distraction is effective for acute and chronic pain relief.
    b. Distraction directly influences the cause of pain.
    c. Distraction should be used instead of other pain control measures.
    d. Distraction alters the perception of pain.

Matching. *Match the action or use with the corresponding adjuvant analgesic.*

Adjuvant Analgesics
a. Topical preparations such as Biofreeze gel
b. Oral local anesthetics such as mexiletine (Mexitil)
c. Antianxiety agents such as clonazepam (Klonopin)
d. Antiepileptic drugs such as gabapentin (Neurontin)
e. Cannabinoids (medical marijuana)

Actions/Uses
_____ 47. Used for neuropathy associated with diabetes mellitus

_____ 48. Not currently available in all states, used primarily for chronic pain

_____ 49. Used for certain types of nerve injury pain

_____ 50. Used for electric, shocklike, continuous pain

_____ 51. Provides cryotherapy for muscle aches and pain

52. The nurse is teaching a patient about acupuncture as an alternative therapy for pain relief. Which statement by the patient indicates the nurse's teaching was effective?
    a. "Acupuncture is used for pain control and anesthetic purposes."
    b. "Acupuncture is commonly used to relieve pain and inflammation."
    c. "A local anesthetic is injected which decreases pain perception."
    d. "Needles are inserted into the body to temporarily deaden the nerve."

53. What is the drug category of choice for the treatment of mild to moderate bone pain?
    a. NSAIDs
    b. Opioids
    c. Anticonvulsants
    d. Antianxiety agents

Matching. Match the descriptions with their associated strategies for coping with pain. Answers may be used more than once.

Associated Strategies

a. Imagery
b. Relaxation
c. Hypnosis
d. Distraction

Descriptions

_____ 54. Massage

_____ 55. Deep-breathing exercises

_____ 56. Going for a walk

_____ 57. Mental experience of sensations or events

_____ 58. Altered state of consciousness

_____ 59. Focusing on pleasant or desirable feeling, sensation, or event

_____ 60. Losing an overall sense of reality

61. Which method would be the recommended route for controlling the pain of a hospice patient with cancer who is unable to take oral medication?
    a. Intramuscular injection
    b. Continuous subcutaneous infusion
    c. Sublingual tablet
    d. Transdermal patch

CASE STUDY: THE PATIENT WITH PAIN

Use a separate sheet of paper to answer the questions in this Case Study, or go to the "Prepare for Class" folder on your Evolve website at http://evolve.elsevier.com/Iggy/ to download and complete as a word processing file. Answer guidelines for this Case Study are also available on your Evolve website.

The nurse is admitting the patient to a medical unit. She is 68 years of age and has a history of ovarian cancer. She had surgery 5 months ago and has had pain ever since the surgery. She reports that she has been taking Tylox tablets at home but that the pain is "never gone."

1. The patient describes her pain as a "10" on a scale of 0 to 10, deep, occasionally cramping, and sharp or stabbing. She waves her hand over her chest and abdomen when asked to pinpoint the location of the pain. How should the nurse document this assessment of pain?

2. During a discussion with the pain management nurse, it is suggested that the patient be given a Duragesic transdermal patch for pain management. She comments, "Oh, good! I know that will help make my pain go away quickly." What would be the best response by the nurse?

3. After consideration of her history and her pain, the pain management specialist recommends that the patient should receive patient-controlled analgesia (PCA). After discussing PCA therapy with her, an infusion is started with morphine as a basal infusion as well as interval self-dosing. The next morning while reviewing the infusion notes, the nurse sees that the patient dosed herself four times during the night. She is awake and states that her pain is now at a "5" and that she feels "a bit of relief now." Later that afternoon during rounds after lunch, the nurse sees that she is asleep and has not touched her meal. Her respiratory rate is 12, but she does not answer when the nurse calls her name. What would the priority action by the nurse be? What additional actions should be taken?

4. During evening rounds, the patient is found to be unresponsive, with respiratory rate of 7 breaths/min. Her son, who was staying with her, said that he "pushed the button a few times" while she was asleep because earlier she was complaining of hurting but wouldn't push it herself. What would be the priority actions by the nurse?

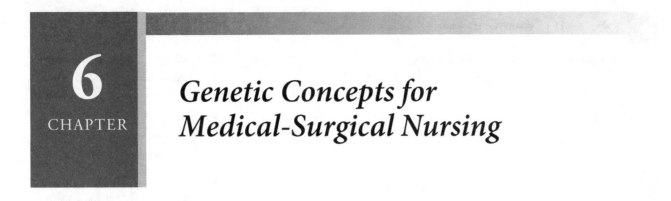

6 CHAPTER

Genetic Concepts for Medical-Surgical Nursing

STUDY/REVIEW QUESTIONS

1. **Crossword Puzzle.** *Complete each item by placing the correct answer in the appropriate number (across or down) in the puzzle.*

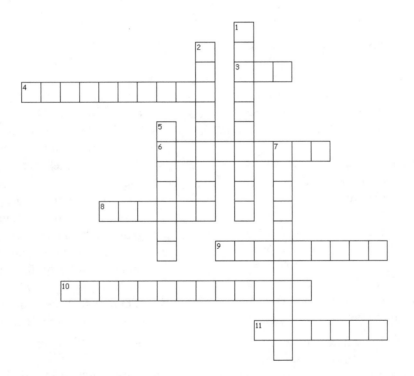

Across

3. Ribonucleic acid
4. The "pinched in" area of a chromosome where the two chromatids are joined
6. The 22 pairs of human chromosomes that do not code for the sexual differentiation of the individual
8. The complete set of genes for a species
9. _____ siblings; two siblings who share a womb and are born at the same time, but are the result of different fertilized eggs
10. The process of making a new strand of DNA
11. The complete set of chromosome pairs found in all of the individual's somatic cells

Down

1. Cellular DNA tightly condensed and coiled into a dense body
2. The observed expression of any given single gene trait (such as blood type, hair color)
5. A set of chromosomes consisting of half of each pair
7. _____ siblings; the product of one fertilized egg that split into two or more equal parts during embryogenesis

2. Describe the term *genomic health care*.

3. Humans have _____ chromosomes that are divided into _____ pairs.

4. What are autosomes?
   a. Chromosomes not involved in gender determination
   b. The organized arrangement of chromosomes in one cell
   c. The proteins needed to generate chromosome pairs
   d. Structures composed of two Xs as the sex chromosomes

5. When a person has homozygous alleles for a particular trait, the genotype and phenotype are the <u>same/different</u> *(circle one)*.

6. When a person has heterozygous alleles for a particular trait, the phenotype and the genotype are the <u>same/different</u> *(circle one)*.

7. For recessive traits, the phenotype and genotype are the <u>same/different</u> *(circle one)*.

8. Specify whether each characteristic is an autosomal dominant (AD) or autosomal recessive (AR) pattern of inheritance, or both (B).

   _____ a. In order for a trait to be expressed, both alleles must be present.

   _____ b. A trait is expressed even when only one allele of the pair is dominant.

   _____ c. The trait is found equally in males and females.

   _____ d. The trait is found in every generation with no skipping.

   _____ e. The trait may not appear in all generations of any one branch of a family.

   _____ f. The risk for an affected person to pass the trait to his or her children is 50% with each pregnancy.

   _____ g. The children of an affected mother and an affected father will always be affected (100% risk).

   _____ h. The trait can be transmitted to children if one parent is an unaffected carrier and the other parent is either a carrier or is affected.

9. Briefly discuss how patterns of inheritance are determined in a family.

10. Which statement best reflects the correct actions of the health care professional who is providing genetic counseling?
    a. "This test will tell us everything about you!"
    b. "We are going to perform this testing because you asked for it and it won't affect your family in any way."
    c. "The results of this genetic testing will be sent to your health insurance carrier immediately."
    d. "I'm here to provide information so that you can make an informed decision about genetic testing."

11. When assessing for genetic risks, which factors indicate that a patient may have an increased genetic risk for a disease or disorder? *(Select all that apply.)*
    a. A close family member has an identified genetic problem.
    b. A patient tells you that he was exposed to a carcinogenic substance during a war.
    c. A patient has been diagnosed with two different types of cancer.
    d. A patient's sister had breast cancer at age 24.
    e. A patient's father was diagnosed with rheumatic fever at 10 years of age.

12. Which disorders have a genetic pattern of inheritance? *(Select all that apply.)*
    a. Malignant hyperthermia
    b. Gallstones
    c. Cystic fibrosis
    d. Acute lymphocytic leukemia
    e. Polycystic kidney disease
    f. Sickle cell disease

13. Write "SLR" for the disorders that have a sex-linked recessive pattern of inheritance, and write "FC" for those that have familial clustering.

    _____ a. Hemophilia

    _____ b. Hypertension

    _____ c. Alzheimer's disease

    _____ d. Red-green color blindness

    _____ e. G6PD deficiency

    _____ f. Schizophrenia

7 CHAPTER

Evidence-Based Practice in Medical-Surgical Nursing

STUDY/REVIEW QUESTIONS

1. Define *evidence-based practice.*

Matching. *Match each term with its correct definition.*

Terms

a   Quantitative question
b. Background question
c. Evidence-based practice
d. Clinical practice guideline
e. Qualitative question
f. CINAHL

Definitions

_____ 2. Collaborative process which helps to answer "burning" clinical questions and involves all members of the health care team

_____ 3. Type of question that asks for a statement on which most authorities or experts would agree

_____ 4. Official recommendation based on evidence to diagnose or manage a health problem

_____ 5. One of the "fantastic four" databases that are searched to find information regarding a question

_____ 6. Type of question that focuses on the meaning and interpretation of human phenomena

_____ 7. Type of question that asks about the relationship between defined or measurable phenomena

8. Which components are included in the process of evidence-based practice (EBP)? *(Select all that apply.)*
   a. Developing and evaluating outcomes
   b. Answering a clinical question
   c. Critically appraising and synthesizing the relevant evidence
   d Developing recommendations to improve current practice
   e. Conducting quantitative research

9. On which levels do most clinically based "burning questions" need to be answered? *(Select all that apply.)*
   a. The individual patient level
   b. A small group of patients
   c. The level of the patient care unit
   d. A global level
   e. The organizational level

10. What are the steps of formulating a clinical question using the PICO(T) format?

11. Which factors have been identified as barriers for nurses to participate in evidence-based practice? *(Select all that apply.)*
    a. Limited timeframe to participate
    b. Difficulty in accessing research materials
    c. Lack of understanding of organization of electronic databases
    d. Difficulty understanding research articles
    e. Lack of value for research in practice

12. How does the Reavy and Tavernier Model of implementing evidence-based practice in the clinical setting see the role of the nurse researcher? *(Select all that apply.)*
    a. A role model
    b. Support in identifying areas for improvement
    c. An extra pair of hands for patient care
    d. A clinical expert ready with all of the answers
    e. An aid with literature review

8
CHAPTER

Rehabilitation Concepts for Chronic and Disabling Health Problems

STUDY/REVIEW QUESTIONS

Matching. *Match the interdisciplinary team member with the example of the type of work performed. Answers may be used more than once, and there may be more than one answer for each example.*

Interdisciplinary Team Members

a. Physiatrist
b. Rehabilitation nurses
c. Physical therapist
d. Occupational therapist
e. Speech-language pathologist
f. Recreational/activity therapist
g. Cognitive therapist
h. Social worker
i. Clinical psychologist
j. Vocational counselor
k. Spiritual care counselor
l. Patient

Types of Work Performed

_____ 1. Screens, tests, and recommends feeding techniques for dysphagia

_____ 2. Assists in job placement and seeking work-related training

_____ 3. Works with patients in learning to feed, bathe, and dress themselves

_____ 4. Teaches patients skills related to coordination such as picking up coins from a table

_____ 5. Specializes in rehabilitation medicine

_____ 6. Involved in patient and family coping skills

_____ 7. Identifies community resources

_____ 8. Coordinates the team's plan of care

_____ 9. Teaches patient skills to achieve mobility

_____ 10. Specializes in spiritual assessments and care

_____ 11. Works directly with patients who have experienced head injuries and have difficulty with memory

_____ 12. Assists patients in learning new interests or hobbies

_____ 13. Coordinates efforts of health care team members and functions as case manager creating a rehabilitation milieu

_____ 14. Teaches patients how to talk again and works with swallowing problems

_____ 15. Performs comprehensive physical, psychosocial, and spiritual assessments

_____ 16. Discharge planning to determine adequacy of current situation and potential needs and how care will be provided to meet those needs

_____ 17. Has final authority regarding teaching plan

18. As a result of a car accident, an adult patient is unable to perform certain activities of daily living (ADLs) such as bathing without assistance. This is an example of which concept listed below?
    a. Rehabilitation
    b. Impairment
    c. Disability
    d. Handicap

19. Which problem is the leading cause of disabling conditions in young adults and the third leading cause of death in young and middle-aged adults?
    a. Stroke
    b. Cancer
    c. Arthritis
    d. Accidents

20. What best describes the primary goal of the rehabilitation team?
    a. To rely on a specific plan of care standardized to the medical diagnosis
    b. To identify and use one conceptual framework to serve as the sole model for the practice of rehabilitation nursing
    c. To restore and maintain the patient's function to the best extent possible
    d. To enable patients and their families to identify strategies to successfully meet short-term goals

21. What are the nurse's responsibilities regarding the skin care assessment of the rehabilitation patient? *(Select all that apply.)*
    a. Identification of actual or potential interruptions of skin integrity
    b. Assisting the patient with hygiene after voiding or bowel movements
    c. Assessment of the skin for all patients under his or her care
    d. Education of the patient in how to inspect his or her own skin
    e. Thorough documentation of the integrity of the skin

22. Which factors does the nurse assess when implementing a position change schedule for an older adult? *(Select all that apply.)*
    a. Ability of the patient to change positions
    b. Condition of the patient's skin with each position change
    c. Nutritional status of the patient
    d. Type of injury the patient sustained
    e. Age of the patient

23. A patient with decreased cardiac output is entering a rehabilitation program. What will the nurse expect to find during the assessment of this patient?
    a. Shortness of breath on activity
    b. Ability to ambulate without angina
    c. Feeling rested upon awakening from sleep
    d. Ability to move from sitting to standing position easily

24. A paraplegic patient is entering a rehabilitation program. What does the nurse focus on first in assessing this patient?
    a. Family and cultural background
    b. Baseline hemoglobin and hematocrit measurements
    c. Habits of bowel elimination before illness
    d. Manual dexterity, muscle control, and mobility

25. A patient with a neurogenic bladder is to be taught how to perform intermittent self-catheterization. Before beginning the teaching-learning sessions, what will the nurse assess in this patient first?
    a. Motor function of both upper extremities
    b. Type of neurogenic bladder the patient has
    c. Patient's gender
    d. Age of the patient

26. To maintain skin integrity of a patient in a rehabilitation unit, what does the nurse assess? *(Select all that apply.)*
    a. Sensation of the skin
    b. Depth and diameter of an open lesion
    c. Ability to move extremities
    d. Presence or absence of exudate and odor
    e. Ability to change position as needed

27. Which statements correctly describe the Functional Independence Measure (FIM)? *(Select all that apply.)*
    a. It is a basic indicator of the severity of a disability.
    b. It tries to measure what a person should do, whatever the diagnosis or impairment.
    c. It tries to measure what a person actually does, whatever the diagnosis or impairment.
    d. The assessment may be performed by various health care disciplines.
    e. Categories for assessment are self-care, sphincter control, mobility and locomotion, communication, and cognition.
    f. Evaluations may be done at specified times during therapy to determine patient progress.

Matching. For each of the activities listed, specify whether it is an activity of daily living or independent living skill.

Type
a. Activity of daily living
b. Independent living skill

Activity
_____ 28. Bathing
_____ 29. Using the telephone
_____ 30. Dressing
_____ 31. Ambulating
_____ 32. Shopping
_____ 33. Preparing food
_____ 34. Feeding self
_____ 35. Housekeeping

36. What best describes the purpose of a vocational assessment for a patient in rehabilitation?
    a. Assist the patient to find meaningful training, education, or employment after discharge from a rehabilitation setting.
    b. Evaluate and retrain patients with deficits that distort consonant and vowel sound production.
    c. Identify resources to assist with patient injuries that cause deficits in cognition.
    d. Demonstrate improvements in physical, social, cognitive, and emotional functions.

37. The nurse reviews with a patient the results of manual muscle testing performed by physical therapy. What ability of the patient does this procedure determine?
    a. Body flexibility and muscle strength
    b. Range of motion and resistance against gravity
    c. Muscle strength and amount of pain on movement
    d. Voluntary versus involuntary muscle movement

38. When assisting a patient with a hemiparesis to transfer or ambulate, what does the nurse instruct the patient to do?
    a. Lean the body weight backward.
    b. Use the weaker hand to assist.
    c. Lean the body weight toward the nurse.
    d. Use the strong hand to assist.

39. The nurse's facility follows a no-lift policy to prevent musculoskeletal injury to staff. Which methods for patient transfer can the nurse use? *(Select all that apply.)*
    a. Independent movement of the patient when he or she is able
    b. Mechanical full-body lift
    c. Following facility guidelines for safe patient transfer
    d. No transfers for patients who are unable to move independently
    e. Multiple staff assistance

40. A patient with impaired physical mobility must be monitored for which early potential complication?
    a. Pressure ulcers
    b. Renal calculi
    c. Osteoporosis
    d. Fractures

41. Which methods to prevent pressure ulcers resulting from immobility are best to teach patients and their significant others? *(Select all that apply.)*
    a. Change position often to relieve pressure on all bony prominences.
    b. Maintain good skin care by keeping the skin clean and dry.
    c. Inspect the skin at least once a day for problems such as reddened areas that do not fade readily.
    d. Use pressure-relieving devices as a substitute for changing position.
    e. Eat foods high in protein, carbohydrates, and vitamins for sufficient nutrition.

42. When assessing a patient who is to perform resistive exercises, what must be present in order for the exercises to be productive?
    a. Limited range of motion
    b. Full range of motion
    c. Full strength
    d. Ability to exercise to the point of pain

43. Which assistive-adaptive device would be recommended for a patient with a weak hand grasp?
    a. Gel pad
    b. Foam buildups
    c. Hook and loop fastener straps
    d. Buttonhook

44. When teaching a patient with hemiplegia about energy conservation techniques, which method does the nurse include?
    a. Using a walker instead of a cane
    b. Scheduling physical therapy immediately before eating
    c. Using a bedside commode
    d. Scheduling recreational activities in afternoon or evening

45. Which statement is true about the use of mechanical pressure-relieving devices?
    a. They effectively eliminate the need to turn patients.
    b. Patients still require regular repositioning.
    c. They prevent pressure ulcers in debilitated patients.
    d. They have been shown to be ineffective against pressure ulcers.

46. A patient has a lower motor neuron injury below T12. This injury results in which type of neurogenic bladder?
    a. Reflex or spastic
    b. Flaccid
    c. Uninhibited
    d. Inhibited

47. A patient with a flaccid bladder will have which urinary elimination problem?
    a. Incontinence and inability to empty the bladder completely
    b. Incontinence caused by inability to wait until on a commode or bedpan
    c. Urinary retention and dribbling because of overflow of urine
    d. Incontinence due to loss of sensation

48. Which statements are correct principles for performing an intermittent catheterization? *(Select all that apply.)*
    a. A catheter is inserted every few hours.
    b. It is usually performed after the Valsalva or Credé maneuver.
    c. A residual of less than 100-150 mL increases the interval between catheterization.
    d. The maximum time interval between catheterizations is 4 hours.
    e. The patient uses sterile technique at home.

49. Which medication would a patient with a mild overactive bladder most likely be given?
    a. Dantrolene sodium (Dantrium)
    b. Bethanechol chloride (Urecholine)
    c. Flavoxate hydrochloride (Urispas)
    d. Trimethoprim (Trimpex)

50. Which patient is most likely to have a flaccid bowel dysfunction?
    a. 28-year-old man with a crushed pelvis
    b. 54-year-old man with Guillain-Barré syndrome
    c. 18-year-old woman with a displaced cervical fracture
    d. 48-year-old woman who has multiple sclerosis

51. In which patients with constipation does the nurse avoid performing digital stimulation? *(Select all that apply.)*
    a. Patient with myocardial infarction who is starting cardiac rehabilitation
    b. Patient with chronic diarrhea resulting from radiation to the bowel
    c. Patient with bowel incontinence resulting from a cerebrovascular accident
    d. Patient with a spinal cord injury resulting from a diving accident
    e. Patient with a spinal cord injury resulting from a motor vehicle accident

52. Which drug might be included in a bowel training program?
    a. Milk of magnesia
    b. Senna concentrate (Senokot)
    c. Dulcolax or glycerin suppository
    d. Psyllium (Metamucil)

53. Lower motor neuron disease or injury results in which bowel dysfunction?
    a. Flaccid bowel pattern
    b. Reflex (spastic) bowel pattern
    c. Uninhibited bowel pattern
    d. Inhibited bowel pattern

54. Which description characterizes the uninhibited bowel pattern dysfunction?
    a. Defecation occurring suddenly and without warning.
    b. Defecation occurring infrequently and in small amounts.
    c. Frequent defecation, urgency, and complaints of hard stool.
    d. Intermittent constipation and diarrhea.

Matching. Match each intervention with the appropriate condition. The conditions may be used more than once.

Conditions

a. Total urinary incontinence
b. Constipation
c. Risk for impaired skin integrity
d. Decreased cardiac output
e. Impaired physical mobility

Interventions

_____ 55. Perform major tasks in the morning

_____ 56. Complete the Braden Scale

_____ 57. Credé maneuver

_____ 58. Perform gait training

_____ 59. Wheelchair "push-ups"

_____ 60. Use a tilt table

_____ 61. Digital stimulation

9 CHAPTER

End-of-Life Care

STUDY/REVIEW QUESTIONS

Matching. *Match each term related to loss with its correct definition.*

Terms
a. Death
b. Dying
c. Grieving
d. Mourning

Definitions

_____ 1. Reaction to loss

_____ 2. Termination of life

_____ 3. The outward social expression of loss

_____ 4. A process leading to the end of life

5. Which statement regarding the approach to hospice/end-of-life care is correct?
   a. Hospice programs only include provision of care in the home.
   b. Admission to hospice is involuntary and directed by a physician's order.
   c. The focus is on facilitating quality of life just for the dying patient.
   d. An interdisciplinary team approach is used for the care of the patient and family.

6. A patient receiving nursing care in a home hospice program can expect which kind of care?
   a. The use of high-technology equipment such as ventilators until time of death.
   b. Around-the-clock skilled direct nursing patient care until time of death.
   c. Pain and symptom management that will achieve the best quality of life.
   d. Complete relief of only distressing physical symptoms.

7. To qualify for hospice benefits, a criterion for admission is that the patient's prognosis must be limited to what amount of time?
   a. 2 weeks or less
   b. 3 months or less
   c. 6 months or less
   d. 1 year or less

8. Which items are relevant to the concept of hospice? *(Select all that apply.)*
   a. Unit of care is the patient and family.
   b. Preferred location is in the hospital setting.
   c. Interdisciplinary team approach is used.
   d. Focus is on alleviating pain and suffering.
   e. Hospice care does not hasten death.

9. Place in correct sequence, using the numbers 1 through 3, the events that occur with multiple organ dysfunction syndrome (MODS).

   _____ a. Anaerobic metabolism, acidosis, hyperkalemia, and tissue ischemia

   _____ b. Release of toxic metabolites and destructive enzymes

   _____ c. Inadequate blood flow to body tissues and cells

10. Which statements about the assessment of a terminally ill patient are true? *(Select all that apply.)*
    a. Assess only the patient; do not include the family's perception of the patient's symptoms.
    b. When the patient is unable to communicate, there is no need to assess symptoms of distress any longer.
    c. Assess patients who are unable to communicate distress by observing for objective signs of discomfort.
    d. Assesses the patient for dyspnea, agitation, nausea, and vomiting only.
    e. Identify alternative methods to assess for symptoms of distress.
    f. The family can help identify patient habits and preferences which may aid in the overall assessment.

11. Which intervention should be done when performing postmortem care?
    a. Place the head of the bed at 30 degrees.
    b. Remove pillows from under the head.
    c. Leave a Foley (indwelling) catheter in place in the bladder.
    d. Place pads under the hips and around the perineum.

12. Which interventions after a patient's death are appropriate to perform? *(Select all that apply.)*
    a. Remove the body to the morgue or funeral home immediately after death.
    b. Follow agency policies to remove all tubes and lines from the body.
    c. A death certificate may accompany the body to the funeral home.
    d. Provide privacy for the family and significant others with the deceased.
    e. Allow family and/or significant other to perform religious and cultural customs.

Matching. *Match the term with its correct definition.*

Terms
a. Living will
b. Durable power of attorney for health care
c. Patient Self-Determination Act
d. Do not resuscitate (DNR)

Definitions

_____ 13. A legal document that appoints a person to make decisions regarding health care for someone else who becomes unable to make his or her own decisions

_____ 14. A physician's order that specifies that a patient has indicated that he or she does not want CPR

_____ 15. A legal document that instructs health care providers and family members of what life-sustaining treatment one wants or does not want if that person becomes unable to make these decisions

_____ 16. Requires that all patients admitted to health care agencies be asked if they have written advance directives

17. A hospice patient is deteriorating and the family is concerned about his restlessness and confusion. Which intervention is the nurse prepared to perform?
    a. Notify the primary health care provider and request orders for transfer to the hospital.
    b. Provide analgesics and oxygen as ordered, and make the patient as comfortable as possible.
    c. Initiate IV hydration to provide the patient with necessary fluids.
    d. Encourage the family to assist the patient to eat in order to gain energy.

18. The most common treatment of pain in a terminally ill patient is administration of which kind of therapy?
    a. Opioids
    b. Steroids
    c. Nonsteroidal anti-inflammatory agents
    d. Radiation treatments

19. Which phrase correctly describes palliative care?
    a. Care for patients with a prognosis of 6 months or less
    b. Diagnoses and treatment for patients with a life-threatening illness
    c. Patient care with a focus on treatment of symptoms
    d. Patient education about relevant treatment alternatives

20. While caring for a Native American/American Indian patient who is dying, what cultural concept should the nurse keep in mind?
    a. Traditional Native American/American Indian families are male-dominated.
    b. Expression of grief is open, especially among women.
    c. Families will not allow the patient to die alone.
    d. Family members are likely to avoid visiting the terminally ill family member.

21. Which statements about pain management in a patient who is dying are true? *(Select all that apply.)*
    a. The patient's pain may come from many areas.
    b. Patients who are dying should discontinue long-acting opioids.
    c. Alternative therapies have been shown to be useful when integrated into a pain management plan of care.
    d. When using massage for patients with cancer, deep pressure is the preferred method.
    e. Aromatherapy, massage, music therapy, and therapeutic touch are a few alternative therapies that have been shown to be useful.

22. Which statements about caring for a patient with dyspnea are true? *(Select all that apply.)*
    a. Pharmacologic interventions should begin early in the course of dyspnea.
    b. Nonpharmacologic, alternative treatments may be used successfully in the place of pharmacologic interventions.
    c. Dyspnea may be caused by the primary diagnosis or its treatments.
    d. Diagnostic testing must be used to determine the cause of dyspnea before beginning treatment.
    e. Oropharyngeal suctioning is appropriate for patients with loud, wet respirations nearing death.

23. Which end-of-life interventions must the nurse be prepared to perform for a dying patient and his or her family? *(Select all that apply.)*
    a. Allow the family to verbalize fears and concerns about the impending loss of their loved one.
    b. Listen and acknowledge the legitimacy of the family's pain.
    c. Minimize the family's loss by using statements such as "don't be upset."
    d. Assist the patient and family with reminiscence or storytelling.
    e. Work to determine the patient's and family's spiritual needs.

Short Answer. *Define and explain the differences between the following two terms.*

24.   Passive euthanasia:

25.   Active euthanasia:

10 CHAPTER

Concepts of Emergency and Trauma Nursing

STUDY/REVIEW QUESTIONS

Matching. *Match the job descriptions with the interdisciplinary team members.*

Interdisciplinary Team Members
a. Forensic nurse examiner
b. Paramedic
c. Emergency medical technician
d. Psychiatric crisis nurse team
e. Emergency medicine physician

Job Descriptions

_____ 1. May work with patients involved with a sudden serious illness or the death of a loved one

_____ 2. Advanced life support provider who can perform advanced techniques, such as cardiac monitoring, advanced airway management and intubation, or giving intravenous drugs en route to the hospital

_____ 3. Offers basic life support interventions such as oxygen, basic wound care, splinting, spinal immobilization, and may carry automated external defibrillators (AEDs)

_____ 4. Obtains patient histories, collects abuse and domestic violence evidence, and offers counseling and follow-up for victims of rape and child abuse

_____ 5. Physician with specialized education and training in emergency patient management

6. The emergency department (ED) nurse is preparing a report on a patient being admitted for bacterial meningitis. Which points are included in the ED nurse's report to the medical-surgical nurse? *(Select all that apply.)*
   a. "Patient reports severe headache with high fever that started 4 days ago."
   b. "Patient currently alert and oriented x 2; speech clear, but rambling."
   c. "Patient is divorced and currently does not have any health insurance."
   d. "IV normal saline into left anterior forearm; received first dose of IV ceftriaxone (Rocephin) at 0700."
   e. "Past history of chronic obesity and fractured femur at age 5."
   f. "Lumbar puncture results are pending, but meningococcal meningitis is suspected."
   g. "Received 1000 mg acetaminophen for pain (9/10) and fever 103° F at 0400; pain continues (7/10), temperature now 100.9° F."

7. A patient received in the ED is diagnosed with stroke. Upon assessment, the patient exhibits difficulty swallowing. When taking a sip of water, the patient coughs and chokes. What priority safety measure does the nurse implement for this patient?
   a. Keep the head of the bed less than 30 degrees.
   b. Set up seizure precautions for the bed.
   c. Intermittently offer ice chips to reassess swallowing.
   d. Set oral suction device.

8. The ED nurse is attempting to transfer a patient to the medical-surgical unit. When the receiving nurse answers the phone, he says, "You people always dump these admissions on us during shift change." Which response by the ED nurse represents the best attempt at respectful negotiation?
   a. "I am sorry. I realize you are busy, but we are busy too."
   b. "When would you be willing to take our patients?"
   c. "I apologize for the timing. I will call back in 15 minutes."
   d. "I apologize. We just received the bed assignment."

9. The nurse is interviewing a psychiatric patient who has been verbally aggressive for the past several hours according to the family. The family states, "He won't hurt anybody." However, the patient is pacing and appears suspicious and angry. Which strategy does the nurse use to conduct the interview?
   a. Sit at eye level with the patient in a quiet, secluded room.
   b. Conduct the interview standing near the door in a quiet room.
   c. Bring the entire family in and have everyone sit in comfortable chairs.
   d. Have the security guard stand by the patient during the interview.

10. The nurse is working alone in triage. It is a busy night and the waiting room is full of people who are restless and unhappy about having to wait. Which situation warrants the nurse to activate the panic button under the triage desk?
    a. The line for patients waiting to be triaged becomes overwhelmingly long.
    b. EMS calls to announce they are en route with a patient in full arrest.
    c. Several patients in the waiting room start to complain very loudly.
    d. A person walks in and starts threatening the registration staff with a weapon.

11. The ED nurse is caring for a patient who was found in an alley with no identification and no known family. The nurse must give medication to the patient. What is the correct procedure?
    a. Emergent conditions prevent identification, so the nurse gives the medication as ordered.
    b. The patient is designated as John Doe and the nurse uses two unique identifiers.
    c. The nurse validates the order with another nurse and both verify that the patient is unidentified.
    d. The nurse gives the medication and identification is made as soon as possible.

12. The nurse is working in the ED with an emergency physician, but the physician is currently involved in the care of several critical patients. The ED nurse must initiate care for patients under interdisciplinary and medical protocols. Which intervention is the *least* likely to be covered by a standing protocol?
    a. Give 50% dextrose IV push for low blood sugar.
    b. Obtain an arterial blood gas and start oxygen therapy.
    c. Ventilate per Ambu bag with 100% oxygen and intubate.
    d. Start a peripheral IV with normal saline at 125 mL/hour.

13. An older adult patient had been waiting in the ED for over 48 hours due to extremely high volume. Risk for Impaired Skin Integrity is identified and the charge nurse delegates turning the patient every 2 hours to the nursing assistants. Since the ED is busy, the patient is not turned and begins to develop a pressure ulcer. What does the charge nurse do to prevent a recurrence of this type of problem for future patients? *(Select all that apply.)*
    a. Nothing; in the overall priorities of the ED, the situation is inevitable.
    b. Make anecdotal notes and counsel all the involved nursing assistants.
    c. Delegate the duty of turning and repositioning to the physical therapist.
    d. File an incident report and seek resolution at the systems level.
    e. Re-educate staff on the need to turn patients at risk for skin breakdown.

14. An older couple on vacation comes to the ED. The man appears to be having a stroke and is unable to speak clearly or coherently. His wife is very distraught and states, "He has many allergies and takes many medications, but I can't remember anything right now!" What does the nurse do to quickly obtain accurate drug and allergy information? *(Select all that apply.)*
    a. Call the patient's family physician for a phone report about his drugs and allergies.
    b. Call one of the patient's children and stress the urgency and importance for accurate information.
    c. Call the pharmacy where the patient obtains his medications.
    d. Check for a medical alert bracelet; help the wife to look in the patient's suitcase.
    e. Instruct the wife to keep a list of the patient's drugs and allergies in her purse.

Matching. Match the types of trauma with their descriptions.

Trauma Types
a. Penetrating trauma
b. Blast effect
c. Rapid acceleration-deceleration forces
d. Blunt trauma

Descriptions
_____ 15. Impact forces such as with fists, kicks, or a baseball bat

_____ 16. Energy from an exploding bomb

_____ 17. High-speed crashes; produces tearing and shearing of anatomic structures

_____ 18. Injury from sharp objects and projectiles such as knives or icepicks

19. A patient is brought to the ED by friends who report "he probably overdosed on downers." The patient has a decreased level of consciousness and a decreased gag reflex; his face and chest are covered with emesis; he demonstrates spontaneous sonorous respirations; and pulse oximetry is 87% on room air. What type of airway management does the nurse expect this patient to receive?
    a. Supplemental oxygen per nasal cannula at 4-6 L/min
    b. Bag-valve-mask and 100% oxygen to assist with ventilatory effort
    c. Non-rebreather mask with high-flow oxygen
    d. Endotracheal intubation with initial high-concentration oxygen

20. The ED nurse is caring for several patients, all of whom are currently lying on stretchers either pending discharge or awaiting transfer to a hospital bed. Which patients are at risk for falls? *(Select all that apply.)*
    a. Patient with chronic pain who received 10 mg PO oxycodone for myalgia
    b. Opioid-naive teenager with a fracture who received 3 mg IV morphine for pain
    c. Middle-aged woman with severe vomiting and frequently watery stools
    d. Child with a fever of 102° F, crying, with an ear infection
    e. Older adult patient with acute dementia secondary to infection

21. A patient was involved in a high-speed motor vehicle crash. The physician instructs the nurse to prepare for several urgent procedures because of severe injury and physical compromise. Which procedure does the nurse prepare for first?
    a. Central line insertion
    b. Peritoneal lavage
    c. Chest tube insertion
    d. Endotracheal intubation

22. For the each patient listed, indicate whether they should be triaged as emergent (E), urgent (U), or nonurgent (N).
    _____ a. 56-year-old man with severe unilateral back pain and previous history of kidney stones
    _____ b. 23-year-old woman with severe abdominal pain; positive home pregnancy test; BP 90/50 mm Hg
    _____ c. 35-year-old man with chest pain and diaphoresis
    _____ d. 10-year-old girl with vomiting, diarrhea, and abdominal pain onset 4 hours after eating fish
    _____ e. 6-year-old with a temperature of 101° F and flu-like symptoms
    _____ f. 44-year-old man with a dislocated elbow
    _____ g. 85-year-old man with new onset of confusion; BP elevated compared to his usual reading
    _____ h. 65-year-old woman with redness and swelling on the forearm associated with a bee sting

23. A patient is brought to the ED by the family because he has verbally threatened others and attempted to stab the neighbor's dog. What does the nurse do in order to ensure the safety of the patient and others? *(Select all that apply.)*
    a. Search the patient's belongings and secure personal effects.
    b. Instruct the patient's family to stay with him and call for help as necessary.
    c. Remove dangerous equipment from the room, such as sharps containers or portable instruments.
    d. Escort the patient to the waiting area where he can readily be observed by the triage nurse.
    e. Use a metal detector to search for objects that could be used as weapons.
    f. Instruct nursing students to avoid wearing a stethoscope around their necks.

24. Identify the following patients in order of greatest to least need for the nurse to advocate for a social services consult. *(Select in order of priority.)*
    a. Toddler who bumped her head on a table; observation for 24 hours is required
    b. Homeless woman who has a urinary tract infection and a vaginal yeast infection
    c. Woman who was punched and beaten by her husband and sustained a broken jaw
    d. Man who drove himself to the ED for a dressing change of an infected wound on his back
    e. Preteen admitted for vaginal bleeding and sexually transmitted disease

25. Which functions represent appropriate referrals to the case manager? *(Select all that apply.)*
    a. Facilitate a referral to a primary care provider who is taking new patients.
    b. Contact the peripherally inserted central catheter (PICC) line nurse to start an IV because the patient has bad veins.
    c. Investigate whether the patient is abusing and overusing ED services.
    d. Follow the patient into the community setting and evaluate the home environment.
    e. Facilitate a referral to a psychiatrist to evaluate a woman who alleges abuse.

26. A patient died in the ED after sustaining multiple injuries that occurred during an aggravated assault. The family arrives after the patient is pronounced dead and they ask to see the body. What does the nurse do?
    a. Explain that viewing the body would be too traumatic because all the tubes must remain in place for the forensic exam.
    b. Remove any tubes or debris that are near the patient's face and then cover the rest of the body with a blanket.
    c. Explain what they will see; dim the lights; leave the patient's face exposed, but cover the rest of the body with a blanket.
    d. Suggest that the family could spend time with their loved one at the mortuary after the medical examiner is finished.

27. Three people who came to the ED with a patient have become verbally argumentative and threatening towards each other. Which actions does the ED nurse take to ensure staff safety? *(Select all that apply.)*
    a. Ask the individuals to sit down and offer them coffee and a snack.
    b. Follow the hospital's security plan.
    c. Attempt to de-escalate the situation.
    d. Quietly ask the individuals to leave.
    e. Look for an escape route.

28. The nurse is evaluating the lower extremities of several patients. Which description represents the *least* serious physical presentation?
    a. Pain in calf; lower leg is swollen and red.
    b. Progressively increasing pain; distal portion is cool and bluish.
    c. Decreased sensation; lower leg has widespread brownish discoloration.
    d. Tight sensation in ankle; skin appears tight, shiny, and edematous.

Matching. *Match the interventions with the primary survey categories. Answers may be used more than once.*

Categories

a. Airway/cervical spine
b. Breathing
c. Circulation
d. Disability
e. Exposure

Interventions

_____ 29. Maintain alignment of cervical spine.

_____ 30. Re-evaluate level of consciousness frequently.

_____ 31. Use direct pressure for external bleeding.

_____ 32. After removing clothing, observe for chest expansion.

_____ 33. Establish patent airway.

_____ 34. Remove all clothing to allow for thorough assessment.

_____ 35. Maintain vascular access with a large-bore catheter.

36. The ED trauma team is preparing to receive a motor vehicle crash victim with severe chest trauma with coughing of blood and a crush injury to the right leg. What type of personal protective equipment (PPE) does the nurse assigned to be the recorder put on?
    a. No PPE is necessary because the nurse is only recording and not giving direct care
    b. Gloves
    c. Gown, gloves, eye protection, face mask, a cap, and shoe covers
    d. The patient situation must first be assessed before determining what PPE to wear

37. A parent brings her 2-year-old child to the ED, stating, "She fell and bumped her head and forearm." Which behavior by the child causes the nurse the *least* concern during the initial triage interview?
    a. Crying and reaching for the parent as the nurse approaches
    b. Alert and still, quietly watching as the nurse approaches
    c. Asleep, limp, with even and unlabored respirations
    d. Crying loudly and inconsolably since she was brought in

38. A 61-year-old patient is brought to the ED reporting difficulty breathing and fatigue. The patient is currently receiving radiation treatments for lung cancer. The physician diagnosis is cardiac tamponade. Which assessment finding does the nurse expect the patient to exhibit?
    a. Decreased cardiac output
    b. Flat jugular veins
    c. Pulse paradoxical not present
    d. Elevated blood pressure of 189/95 mm Hg

39. What is the fastest way for the nurse to estimate the systolic blood pressure in a patient who is being resuscitated?
    a. Palpate for presence of a radial pulse.
    b. Use the automated blood pressure cuff.
    c. Place the patient on a cardiac monitor.
    d. Check for the presence of capillary refill.

40. A patient comes to the ED after falling off a roof. He displays absent breath sounds over the left chest, severe respiratory distress, hypotension, jugular vein distention, and tracheal deviation. Based on these assessment findings, for which condition does the nurse anticipate the patient must receive immediate treatment?
    a. Tension pneumothorax
    b. Cardiac arrest
    c. Airway obstruction
    d. Multiple fractured ribs

41. The nurse is helping the physician treat a patient with a tension pneumothorax. What type of equipment does the nurse obtain to immediately alleviate this life-threatening condition?
    a. Large adult endotracheal tube
    b. 14-gauge IV catheter 3-6 cm long
    c. Chest tube insertion tray
    d. Tracheostomy tray

42. The nurse's next-door neighbor has sustained a deep laceration to the right upper arm and there is active bright red bleeding. What does the nurse do to immediately control the bleeding? *(Select all that apply.)*
    a. Apply a tourniquet just above the laceration.
    b. Have the neighbor lie flat and elevate the arm.
    c. Apply direct pressure with a thick, dry towel.
    d. Apply a sterile gauze and wrap the wound with an Ace bandage.
    e. Rinse the wound gently with tepid water and apply direct pressure with a towel.

43. A patient who sustained multiple injuries in a job site accident has a BP of 100/60 and pulse of 120/min. Two large-bore IVs are established and IV fluid resuscitation is initiated. After receiving IV fluid, repeat vital signs are BP 94/56, pulse 135/min; then BP 80/50, pulse 150/min. With these vital signs, the patient is likely to require blood products after how many liters of IV fluid?
    a. 1
    b. 2
    c. 4
    d. 5

44. The nurse is caring for a patient with a head injury whose Glasgow Coma Scale score is 3. This score indicates the patient is most likely to do what?
    a. Withdraw from painful stimuli
    b. Open eyes spontaneously
    c. Moan with incoherent speech
    d. Be totally unresponsive

45. A patient involved in a boating accident has extensive injuries and comes to the ED in wet clothes. The nurse identifies a risk for hypothermia. Which interventions does the nurse implement? *(Select all that apply.)*
    a. Remove wet clothing.
    b. Infuse warm IV solutions.
    c. Set the room temperature at 90° F.
    d. Give sips of warm fluid.
    e. Use a heat lamp.

46. Each patient listed below has entered the ED's waiting area. Place them in order of priority, with 1 being the highest priority and 4 being the lowest priority.
    _____ a. 3-year-old child with inconsolable high-pitched crying, high fever, headache, and nuchal rigidity
    _____ b. 65-year-old man having diaphoresis with left anterior crushing chest pain
    _____ c. 32-year-old woman reporting upper abdominal pain and vomiting green bile emesis
    _____ d. 16-year-old boy with a broken arm from skateboarding, pulse and sensation intact

47. A patient comes to the ED with severe respiratory distress. He has a long history of chronic respiratory disease and now requires endotracheal intubation. How does the nurse assess this patient's lung compliance?
    a. Auscultate the lung fields, especially for coarse crackles.
    b. Sense the degree of difficulty in ventilating with a bag-valve-mask.
    c. Monitor the pulse oximeter for decreasing saturation levels.
    d. Count the respiratory rate and observe the respiratory effort.

48. A patient admitted to the ED has a closed tibia fracture from a fall. Which question is essential to the requirement of the continuum of care?
    a. Establish the patient's insurance coverage.
    b. Provide physician referral resources.
    c. List the patient's home medications.
    d. Determine any medical equipment the patient may need at home.

49. A patient has been admitted to the ED following a motor vehicle crash and has a history of substance abuse. What must be a priority for the nurse to include in the assessment?
    a. Assess the time the patient last ate.
    b. Assess the patient's risk factors for suicide.
    c. Evaluate the patient's spiritual beliefs.
    d. Identify the primary family or individual who is supportive of patient.

50. A patient in the ED has been diagnosed with a flail chest following a three-story fall from a ladder. Which interventions does the nurse include for this patient? *(Select all that apply.)*
    a. Requesting pain medication
    b. Placing the patient in a supine position
    c. Promoting deep breathing
    d. Providing humidified oxygen
    e. Placing an elastic binder around the chest

True or False? Read each statement and write T for true or F for false in the blanks provided. If the statement is false, correct the statement to make it true.

_____ 51. It is illegal to search a patient and his or her belongings even if the nurse believes that the patient may be seriously mentally ill.

_____ 52. Educational materials and discharge instructions should be available at the 6th grade reading level or lower.

53. A patient in the ED has been diagnosed with a flail chest following a fall from a two-story height. What findings does the nurse expect to see upon assessment? *(Select all that apply.)*
    a. Bradycardia
    b. Dyspnea
    c. Expiratory wheezes
    d. Elevated blood pressure of 188/97 mm Hg
    e. Paradoxic chest movement

54. The nurse is caring for a patient admitted to the ED with cardiac tamponade. What assessment findings does the nurse expect to see? *(Select all that apply.)*
    a. Coarse lung sounds
    b. Jugular vein distention
    c. Slow respiratory rate
    d. Decreased cardiac output
    e. Muffled heart sounds
    f. Blood pressure less than 10 mm Hg lower on expiration than on inspiration

55. A patient in the ED has sustained a closed fracture after falling 50 feet while rock climbing. What are the assessments and interventions the nurse would perform for this patient in priority order? *(Select in order of priority.)*
    a. Evaluate the neuromuscular status of the left lower extremity.
    b. Assess the head, chest, and abdomen for injuries.
    c. Assess airway, breathing, and circulation.
    d. Immobilize the injured extremity.
    e. Monitor the degree of pain or discomfort.

CASE STUDY: THE PATIENT WITH A SPINAL CORD INJURY

Use a separate sheet of paper to answer the questions in this Case Study, or go to the "Prepare for Class" folder on your Evolve website at http://evolve.elsevier.com/Iggy/ to download and complete as a word processing file. Answer guidelines for this Case Study are also available on your Evolve website.

The patient is a 17-year-old male who has just been transported by EMS to the ED. He sustained a spinal cord injury from a diving accident at the lake. EMS brought the patient in on a backboard and a cervical collar is in place.

The patient is drowsy, but will answer most questions appropriately. A urine specimen for drug screen reveals he is positive for alcohol but no other drugs. He says he has no sensation when touched during assessment from the nipple line down. Flaccid paralysis is noted of the bilateral upper extremities and bilateral lower extremities. In addition, there is a loss of reflexes from the neck down.

Respirations are shallow with diminished breath sounds throughout, but are notable in the bases of the lungs anteriorly and posteriorly. The pulse oximetry reading is 87% on 2 L O_2 via nasal cannula. The ED physician and anesthesiologist inserted an endotracheal tube and started the patient on mechanical ventilation. A right forehead superficial laceration has a small amount of bleeding noted on the 4x4 gauze dressing over the injury. The edges are approximated.

Vital signs are: temp 37.9° C (100.2° F); BP 88/50 mm Hg; heart rate 130/min, sinus tachycardia; respiratory rate per mechanical ventilation is 22/min; pulse oximetry 95% on 40% Fio_2.

Family and friends are in the waiting room. A chaplain has been paged to stay with them until the physician gives them a report on the patient's condition.

1. What are the top three priority problems for this patient from the selection below?
   - Risk for Infection, altered skin integrity
   - Risk for respiratory insufficiency
   - Potential for spinal shock, related to injury
   - Risk for Ineffective Airway Clearance

2. Document a nursing note for this patient using the three patient problems chosen from question #1.

3. How can the patient's family or significant others be included in the patient's care?

CASE STUDY: THE TRAUMA PATIENT

Use a separate sheet of paper to answer the questions in this Case Study, or go to the "Prepare for Class" folder on your Evolve website at http://evolve.elsevier.com/Iggy/ to download and complete as a word processing file. Answer guidelines for this Case Study are also available on your Evolve website.

The patient is a 37-year-old man who was the driver in a high-speed motor vehicle accident. EMS reports that his vehicle was struck on the driver's side by a truck and the victim had to be extracted using the "jaws of life." The patient was wearing a seatbelt and he was unconscious when EMS arrived, but he has intermittently aroused reporting extreme pain in the chest and pelvis area. He arrives secured to a backboard with a C-collar in place. His breathing is uneven and becomes increasingly more labored as he is transferred to the ED stretcher. Vital signs are respirations 35/min; pulse 125/min; blood pressure 86/40 mm Hg; cardiac monitor shows sinus tachycardia. The resuscitation team includes an ED physician, primary nurse, secondary nurse, respiratory therapist, and a nursing assistant.

1. During the primary survey, what is the *highest* priority intervention?
2. When assessing breathing during the primary survey, what is included in this assessment?
3. Discuss interventions that accompany the ABCDE of the primary survey.
4. Discuss with a classmate several ways that assessment, interventions, and responsibilities could be divided between the primary and secondary nurse. (Use your critical thinking skills and discuss your answer with your instructor.)
5. What duties would be appropriate to delegate to the nursing assistant?
6. What is the purpose of the secondary survey?
7. Why is the mechanism of injury (MOI) important in trauma cases? In the scenario above, speculate about the relationship of the mechanism of injury and the EMS report on the patient's complaints and injuries.
8. Explain why the patient is likely to have a nasogastric tube and a Foley catheter inserted.

11 CHAPTER

Care of Patients with Common Environmental Emergencies

STUDY/REVIEW QUESTIONS

1. Which of the following are predisposing factors associated with heat-related illness? *(Select all that apply.)*
   a. High humidity
   b. Low humidity
   c. Obesity
   d. Anemia
   e. Seizures
   f. Dehydration
   g. Beta-adrenergic blockers

2. The nurse is providing patient education about the prevention of heat-related illness. Which statements are correct? *(Select all that apply.)*
   a. "Wear lightweight, dark-colored clothing when working outside."
   b. "Plan to limit activities at the hottest time of day."
   c. "Avoid fluids with electrolytes before, during, and after exercise."
   d. "Wear loose-fitting clothing."
   e. "Rest frequently when working in a hot environment."

3. A television meteorologist has been doing a photo shoot during a day when temperatures reached 110° F. Later in the day, he reports that he feels weak, has a headache, and feels nauseated and dizzy. He states that he had water with him but often forgot to drink it. His body temperature is 98.9° F. What is this patient suffering from?
   a. Classic heat stroke
   b. Exertional heat stroke
   c. Heat exhaustion
   d. Fluid overload

4. Which nursing interventions apply to the meteorologist in the question number 3? *(Select all that apply.)*
   a. Provide salted snacks for him to eat.
   b. Call for emergency medical services.
   c. Provide oral hydration such as a sports drink.
   d. Fan or spray water on his skin.
   e. Avoid giving him salt tablets.

5. During a summer marathon at a beach resort city, a runner suddenly collapses after running in the race for 1 hour. The weather has been extremely hot during the race day, with temperatures of almost 100° F and high humidity. The runner's body temperature is 105.2° F, she is confused and sweating. What is this patient suffering from?
   a. Classic heat stroke
   b. Exertional heat stroke
   c. Heat exhaustion
   d. Dehydration

6. For the runner in question number 5, what first-aid interventions would be performed while waiting for an ambulance to arrive? *(Select all that apply.)*
   a. Placing ice packs on the neck, axillae, chest, and groin
   b. Immersion in ice
   c. Removal of clothing
   d. Wetting the body with tepid water, then fanning rapidly to cool by evaporation
   e. Oral antipyretics, such as acetaminophen or aspirin

7. The nurse is participating in a local community sports day. The day is hot and humid and older adults are walking around. Prevention of heat-related injuries would include which intervention?
   a. Encouraging participants to eat high-energy snacks, such as sports bars
   b. Advising that people with disabilities should not participate
   c. Setting up a shade tent with areas for rest and relaxed activity
   d. Limiting direct sun exposure to 2 hours during the hottest time of the day

8. The nurse is volunteering at the first-aid station at a local community fair. The weather is predicted to be hot and humid. In planning care for people who may experience heat-related illness in this setting, what should the nurse obtain?
   a. Supply of salt tablets and bottles of water
   b. Bags of IV normal saline and IV insertion equipment
   c. Several water spray bottles and a portable fan
   d. Supply of educational pamphlets and sunscreen samples

9. It is the middle of summer and the weather has been hot and humid for several weeks. Which patient has the highest risk for severe heat-related illness?
   a. Older adult woman who lives alone in an apartment with no air conditioning
   b. Well-conditioned athlete who is participating in a marathon
   c. Experienced construction worker who is working on an outdoor structure
   d. Young child who is participating in an organized team sport

10. The nurse has received reports on several patients who were admitted for heat-related illnesses. The patient who has the most severe case of heat-related illness exhibits which signs/symptoms?
   a. Headache; heavy perspiration; temperature of 101° F
   b. Feeling of illness; nausea and vomiting
   c. Significant sunburn to extremities, face, and neck; temperature of 102° F
   d. Hot and dry skin; alert and oriented to person; pulse of 110

11. A homeless man is found lying in a vacant lot in the middle of July. He is lethargic and confused and he has sustained severe sunburns on the exposed areas of his skin. His core temperature is 106° F. What do prehospital emergency cooling measures include for this patient? (Select all that apply.)
   a. Administering cold IV fluid
   b. Stripping off all clothing
   c. Packing the axilla and groin with ice
   d. Encouraging sips of cool water
   e. Sponging with tepid water and fanning

12. A young migrant worker who has been living in a garden shed for several months is brought to the ED. He is alert and conversant, but appears fearful and somewhat confused. His skin is hot and dry and his lips are cracked and bleeding. His skin turgor is poor and he appears malnourished. His blood pressure is 96/60 mm Hg, pulse is 120, respirations 30, temperature is 105° F. In addition to high-flow oxygen, what does the nurse anticipate the ED physician will initially order?
   a. IV normal saline and a Foley catheter
   b. IV Ringer's lactate and an NG tube
   c. IV 5% dextrose and acetaminophen (Tylenol)
   d. IV 45% saline and chlorpromazine (Thorazine)

13. An older adult man in the ED has sustained a snakebite. What key questions does the nurse ask to assess the risk for envenomation? *(Select all that apply.)*
    a. Did the snake have a depression between each eye?
    b. Did the snake have an oval-shaped head?
    c. Did the bite cause swelling at the site?
    d. Did the bite leave any secretions on the skin?
    e. Did the snake have curved fangs?

14. A patient sustained a bite from a pit viper and is admitted for observation. Which potential complications does the nurse observe for? *(Select all that apply.)*
    a. Local tissue necrosis
    b. Diarrhea
    c. Massive tissue swelling
    d. Renal failure
    e. Hypovolemic shock
    f. Increased intracranial pressure

15. The nurse is participating in a summer hike with a group of children. Suddenly the children start screaming, "Snake! Snake!" One little girl is sitting in a tall grassy area, clutching her ankle and crying. What is the first priority in the field care of this child?
    a. Remove any constricting clothing.
    b. Maintain the extremity below the level of the heart.
    c. Move the child to a safe area and encourage rest.
    d. Keep the child warm and provide calm reassurance.

16. The nurse is on a backpacking trip. One of the hikers sustains a pit viper bite to the lower leg. Transportation to the hospital will be delayed by several hours while others go for help. The nurse decides that the circumstances warrant which first-aid measure?
    a. Elevating the leg and applying cool packs
    b. Incising the fang marks with a pocket knife
    c. Checking the puncture site for swelling and pain
    d. Applying a constricting band proximal to the fang marks

17. A patient arrives in the ED after sustaining a cottonmouth snakebite. What are the immediate interventions for this patient?
    a. Establishing a central line with normal saline
    b. Applying a pressure bandage
    c. Monitoring blood pressure and cardiac function
    d. Administering antivenin

18. A patient is admitted for a poisonous snakebite. The nurse observes that the patient has hematuria, hemoptysis, petechiae, and extensive bruising. These clinical observations indicate to the nurse that the patient may be experiencing which hemorrhagic complication associated with snakebite?
    a. Disseminated intravascular coagulation
    b. Agranulocytosis
    c. Thrombocytopenia
    d. Aplastic anemia

19. Antivenin polyvalent is given to patients with caution when they exhibit which preexisting factors? *(Select all that apply.)*
    a. Previous allergic reaction to antivenom therapy
    b. An older adult likely to have an adverse reaction
    c. Sensitivity to mercury-containing products
    d. Pregnancy
    e. Hypersensitivity to bovine protein

20. A patient is to receive antivenin (*Crotalidae*) polyvalent (ACP) for treatment of a rattlesnake bite 10 days ago. Which symptoms indicate that the patient may have the beginning of serum sickness?
    a. Skin rash with pruritus
    b. Nausea and vomiting
    c. Dizziness and lightheadedness
    d. Malaise and excessive fatigue

21. A patient is transported to the ED by a family member after sustaining a snakebite on a hiking trip. The patient may be a potential candidate for *Crotalidae* Polyvalent Immune Fab (CroFab). In order to safely administer therapy, which question would the nurse ask?
    a. "What type of snake inflicted the bite?"
    b. "How much time has passed since the snakebite occurred?"
    c. "Do you have a history of DVT or do you take Coumadin?"
    d. "Do you have allergies to papaya or pineapple?"

22. A patient sustained a snakebite 2 hours ago and the health care provider orders *Crotalidae* Polyvalent Immune Fab (CroFab). What is the priority nursing intervention in administering this medication to the patient?
    a. Monitor for symptom control after the first dose.
    b. Monitor the patient closely for hives, rash, or difficulty breathing.
    c. Give the bolus dose slowly over 10 minutes.
    d. Give the medication within 3 hours of the snakebite.

23. A patient sustained a coral snakebite on the forearm approximately 12 hours ago and he has been admitted for observation. He reported a mild transient pain, but was otherwise asymptomatic on admission. Which clinical manifestations are early signs of envenomation?
    a. Nausea, vomiting, and pallor
    b. Difficulty speaking and swallowing
    c. Total flaccid paralysis
    d. Severe pain and swelling at the site

24. A patient sustained a coral snakebite and developed severe complications. Which diagnostic test results reveal the physiologic insufficiency and/or damage that occurs with envenomation? *(Select all that apply.)*
    a. Complete blood count (CBC)
    b. Electrocardiogram (ECG)
    c. Creatinine kinase
    d. Electrolytes
    e. Coagulation profile

25. A patient is admitted for a coral snakebite and is to receive antivenin *Micrurus fulvius*. While waiting for the arrival of the antivenin, which equipment does the nurse prepare in case the most significant risk associated with the administration of the antivenin should occur?
    a. Resuscitation equipment, epinephrine, and antihistamines
    b. Cooling blanket, cool mist humidifier, and antipyretics
    c. Padding for side rails, oral suction equipment, and anticonvulsants
    d. Oral suction equipment, emesis basin, and antiemetics

26. A patient is receiving an infusion of antivenin *Micrurus fulvius*. He reports subjective itching at the infusion site that radiates up the arm, and the nurse notes a raised red welt in the axillary area of the same arm. What is the priority nursing action for this patient?
    a. Slow the infusion and reassess the site.
    b. Stop the infusion and give epinephrine or antihistamine.
    c. Flush the line with saline and call the provider.
    d. Discontinue the IV and reestablish the IV at another site.

27. To avoid the reaction experienced by the patient in the previous question, what could the nurse have done differently?
    a. Performed an intradermal skin test.
    b. Evaluated the patency of the IV before administering *Micrurus fulvius*.
    c. Assessed for pain or itching in the extremity before administering antivenin.
    d. Applied cortisone topical ointment to the skin before administering *Micrurus fulvius*.

28. The nurse's next-door neighbor calls because he has just killed a snake that has bitten him on the arm while he was gardening. He does not know how to identify the snake. What features lead the nurse to believe that this snake is poisonous? *(Select all that apply.)*
    a. Triangular head
    b. Two fangs that are curved
    c. The snake hissed before biting
    d. Depression in the skin between each eye and nostril
    e. Diamond pattern on its back
    f. Black, red, and yellow bands of color on the snake (red bands next to black bands)
    g. Black, red, and yellow bands of color on the snake (red bands next to yellow bands)

29. A patient sustained a coral snakebite and calls the ED for instructions. Besides calling for an ambulance, what does the nurse instruct the patient to do?
    a. Apply ice to the wound.
    b. Incise the wound to allow the blood to flow freely.
    c. Place a constricting band proximal to the wound that impedes lymphatic flow but does not impair arterial flow.
    d. Place a constricting band proximal to the wound that is tight enough to reduce arterial flow of the venom.

Matching. Match the type of envenomation with its physical manifestations.

Type of Envenomation
a. Pit viper envenomation
b. Coral snake envenomation
c. Both types

Manifestation
_____ 30. Mild and transient pain at the bite site
_____ 31. Severe pain, swelling, and bruising at the bite site
_____ 32. Formation of vesicles or hemorrhagic bullae
_____ 33. Cranial and peripheral nerve deficits
_____ 34. Nausea and vomiting
_____ 35. Coagulopathy
_____ 36. Total flaccid paralysis
_____ 37. Minty, rubbery, or metallic taste in the mouth

38. When administering antivenin, the nurse needs to monitor closely for which common complication?
    a. Hemorrhage
    b. Neurologic impairment
    c. Anaphylactic shock
    d. Seizures

39. **Crossword Puzzle.** *Complete the crossword puzzle using the clues listed below.*

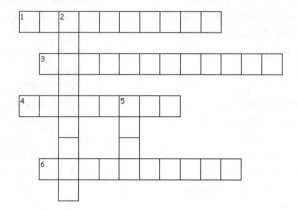

Across

1. The type of hairs launched by the spiders in 2 down that may induce a severe inflammatory reaction if they penetrate the eyes or skin.
3. This type of spider hides in areas that are dark and secluded, and are also known as fiddle-backs or violin spiders *(two words)*.
4. The type of bee that cannot sting repeatedly when disturbed.
6. This type of spider is often found in cool, damp areas such as outdoor log piles, under rocks, or in sheds or garages. The female has a red hourglass pattern on her ventral abdomen *(two words.)*

Down

2. The largest spiders in the arachnid class.
5. The venom of this type of scorpion is neuro-toxic.

Matching. *Match the first aid and hospital interventions with the appropriate spider bite. Some interventions may be appropriate for both types of spider bites.*

Spider Bites

a. Brown recluse spider
b. Black widow spider

Interventions

_____ 40. Apply cold compresses.

_____ 41. Elevate extremity.

_____ 42. Administer opioid pain medications.

_____ 43. Administer muscle relaxants.

_____ 44. Administer oral dapsone.

_____ 45. Administer tetanus prophylaxis.

_____ 46. Monitor for seizures and rapidly rising BP.

_____ 47. Antivenin is available for use.

_____ 48. Débridement and skin grafting may be needed later for severe wounds to heal.

49. A patient calls the health care provider's office after sustaining a spider bite on the arm 3 hours ago asking for advice about whether to come into the office or hospital for evaluation. She denies any allergic reactions or shortness of breath. Which question would be the most relevant in helping the patient to make the decision?
    a. "Do you have Benadryl at the house?"
    b. "Is your arm painful or swollen?"
    c. "Were you able to capture or identify the spider?"
    d. "Was the spider hiding in a dark secluded area?"

50. A patient calls the ED for advice on immediate first aid for a brown recluse spider bite on his hand. He denies allergic response or shortness of breath and states that he plans to see his health care provider, but is currently about 2 to 3 hours away. What does the nurse advise the patient to do?
    a. Apply a warm pack and elevate the extremity.
    b. Wash the bite area several times with soap and water.
    c. Apply ice and rest as much as possible.
    d. Apply a snug constricting band at the wrist level.

51. A patient sustained a brown recluse bite and has been admitted for IV antibiotics and wound management. Which laboratory value indicates that the patient may be developing a serious complication from the bite?
    a. Increased red blood count
    b. Increased platelet count
    c. Decreased white blood count
    d. Decreased blood urea nitrogen

52. A patient was bitten by a brown recluse spider 4 days ago. The nurse observes petechiae, reddish bruising, ecchymoses, and prolonged bleeding after venipunctures. The patient also has a platelet count of 10,000/μL. What do these findings indicate?
    a. Thrombocytopenia
    b. Hemolytic anemia
    c. Aplastic anemia
    d. Agranulocytosis

53. Which complications are related to a black widow spider bite? *(Select all that apply.)*
    a. Muscle rigidity and spasms of large muscles
    b. Severe dizziness and tinnitus
    c. Severe abdominal pain
    d. Latrodectism
    e. Hypertension

54. The nurse is assessing a patient who reports being bitten by a black widow spider. The patient may have clinical signs and symptoms that mimic which disorder?
    a. Myocardial infarction
    b. Peritonitis
    c. Small bowel obstruction
    d. Deep vein thrombosis

55. A patient who has been bitten by a black widow spider requires the following interventions in which priority order? *(Select in order of priority.)*

    _____ a. Administration of antivenin for severe reaction (respiratory arrest and uncontrolled hypertension)

    _____ b. Application of an ice pack to the site

    _____ c. Monitoring of vital signs

    _____ d. Administration of diazepam (Valium) for seizures

56. A patient reports severe skin inflammation after sustaining a tarantula bite. On close inspection, the nurse observes that the skin area is covered with fine hairs. What is the first intervention for this skin irritation?
    a. Flush the skin with sterile normal saline
    b. Wash the area thoroughly with soap and water
    c. Apply sticky tape to the skin and pull off to remove hairs
    d. Gently scrape the skin with a rigid plastic card

57. A patient reports a scorpion sting to the back of the hand. There is no obvious redness or inflammation at the suspected sting site. Which assessment technique does the nurse use to confirm a bark scorpion sting?
   a. Raise the arm and observe for blanching.
   b. Observe for the stinger embedded in the skin.
   c. Look for puncture marks surrounded by fine hairs.
   d. Gently tap at the suspected area to elicit pain.

58. A patient is admitted for observation following a bark scorpion sting. The nurse monitors the patient for which type of systemic complications? *(Select all that apply.)*
   a. Gastrointestinal disorders
   b. Tachycardia
   c. Hypotension
   d. Temperature of 100.7° F (38.2° C)
   e. Pulmonary edema

59. A patient is being treated for a bark scorpion sting. He is currently alert, but somewhat confused. He complains of localized pain (5/10) at the site and requires frequent oral suction. Vital signs are temperature 102° F, pulse 95, respirations 12, and BP 140/85. Which medication order does the nurse question?
   a. Acetaminophen 650 mg PRN for fever
   b. Tetanus toxoid 0.5 mL intramuscularly x 1 dose
   c. Morphine 20 mg intravenous push for severe pain
   d. Atropine 0.4 mg subcutaneously for hypersalivation

60. A patient sustained a bark scorpion sting and the health care provider considers the administration of *Centruroides exilicauda* antivenin if the patient's condition worsens. Which chronic health condition does the nurse assess for that could potentiate a hypersensitivity reaction?
   a. Hypertension
   b. Asthma
   c. Diabetes mellitus
   d. Cardiac disease

61. A person is stung by a wasp at a picnic. The person has no difficulty breathing and no history of allergic reaction to bee or wasp stings. What is the priority first-aid action for this person?
   a. Place a tourniquet proximal to the sting.
   b. Gently scrape the stinger off with the edge of a credit card.
   c. Apply an ice pack to the area and elevate.
   d. Observe the area for signs of inflammation prior to taking any action.

62. A teenager is brought to the ED with a reported bee sting. The nurse observes facial swelling, an audible wheeze, and labored rapid breathing. The teen's girlfriend reports he has been vomiting and having trouble speaking and breathing. What does the nurse anticipate the priority medication order will be?
   a. IV normal saline bolus of 400 mL
   b. 50 mg diphenhydramine (Benadryl) PO
   c. 0.5 mL of 1:1000 epinephrine IM
   d. 100 mg methylprednisolone sodium succinate (Solu-Medrol) IV infusion

63. The health care provider orders IV infusion of epinephrine for an older adult patient who is not responding to the IM epinephrine that was administered for an allergic reaction to a bee sting. In conjunction with the epinephrine administration, which action does the nurse take?
   a. Place the patient on a cardiac monitor.
   b. Place the patient on continuous pulse oximetry.
   c. Obtain an order for an ECG.
   d. Obtain an order for an arterial blood gas.

64. The school nurse is preparing for an outside field trip to a farm with middle school–aged children. What instructions does the nurse provide to the children for bee and wasp sting prevention? *(Select all that apply.)*
   a. Place all jackets or sweaters in a pile on the ground.
   b. Do not try to outrun bees if attacked by a swarm.
   c. Keep food in closed containers.
   d. Wear light-colored clothing and shoes.
   e. Do not swat at bees or wasps close to you.

65. A patient calls the health care provider's office asking for advice about whether to seek immediate medical attention for a bee sting. She has no shortness of breath or swelling to the face, throat, or lips. Which question will elicit information to assist the patient in making the decision?
    a. "Were you stung by an African 'killer bee'?"
    b. "Is the affected area red, painful, or swollen?"
    c. "Did you receive multiple stings?"
    d. "Were you able to remove the stinger?"

66. A mother of a toddler asks the nurse on a routine appointment what first-aid treatment would be for a bee or wasp sting. What instruction by the nurse is correct?
    a. Apply a warm compress immediately over the area.
    b. Immediately remove the stinger with a tweezer.
    c. Apply an ice pack before removing the stinger.
    d. Place a bandage over the stinger and go immediately to the ED.

67. A 37-year-old woman was stung by a bee while gardening. What will cause her to develop a systemic effect?
    a. Multiple bee stings
    b. Allergy to the venom
    c. Desensitization to the venom
    d. No prior allergic reaction to bee stings

68. An anaphylactic reaction to a wasp or bee sting manifests as which conditions? *(Select all that apply.)*
    a. Hypertension
    b. Respiratory distress
    c. Hypoglycemia
    d. Laryngeal edema
    e. Deterioration in mental status

69. A patient with which situation would best benefit from always carrying an EpiPen?
    a. No prior allergic reaction to bee or wasp stings
    b. Allergy to poison ivy and grass
    c. Previous allergic reaction to a wasp sting
    d. No history of being stung by a bee or wasp

70. The nurse is administering an ordered dose of epinephrine to a patient with laryngeal edema after a bee sting. Which route of administration is recommended?
    a. Subcutaneous
    b. Intramuscular
    c. Intravenous
    d. Mucosal

71. A man who was stung by a wasp while painting the outside of his house has developed urticaria and pruritus. What will the nurse likely administer first?
    a. Epinephrine
    b. Diphenhydramine
    c. 2 L oxygen via nasal cannula
    d. Oral placement of airway

72. The nurse is instructing a patient who has a history of allergic reaction to bee stings how to prepare if he or she experiences a bee sting in the future. What information does the nurse relay to the patient? *(Select all that apply.)*
    a. Wear a medical alert bracelet.
    b. Take an antihistamine before administering an EpiPen injection.
    c. Administer epinephrine immediately.
    d. Call 911 to be transported to a medical facility.
    e. Take an aspirin immediately.

73. A patient treated for a severe allergic reaction to a bee sting tells the nurse, "The doctor told me that I had to be careful about getting bee stings in the future, because I could have another allergic reaction." Based on the patient's statement, what is the nurse's first action?
    a. Repeat the information that the physician gave her.
    b. Assess the patient's understanding of allergic reactions and first aid.
    c. Advise the patient to obtain a medical alert bracelet.
    d. Ensure that the patient has a prescription for an EpiPen.

74. Which person has the greatest risk for injury from lightning strike?
    a. Jogger in the park at mid-morning in December
    b. Deer hunter walking through the woods in the evening in October
    c. Golfer out on the green in the late afternoon in June
    d. Camper walking on the beach during the early morning in April

75. Which lightning-strike victim should receive attention first?
    a. Teenager who is motionless except for shallow respirations; he has a weak pulse
    b. Middle-aged man, unconscious, with no palpable pulse
    c. Confused older adult woman with apparent paralysis in lower extremities
    d. Child crying, bleeding from ears, mottled skin, and decreased pulses in left leg

76. A construction worker who was struck by lightning is brought to the ED. He was reported to be unconscious, but CPR was started immediately and he awoke just before the arrival of EMS personnel. In the ED, he is alert and confused, and reports pain to his right hand and foot with fernlike marks. Which assessment tool is the priority for this patient?
    a. Glasgow Coma Scale
    b. Pulse oximeter
    c. Cardiac monitor
    d. Rule of Nines chart

77. The nurse receives a phone call from a child who says, "Mommy was hit by lightning! She's outside. I'm afraid to touch her! I'll get shocked too!" How does the nurse advise the child?
    a. "There is no danger in touching your mom. You won't get hurt."
    b. "It will be okay, just quickly run outside and see if she is breathing."
    c. "Is there anybody at home with you? Let me speak to an adult."
    d. "You stay in the house and someone will come to help very soon."

78. A patient reports that several weeks ago she and a friend were at the beach. The friend was struck by lightning and had cardiac arrest and now has severe cognitive impairment. The patient now reports headache, chronic pain, and extreme fatigue. What are these symptoms and this situation consistent with?
    a. Generalized anxiety disorder
    b. Delayed response lightning strike injury
    c. Post-traumatic stress disorder
    d. Occult lightning strike injury

79. The nurse is caring for a patient who had cardiac and respiratory arrest after being struck by lightning. The patient was resuscitated, and he is now alert and appears to be progressing toward recovery. The nurse observes tea-colored urine in the Foley drainage bag. What does the nurse suspect?
    a. This is a normal finding associated with trauma and resuscitation
    b. Dehydration
    c. Urinary tract infection
    d. Excessive muscle damage affecting the kidneys

80. The nurse is advising parents who are trying to organize a winter cross-country skiing trip. In assisting the parents to develop an appropriate winter clothing list, which articles should be taken on the trip? *(Select all that apply.)*
    a. Synthetic socks
    b. Cotton underwear
    c. Polyester fleece shirt
    d. Windproof outer jacket
    e. Hat made from Gore-Tex
    f. Sunglasses

81. The day camp nurse is with a group of children who have been participating in hiking, swimming, and crafts. The nurse sees a child who is soaking wet, stumbling, and taking off all of her clothes. What does the nurse suspect is wrong with this child?
    a. Snakebite
    b. High-altitude sickness
    c. Hypothermia
    d. Cold diuresis

82. The nurse is conducting a community presentation on cold weather safety. Which point is the nurse sure to include in the presentation?
    a. Hydration and water intake are not an issue, so pack extra clothes, not extra water.
    b. Wear multiple layers of socks when participating in winter sports.
    c. When driving in cold winter weather, carry extra clothes, food, and fluids.
    d. Hypothermia occurs only in the winter months in the United States.

83. Which signs/symptoms indicate the most severe case of hypothermia? *(Select all that apply.)*
    a. Tachycardia
    b. Depressed respiratory rate
    c. Decreased pain response
    d. Acid-base imbalance
    e. Dysarthria

84. The nurse is caring for a patient who suffered prolonged cold exposure during a hunting trip. The health care provider instructs the nurse to observe for "cold diuresis" and to administer a 400 mL fluid bolus if symptoms occur. What does the nurse monitor for?
    a. Bradycardia
    b. Increased urine output
    c. Increased respiratory rate
    d. Decreased metabolic rate

85. Several people on a cross-country ski trip experience mild hypothermia. Which items does the nurse offer or obtain for the hypothermia victims? *(Select all that apply.)*
    a. Synthetic-fiber hat
    b. Warm broth
    c. Caffeinated beverage
    d. Polyester fleece shirt
    e. Dry socks and gloves

86. A patient arrives at the ED after a prolonged cold exposure. The nursing assistant handles the patient with rough and vigorous movements during the transfer from stretcher to bed. Which complication has the nursing assistant's actions placed the patient at risk for?
    a. Ventricular fibrillation related to rough handling
    b. Third-degree heart block related to cold autotransfusion
    c. Tissue damage related to frostbite of the extremities
    d. Pulmonary emboli related to dislodgment of a clot

87. The health care provider orders core warming methods for a patient who has moderate hypothermia. What equipment would the nurse obtain in order to provide this therapy?
    a. Three-way Foley with warmed lavage fluid
    b. Axillary thermometer to monitor core temperature
    c. Ambu bag with warmed humidified oxygen
    d. Several warm blankets and warming pads

88. A man is found lying in an alley in cold weather for an unknown length of time. His hands, toes, and face show evidence of frostbite; otherwise there are no obvious injuries. He is severely obtunded with a pulse of 43 beats/min, respirations of 9/min, and a core temperature of 27° C. What is this patient's most immediate physiologic risk?
    a. Acute respiratory distress syndrome
    b. Pulmonary edema
    c. Cardiac arrest
    d. Acute renal failure

89. The nurse has volunteered at a storm shelter to identify potential problems related to cold-related injuries. Which conditions predispose people to a greater risk for cold injury? *(Select all that apply.)*
    a. Hypothyroidism
    b. Old age
    c. Crohn's disease
    d. Osteoarthritis
    e. Malnutrition

90. The nurse is working in a mountain clinic where there is a high incidence of cold-related injuries. Which signs/symptoms indicate the most severe case of frostbite?
    a. Large fluid-filled blisters with partial thickness skin necrosis
    b. Numbness, coldness, and bloodlessness of affected area
    c. Small blisters that contain dark fluid; skin is cool
    d. Pain, numbness, and pallor of the affected area

91. Which measures are *correct* when rewarming a victim of deep frostbite? *(Select all that apply.)*
    a. Rubbing the area helps speed the warming process.
    b. Rapid rewarming in a 38° C to 41° C water bath will be required.
    c. Rapid rewarming is avoided due to the possibility of seizures.
    d. Rewarming does not cause pain due to damage to the peripheral nerves.
    e. An opioid analgesic may be given because of the pain associated with rewarming.
    f. Dry heat may be applied as needed to assist in the rewarming process.
    g. After rewarming, the extremity should be elevated above the heart level.
    h. Immunization for tetanus prophylaxis will be needed.

92. The nurse is conducting a class about cold-weather hiking. To recognize early signs of frostbite, what should hiking partners observe each other frequently for?
    a. White, waxy appearance to exposed skin on the ears, nose, and cheeks
    b. Edema and redness over the exposed skin
    c. Mottled coloring of the skin
    d. Small blisters that contain dark fluid and areas that do not blanch

93. The ED nurse receives a phone call from someone stating that he and his friend have been out in the cold weather and his friend's fingers 3 through 5 appear white and waxy. What does the nurse direct the caller to do?
    a. Seek shelter immediately and massage and briskly rub the fingers.
    b. Seek shelter immediately and place the hands under the armpits.
    c. Seek medical attention immediately and intermittently apply dry heat while en route.
    d. Seek medical attention immediately and place fingers in cool water while en route.

94. A patient has sustained severe frostbite to the toes and lower legs. He received rewarming therapy in the ED and arrives to the medical-surgical unit with a splint on both legs. IV normal saline is infusing at 125 mL/hr. He reports severe pain in the lower extremities. Which health care provider order does the nurse question?
    a. Morphine 1-2 mg IV push PRN for pain in extremities
    b. Elevate bilateral lower extremities above the level of the heart
    c. Neurologic and circulation checks every 1 hour to bilateral lower extremities
    d. Apply compression bandage to bilateral lower extremities

95. The nurse is reviewing the CBC results for a patient who lives in a high mountain town. The patient's RBC is 6.8 million/mm^3. What does this lab value indicate?
    a. Anemia related to a decreased production of erythropoietin
    b. Polycythemia related to chronic hypoxia
    c. Pernicious anemia related to a regional dietary deficiency
    d. Cold antibody anemia related to cold temperature

96. A patient reports having a throbbing headache with nausea and vomiting "like the worst hangover of my life" after recently returning from a hiking trip to the mountains. The nurse suspects that the patient could be suffering from a high-altitude illness. Which question helps the nurse gather relevant information about this condition?
    a. "Did you experience any episodes of hypothermia during your trip?"
    b. "How quickly did you ascend to the top of the mountain range?"
    c. "Did you go skiing or hiking in a high-altitude area?"
    d. "Did you have trouble sleeping while you were in the mountains?"

97. A patient is admitted to the ED for high-altitude sickness. In the morning, he appears apathetic and declines to perform basic ADLs. Later in the shift, the patient is unable to move himself in bed or to independently sit upright. What condition does the nurse suspect?
    a. High-altitude cerebral edema (HACE)
    b. Severe hypoxemia
    c. Acute mountain sickness (AMS)
    d. Severe hypothermia

98. Which most common signs/symptoms indicate high-altitude pulmonary edema (HAPE)? *(Select all that apply.)*
    a. Dyspnea at rest
    b. Persistent, dry cough
    c. Abdominal pain and cramping
    d. Pale lips and nail beds
    e. Cyanotic lips and nail beds

99. A foreign service employee must take an emergency trip to a high mountain area. He normally lives in a coastal area and there is no time for him to acclimate. He asks the nurse what he can do if acute mountain sickness occurs when he is at a high altitude. What does the nurse instruct the patient to do? *(Select all that apply.)*
    a. Stay at a higher altitude if a throbbing headache occurs.
    b. If available, administer oxygen.
    c. Take the oral form of furosemide (Lasix).
    d. Descend to a lower altitude.
    e. Take the oral form of acetazolamide (Diamox).

100. Which occurrence in the patient treated for AMS indicates that treatment with acetazolamide (Diamox) was effective?
    a. Decreased pulse rate and decreased urine output
    b. Increased urine output and an increased respiratory rate
    c. Periodic respirations during sleep and decreased pulse
    d. Decreased sleep disturbance and decreased respiratory rate

101. A rescue team is attempting to take the patient to the hospital for symptoms of HAPE. The descent to the hospital is delayed due to severe weather conditions. What is the most important treatment for this patient during the delay?
    a. Dexamethasone (Decadron)
    b. Furosemide (Lasix)
    c. Oxygen administration
    d. Avoidance of cold stress

102. Two teenagers bring their friend to the ED because "he was drowning." The patient is unconscious but shows spontaneous breathing, and he is immediately taken to the resuscitation area. Which question is most important for the nurse to ask the patient's friends in determining the outcomes for the patient?
    a. "Was this a fresh water or salt water drowning?"
    b. "Does he have any medical conditions, such as seizures?"
    c. "Was the water contaminated with chemicals or algae?"
    d. "How long was he under the water and not breathing?"

103. What responses does the "diving reflex" cause in the body? *(Select all that apply.)*
    a. Tachycardia
    b. Metabolic alkalosis
    c. Bradycardia
    d. Increased cardiac output
    e. Vasoconstriction of vessels in the intestines and kidneys

104. At the lake, several people are looking out across the lake and pointing to a swimmer in the distance who appears to be struggling to stay afloat. What is the correct sequence of emergency steps to take? *(Select in order of priority.)*

_____ a. Stabilize the spine with a board.

_____ b. Safely rescue the victim.

_____ c. Begin immediate cardiopulmonary resuscitation (CPR).

_____ d. Assess neurologic status.

_____ e. Assess airway patency.

CASE STUDY: THE PATIENT WITH MULTIPLE WASP STINGS

Use a separate sheet of paper to answer the questions in this Case Study, or go to the "Prepare for Class" folder on your Evolve website at http://evolve.elsevier.com/Iggy/ to download and complete as a word processing file. Answer guidelines for this Case Study are also available on your Evolve website.

A young adult arrives in the ED with reported multiple wasp stings. The nurse assesses the patient to have audible wheezes, rapid breathing, and hypotension. The ED physician has ordered epinephrine 0.5 mg of 1:1000 IM and albuterol via nebulizer administered by the respiratory therapist. The patient is able to state his name, where he is, and the month and year. When asked to stand, he demonstrates that he can stand up next to the exam table without assistance, though he is slightly short of breath.

Vital signs are: temp 37.2° C (98.9° F); blood pressure 92/70 mm Hg; heart rate 80/min sinus arrhythmia; respirations 30/min; pulse oximetry 92% on 2 L of oxygen via nasal cannula.

1. Of the following, what is the priority problem for this patient?
   - Ineffective Airway Clearance
   - Autonomic Dysreflexia
   - Impaired oxygenation

2. Of the following, what nursing protocol is indicated for the patient?
   - Allergy management
   - Assess and maintain respiratory status and airway patency
   - Monitor vital signs and pulse oximeter readings

12 CHAPTER

Concepts of Emergency and Disaster Preparedness

STUDY/REVIEW QUESTIONS

Fill in the Blank. Identify the terms in each of the statements below.

1. Nuclear, chemical, or biological agents that can cause devastating results and indiscriminate death on a large scale are called _____ of _____ _____.

2. The training that ED physicians and nursing staff take to learn to identify patterns of illness in patients is called _____ _____ training.

3. When there is a national catastrophe, _____ _____ _____ _____ teams are set up to manage mass fatalities.

4. A common organizational model for disaster management in the hospital is the _____ _____ _____ system.

5. The goal of _____ [acronym] training is to decontaminate and manage victims of hazardous materials incidents.

6. A designated location in the hospital with accessible communication to manage requests for additional personnel and resources is known as the _____ _____ center.

7. For which event would the hospital's disaster plan typically be activated?
   a. Three-car collision on the freeway
   b. Fight between two local street gangs
   c. School bus involved in an accident
   d. Explosion at a chemical factory

8. The hospital in a small mountain town is updating their disaster plan to incorporate the "all hazards approach" and to address all credible threats to the area. Which disaster events are the likely priorities in this community's disaster plan? *(Select all that apply.)*
   a. Avalanches
   b. Floods
   c. Burns
   d. Car accidents
   e. Tornados
   f. Bioterrorism
   g. Blizzards

9. The hospital committee is reviewing the disaster plan of their small community hospital in a suburban area of a large city. What is a priority to include in this hospital's disaster plan?
   a. Plan for evacuation routes out of the city
   b. Plan for transporting patients to other hospitals
   c. Method to contact the National Disaster Medical System
   d. Stockpiling postexposure prophylactic antibiotics

10. The hospital staff is participating in a disaster drill and the nurse is assigned to organize personnel who are called in from home. Which task would be appropriate to delegate to a nursing assistant who usually works in the labor and delivery area?
    a. Stay with "black tag" patients in the holding area.
    b. Talk to the families of the "red tag" patients.
    c. Care for and support the "green tag" patients.
    d. Obtain vital signs of the "yellow tag" patients.

11. The emergency nurse is instructing a recently hired registered nurse to the ED about the protective attire that is required for the ED's hazardous materials decontamination plan. What materials does the emergency nurse include? *(Select all that apply.)*
    a. Facemask
    b. Socks
    c. Impervious gown
    d. Eye protection
    e. Protective head cover

Matching. *Several individuals have been injured in a major explosion at an assembly plant. Classify the triage priority according to the color-coded disaster triage tag system (green, yellow, red, or black tag).*

Triage Tags
a. Black tag
b. Green tag
c. Red tag
d. Yellow tag

Triage Priorities
_____ 12. Patient who has died of his injuries
_____ 13. Patient with a fractured ankle
_____ 14. Patient who is short of breath and has broken ribs and a hemothorax
_____ 15. Patient with an open fracture of the femur and a distal pulse
_____ 16. Patient who has a weak pulse and is bleeding profusely from a severe arm laceration
_____ 17. Patient who has a 4-inch leg laceration that is oozing blood slowly
_____ 18. Patient who has fallen and sprained her shoulder

19. The nurse based in Iowa is a volunteer member of the Medical Reserve Corps (MRC) and has been called to serve in Ohio where he does not hold an active nursing license. What should the nurse do?
    a. Determine if Ohio has reciprocity with Iowa before accepting deployment.
    b. Decline deployment because his nursing license will not allow him to practice in Ohio.
    c. Prepare for deployment because he will be considered a federal employee with valid licensure.
    d. Delay deployment until he has reviewed the nurse practice act that is specific to Ohio.

20. The nursing director of a long-term care facility is designated as the "incident commander" for the facility's disaster plan. What is the priority action for the incident commander?
    a. Call all the off-duty staff and ask them to come into work.
    b. Take inventory of available supplies according to the disaster plan.
    c. Activate the disaster management process according to the plan.
    d. Call the National Guard to move all the patients to other facilities.

21. The nurse is assigned to assist the "hospital incident commander" during a disaster drill. Which responsibility is appropriate for the nurse in this capacity?
    a. Call all nursing units to determine the number of patients who could potentially be discharged.
    b. Call the physical therapy department and direct therapists to assist in the operating room or the ICU.
    c. Go to the emergency department (ED) and assist with the triage of disaster victims to appropriate clinical areas.
    d. Contact the security department and instruct them to control the number of people who attempt to enter the hospital.

22. The nurse serves on a committee that is tasked to develop tools and aids that the "medical command physician" could use during a disaster event. What is an appropriate project for this purpose?
    a. Make a current list, including contact information, of trauma and orthopedic surgeons.
    b. Make a telephone tree for contacting the nursing and ancillary staff.
    c. Design a triage algorithm that addresses different types of disaster events.
    d. Design an algorithm for contacting the Federal Emergency Management Agency.

23. At 3:00 AM, the ED charge nurse of a large suburban hospital receives notification that a commercial plane has just crashed outside the city limits. What does the nurse do? *(Select all that apply.)*
    a. Collaborate with the medical command physician.
    b. Activate the hospital's disaster plan.
    c. Initiate the staff telephone tree.
    d. Collaborate with the triage officer.
    e. Organize nursing and ancillary services.

24. A local news station calls the hospital seeking permission to verify the number of victims and details of a local disaster. What is the nurse's best response?
    a. "Please don't bother us now. We are swamped with victims."
    b. "We have a lot of stable victims and two people have died."
    c. "Please hold and I will connect you to the public information officer."
    d. "I will connect you with the Emergency Command Center."

25. During a mass casualty, a _____ _____ rapidly evaluates each patient who presents to the hospital, even those already with triage tags.

26. During a disaster event, several nurses from the quality assurance department are reassigned to clinical roles. Which area is the most appropriate assignment for these nurses?
    a. Operating room to scrub in for emergency surgeries
    b. ED to take vital signs and transport patients
    c. ED to assist in the triage of incoming patients
    d. Clinic area to provide care for "green tag" patients

27. A city committee reviews possible scenarios related to a disaster event. Which is an example of the "greatest good for the greatest number of people?"
    a. The city's supply of antibiotics is sent to one hospital that has 25 victims with exposure to a bioterrorism agent.
    b. Twenty victims infected by a bioterrorism agent are placed on life support and mechanical ventilation.
    c. Thirty people with possible exposure to a bioterrorism agent are quarantined including five children who are asymptomatic.
    d. Elderly community members are treated with prophylactic antibiotics for a bioterrorism agent.

28. The nurse is making a personal emergency preparedness plan. What is the nurse sure to include in the plan?
    a. Make a disaster supply kit with clothing and basic survival supplies.
    b. Resolve the ethical conflicts of family and professional obligations.
    c. Stockpile antibiotics, first-aid supplies, and resuscitation equipment.
    d. Teach family members about radiation and HAZMAT safety issues.

29. A patient comes to the ED worried that he has been exposed to anthrax after opening a box that contained a white powder. The patient has brought the box with him. What priority actions does the ED nurse take in order of importance? *(Select in order of priority.)*

    _____ a. Activate the ED hazardous materials decontamination plan.

    _____ b. Have the patient place the box on the ground.

    _____ c. Call local police and the Department of Public Health.

    _____ d. Notify security and escort the patient out of the building.

    _____ e. Ask the security guard to place a sheet over the box.

30. The nurse is assigned to assist the incident commander who is evaluating the feasibility of deactivating the emergency response plan. The commander directs the nurse to accomplish certain tasks. Which task is the priority?
    a. Contact all hospital departments and determine if needs have been met.
    b. Go to the ED and supervise the inventory and restocking of supplies.
    c. Arrange for temporary sleeping quarters for exhausted staff members.
    d. Assist in the preparations of the critical incident stress debriefing.

31. A patient comes to the ED worried about possible exposure to a hazardous substance. He presents with periorbital swelling and redness on exposed skin areas (i.e., face and hands). The triage nurse elects to activate the hazardous materials decontamination plan. What precautions does this plan entail? *(Select all that apply.)*
    a. Staff wear protective gowns, gloves, masks, and protective eyewear.
    b. Patient is taken immediately to the closest available shower room.
    c. Patient is directed to remove all of his own clothing.
    d. Patient is directed to wash with soap and water and rinse liberally.
    e. Patient is instructed to wear gown, mask, gloves, and eyewear.
    f. Staff confiscate the patient's clothes and place them in a hazardous waste bag.

32. The nurse is working in the ED where several local gang members are being treated for gunshot and knife wounds. The nurse hears gunshots in the waiting room, followed by screaming and cries for help. What does the nurse do?
    a. Grab the resuscitation box and run to the waiting room.
    b. Assist all the ambulatory patients to leave through a back entrance.
    c. Alert the ED physician that additional trauma victims need care.
    d. Assess the level of threat to self and others and call for help.

33. A multiple-car accident with mass casualties has occurred near an urban hospital. The hospital's emergency preparedness plan is activated. For what purposes is the post-plan administrative review conducted? *(Select all that apply.)*
    a. To identify only the things that went wrong during the plan
    b. To regroup after the plan is discontinued
    c. To establish a social networking system for the employees
    d. To provide all employees the opportunity to express positive and negative comments
    e. To solicit written critique forms for additional information

34. To prevent the development of post-traumatic stress disorder (PTSD) in hospital staff, what action is likely to be taken by the facility?
    a. Conducting administrative debriefings
    b. Providing employees with information on PTSD
    c. Offering employees psychological counseling
    d. Conducting critical incident stress debriefings

35. To protect hospital staff from experiencing post-traumatic stress disorder (PTSD), what are appropriate recommendations by the facility to its employees? *(Select all that apply.)*
    a. Drink plenty of water
    b. Limit verbalizing feelings to family and friends
    c. Use available counseling
    d. Encourage and support coworkers
    e. Do not work more than 14 hours per day

36. To promote effective coping for survivors of a mass-casualty event, the nurse practices which principles while interacting with patients in crisis? *(Select all that apply.)*
    a. Listening to patients
    b. Encouraging patients to have solitude
    c. Promoting relaxation
    d. Allowing unstructured routines
    e. Facilitating community cohesion

37. A gang-related incident has occurred involving major casualties from gunshot wounds to 11 victims. Which type of debriefing is utilized by the hospital after handling this event?
    a. Critical incident stress
    b. Post-traumatic stress
    c. Administrative stress
    d. Restoring normalcy

38. A community hospital is reviewing the activation and implementation of its emergency preparedness plan after a recent mass-casualty event. What is the appropriate type of debriefing that will effectively evaluate these procedures?
    a. Hospital incident command
    b. Event resolution
    c. Administrative
    d. Critical incident

39. After a major crisis, which type of debriefing is most appropriate for hospital staff?
    a. Administrative debriefing
    b. Critical incident stress debriefing
    c. Discussion within small groups that can be shared with close family and friends
    d. Referrals for mental health counseling

40. The triage method for multi-casualty or mass response utilizes what sorting methods? *(Select all that apply.)*
    a. Patients are alphabetized by name
    b. Physicians triage most critical patients
    c. Patients are labeled by number
    d. Patients are ranked by assessment scores
    e. Patients are ranked using color labels

CASE STUDY: DISASTER PREPAREDNESS

Use a separate sheet of paper to answer the questions in this Case Study, or go to the "Prepare for Class" folder on your Evolve website at http://evolve.elsevier.com/Iggy/ to download and complete as a word processing file. Answer guidelines for this Case Study are also available on your Evolve website.

A nurse is working in the ED of a large metropolitan city that experienced severe flooding in the last 24 hours. The ED has received numerous patients who have sustained various types of injuries such as near-drowning, lightning strikes, head injuries, abrasions, and lacerations. The medical command physician is working with the triage officer to examine patients for appropriate disposition for care in either the ED or another area of the hospital that best meets each patient's needs.

The most recent casualties who have come into the ED for triage are:
- A woman receiving CPR for asystole following a lightning strike
- An 11-year-old boy with mild burns on his right shoulder from a reported lightning strike
- A confused older man who is not able to provide his wife's name or state the present month. His wife states that the confusion is new and says he has a history of chronic obstructive pulmonary disease (COPD) and insulin-dependent diabetes.
- A teenager with an occipital laceration and small amount of bleeding. His family reports a blunt object hit him in the head before they pulled him out of the water. The patient denies any loss of consciousness.

1. List which patients would be seen in the order of priority.
2. Identify two to three potential complications for each patient.

Assessment and Care of Patients with Fluid and Electrolyte Imbalances

STUDY/REVIEW QUESTIONS

Fill in the Blank. *Complete the sentences below using the terms listed. Not all terms will be used.*

Terms
Diffusion
Excess fluid
Filtration
Fluid loss
Hydrostatic pressure
Osmolality
Osmolarity
Osmosis

1. The free movement of solutes (electrolytes) across a membrane is called _____.

2. In _____, water moves down its pressure gradient through a semipermeable membrane from diluted fluid to a more concentrated fluid until equilibrium occurs.

3. _____ occurs when water crosses the capillary membrane into the interstitial space.

4. _____ _____ in the vascular system is the blood pressure created in the vessels by the contraction of the heart.

5. _____ is the number of milliosmoles in a liter of solution.

6. _____ is the number of milliosmoles in a kilogram of solution.

7. Which findings indicate that a patient may have hypervolemia? *(Select all that apply.)*
   a. Increased, bounding pulse
   b. Jugular venous distention
   c. Diminished peripheral pulses
   d. Presence of crackles
   e. Excessive thirst
   f. Elevated blood pressure
   g. Orthostatic hypotension
   h. Skin pale and cool to touch

8. The difference in concentration of particles that is greater on one side of a permeable membrane than on the other side is known as what?
   a. Hydrostatic pressure
   b. Concentration gradient
   c. Passive transport
   d. Active transport

9. A patient's blood osmolarity is 302 mOsm/L. What manifestation does the nurse expect to see in the patient?
   a. Increased urine output
   b. Thirst
   c. Peripheral edema
   d. Nausea

10. A patient is at risk for hypervolemia. For self-management at home, what does the nurse teach the patient to do? *(Select all that apply.)*
    a. Call the physician if swelling occurs.
    b. Monitor skin turgor and record daily.
    c. Limit the amount of free water intake.
    d. Weigh self each day on the same scale.
    e. Avoid high-sodium foods.

11. An older adult patient at risk for fluid and electrolyte problems is vigilantly monitored by the nurse for the first indication of a fluid balance problem. What is this indication?
    a. Fever
    b. Mental status changes
    c. Poor skin turgor
    d. Dry mucous membranes

12. Which intake-output record represents the norm for the average adult?
    a. 500 mL of fluid per day, ingesting an additional 200 mL of fluid from food
    b. 1500 mL of fluid per day, ingesting an additional 800 mL of fluid from food
    c. 3000 mL of fluid per day, ingesting an additional 500 mL of fluid from food
    d. 5000 mL of fluid per day, ingesting an additional 100 mL of fluid from food

13. What are the consequences for a patient who does not meet the obligatory urine output? *(Select all that apply.)*
    a. Lethal electrolyte imbalances
    b. Alkalosis
    c. Urine becomes diluted
    d. Toxic buildup of nitrogen
    e. Acidosis

14. What is the minimum amount of urine per day needed to excrete toxic waste products?
    a. 200 to 300 mL
    b. 400 to 600 mL
    c. 500 to 1000 mL
    d. 1000 to 1500 mL

15. A patient who loses a lot of fluid and sodium is likely experiencing an increase in _____ secretion.

16. Patients with which conditions are at great risk for deficient fluid volume? *(Select all that apply.)*
    a. Fever of 103° F
    b. Extensive burns
    c. Thyroid crisis
    d. Water intoxication
    e. Continuous fistula drainage
    f. Diabetes insipidus

17. The nurse is working in a long-term care facility where there are numerous patients who are immobile and at risk for dehydration. Which task is best to delegate to the unlicensed assistive personnel (UAP)?
    a. Offer patients a choice of fluids every 1 to 2 hours.
    b. Check patients at the beginning of the shift to see who is thirsty.
    c. Give patients extra fluids around medication times.
    d. Evaluate oral intake and urinary output.

18. The nurse is assisting a community group to plan a family sports day. In order to prevent dehydration, what beverage does the nurse suggest be supplied?
    a. Iced tea
    b. Light beer
    c. Diet soda
    d. Bottled water

19. The nurse is assessing the weight of a patient with chronic renal failure. The patient shows a 2 kg weight gain since the last clinic appointment. This is equivalent to _____ liters of fluid.

20. Which factors affect the amount and distribution of body fluids? *(Select all that apply.)*
    a. Race
    b. Age
    c. Gender
    d. Height
    e. Body fat

21. The nurse is caring for a patient with hypovolemia secondary to severe diarrhea and vomiting. In evaluating the respiratory system for this patient, what does the nurse expect to assess?
    a. No changes, because the respiratory system is not involved
    b. Hypoventilation, because the respiratory system is trying to compensate for low pH
    c. Increased respiratory rate, because the body perceives hypovolemia as hypoxia
    d. Normal respiratory rate, but a decreased oxygen saturation

22. The nurse is assessing skin turgor in a 65-year-old patient. What is the correct technique to use with this patient?
    a. Pinch the skin over the sternum and observe for tenting and resumption of skin to its normal position after release.
    b. Observe the skin for a dry, scaly appearance and compare it to a previous assessment.
    c. Pinch the skin over the back of the hand and observe for tenting; count the number of seconds for the skin to recover position.
    d. Observe the mucous membranes and tongue for cracks, fissures, or a pasty coating.

23. The emergency department (ED) nurse is caring for a patient who was brought in for significant alcohol intoxication and minor trauma to the wrist. What will serial hematocrits for this patient likely show?
    a. Hemoconcentration
    b. Normal and stable hematocrits
    c. Progressively lower hematocrits
    d. Decreasing osmolality

24. The nurse is caring for a child at risk for dehydration secondary to diarrhea, vomiting, and fever. The child is alert, quiet, and clinging to the parent. What is the best nursing intervention to rehydrate this patient?
    a. Give an oral rehydration solution such as Oralyte or Rehydralyte.
    b. Have the parent give small sips of preferred diluted fluids every 5 to 10 minutes.
    c. Obtain an order for IV access and an isotonic solution such as normal saline.
    d. Encourage the child to take as much water as possible and offer popsicles.

25. Which statements about the function of the lymphatic system are true? *(Select all that apply.)*
    a. Lymph fluid contains more protein than plasma.
    b. Lymph flow is slower than blood flow.
    c. Lymph flow is enhanced by a pump system.
    d. Lymphatic vessels carry lymph fluid toward the heart.
    e. Lymph fluid is filtered by lymph nodes.
    f. The lymphatic system takes lymph to the kidneys for excretion.

26. The nurse is caring for several older adult patients who are at risk for dehydration. Which task can be delegated to the UAP?
    a. Withhold fluids if patients are incontinent of bowels or bladder.
    b. Assess for and report any difficulties that patients are having in swallowing.
    c. Stay with patients while they drink and note the exact amount ingested.
    d. Divide the total amount of fluids needed over a 24-hour period and post a note.

27. The nurse assessing a patient notes a bounding pulse quality, neck vein distention when supine, presence of crackles in the lungs, and increasing peripheral edema. These findings reflect a condition of fluid _____.

28. A patient is at risk for fluid volume excess and dependent edema. Which task does the nurse delegate to the UAP?
    a. Massage the legs and heels to stimulate circulation.
    b. Evaluate the effectiveness of a pressure-reducing mattress.
    c. Assess the coccyx, elbows, and hips daily for signs of redness.
    d. Assist the patient to change position every 2 hours.

29. The nurse is reviewing orders for several patients who have risk for fluid volume excess. For which patient condition does the nurse question an order for diuretics?
    a. Pulmonary edema
    b. Congestive heart failure
    c. End-stage renal disease
    d. Ascites

30. The UAP reports to the nurse that a patient being evaluated for kidney problems has produced a large amount of pale yellow urine. What does the nurse do next?
    a. Instruct the UAP to measure the amount carefully and then discard the urine.
    b. Instruct the UAP to save the urine in a large bottle for a 24-hour urine specimen.
    c. Assess the patient for signs of fluid imbalance and check the specific gravity of the urine.
    d. Compare the amount of urine output to the fluid intake for the previous 8 hours.

31. On admission, a patient with pulmonary edema weighed 151 lbs; now the patient's weight is 149 lbs. Assuming the patient was weighed both times with the same clothing, same scale, and same time of day, how many milliliters of fluid does the nurse estimate the patient has lost?
    a. 500
    b. 1000
    c. 2000
    d. 2500

32. The nurse is giving discharge instructions to the patient with advanced congestive heart failure who is at continued risk for fluid volume excess. For which physical change does the nurse instruct the patient to call the health care provider?
    a. Greater than 3 lbs gained in a week or greater than 1 to 2 lbs gained in a 24-hour period
    b. Greater than 5 lbs gained in a week or greater than 1 to 2 lbs gained in a 24-hour period
    c. Greater than 15 lbs gained in a month or greater than 5 lbs gained in a week
    d. Greater than 20 lbs gained in a month or greater than 5 lbs gained in a week

33. The nurse is caring for several patients at risk for falls because of fluid and electrolyte imbalances. Which task related to patient safety and fall prevention does the nurse delegate to the UAP?
    a. Assess for orthostatic hypotension.
    b. Orient the patient to the environment.
    c. Help the incontinent patient to toilet every 1 to 2 hours.
    d. Encourage family members or significant other to stay with the patient.

34. The nurse is assessing a patient's urine specific gravity. The value is 1.035. How does the nurse interpret this result?
    a. Overhydration
    b. Dehydration
    c. Normal value for an adult
    d. Renal disease

Matching. Match each electrolyte with its corresponding lab value and description. Answers can be used more than once.

Electrolytes

a. Sodium
b. Potassium
c. Calcium
d. Phosphorus
e. Magnesium
f. Chloride

Normal Lab Values and Descriptions

_____ 35. Normal plasma value is 3.5 to 5.0 mEq/L

_____ 36. Major anion of extracellular fluid (ECF)

_____ 37. Normal value is 98 to 106 mEq/L

_____ 38. Main cation in ECF of the cell that maintains ECF osmolarity

_____ 39. Works in balance with calcium

_____ 40. Normal plasma value is 136 to 145 mEq

_____ 41. Has more activity in the cell than in the blood

_____ 42. Major cation of intracellular fluid (ICF) in the cell

_____ 43. Maintains action potentials in excitable membranes

_____ 44. Functions include contraction of skeletal and cardiac muscle

_____ 45. Normal value is 3.0 to 4.5 mg/dL

_____ 46. Major intracellular anion

_____ 47. Free form is physiologically active in the body

_____ 48. Normal value is 1.3 to 2.1 mEq/L

49. What are the functions of potassium in the body? *(Select all that apply.)*
    a. Regulates hydration status
    b. Regulates protein synthesis
    c. Stimulates the secretion of antidiuretic hormone (ADH)
    d. Regulates glucose use and storage
    e. Helps maintain normal cardiac rhythm

50. Which statements are true about the electrolyte chloride and its role in the cellular environment of the body? *(Select all that apply.)*
    a. It is a major cation in extracellular fluid (ECF).
    b. It maintains plasma acid-base balance.
    c. It provides electroneutrality in relation to sodium.
    d. Chloride imbalances occur with alterations in body water volume.
    e. Chloride concentration varies inversely with changes in bicarbonate concentration.

51. What impacts does sodium have on body function? *(Select all that apply.)*
    a. Maintains electroneutrality
    b. Maintains electrical membrane excitability
    c. Aids in carbohydrate and lipid metabolism
    d. Regulates water balance
    e. Regulates plasma osmolality

52. What impacts does phosphorus have in the body? *(Select all that apply.)*
    a. Activates B-complex vitamins
    b. Adds strength/density to bones and teeth
    c. Aids in blood-clotting cascade
    d. Assists in the formation of adenosine triphosphate (ATP)
    e. Stabilizes excitable membranes

53. The electrolyte magnesium is responsible for which functions? *(Select all that apply.)*
    a. Formation of hydrochloric acid
    b. Carbohydrate metabolism
    c. Contraction of skeletal muscle
    d. Regulation of intracellular osmolarity
    e. Formation of adenosine triphosphate (ATP)

54. _____ is a major cation of intracellular fluid (ICF) in the cell.

55. A patient is talking to the nurse about sodium intake. Which statement by the patient indicates an understanding of high-sodium food sources?
    a. "I have bacon and eggs every morning for breakfast."
    b. "We never eat seafood because of the salt water."
    c. "I love Chinese food, but I gave it up because of the soy sauce."
    d. "Pickled herring is a fish and my doctor told me to eat a lot of fish."

56. Which statement best explains how antidiuretic hormone (ADH) affects urine output?
    a. It increases permeability to water in the tubules causing a decrease in urine output.
    b. It increases urine output as a result of water being absorbed by the tubules.
    c. Urine output is reduced as the posterior pituitary decreases ADH production.
    d. Increased urine output results from increased osmolarity and fluid in the extracellular space.

57. A patient with hyponatremia would have which gastrointestinal findings upon assessment? *(Select all that apply.)*
    a. Hyperactive bowel sounds on auscultation, mostly in the left lower quadrant
    b. Hard, dark brown stools
    c. Hypoactive bowel sounds on auscultation
    d. Bowel movements that are frequent and watery
    e. Abdominal cramping

58. The nurse is caring for a patient with severe hypocalcemia. What safety measures does the nurse put in place for this patient? *(Select all that apply.)*
    a. Encourage the patient to use a cane when ambulating.
    b. Turn on a bed alarm when the patient is in bed.
    c. Obtain an order for zolpidem (Ambien) to ensure the patient sleeps at night.
    d. Place the patient on a low bed.
    e. Ensure the side rails are up when the patient is in bed.

59. Which patients are at risk for developing hyponatremia? *(Select all that apply.)*
    a. Postoperative patient who has been NPO for 24 hours with no IV fluid infusing
    b. Patient with decreased fluid intake for several days
    c. Patient with excessive intake of 5% dextrose solution
    d. Diabetic patient with blood glucose of 250 mg/dL
    e. Patient with overactive adrenal glands
    f. Tennis player in 100° F weather who has been drinking water

60. The nurse is evaluating the lab results of a patient with hyperaldosteronism. What abnormal electrolyte finding does the nurse expect to see?
    a. Hyponatremia
    b. Hyperkalemia
    c. Hypocalcemia
    d. Hypernatremia

61. The nurse assistant informs the nurse that a patient with hypernatremia who was initially confused and disoriented on admission to the hospital is now trying to pull out the IV access and Foley catheter. Which actions, in order of priority, does the nurse take? *(Select in priority order.)*
    _____ a. Place bilateral soft wrist restraints.
    _____ b. Inform the physician of the patient's change in behavior and obtain an order for restraints.
    _____ c. Assess the patient.
    _____ d. Offer the patient oral fluids.

62. Patients with which conditions are at risk for developing hypernatremia? *(Select all that apply.)*
    a. Chronic constipation
    b. Heart failure
    c. Severe diarrhea
    d. Severe vomiting
    e. Profound diaphoresis

63. The physician has ordered therapy for a patient with low sodium and signs of hypervolemia. Which diuretic is best for this patient?
    a. Conivaptan (Vaprisol)
    b. Furosemide (Lasix)
    c. Hydrochlorothiazide (HydroDIURIL)
    d. Bumetanide (Bumex)

64. The nurse is assessing a patient with a mild increase in sodium level. What early manifestation does the nurse observe in this patient?
    a. Muscle twitching and irregular muscle contractions
    b. Inability of muscles and nerves to respond to a stimulus
    c. Muscle weakness occurring bilaterally with no specific pattern
    d. Reduced or absent deep tendon reflexes

65. The nurse is caring for a patient with hypernatremia caused by fluid and sodium losses. What type of IV solution is best for treating this patient?
    a. Hypotonic 0.225% sodium chloride
    b. Small-volume infusions of hypertonic (2% to 3%) saline
    c. Isotonic sodium chloride (NaCl)
    d. 0.45% sodium chloride

66. Which serum value does the nurse expect to see in a patient with hyponatremia?
    a. Sodium less than 136 mEq/L
    b. Chloride less than 95 mEq/L
    c. Sodium less than 145 mEq/L
    d. Chloride less than 103 mEq/L

67. A patient having watery diarrhea with abdominal cramping has the electrolyte imbalance of
    _____.

68. The nurse is caring for a psychiatric patient who is continuously drinking water. The nurse monitors for which complication related to potential hyponatremia?
    a. Proteinuria/prerenal failure
    b. Change in mental status/increased intracranial pressure
    c. Pitting edema/circulatory failure
    d. Possible stool for occult blood/gastrointestinal bleeding

69. What interventions are appropriate for a patient with mild hypernatremia caused by excessive fluid loss? *(Select all that apply.)*
    a. Hypotonic intravenous infusion
    b. 0.45% sodium chloride intravenous infusion
    c. D_5W intravenous infusion
    d. Administration of bumetanide (Bumex)
    e. Gradual reduction of serum sodium to establish to normal level

70. The nurse is caring for several patients at risk for fluid and electrolyte imbalances. Which patient problem or condition can result in a relative hypernatremia?
    a. Use of a salt substitute
    b. Diarrhea
    c. Drinking too much water
    d. NPO status

71. The nurse is caring for an older adult patient whose serum sodium level is 150 mEq/L. The nurse assesses the patient for which common manifestations associated with this sodium level? *(Select all that apply.)*
    a. Intact recall of recent events
    b. Increased pulse rate
    c. Rigidity of extremities
    d. Hyperactivity
    e. Muscle weakness

72. Which conditions cause a patient to be at risk for hypernatremia? *(Select all that apply.)*
    a. Renal failure
    b. Immobility
    c. Use of corticosteroids
    d. Watery diarrhea
    e. Cushing's syndrome

73. An older adult patient with decreased sensitivity to thirst is most at risk for developing the imbalance of _____.

74. Which precaution or intervention does the nurse teach a patient at continued risk for hypernatremia?
    a. Avoid salt substitutes
    b. Avoid aspirin and aspirin-containing products
    c. Read labels on canned or packaged foods to determine sodium content
    d. Increase daily intake of caffeine-containing foods and beverages

75. The nurse identifies the priority problem of "potential for injury" for a patient with hyponatremia. What is the etiology of this priority patient problem?
    a. Altered mental capabilities
    b. Fragility of bones
    c. Immobility
    d. Altered senses

76. A patient with renal failure that results in hypernatremia will require which interventions? *(Select all that apply.)*
    a. Administration of furosemide (Lasix)
    b. Hemodialysis
    c. IV infusion of 0.9% sodium chloride
    d. IV infusion of 0.45% sodium chloride
    e. Administration of bumetanide (Bumex)

77. The nurse is teaching a patient to recognize foods that are high in sodium. Which food items does the nurse use as examples? *(Select all that apply.)*
    a. Egg roll with soy sauce
    b. White rice
    c. Salad with oil and vinegar dressing
    d. Bacon and eggs
    e. Cottage cheese and tomato
    f. Steak
    g. Soup with saltine crackers
    h. Steamed vegetables

Matching. Identify which patient conditions cause the patient to be at risk for developing hyperkalemia or hypokalemia.

Disorder
a. Hyperkalemia
b. Hypokalemia

Patient Conditions

_____ 78. Severe malnutrition in an older adult man

_____ 79. Chronic obstructive pulmonary disease (COPD) managed with prednisone

_____ 80. Short bowel syndrome with use of total parenteral nutrition

_____ 81. Multiple transfusions of packed red cells

_____ 82. End-stage kidney disease

_____ 83. Hypertension managed with Aldactone

_____ 84. Metabolic alkalosis

_____ 85. Ileostomy

_____ 86. Early stage of severe burns

_____ 87. Respiratory acidosis

_____ 88. Diabetes insipidus

_____ 89. Uncontrolled diabetes mellitus

_____ 90. Trauma patient with crushed extremities

_____ 91. Congestive heart failure managed with loop diuretics

92. A hospitalized patient who is known to be homeless has been diagnosed with severe malnutrition, end-stage renal disease, and anemia. He is transfused with 3 units of packed red blood cells. Which potential electrolyte imbalance does the nurse anticipate to occur in this patient?
    a. Hypernatremia
    b. Hyperkalemia
    c. Hypercalcemia
    d. Hypermagnesemia

93. A newly admitted patient with congestive heart failure has a potassium level of 5.7 mEq/L. How does the nurse identify contributing factors for the electrolyte imbalance? *(Select all that apply.)*
    a. Assess the patient for hypokalemia.
    b. Obtain a list of the patient's home medications.
    c. Assess the patient for hyperkalemia.
    d. Ask about the patient's method of taking medications at home.
    e. Evaluate the patient's appetite.

94. A young adult patient is in the early stages of being treated for severe burns. Which electrolyte imbalance does the nurse expect to assess in this patient?
    a. Hypernatremia
    b. Hypokalemia
    c. Hypercalcemia
    d. Hyperkalemia

95. A patient with hypokalemia is likely to have which conditions? *(Select all that apply.)*
    a. Ileus
    b. Metabolic alkalosis
    c. Chronic obstructive pulmonary disease
    d. Hypothyroidism
    e. Short bowel syndrome

96. The nurse is taking care of a trauma patient who was in a motor vehicle accident. The patient has a history of hypertension which is managed with spironolactone (Aldactone). This patient is at risk for developing which electrolyte imbalance?
    a. Hyperkalemia
    b. Hypernatremia
    c. Hypokalemia
    d. Hypocalcemia

97. A patient with lung cancer is admitted to the hospital for respiratory distress. Which imbalances does the nurse expect this patient to have? *(Select all that apply.)*
    a. Metabolic alkalosis
    b. Hypokalemia
    c. Hyperkalemia
    d. Hypermagnesemia
    e. Respiratory acidosis

98. The nurse is caring for a patient who has recently emigrated from Mexico to the U.S. The patient had been diagnosed with type 1 diabetes and placed on insulin one month before. Which nursing interventions are best for this patient? *(Select all that apply.)*
    a. Have a social worker evaluate the patient's financial needs for purchasing insulin and food.
    b. Consult a registered dietitian for meal planning.
    c. Ask the physician to address the education needs of the patient and family.
    d. Ask the patient how he manages his diabetes at home and work.
    e. Provide information based on what the patient requests.

99. Which serum laboratory value does the nurse expect to see in the patient with hypokalemia?
    a. Calcium less than 8.0 mg/dL
    b. Potassium less than 5.0 mEq/L
    c. Calcium less than 11.0 mg/dL
    d. Potassium less than 3.5 mEq/L

100. The patient's potassium level is 2.5 mEq/L. Which clinical findings does the nurse expect to see when assessing this patient? *(Select all that apply.)*
    a. General skeletal muscle weakness
    b. Moist crackles and tachypnea
    c. Lethargy
    d. Increased specific gravity and decreased urine output
    e. Weak hand grasps

101. The nurse administering potassium to a patient carefully monitors the infusion because of the risk for which condition?
    a. Pulmonary edema
    b. Cardiac dysrhythmia
    c. Postural hypotension
    d. Renal failure

102. Which changes on a patient's electrocardiogram (ECG) reflect hyperkalemia?
    a. Tall peaked T waves
    b. Narrow QRS complex
    c. Tall P waves
    d. Normal P-R interval

103. The nurse is teaching the patient about hypokalemia. Which statement by the patient indicates a correct understanding of the treatment of hypokalemia?
    a. "My wife does all the cooking. She shops for food high in calcium."
    b. "When I take the liquid potassium in the evening, I'll eat a snack beforehand."
    c. "I will avoid bananas, orange juice, and salt substitutes."
    d. "I hate being stuck with needles all the time to monitor how much sugar I can eat."

104. The nurse is caring for a patient who takes potassium and digoxin. For what reason does the nurse monitor both laboratory results?
    a. Digoxin increases potassium loss through the kidneys.
    b. Digoxin toxicity can result if hypokalemia is present.
    c. Digoxin may cause potassium levels to rise to toxic levels.
    d. Hypokalemia causes the cardiac muscle to be less sensitive to digoxin.

105. Which serum laboratory value does the nurse expect to see in a patient with hyperkalemia?
    a. Calcium greater than 8.0 mg/dL
    b. Potassium greater than 3.5 mEq/L
    c. Calcium greater than 11.0 mg/dL
    d. Potassium greater than 5.0 mEq/L

106. A patient has an elevated potassium level. Which assessment findings are associated with hyperkalemia? *(Select all that apply.)*
    a. Wheezing on exhalation
    b. Numbness in hands, feet, and around the mouth
    c. Frequent, explosive diarrhea stools
    d. Irregular heart rate and hypotension
    e. Circumoral cyanosis

107. The nurse is teaching a patient with hypokalemia about foods high in potassium. Which food items does the nurse recommend to this patient? *(Select all that apply.)*
    a. Soybeans
    b. Lettuce
    c. Cantaloupe
    d. Potatoes
    e. Peaches

108. A patient's serum potassium value is below 2.8 mEq/L. The patient is also on digoxin. The nurse quickly assesses the patient for which cardiac problem before notifying the physician?
    a. Cardiac murmur
    b. Cardiac dysrhythmia
    c. Congestive heart failure
    d. Cardiac tamponade

109. Which potassium levels are within normal limits? *(Select all that apply.)*
    a. 2.0 mmol/L
    b. 3.5 mmol/L
    c. 4.5 mmol/L
    d. 5.0 mmol/L
    e. 6.0 mmol/L

110. A patient has hyperkalemia resulting from dehydration. Which additional laboratory findings does the nurse anticipate for this patient?
    a. Increased hematocrit and hemoglobin levels
    b. Decreased serum electrolyte levels
    c. Increased urine potassium levels
    d. Decreased serum creatinine

111. A 65-year-old patient has a potassium laboratory value of 5.0 mEq/L. How does the nurse interpret this value?
    a. High for the patient's age
    b. Low for the patient's age
    c. Normal for the patient's age
    d. Dependent upon the medical diagnosis

112. A patient's potassium level is low. What change in the cardiovascular system does the nurse expect to see related to hypokalemia?
    a. Tall, peaked T waves
    b. Weak, thready pulse
    c. Malignant hypertension
    d. Distended neck vein

113. Plasma is part of which components? *(Select all that apply.)*
    a. The intracellular compartment
    b. The extracellular compartment
    c. All fluid within the cells
    d. Interstitial fluid
    e. Intravascular fluid

114. Which fluid has the highest corresponding electrolyte content?
    a. Intracellular fluid is highest in potassium.
    b. Extracellular fluid is highest in sodium.
    c. Extracellular fluid is highest in sodium and chloride.
    d. Intracellular fluid is highest in magnesium and sodium.

115. Which component has a high content of potassium and phosphorus?
    a. Extracellular fluid
    b. Intracellular fluid
    c. Extracellular fluid and the intravascular space
    d. Intracellular fluid and lymph fluid

116. A patient with low potassium must have an IV potassium infusion. The pharmacy sends a 250-mL IV bag of dextrose in water with 40 mEq of potassium. The label is marked "to infuse over 1 hour." What does the nurse do?
    a. Obtain a pump and administer the solution.
    b. Double-check the physician's order and call the pharmacy.
    c. Hold the infusion because there is an error in labeling.
    d. Recalculate the rate so that it is safe for the patient.

117. An older adult patient needs an oral potassium solution, but is refusing it because it has a strong and unpleasant taste. What is the best strategy the nurse uses to administer the drug?
    a. Tell the patient that failure to take the drug could result in serious heart problems.
    b. Ask the patient's preference of juice and mix the drug with a small amount.
    c. Mix the solution into food on the patient's meal tray and encourage the patient to eat everything.
    d. Offer the drug to the patient several times and then document the patient's refusal.

118. A patient has a low potassium level and the physician has ordered an IV infusion. Before starting an IV potassium infusion, what does the nurse assess?
    a. Adequate urine output
    b. Oxygen saturation level
    c. Baseline mental status
    d. Apical pulse

119. Which foods will the nurse instruct a patient with kidney disease and hyperkalemia to avoid? *(Select all that apply.)*
    a. Canned apricots
    b. Dried beans
    c. Potatoes
    d. Cabbage
    e. Cantaloupe

120. Which assessment findings are related to hypercalcemia? *(Select all that apply.)*
    a. Bradycardia
    b. Paresthesia
    c. Leg cramping
    d. Hyperactive bowel sounds
    e. Ineffective respiratory movements
    f. Shortened QT interval
    g. Impaired blood flow
    h. Profound muscle weakness

121. Which nursing interventions apply to patients with hypercalcemia? *(Select all that apply.)*
    a. Administer IV normal saline (0.9% sodium chloride).
    b. Assess the patient for a positive Homans' sign.
    c. Measure the abdominal girth.
    d. Massage calves to encourage blood return to the heart.
    e. Monitor for ECG changes.
    f. Provide adequate intake of vitamin D.
    g. During treatment, monitor for tetany.

122. The nurse is reviewing the laboratory calcium level results for a patient. Which value indicates mild hypocalcemia?
    a. 5.0 mg/dL
    b. 8.0 mg/dL
    c. 10.0 mg/dL
    d. 12.0 mg/dL

123. A patient with a recent history of anterior neck injury reports muscle twitching and spasms with tingling in the lips, nose, and ears. The nurse suspects these symptoms may be caused by which condition?
    a. Hypocalcemia
    b. Hypokalemia
    c. Hyponatremia
    d. Hypomagnesemia

124. Which conditions cause a patient to be at risk for hypocalcemia? *(Select all that apply.)*
    a. Crohn's disease
    b. Acute pancreatitis
    c. Removal or destruction of parathyroid glands
    d. Immobility
    e. Use of digitalis

125. The nurse is assessing the patient with a risk for hypocalcemia. What is the correct technique to test for Chvostek's sign?
    a. Patient flexes arms against the chest and examiner attempts to pull the arms away from the chest.
    b. Place a blood pressure cuff around the upper arm and inflate the cuff to greater than the patient's systolic pressure.
    c. Tap the face just below and in front of the ear to trigger facial twitching of one side of the mouth, nose, and cheek.
    d. Lightly tap the patellar and Achilles tendons with a reflex hammer and measure the movement.

126. The nurse is caring for several patients with electrolyte imbalances. Which interventions are included in the plan of care for a patient with hypocalcemia?
    a. Implementing an oral fluid restriction of 1500 mL/day
    b. Implementing a renal diet
    c. Providing moderate environmental stimulation with music
    d. Placing the patient on seizure precautions

127. Which clinical condition can result from hypocalcemia?
    a. Stimulated cardiac muscle contraction
    b. Increased intestinal and gastric motility
    c. Decreased peripheral nerve excitability
    d. Increased bone density

128. Which patient is at greatest risk of developing hypocalcemia?
    a. 30-year-old Asian woman with breast cancer
    b. 45-year-old Caucasian man with hypertension and diuretic therapy
    c. 60-year-old African-American woman with a recent ileostomy
    d. 70-year-old Caucasian man on long-term lithium therapy

129. Which is a preventive measure for patients at risk for developing hypocalcemia?
    a. Increase daily dietary calcium intake to 1000 mg.
    b. Increase intake of phosphorus.
    c. Apply sunblock and wear protective clothing whenever outdoors.
    d. Administer calcium-containing IV fluids to patients receiving multiple blood transfusions.

130. The patient who has undergone which surgical procedure is most at risk for hypocalcemia?
    a. Thyroidectomy
    b. Adrenalectomy
    c. Pancreatectomy
    d. Gastrectomy

131. Which medication order does the nurse clarify before administering the drug to a patient with hypomagnesemia?
    a. Magnesium sulfate 1 g IM every 6 hours for four doses
    b. Aluminum hydroxide (AlternaGEL) 15 mL orally three times a day and at bedtime
    c. Calcium carbonate 1000 mg orally after meals and at bedtime
    d. Calcium gluconate 5 mEq IV PRN for tetany

132. Which are typical nursing assessment findings for a patient with hypocalcemia? *(Select all that apply.)*
    a. Positive Chvostek's sign
    b. Hypertension
    c. Diarrhea
    d. Prolonged ST interval
    e. Elevated T wave

133. Which intervention does the nurse implement for a patient with hypocalcemia?
    a. Encourage activity by the patient as tolerated, including weight-lifting.
    b. Encourage socialization and active participation in stimulating activities.
    c. Include a tracheostomy tray at the bedside for emergency use.
    d. Provide adequate intake of vitamin D and calcium-rich foods.

134. A patient has chronic renal failure (CRF). Which electrolyte imbalance often associated with hypocalcemia and CRF does the nurse monitor for?
    a. Hypophosphatemia
    b. Hyperphosphatemia
    c. Hyperkalemia
    d. Hyponatremia

135. A patient with hypocalcemia is in need of supplemental diet therapy. Which foods does the nurse recommend to provide both calcium and vitamin D? *(Select all that apply.)*
    a. Tofu
    b. Cheese
    c. Eggs
    d. Broccoli
    e. Milk

136. A patient shows a positive Trousseau's or Chvostek's sign. The nurse prepares to give the patient which urgent treatment?
    a. IV calcium
    b. Calcitonin (Calcimar)
    c. IV potassium chloride
    d. Large doses of oral calcium

137. Which is a preventive nursing intervention for a patient at risk for developing hypercalcemia? *(Select all that apply.)*
    a. Administer D$_5$W.
    b. Administer furosemide (Lasix).
    c. Ensure adequate hydration.
    d. Administer plicamycin (Mithracin).
    e. Discourage weight-bearing activity such as walking.

138. The nurse caring for a patient with hypercalcemia anticipates orders for which medications? *(Select all that apply.)*
    a. Magnesium sulfate
    b. Calcitonin (Calcimar)
    c. Furosemide (Lasix)
    d. Plicamycin (Mithracin)
    e. Calcium gluconate
    f. Aluminum hydroxide

139. The nurse instructs the UAP to use precautions with moving and using a lifting sheet for which patient with an electrolyte imbalance?
    a. Young diabetic woman with hyperkalemia
    b. Psychiatric patient with hyponatremia
    c. Older woman with hypocalcemia
    d. Child with severe diarrhea and hypomagnesemia

140. A patient's laboratory results show a decrease in serum phosphorus level. The nurse expects to see a reciprocal increased change in which serum level?
    a. Calcium
    b. Potassium
    c. Sodium
    d. Magnesium

141. _____ is the accompanying and potentially life-threatening electrolyte imbalance that the nurse monitors for in a patient with hyperphosphatemia.

142. Which intervention does the nurse include for a patient with moderate hypophosphatemia?
    a. Aggressive treatment with parenteral phosphorous
    b. Administration of oral vitamin D and phosphorus supplements
    c. Concurrent administration of calcium supplements
    d. Elimination of beef, pork, and legumes from the diet

143. Which manifestations reflect severe hypophosphatemia? *(Select all that apply.)*
    a. Profound muscle weakness
    b. Decreased peristalsis
    c. Elevated T wave
    d. Irritability
    e. Cardiac muscle damage

144. Which factors can cause hyperphosphatemia? *(Select all that apply.)*
    a. Tumor lysis syndrome
    b. Decreased intake of phosphorus
    c. Hypoparathyroidism
    d. Decreased renal excretion
    e. Hyperthyroidism

145. A patient recently admitted to the hospital with malnutrition from alcohol abuse is likely to have the electrolyte imbalance _____.

146. What are common causes of hypophosphatemia? *(Select all that apply.)*
    a. Increased intake of phosphorus
    b. Hypercalcemia
    c. Immobility
    d. Uncontrolled diabetes
    e. Use of magnesium-based antacids

147. A patient with which condition would need priority nursing assessment?
    a. Renal insufficiency
    b. Potassium level of 3.4 mEq/L
    c. Sodium level of 133 mEq/L
    d. Irritability

148. The physician orders magnesium sulfate (MgSO$_4$) for a patient with severe hypomagnesemia. What is the preferred route of administration for this drug?
    a. Oral
    b. Subcutaneous
    c. Intramuscular
    d. Intravenous

149. The nurse is assessing a patient with severe hypermagnesemia. Which assessment findings are associated with this electrolyte imbalance?
    a. Bradycardia and hypotension
    b. Tachycardia and weak palpable pulse
    c. Hypertension and irritability
    d. Irregular pulse and deep respirations

150. A patient in the hospital has a severely elevated magnesium level. What interventions, in order of priority, are performed by the nurse to treat the patient? *(Select in order of priority.)*

    _____ a. Discontinue oral magnesium.

    _____ b. Administer furosemide (Lasix).

    _____ c. Discontinue parenteral magnesium.

    _____ d. Administer calcium to treat bradycardia.

151. A patient has a magnesium level of 0.8 mg/dL. Which treatment does the nurse expect to be ordered for this patient?
    a. Intramuscular magnesium sulfate
    b. Increased intake of fruits and vegetables
    c. Oral preparations of magnesium sulfate
    d. IV magnesium sulfate and discontinuation of diuretic therapy

152. The nurse monitors the effectiveness of magnesium sulfate by assessing which factor every hour?
    a. Deep tendon reflexes
    b. Vital signs
    c. Serum laboratory values
    d. Urine output

153. Which patient condition places a patient at risk for hypocalcemia, hyperkalemia, and hypernatremia?
    a. Hypothyroidism
    b. Diabetes mellitus
    c. Chronic renal failure
    d. Adrenal insufficiency

154. A patient with congestive heart failure is receiving a loop diuretic. The nurse monitors for which electrolyte imbalances? *(Select all that apply.)*
    a. Hypocalcemia
    b. Hypokalemia
    c. Hyponatremia
    d. Hypercalcemia
    e. Hyperkalemia
    f. Hypernatremia

CASE STUDY: THE PATIENT WITH HYPOMAGNESEMIA

Use a separate sheet of paper to answer the questions in this Case Study, or go to the "Prepare for Class" folder on your Evolve website at http://evolve.elsevier.com/Iggy/ to download and complete as a word processing file. Answer guidelines for this Case Study are also available on your Evolve website.

A patient is admitted to the hospital after being found lying on the ground at a street corner. Assessment reveals signs and symptoms of malnutrition and ethanol intoxication. The patient's serum magnesium level is 1.2 mEq/L and serum albumin is 2.3 g/dL. The patient is lethargic and oriented to his name and correct name of the city, but otherwise he is confused. Slight body odor and flat affect of the patient is noted. Abdomen is distended and soft with hypoactive bowel sounds in all four quadrants.

1. Of the following, identify the two priority problems to document for this patient.
   - Risk for Injury
   - Inadequate nutritional intake
   - Abnormal electrolyte balance
   - Altered gastrointestinal function

2. Hypomagnesemia usually occurs with metabolic or nutritional abnormalities. Identify at least three abnormalities for which this patient is at risk.

3. What kinds of magnesium-rich food sources will you recommend to this patient?

CASE STUDY: THE PATIENT WITH HYPOVOLEMIA

Use a separate sheet of paper to answer the questions in this Case Study, or go to the "Prepare for Class" folder on your Evolve website at http://evolve.elsevier.com/Iggy/ to download and complete as a word processing file. Answer guidelines for this Case Study are also available on your Evolve website.

A 78-year-old patient is hospitalized for vomiting and diarrhea that developed 2 days prior to admission. The patient's home medications include diuretics. Temperature is 38.3° C (100.9° F), heart rate 127/min, sinus tachycardia, blood pressure 100/57 mm Hg, respirations 24/min, regular and nonlabored at rest. A Foley catheter is in place to dependent drainage with 110 mL amber, concentrated urine output in the last 5 hours. Tenting of skin is observed when gently pinched over the sternum. The patient can correctly tell the nurse his name and that he is in the hospital because he does not feel well. When asked to stick out his tongue, the nurse notes the surface of the tongue to have deep furrows.

1. Of the following, identify the **two** priority problems to document for this patient.
   - Increased body temperature
   - Dehydration
   - Potential for electrolyte imbalance
   - Risk for altered skin integrity

2. What are at least three clinical manifestations of hypovolemia in this patient?

3. What are at least three risk factors that may have caused the patient to develop hypovolemia?

CASE STUDY: THE PATIENT WITH A FLUID IMBALANCE

Use a separate sheet of paper to answer the questions in this Case Study, or go to the "Prepare for Class" folder on your Evolve website at http://evolve.elsevier.com/Iggy/ to download and complete as a word processing file. Answer guidelines for this Case Study are also available on your Evolve website.

The patient is a 45-year-old man who had GI surgery 4 days ago. He is NPO, has a nasogastric tube, and IV fluids of $D_5 1/2$ normal saline at 100 mL/hr. The nursing physical assessment includes the following: alert and oriented; fine crackles; capillary refill within normal limits (WNL); moving all extremities; complaining of abdominal pain, muscle aches, and "cottony" mouth; dry mucous membranes; bowel sounds hypoactive, last BM was 4 days ago; skin turgor is poor; 200 mL of dark green substance has drained from NG tube in last 3 hours. Voiding dark amber urine without difficulty. Intake for last 24 hours is 2500 mL. Output is 2000 mL including urine and NG drainage. Febrile and diaphoretic; BP 130/80 mm Hg; pulse 88 bpm; urine specific gravity 1.035; serum potassium 3.0 mEq/L; serum sodium 140 mEq/L; Cl 92 mEq/L; Mg 1.4 mg/dL.

1. Analyze the data in the case study. Do the findings indicate a fluid deficit or fluid excess problem? Support your answer with data from this patient.

2. What factors could be contributing to this problem?

3. Evaluate the patient's electrolyte values and give a rationale for the answer.

CASE STUDY: THE PATIENT WITH OVERHYDRATION

Use a separate sheet of paper to answer the questions in this Case Study, or go to the "Prepare for Class" folder on your Evolve website at http://evolve.elsevier.com/Iggy/ to download and complete as a word processing file. Answer guidelines for this Case Study are also available on your Evolve website.

A patient is admitted to the hospital with a decreased serum osmolality and a serum sodium of 126 mEq/L. The nurse recognizes that dehydration or overhydration may accompany hypotonic conditions.

1. Using Gordon's Functional Health Patterns, what questions would the nurse ask to assess the patient?

2. Which assessments would indicate that the patient has fluid volume excess?
   a. Increased, bounding pulse
   b. Jugular venous distention
   c. Presence of crackles
   d. Elevated blood pressure
   e. Skin pale and cool to touch

3. After determining by an in-depth clinical assessment that the patient is not dehydrated, which intervention is best to correct this hypotonic overhydration?
   a. Administration of 0.9% NS
   b. Restriction of free water
   c. Administration of antihypertensives
   d. Restriction of potassium

4. What does the nurse monitor for as evidence of a worsening hypotonic condition?
   a. Mental status changes
   b. Urine output
   c. Skin changes
   d. Bowel sounds

CASE STUDY: THE PATIENT WITH DEHYDRATION

Use a separate sheet of paper to answer the questions in this Case Study, or go to the "Prepare for Class" folder on your Evolve website at http://evolve.elsevier.com/Iggy/ to download and complete as a word processing file. Answer guidelines for this Case Study are also available on your Evolve website.

The patient with a history of vomiting and diarrhea from the flu presents with a rapid pulse, orthostatic hypotension, urine output of 20 mL/hr, skin turgor poor with tenting, and increased respiratory rate.

1. Which type of dehydration does this patient have? Explain your answer.

2. In evaluating the patient's laboratory values, indicate whether the following values are likely to be normal, elevated, or decreased.
   - Urine specific gravity
   - Urine volume
   - Serum sodium
   - Serum hematocrit and hemoglobin
   - Blood urea nitrogen (BUN)
   - Serum osmolality

3. Which increased compensatory mechanism is responsible for the patient's rapid pulse?
   a. Circulation of angiotensin
   b. Sympathetic discharge
   c. Aldosterone production
   d. Renal reabsorption of sodium and water

4. Which immediate intervention will correct this patient's fluid volume imbalance?
   a. Rapid hydration with D_5W
   b. Administration of a loop diuretic
   c. Administration of an osmotic diuretic
   d. Rapid hydration with D_5/0.45% NS

5. What is the most important thing to monitor to determine the patient's response to corrective interventions?
   a. Respiratory rate and depth
   b. Skin turgor
   c. Urinary output
   d. Weight

6. What indicates that the patient is having a negative response to fluid resuscitation?
   a. Increased blood pressure
   b. Urinary output of 40 mL/hr
   c. Presence of crackles
   d. Widening of pulse pressure

CASE STUDY: THE PATIENT WITH A POTASSIUM IMBALANCE

Use a separate sheet of paper to answer the questions in this Case Study, or go to the "Prepare for Class" folder on your Evolve website at http://evolve.elsevier.com/Iggy/ to download and complete as a word processing file. Answer guidelines for this Case Study are also available on your Evolve website.

A male adult patient is admitted for palpitations. His serum potassium level on admission is 5.4 mEq/L. Yesterday he ate two eggs, bacon, and toast for breakfast. For lunch he had a fresh fruit salad, and for dinner he ate baked halibut, baked potatoes, a salad, and spinach. He usually has a cola drink and dried fruit for a snack. He uses a salt substitute regularly. He tells the nurse that he has been taking spironolactone 50 mg once daily for hypertension for 2 months, but missed his 1-month follow-up appointment.

1. Identify the foods in his diet that may be contributing to his hyperkalemia.
2. Which ECG changes would be typical for a patient such as this?
3. This patient states that he has had abdominal cramping and several very loose diarrhea stools since yesterday. The physician orders a sodium polystyrene sulfonate (Kayexalate) retention enema to be given stat. Discuss the etiology of the patient's symptoms.
4. Explain whether the nurse should clarify the physician's order before administering the enema.
5. Will the patient continue to take the spironolactone? Explain.
6. Eventually the patient recovers and is scheduled for discharge. Develop a teaching-learning plan for him including information about his diet.

CASE STUDY: THE PATIENT WITH A SODIUM IMBALANCE

Use a separate sheet of paper to answer the questions in this Case Study, or go to the "Prepare for Class" folder on your Evolve website at http://evolve.elsevier.com/Iggy/ to download and complete as a word processing file. Answer guidelines for this Case Study are also available on your Evolve website.

The nurse is caring for a 77-year-old woman who was admitted after gardening on a hot summer day. Her daughter found her lying on the couch, slightly confused, and unable to get up to the bathroom. She is weak, anxious, and slightly confused to time and place. Her pulse is 110 beats/min; blood pressure is 108/58. Her skin is dry and urine specific gravity is 1.028. The nurse notes that the patient's deep tendon reflexes are slightly reduced.

1. Discuss whether this patient's serum sodium would be elevated, decreased, or normal.
2. What are the signs and symptoms that will occur in hypernatremia?
3. What treatment does the nurse expect this patient to receive at this time?
4. This patient will be discharged to home care. Develop a teaching plan for her.

CHAPTER 14

Assessment and Care of Patients with Acid-Base Imbalances

STUDY/REVIEW QUESTIONS

1. A patient with chronic obstructive pulmonary disease (COPD) has just developed respiratory distress. Vital signs are: pulse oximetry 88% on 2 L nasal cannula oxygen; dyspnea at rest; respirations 32 per minute. The patient reports shortness of breath. Which statements apply to this clinical situation? *(Select all that apply.)*
   a. Interference in alveolar-capillary diffusion results in carbon dioxide retention.
   b. The nurse should instruct the patient to use pursed-lip breathing.
   c. Position the patient with the head of the bed less than 20 degrees up.
   d. Interference in alveolar-capillary diffusion results in acidemia.
   e. The nurse should explain to the patient that the need for rapid breathing will relieve the shortness of breath.

2. In the case of the previous question, what is the priority order of actions the nurse takes to manage this patient? *(Select in order of priority.)*

   _____ a. Page the physician immediately.

   _____ b. Delegate the monitoring of vital signs to unlicensed personnel.

   _____ c. Call the respiratory therapist.

   _____ d. Document the incident in the patient's chart.

3. A patient with bilateral lower lobe pneumonia is diagnosed to have respiratory acidosis based on arterial blood gas results. What is this patient's likely cause of respiratory acidosis?
   a. Underelimination of carbon dioxide from the lungs
   b. Buffering of extracellular fluid by ammonium
   c. Overelimination of carbon dioxide from the lungs
   d. An increased bicarbonate level due to respiratory elimination of acid

4. A patient is admitted to the hospital for diabetic ketoacidosis. What may likely occur with this patient? *(Select all that apply.)*
   a. Metabolic acidosis
   b. Liver produces excess bicarbonate
   c. Metabolic alkalosis
   d. Excessive oxidation of fatty acids
   e. Overproduction of hydrogen ions

5. A patient who recently emigrated to the U.S. from Germany, but speaks fluent English, has been admitted to the ER with diabetic ketoacidosis. On intake assessment, the patient cannot recall the medications she takes. What actions does the nurse take? *(Select all that apply.)*
   a. Instruct the patient to compare a hospital list of medications to her home medications when she is discharged to home.
   b. Ask the patient's significant other to bring the patient's medications from home.
   c. Ask the patient or significant other about the patient's typical 24-hour home meal plan.
   d. Have a social worker assess if the patient has insurance or money to pay for medications.
   e. Have the dietitian give the patient a standardized 24-hour meal plan to use at home.

6. A patient who has pancreatitis with nausea and vomiting will likely have which related alterations in acid-base balance? *(Select all that apply.)*
   a. Overproduction of hydrogen ions
   b. Metabolic acidosis
   c. Serum pH value that is directly related to the concentration of hydrogen ions
   d. Underproduction of bicarbonate
   e. Metabolic alkalosis

7. Which statements correctly apply to acid-base balance in the body? *(Select all that apply.)*
   a. Renal mechanisms are stronger in regulating acid-base balance but slower to respond than respiratory mechanisms.
   b. The immediate binding of excess hydrogen ions occurs primarily in the red blood cells.
   c. Combined acidosis is less severe than either metabolic acidosis or respiratory acidosis alone.
   d. Respiratory acidosis is caused by a patent airway.
   e. Acid-base balance occurs through control of hydrogen ion production and elimination.

Fill in the blank.

8. An increase in the CO_2 level causes the free hydrogen ion level to increase and the pH to decrease, or become more _____.

9. The ratio between carbonic acid and bicarbonate should remain at _____.

10. In the healthy person, the kidneys control _____ levels and the lungs control _____ levels.

Matching. Match the terms with their associated functions and substances. Answers may be used more than once.

Terms
a. Acid
b. Base
c. Buffer
d. pH

Associated Statements

_____ 11. Accepts hydrogen ion

_____ 12. Donates hydrogen ion

_____ 13. Formed in the body as a result of metabolism

_____ 14. Releases or binds hydrogen ions into/from a fluid

_____ 15. Measure of the body's free hydrogen ion level

_____ 16. H_2CO_3

_____ 17. Increases as the amount of base increases

_____ 18. HCO_3^-

_____ 19. Hemoglobin

20. Use arrows to indicate the direction the carbonic anhydrase equation shifts when excess carbon dioxide is produced.

$$CO_2 + H_2O \qquad H_2CO_3 \qquad H^+ + HCO_3^-$$

21. For the conditions listed below, indicate whether plasma pH will increase (I) or decrease (D).

_____ a. Increase in CO_2

_____ b. Decrease in HCO_3^-

_____ c. Increase in lactic acid

_____ d. Increase in HCO_3^-

_____ e. Decrease in CO_2

Matching. Match the buffer systems with their descriptive statements. Answers may be used more than once.

Buffer Systems
a. Chemical
b. Respiratory
c. Renal
d. Protein

Statements

_____ 22. Chemoreceptor response to increase in CO_2

_____ 23. Binding of hydrogen ions to phosphate ions to form H_2PO_4

_____ 24. Reabsorbs HCO_3^-

_____ 25. Binds H^+ with HCO_3^-

_____ 26. Binds H^+ with hemoglobin

_____ 27. Response occurs within minutes

28. Which blood pH value is within normal limits?
    a. 7.27
    b. 7.37
    c. 7.47
    d. 7.5

29. The early stage of incomplete breakdown of glucose occurs whenever cells metabolize under anaerobic conditions to form lactic acid. Based on this knowledge of pathophysiology, which conditions could cause the patient to develop acidosis? *(Select all that apply.)*
    a. Sepsis
    b. Hypovolemic shock
    c. Use of a mechanical ventilator
    d. Prolonged nasogastric suctioning
    e. Hypoventilation

30. Which patient with the highest risk for acidosis must the nurse care for first?
    a. Patient in mild pain with a kidney stone
    b. Patient with chronic obstructive pulmonary disease, pulse oximetry 88% on 2 L oxygen
    c. Patient who just had a seizure with pulse oximetry of 91%
    d. Patient with a rectal tube in place for frequent diarrhea

31. A patient's ABG results show an increase in pH. Which condition is most likely to contribute to this laboratory value?
    a. Mechanical ventilation
    b. Ketoacidosis
    c. Nasogastric suction
    d. Diarrhea

32. Which patient is most likely to have a decrease in bicarbonate?
    a. Patient with pancreatitis
    b. Patient with hypoventilation
    c. Patient who is vomiting
    d. Patient with emphysema

33. A patient has a new onset of shallow and slow respirations. While the patient's body attempts to compensate, what happens to the patient's pH level?
    a. Increases
    b. Decreases
    c. Stabilizes
    d. Fluctuates

34. A patient is at risk for acid-base imbalance. Which laboratory value indicates that the patient is acidotic?
    a. $Paco_2$ = 55 mm Hg
    b. CO_3^- = 25 mEq/L
    c. Lactate = 2.5 mmol/L
    d. pH = 7.30

35. Which type of medication increases an older adult patient's risk for acid-base imbalance?
    a. Antilipemics
    b. Hormonal therapy
    c. Diuretics
    d. Antidysrhythmics

36. The nurse is giving discharge instructions about medication to an older, forgetful patient, and the daughter whom the patient lives with at home. What does the nurse do to facilitate medication compliance? *(Select all that apply.)*
    a. Find out how the patient organizes his or her medications at home.
    b. Give the patient written instructions and a number to call the pharmacy for questions.
    c. Include the daughter in the discharge instructions.
    d. Have the social worker ask the patient about his or her ability to pay for medications.
    e. Suggest that the patient use a weekly pill organizer and have the daughter supervise medication administration.

Matching. *Match the etiologies of metabolic acidosis to their resulting states of pathophysiology. Answers may be used more than once.*

Etiology of Metabolic Acidosis
a. Hydrogen ion production
b. Hydrogen ion elimination
c. Base elimination
d. Base production

Pathophysiology State
_____ 37. Diabetic ketoacidosis

_____ 38. Renal failure

_____ 39. Dehydration

_____ 40. Seizures

_____ 41. Pancreatic insufficiency

_____ 42. Diarrhea

Matching. Match the pathophysiologic causes of respiratory failure with their associated conditions. Answers may be used more than once.

Associated Conditions

a. Respiratory depression
b. Inadequate chest expansion
c. Airway obstruction
d. Altered alveolar capillary diffusion

Pathophysiology

_____ 43. Asthma

_____ 44. Muscular dystrophy

_____ 45. Morphine infusion

_____ 46. Pulmonary embolus

_____ 47. Bronchiolitis

_____ 48. Ascites

_____ 49. Stroke

_____ 50. Flail chest

_____ 51. Hemothorax

_____ 52. Hyperkalemia

_____ 53. Pneumonia

54. Which medication usage could cause metabolic acidosis?
   a. Aspirin overdose
   b. Overuse of antacids
   c. Prolonged use of antihistamines
   d. Vitamin overdose

55. Which nursing assessment finding indicates a worsening of respiratory acidosis?
   a. Decreased respiratory rate
   b. Decreased blood pressure
   c. Use of accessory respiratory muscles
   d. Pale nail beds

56. Which patient is most likely to have respiratory acidosis?
   a. Patient who is anxious and breathing rapidly
   b. Patient with multiple rib fractures
   c. Patient with IV normal saline bolus
   d. Patient with increased urinary output

57. Which patient requires assessment related to inadequate chest expansion, which places the patient at risk for respiratory acidosis? *(Select all that apply.)*
   a. Patient with lordosis
   b. Patient with emphysema
   c. Severely obese patient on prolonged bedrest
   d. Patient in the first trimester of pregnancy
   e. Patient 2 days post-op for cholecysectomy

58. The nurse reviews the ECG and cardiovascular status of a patient. Which findings are early changes associated with mild acidosis?
   a. Decreased heart rate with hypertension
   b. Hypotension and faint peripheral pulses
   c. Increased heart rate and increased cardiac output
   d. Peaked T waves and wide QRS complexes

59. The nurse is assessing a patient with an acid-base imbalance by using Gordon's Functional Health Patterns. What primary areas are affected? *(Select all that apply.)*
   a. Values/Beliefs
   b. Activity-Exercise
   c. Health Perception–Health Management
   d. Elimination
   e. Sleep–Rest
   f. Cognitive–Perceptual
   g. Coping–Stress Tolerance

60. The nurse is testing the muscle strength of a patient at risk for acid-base imbalance. Which technique does the nurse use to test arm strength?
   a. Asks the patient to hold the arms straight out in front and the nurse observes for drift.
   b. The patient flexes the arms against the chest; the nurse tries to pull the arms from the chest.
   c. Asks the patient to pick up an object that weighs at least 10 lbs.
   d. The patient clasps the hands together and pushes as hard as possible.

61. The nurse assesses an acidotic patient's lower extremities for strength as part of the shift assessment. What finding does the nurse expect to see?
   a. Bilateral weakness
   b. Weakness on the dominant side
   c. No change from baseline
   d. Cramping, but no weakness

62. The nurse observes tall peaked T waves on the ECG of a patient with metabolic acidosis. Before notifying the health care provider, the nurse also assesses the results of which laboratory test?
   a. Serum calcium
   b. Serum glucose
   c. Serum potassium
   d. Serum magnesium

Matching. *Match the signs and symptoms to either metabolic acidosis or respiratory acidosis. Answers may be used more than once.*

Acid-Base Condition
a. Metabolic acidosis
b. Respiratory acidosis

Signs and Symptoms
_____ 63. Kussmaul respirations

_____ 64. Shallow, rapid respirations

_____ 65. Warm, flushed skin

_____ 66. Skin pale to cyanotic

_____ 67. Elevated $Paco_2$

_____ 68. Decreased bicarbonate

69. What interventions are included in the plan of care for a patient with metabolic ketoacidosis? *(Select all that apply.)*
   a. Monitor ABG levels for decreasing pH level, as appropriate.
   b. Maintain patent IV access.
   c. Administer fluids as prescribed.
   d. Monitor for irritability and muscle tetany.
   e. Monitor determinants of tissue oxygen delivery, such as hemoglobin.
   f. Monitor loss of bicarbonate through the GI tract such as diarrhea.

70. What is the priority intervention for a patient with diabetic ketoacidosis?
   a. Administer bicarbonate.
   b. Give furosemide.
   c. Administer insulin.
   d. Administer potassium.

71. Which statement made by the patient indicates that he or she may have an alkaline condition?
   a. "I am more and more tired and can't concentrate."
   b. "I have tingling in my fingers and toes."
   c. "My feet and ankles are swollen."
   d. "I am short of breath all of the time."

72. Which patient is most likely to have respiratory alkalosis?
    a. Hypoxic patient
    b. Patient with a body cast
    c. Patient having a panic attack
    d. Morbidly obese patient

73. Which type of electrolyte imbalance does the nurse expect to see in a patient with metabolic alkalosis?
    a. Hyperkalemia
    b. Hypophosphatemia
    c. Hyperchloremia
    d. Hypocalcemia

74. Which patient is most likely to develop metabolic alkalosis as a result of base excess?
    a. Patient taking thiazide diuretics
    b. Patient who is having nasogastric suction
    c. Patient with severe vomiting
    d. Patient who had a massive blood transfusion

75. The nurse is assessing a patient with metabolic alkalosis. Which neuromuscular finding is the most ominous and warrants immediate notification of the health care provider?
    a. Muscle cramps
    b. Muscle twitching
    c. Hyperactive deep tendon reflexes
    d. Tetany

76. The nurse is caring for a patient with metabolic alkalosis secondary to diuretic medication. Which equipment does the nurse obtain to administer the correct therapy to this patient?
    a. Oxygen tubing and cannula or mask
    b. IV catheter and IV start kit
    c. Foley catheter and drainage bag
    d. Antiemetic drug and emesis basin

77. Which occurrence can be a result of hyperventilation?
    a. Hypocalcemia
    b. Anxiety
    c. Respiratory alkalosis
    d. Respiratory acidosis

78. Which patient showing symptoms of an acid-base imbalance must the nurse see first?
    a. Patient who exhibits increased heart rate of 110/min and increased cardiac output
    b. Patient showing activity weakness and lethargy
    c. Patient who has a reduced attention span
    d. Patient who has asymptomatic bradycardia with a heart rate of 59/min

79. A patient has taken antacids for the past 3 days to relieve "heartburn." What alteration in acid-base balance will the nurse likely find in this patient?
    a. Respiratory alkalosis
    b. Metabolic acidosis
    c. Metabolic alkalosis
    d. Respiratory acidosis

80. A patient with anemia has completed a blood transfusion of 2 units of packed red blood cells. Which imbalance will the patient likely have after the blood transfusion?
    a. Metabolic alkalosis
    b. Respiratory acidosis
    c. Metabolic acidosis
    d. Respiratory alkalosis

81. A patient is hospitalized with hyperglycemia and has a blood glucose of 476 mg/dL. Which events does the nurse expect to see in this patient? *(Select all that apply.)*
    a. Hyperventilation
    b. Kussmaul respirations
    c. Respiratory acidosis
    d. Hypotension
    e. Metabolic acidosis

82. A patient having diarrhea for the past 2 days will likely have which abnormalities in acid-base balance? *(Select all that apply.)*
    a. Overelimination of bicarbonate
    b. Respiratory alkalosis
    c. Metabolic acidosis
    d. Underelimination of hydrogen ions
    e. Overproduction of hydrogen ions

83. A patient who has advanced muscular dystrophy will likely have which complications related to their disease? *(Select all that apply.)*
   a. Hyperventilation
   b. Hypoventilation
   c. Underproduction of bicarbonate
   d. Respiratory acidosis
   e. Underelimination of hydrogen ions

84. A patient who has a decreased amount of hydrogen ions and a decreased amount of carbon dioxide in the body will have what response?
   a. Decreased rate and depth of respirations
   b. Decreased renal absorption of hydrogen ions
   c. Increased rate and depth of respirations
   d. Decreased renal excretions of bicarbonate

85. A patient's arterial blood gas reveals respiratory acidosis. How does the body compensate for this imbalance?
   a. Loss of bicarbonate
   b. Regular, unlabored respirations
   c. Hypoventilation
   d. Renal reabsorption of bicarbonate

86. The nurse is caring for a patient with excessive alcohol ingestion and salicylate intoxication. What is the most likely acid-base imbalance this patient will have?
   a. Bicarbonate underelimination
   b. Bicarbonate loss
   c. Metabolic acidosis
   d. Metabolic alkalosis

Matching. *Match the arterial blood gas value to the corresponding acid-base imbalance. Answers may be used more than once.*

Acid-Base Imbalance
a. Metabolic acidosis
b. Respiratory acidosis
c. Metabolic alkalosis
d. Respiratory alkalosis
e. Normal values

ABG Values

_____ 87. pH 7.30, $Paco_2$ 66, bicarbonate 38, Pao_2 70

_____ 88. pH 7.52, $Paco_2$ 45, bicarbonate 36, Pao_2 95

_____ 89. pH 7.55, $Paco_2$ 24, bicarbonate 20, Pao_2 95

_____ 90. pH 7.28, $Paco_2$ 24, bicarbonate 15, Pao_2 95

_____ 91. pH 7.35, $Paco_2$ 24, bicarbonate 15, Pao_2 95

_____ 92. pH 7.45, $Paco_2$ 50, bicarbonate 42, Pao_2 80

_____ 93. pH 7.45, $Paco_2$ 41, bicarbonate 25, Pao_2 97

94. A patient has a low pH level. Which other concurrent change does the nurse expect to see in this patient?
   a. Elevated serum sodium level
   b. Elevated serum potassium
   c. Decreased serum chloride level
   d. Decreased serum calcium level

95. What is the safest way to administer oxygen to a patient with chronic respiratory acidosis?
   a. High-volume intermittent positive pressure
   b. Low-flow oxygen (2 L/min) via nasal cannula
   c. High-flow 40% oxygen via facemask
   d. Positive end-expiratory pressure (PEEP)

96. Which assessment finding indicates that a patient with chronic respiratory acidosis is responding favorably to treatment?
    a. Nail beds pale, extremities cool
    b. Respiratory stridor with inspiration
    c. Expectorating clear, thin mucus
    d. Diffuse crackles auscultated bilaterally

97. In order to ensure the safety of a patient with metabolic alkalosis, which task is best to delegate to the unlicensed assistive personnel (UAP)?
    a. Watch the patient when he or she eats or drinks anything.
    b. Sit with the patient to prevent wandering.
    c. Clean up spills immediately.
    d. Remove all sharp objects from the bedside table.

98. Determine whether the arterial blood values indicate an acid or alkaline condition.
    a. $Paco_2$ = 66 mm Hg _____
    b. Bicarbonate = 16 mEq/L _____
    c. pH = 7.55 _____
    d. pH = 7.32 _____

CASE STUDY: THE PATIENT WITH ACID-BASE IMBALANCE

Use a separate sheet of paper to answer the questions in this Case Study, or go to the "Prepare for Class" folder on your Evolve website at http://evolve.elsevier.com/Iggy/ to download and complete as a word processing file. Answer guidelines for this Case Study are also available on your Evolve website.

A 40-year-old male is admitted to the hospital with a report of severe abdominal pain. The patient has facial grimacing and moans occasionally during the nursing assessment.

Vital signs are: blood pressure 80/47 mm Hg, supine in right arm; heart rate 117/min; respirations 26/min, slightly dyspneic at rest; pulse oximeter reading 92% after being placed on 100% O_2 via facemask. Lungs auscultated: clear upper lobes anterior and posterior, with few crackles in bases anterior and posterior. No productive cough is noted. There is no report of shortness of breath. The patient denies smoking presently and has no smoking history. There is trace edema of the ankles bilaterally, but there is no edema of the arms or trunk of the body.

A Foley catheter is put in place and in the past 5 hours there is a total output of 110 mL of amber, clear urine. The patient says he has vomited 1 to 2 times in the last 2 days and has had no bowel movement in the last 3 days; he normally has a bowel movement daily. Auscultation of the abdomen reveals hypoactive bowel sounds. The skin is intact, slightly moist and pale, with no rash or wounds. The patient is alert and oriented to person, place, and time. He can move all extremities and can follow simple commands.

The patient's laboratory results are as follows:
- Arterial blood gas pH 7.29
- Pao_2 78
- $Paco_2$ 36
- HCO_3 23 mEq/L
- WBC 20/mm^3
- Hgb 11.7 g/dL
- Hct 38%
- Blood glucose 373 mg/dL
- Na 137 mEq/L
- Ca 8.7 mg/dL
- Lipase 117 units/L
- Alanine aminotransferase 90 International Units/L
- Amylase 203 International Units/L

1. What are the top four body systems important to focus on in this patient's assessment?
2. Document a nursing note using the body systems identified in question #1.
3. What likely is the disease process of the patient?
4. What laboratory values indicate the medical condition of the patient?

CASE STUDY: THE PATIENT WITH RESPIRATORY ACIDOSIS

Use a separate sheet of paper to answer the questions in this Case Study, or go to the "Prepare for Class" folder on your Evolve website at http://evolve.elsevier.com/Iggy/ to download and complete as a word processing file. Answer guidelines for this Case Study are also available on your Evolve website.

The patient is a 75-year-old man with a history of emphysema. He comes to the emergency department (ED) reporting a productive cough that causes chest pain and fatigue. "I am having more problems breathing than usual."

1. What should the nurse include in the initial history when a patient is suspected of having an acid-base imbalance?

2. Which assessment indicates that this patient has inadequate oxygenation?
   a. Decreased urine output
   b. Bradycardia
   c. Decreased chest expansion
   d. Hypotension

3. Which ABG value indicates that this patient is retaining carbon dioxide?
   a. $Paco_2$ = 40 mm Hg
   b. $Paco_2$ = 60 mm Hg
   c. Bicarbonate = 42
   d. Pao_2 = 60 mm Hg

4. The patient's baseline ABG values are: pH 7.36; $Paco_2$ 60 mm Hg, Pao_2 52 mm Hg, bicarbonate 42 mEq/L. Which ABG result would most likely indicate that he is having a negative response to the administration of oxygen?
   a. pH 7.35; $Paco_2$ 64, Pao_2 60, bicarbonate 42 mEq/L
   b. pH 7.36, $Paco_2$ 60, Pao_2 60, bicarbonate 42 mEq/L
   c. pH 7.36, $Paco_2$ 60, Pao_2 58, bicarbonate 38 mEq/L
   d. pH 7.33, $Paco_2$ 66, Pao_2 66, bicarbonate 42 mEq/L

5. Based on the answer for question 4, is the patient's respiratory acidosis compensated or uncompensated? Explain your answer.

6. The patient is admitted with a diagnosis of pneumonia. What immediate interventions are needed for this patient?

7. Later in the shift, the nurse notes that his oxygen is set at 5 L/minute. The patient says that he asked the UAP to turn up his oxygen because he was having trouble breathing. What actions, if any, should the nurse take at this time?

CASE STUDY: THE PATIENT WITH METABOLIC ACID-BASE IMBALANCE

Use a separate sheet of paper to answer the questions in this Case Study, or go to the "Prepare for Class" folder on your Evolve website at http://evolve.elsevier.com/Iggy/ to download and complete as a word processing file. Answer guidelines for this Case Study are also available on your Evolve website.

A 65-year-old woman with a recent history of cellulitis is admitted to the hospital with fever, shortness of breath, and hypotension. She has had a 2-day history of diarrhea. Her ABG reveals a pH of 7.30, $Paco_2$ of 28, Pao_2 of 88, and bicarbonate of 17 mEq/L.

1. What additional information could the nurse collect using Gordon's Functional Health Patterns?

2. This patient's symptoms are most likely a result of which condition?
   a. Metabolic acidosis
   b. Metabolic alkalosis

3. The bicarbonate level of 17 mEq/L is the result of which factor?
   a. Respiratory hypoventilation
   b. Overelimination of bicarbonate
   c. Respiratory compensation
   d. Underelimination of hydrogen ions

4. Which finding indicates a worsening acidotic condition?
   a. Increased blood pressure
   b. Anxiety
   c. Decreasing pH
   d. Increased urinary output

5. What does this patient critically need to reverse the condition?
   a. Fluids
   b. Oxygen
   c. Calcium
   d. Potassium

6. Explain whether or not bicarbonate would be given to this patient to correct her condition.

7. What other laboratory values would be important to monitor at this time? Explain your answer.

Infusion Therapy

STUDY/REVIEW QUESTIONS

1. The nurse is preparing to start an infusion of 10% dextrose. Why does the nurse infuse the solution through a central line?
   a. Osmolarity of the solution could cause phlebitis or thrombosis.
   b. The patient could be at risk for fluid overload.
   c. Viscosity of the solution would slow the infusion.
   d. The solution should not be mixed with other drugs or solutions.

2. A patient is in the hospital for his first chemotherapy treatment for lung cancer. Which IV access methods are appropriate for this patient? *(Select all that apply.)*
   a. Peripheral IV access
   b. Peripherally inserted central catheter (PICC)
   c. Dialysis catheter
   d. Tunneled central venous catheter
   e. Implanted port

3. A patient has a peripherally inserted central catheter (PICC) inserted and is ordered to receive IV cisplatin (Platinol). The drug has infiltrated into the tissue and redness is observed in the right lower side of the neck. What interventions, in order of priority, will the nurse perform? *(Select in order of priority.)*
   a. Apply cold compresses to the site of swelling.
   b. Stop the infusion and disconnect the IV line from the administration set.
   c. Aspirate the drug from the IV access device.
   d. Monitor the patient and document.

4. The nurse is preparing to give a patient IV drug therapy. What information does the nurse need before administering the drug? *(Select all that apply.)*
   a. Indications, contraindications, and precautions for IV therapy
   b. Appropriate dilution, pH, and osmolarity of solution
   c. Rate of infusion and dosage of drugs
   d. Generic, chemical, and brand name of the drug
   e. Compatibility with other IV medications
   f. Percentage of adverse events for the drug
   g. Specifics of monitoring because of immediate effect

5. The charge nurse is reviewing IV therapy orders. What information is included in each order? *(Select all that apply.)*
   a. Specific type of solution
   b. Rate of administration
   c. Specific drug dose to be added to the solution
   d. Method for diluting drugs for the solution
   e. Specific type of administration equipment

6. The nurse must insert a short peripheral IV catheter. In order to decrease the risk of deep vein thrombosis or phlebitis, which vein does the nurse choose for the infusion site?
   a. Wrist
   b. Foot
   c. Forearm
   d. Antecubital

7. A patient requires IV therapy via a peripheral line. What considerations does the nurse use when inserting the peripheral IV? *(Select all that apply.)*
   a. Use either an upper or lower extremity for the insertion site.
   b. Start with more distal sites, such as the hand veins.
   c. Start with more proximal sites, such as the forearm.
   d. Choose the patient's nondominant arm.
   e. Do not use the arm if the patient had a mastectomy on that side.
   f. If the vein is hard and cordlike, use an indirect approach.
   g. Avoid placing an IV over the palm side of the wrist.

8. The nurse is assessing a patient's IV site and identifies signs and symptoms of infiltration. What are the nursing actions, in order of priority, the nurse implements for this patient? *(Select in order of priority.)*
   a. Elevates the extremity
   b. Applies a sterile dressing if weeping from the tissue has occurred
   c. Removes the IV access
   d. Stops the infusion

9. Which items does the nurse include in the documentation after completing the insertion of a peripherally inserted central catheter (PICC)? *(Select all that apply.)*
   a. Type of dressing applied
   b. Response of the family to IV access
   c. Type of IV access device used
   d. How long it took to place the IV access
   e. Location and vein that was used for insertion

10. The nurse is selecting a site for peripheral IV insertion. Which patient condition influences the choice of left versus right upper extremity?
    a. Pneumothorax with a chest tube on the right side
    b. Myocardial infarction with pain radiating down the left arm
    c. Right hip fracture with immobilization and traction in place
    d. Regular renal dialysis with a shunt in the left upper forearm

11. The nurse is attempting to insert a peripheral IV when the patient reports tingling and a feeling like "pins and needles." What does the nurse do next?
    a. Change to a short-winged butterfly needle.
    b. Stop immediately, remove the catheter, and chose a new site.
    c. Ask the patient to wiggle the fingers to stimulate circulation.
    d. Pause the procedure and gently massage the fingers.

12. A patient has been on prolonged steroid therapy. In assessing the patient for IV insertion, what finding does the nurse expect to see?
    a. Skin and vein fragility that makes repeated venipuncture difficult
    b. Skin that is thick, tough, dry, and difficult to puncture
    c. Edema or puffiness making visualization of veins difficult
    d. Rash with excoriation from scratching which limits site selection

13. Under what circumstances does the nurse elect to use only one secondary set rather than a secondary set for each medication?
    a. When multiple intermittent medications are required
    b. To eliminate the cost of using multiple secondary sets
    c. When the nurse is using the backpriming method
    d. When the medications are compatible

14. When using an intermittent administration set to deliver medications, how often does the Infusion Nurse's Society recommend that the set be changed?
    a. Every 24 hours
    b. Every shift
    c. Every morning
    d. After every dose

15. The nurse is supervising a student nurse who is preparing an IV bag with IV administration tubing. Which action by the student nurse causes the nurse to intervene?
    a. The student touches the drip chamber.
    b. The sterile cap from the distal end of the set is removed.
    c. The distal end is attached to a needleless connector.
    d. The student touches the tubing spike.

16. The nurse is caring for a patient with a Groshong catheter. According to the manufacturer's recommendations, which technique does the nurse use in maintaining this type of catheter?
    a. Flush the catheter with heparin.
    b. Flush the catheter with saline.
    c. Avoid flushing the catheter.
    d. Aspirate the catheter to remove clots.

17. A patient has a peripherally inserted central catheter (PICC) line placed by an advanced-practice nurse at the bedside. Before using the catheter, how is its placement verified?
    a. The physician who ordered the procedure verifies placement.
    b. The line is aspirated gently and the nurse watches for blood return.
    c. A chest x-ray is taken which shows the catheter tip in the lower superior vena cava.
    d. The line is slowly flushed with 10 mL of saline while the nurse notes the ease of flow.

18. A patient requires a nontunneled percutaneous central catheter. What is the nurse's role in this procedure?
    a. Insert the catheter using sterile technique.
    b. Place the patient in Trendelenburg position.
    c. Read the chest x-ray to validate placement.
    d. Select and prepare the insertion site.

19. A patient requires an infusion of packed red blood cells (PRBCs). Which factor allows the nurse to infuse the PRBCs through the patient's PICC line?
    a. Length of the PICC allows infusion within 6 hours.
    b. The nurse is unable to obtain an infusion pump.
    c. Lumen size of the PICC is 4 Fr or larger.
    d. PRBCs can be warmed before infusion.

20. Which patient is the most likely candidate for a tunneled central venous catheter?
    a. Patient with trauma from a motor vehicle accident
    b. Patient in need of IV antibiotics for several weeks
    c. Patient in need of permanent parental nutrition
    d. Patient in need of intermittent chemotherapy

21. Which nursing interventions are implemented when caring for a patient with an implanted port? *(Select all that apply.)*
    a. Before puncture, palpate the port to locate the septum.
    b. Use a large-bore needle to access the port.
    c. Flush the port before each use.
    d. Use a noncoring needle to access the port.
    e. Flush the port at least once a month.

22. A 65-year-old patient has been receiving IV fluids at 100 mL/hr of $D_5 1/2\%$ NS for the past 3 days, along with IV antibiotic therapy. After receiving the new antibiotic, the patient reports general itching and difficulty catching his breath. The nurse notes audible wheezing and rhonchi over the lung fields bilaterally and a rash over his back and chest. What complication do these assessment findings indicate?
    a. Infection in the blood
    b. Allergic reaction
    c. Speed shock
    d. Circulatory overload

23. A patient has a central line inserted in the vena cava. The nurse assesses the patient for which potential complications related to the procedure? *(Select all that apply.)*
    a. Phlebitis
    b. Hemothorax
    c. Air embolism
    d. Cardiac tamponade
    e. Arterial puncture

24. The nurse is helping the physician insert a central line when the patient develops chest pain and shortness of breath with decreased breath sounds and restlessness. What does the nurse do next?
    a. Tell the patient "Relax, the procedure will soon be over" and administer pain medication.
    b. Administer pain medication to minimize the pain of insertion and order a stat chest x-ray.
    c. Administer oxygen, remove the catheter, place an occlusive dressing, and order a stat chest x-ray.
    d. Monitor ongoing pulse oximetry and respiratory changes after placing an occlusive dressing over the catheter site.

25. A triple lumen catheter central line is inserted in a patient. What does the nurse do immediately after the procedure?
    a. Start IV fluids but at a slower rate to prevent any fluid overload.
    b. Watch and wait for any complications before using the site.
    c. Get a portable chest x-ray immediately and hold IV fluids until results are obtained.
    d. Assess vital signs and assess the patient; if patient is stable, start IV fluids.

26. After a tubing change to a patient's central line, the line is later found to be disconnected from the catheter. The patient develops chest pain and restlessness, heart rate of 120 beats/min, blood pressure drops to 90/40, and pulse oximetry is 89%. What does the nurse do next?
    a. Place the patient in Trendelenburg position on the left side, clamp the catheter, and notify the physician.
    b. Assess for patency of the catheter, change the tubing, and resume IV fluids.
    c. Notify the physician, remove the central line, apply pressure, and place the patient in a semi-Fowler's position.
    d. Notify the physician and administer urokinase to unclot the catheter.

27. Which nursing interventions are key in preventing an infection in a patient with a central line? *(Select all that apply.)*
    a. Assess the dressing and insertion site of the central line.
    b. Use aseptic technique when administering medications and changing tubing.
    c. Change the catheter every 72 hours and tubing every 24 hours.
    d. Monitor the patient's temperature for any elevation and give acetaminophen as needed.
    e. Use sterile technique when inserting a central line.
    f. Use proper handwashing and nonsterile gloves before coming into contact with a central line.

28. A patient with an implanted port is discharged to home and will receive long-term therapy on an outpatient basis. How frequently must the port be flushed between courses of therapy?
    a. Daily
    b. Weekly
    c. Monthly
    d. When therapy resumes

29. The nurse is preparing to deliver IV infusion therapy through an implanted port. What technique does the nurse use to access the port?
    a. Palpate the port to locate the septum, scrub, and access with a Huber needle.
    b. Scrub the port with alcohol and access with a needleless device.
    c. Scrub the port with Betadine and flush using a 10 mL syringe.
    d. Palpate the port, scrub, and access with a winged butterfly needle.

30. A patient is to be discharged to home with an implanted port and needs discharge instructions on prescribed medication administration. Which instructions does the nurse give to the patient and family member who will be assisting the patient? *(Select all that apply.)*
    a. The device must be flushed every 24 hours.
    b. When the port is not accessed an occlusive dressing should be applied.
    c. The skin will be punctured over the port when the port is accessed.
    d. When the port is not accessed, no dressing needs to be applied.
    e. The port must be flushed after each use.

31. The nurse is preparing to give IV infusion therapy to a patient. When is the choice of using a glass container appropriate?
    a. When the patient needs a rapid infusion of fluids
    b. When the patient needs emergency transportation
    c. When the nurse must accurately read the container
    d. When the drug is incompatible with a plastic container

32. A patient requires a 2-month course of antibiotics to treat a resistant infection. Which device is chosen for this therapy?
    a. Short peripheral catheter
    b. Midline catheter
    c. Nontunneled percutaneous central catheter
    d. PICC

33. The nurse is attaching an administration set to a central venous catheter. Which type of equipment decreases the risk of accidental disconnection or leakage?
    a. Slip lock connector
    b. Luer-Lok connector
    c. Extension set
    d. Needleless connector

34. The nurse is adding a filter to an IV administration setup. Where is the best place to add the filter to the IV line?
    a. As close to the solution container as possible
    b. Immediately below the infusion pump
    c. At any convenient connection point
    d. As close as possible to the catheter hub

35. Which safety measures does the nurse apply to decrease the risk of catheter-related bloodstream infection (CR-BSI) related to needleless systems? *(Select all that apply.)*
    a. Clean needleless system connections vigorously every 24 hours.
    b. Do not tape connections between tubing sets.
    c. Use evidence-based hand hygiene guidelines from the Centers for Disease Control and Prevention (CDC) and the Occupational Safety and Health Administration (OSHA).
    d. Attend educational offerings to prevent or minimize CR-BSI.
    e. Use needleless systems only when necessary.
    f. Discard needleless equipment in a biohazard container.

36. A patient is receiving IV therapy via an infusion pump. What is a nursing responsibility related to the therapy and equipment?
    a. Count the number of drops per minute.
    b. Monitor the patient's infusion site and rate.
    c. Check the equipment at the end of the infusion.
    d. Position the container for gravity flow.

37. Identify whether each characteristic relates to a pump (P) or a controller infusion device (CID).

    _____ a. Delivers fluids under pressure

    _____ b. Relies on gravity to create fluid flow

    _____ c. Is pole-mounted or ambulatory and portable

    _____ d. Is best for accurate infusion

    _____ e. Counts drops to regulate flow

38. The nurse is assessing a patient's IV insertion site. What features does the nurse look for in the assessment? *(Select all that apply.)*
    a. Observe for redness and swelling.
    b. Check that the dressing is clean and dry.
    c. Ensure that the dressing is adherent to the skin.
    d. Observe for yellow discoloration.
    e. Observe for hardness or drainage.

39. A patient's central venous IV site is covered with a transparent membrane dressing. How often does the nurse change this dressing?
    a. Every 24 hours
    b. Every 48 hours
    c. At least every 7 days
    d. The dressing does not need changing

40. A patient is ordered to receive peripheral parenteral nutrition (PPN). What type of access device is appropriate for this patient?
    a. Peripheral 20 gauge IV needle
    b. Nontunneled percutaneous central catheter
    c. Peripheral 22 gauge IV needle
    d. Peripherally inserted central catheter (PICC)

41. An external long-term IV catheter is required for hemodialysis of a hospitalized patient. Which statements are true about this patient's venous access device? *(Select all that apply.)*
    a. It should not be used for administration of other fluids or medications except in an emergency.
    b. A nontunneled catheter with large lumen is required for hemodialysis.
    c. Vein thrombosis is a common problem with hemodialysis access.
    d. A device for hemodialysis has a port to access the catheter.
    e. A tunneled catheter with large lumen is required for hemodialysis.

42. The nurse has removed the dressing from a patient's central venous catheter site. In order to monitor the catheter position, what does the nurse do?
    a. Gently push the catheter into the insertion site.
    b. Slightly retract the catheter and observe the position.
    c. Mark the catheter with a pen to monitor the length.
    d. Note the length of the catheter which is external to the insertion site.

43. The nurse is caring for a patient with a central venous catheter. What measures does the nurse use to prevent air emboli when changing the administration set or connectors? *(Select all that apply.)*
    a. The patient lies flat so the catheter site is below the heart.
    b. Use the pinch clamp that can be closed during the procedure.
    c. Use sterile technique when handling the equipment.
    d. Have an assistant apply pressure at the insertion site.
    e. Ask the patient to perform the Valsalva maneuver by holding the breath and bearing down.

44. After assessing the patency of a patient's IV catheter, the nurse attempts to flush the catheter and meets resistance. What does the nurse do next?
    a. Get a larger-sized syringe and repeat the flush attempt.
    b. Use a heparinized solution and repeat the flush attempt.
    c. Gently force-flush the catheter using the push-pause method.
    d. Stop the flush attempt and discontinue the IV.

45. A patient is admitted with a small bowel obstruction and is on a mechanical ventilator with a tracheostomy for respiratory failure. A resident physician orders placement of a right internal jugular central line for total parenteral nutrition infusion. What is the nurse's response to this order?
    a. Notify the physician that placement of a line in the femoral vessel will increase the risk of infection.
    b. Place the line as ordered and keep the dressing clean.
    c. Suggest that a peripheral line be placed in the antecubital site of the upper extremity.
    d. Page the physician and suggest that a peripherally inserted central catheter (PICC) line be placed in the upper extremity.

46. The nurse is preparing to draw blood from a patient who has a central line. The patient's spouse asks, "Why can't you just take the blood out of that big IV line?" What information does the nurse use to explain why the central line is not used for blood draws? *(Select all that apply.)*
    a. Additional hub manipulation is a major cause of CR-BSI.
    b. Heparin used in flushing can interfere with coagulation studies.
    c. Electrolytes in the IV fluid may alter the results of serum electrolytes.
    d. Infusion of antibiotics can interfere with peak serum levels of the drug.
    e. The blood vacutainer may cause the catheter to temporarily collapse.

47. The nurse is flushing a patient's short peripheral IV catheter. What does the nurse typically use for this procedure?
    a. 3 mL of normal saline
    b. 5 mL of heparin
    c. 10 mL of normal saline
    d. 30 mL of bacteriostatic saline

48. Place the steps of removing a peripheral catheter in the proper order using the numbers 1 through 7.
    _____ a. Hold pressure on the site until hemostasis is achieved.
    _____ b. Immediately cover the puncture site with dry gauze.
    _____ c. Assess the catheter tip to make sure it is intact and completely removed.
    _____ d. Slowly withdraw the catheter from the skin.
    _____ e. Lift opposite sides of the transparent dressing.
    _____ f. Document catheter removal and the appearance of the IV site.
    _____ g. Pull laterally to remove the dressing from the site while stabilizing the catheter.

49. The nurse is attempting to remove a PICC line and feels resistance. What technique does the nurse use first to attempt to resolve this problem?
    a. Gently pull on the catheter while the patient holds his or her breath.
    b. Place a cold pack on the extremity and give the patient a cold drink.
    c. Use simple distraction techniques and deep breathing.
    d. Place the patient in Trendelenburg position.

50. The nurse is assessing a short peripheral catheter after removal and it appears that the catheter tip is missing. What does the nurse do next?
    a. Notify the health care provider.
    b. Assess the patient for symptoms of emboli.
    c. Apply firm pressure to the insertion site.
    d. Assess the extremity for coldness, cyanosis, or numbness.

51. A patient has a local complication from a peripheral IV access with 0.9% normal saline infusing at 100 mL/hour. What does the nurse assess at the insertion site? *(Select all that apply.)*
    a. Blood returns in the catheter when nurse draws back on the IV access.
    b. A red streak is present proximal to the site.
    c. Edema is present proximal to the site.
    d. A scant amount of blood is noted beneath the clear dressing at the site.
    e. The IV fluids are not infusing.

52. The nurse is caring for the patient receiving arterial therapy via the carotid artery. What important nursing action is specific to this therapy?
    a. Assess the extremities for sensation and pulses.
    b. Monitor respirations for rate and regularity.
    c. Perform frequent neurologic assessments.
    d. Place antiembolic stockings on the patient's lower extremities.

53. Which statements are correct about intraperitoneal infusion (IP)? *(Select all that apply.)*
    a. Sterile technique is used with IP access and supplies.
    b. IP can be accessed by a catheter with an implanted port and large internal lumens.
    c. Strict aseptic technique is used with IP access and supplies.
    d. IP is used for patients who are receiving medications for diagnostic tests.
    e. IP can be accessed by a tunneled catheter with capped ports and large internal lumens.
    f. IP is used for patients who are receiving chemotherapy agents.

54. During intraperitoneal therapy, a patient reports nausea and vomiting. What does the nurse do next?
    a. Help the patient move from side to side.
    b. Flush the catheter with normal saline.
    c. Reduce the flow rate and give antiemetics.
    d. Obtain an order for an abdominal x-ray.

55. In what position does the nurse place a patient before starting intraperitoneal therapy?
    a. Semi-Fowler's
    b. Prone
    c. Supine
    d. Side-lying

56. Hypodermoclysis can be used for a patient under which types of circumstances? *(Select all that apply.)*
    a. If the patient requires palliative care
    b. For IV fluid replacement that is less than 2000 mL
    c. When a subcutaneous IV infusion is warranted
    d. If the patient requires acute care
    e. When short-term fluid volume replacement is warranted

57. The nurse is preparing to start a hypodermoclysis treatment on a patient. What is the preferred insertion site?
    a. Anterior forearm
    b. Anterior tibial area
    c. Lateral aspect of the upper arm
    d. Area under the clavicle

58. The home health nurse is adjusting the rate for a hypodermoclysis treatment. What is the usual maximum rate for this therapy?
    a. 2 mL/hr
    b. 30 mL/hr
    c. 80 mL/hr
    d. 125 mL/hr

59. The home health nurse is caring for a patient receiving hypodermoclysis therapy. How often are the subcutaneous sites rotated?
    a. Every 4 hours
    b. Every 24 hours
    c. At least every 3 days
    d. At least once a week

60. The nurse is caring for a patient receiving intrathecal pain medication. Which agent is preferred for cleaning the access site?
    a. Alcohol
    b. Soap and water
    c. Povidone iodine
    d. Chlorhexidine gluconate

61. A patient is receiving epidural medication therapy. The nurse assesses for which potential problem specific to this type of therapy?
    a. Meningitis
    b. Loss of bowel function
    c. Respiratory distress
    d. Cardiac dysrhythmias

62. A patient is brought to the emergency department (ED) after a serious motor vehicle accident. Which factor makes the patient a candidate for intraosseous (IO) therapy?
    a. Patient has a history of chronic renal failure.
    b. Endotracheal intubation is difficult to accomplish.
    c. Patient is an older adult and very thin.
    d. IV access cannot be achieved within a few minutes.

63. A patient has an IO needle in place. Why does the nurse advocate for removal of the device within 24 hours after insertion?
    a. There is an increased risk for osteomyelitis.
    b. There is an increased risk for arterial insufficiency.
    c. The device hinders patient mobility.
    d. The device is unstable and easily dislodged.

64. **Crossword Puzzle.** Complete the crossword puzzle below by answering the questions about complications of IV therapy.

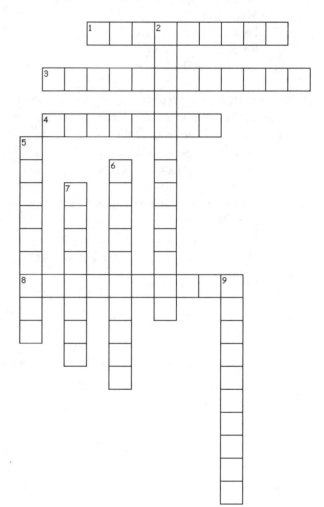

Across

1. During a central line dressing change, the nurse notes redness and swelling at the catheter insertion site, and a small amount of purulent drainage. The nurse suspects _____ at the insertion site.

3. During rounds, the nurse notes that the patient's IV site is swollen, cool, and that the IV has stopped infusing. The patient reports tenderness at the IV site. The nurse suspects _____.

4. The patient is receiving an infusion of chemotherapy, and the nurse monitors the IV infusion and site closely because the medication may cause tissue damage if it escapes into the subcutaneous tissue. The medication is known as a(n) _____.

8. After multiple IV start attempts, the nurse finally starts a peripheral IV infusion. However, that evening, the area is swollen, tender, red at the site, and the vein looks engorged. The infusion has stopped. The nurse suspects a(n) _____ at the IV site.

Down

2. Medication infuses into the subcutaneous tissue and may result in tissue sloughing. This is known as _____.

5. Two days after a peripheral IV infusion has been discontinued, the patient calls the clinic because he noticed a red, cordlike vein on his forearm above the old IV site. The nurse suspects _____.

6. The patient receiving heparin has accidentally dislodged his IV catheter. A new IV has been started, but the old site is slightly swollen, bruised, and very tender. The skin condition would be documented as _____.

7. After a dose of IV penicillin, the patient reports itching and has a rash across his back. Slight wheezes are audible. This is a(n) _____ reaction.

9. After hanging an IVPB antibiotic, the nurse steps out when called by another patient. The nurse returns after a few minutes to find that the IV antibiotic has completely infused. The patient reports dizziness, chest tightness, and has an irregular pulse and a flushed face. The nurse suspects _____.

CASE STUDY: THE PATIENT WITH A CENTRAL LINE

Use a separate sheet of paper to answer the questions in this Case Study, or go to the "Prepare for Class" folder on your Evolve website at http://evolve.elsevier.com/Iggy/ to download and complete as a word processing file. Answer guidelines for this Case Study are also available on your Evolve website.

A patient was admitted to the hospital 3 days ago for a right ischemic stroke resulting in expressive aphasia, left hemiparesis, and respiratory failure. In addition to this, the patient developed a gastrointestinal bleed. A left subclavian central line was inserted for monitoring and to administer IV medication. The dressing over the IV access site 2 days ago was clean and dry.

On the third day of hospitalization, the patient was ordered to receive total parenteral nutrition (TPN). Accuchecks are done every 6 hours. The last accucheck reading taken at 8:00 AM was 187 mg/dL. Using the sliding insulin scale, the patient was treated with 4 units of subcutaneous insulin in the right lateral abdomen. It is noted that the patient is in bed with his eyes open when the nurse enters the room. He nods his head appropriately to simple yes and no questions. He also moves his right upper and lower extremities on command, but both his left extremities are flaccid.

When the patient is repositioned, a reported stage 2 wound on the sacral area is measured and assessed by turning back one corner of the dressing. The wound measures 2 cm × 3 cm, and 90% of the wound is pink and has a slightly wet appearance, and 10% of the wound is white. A scant amount of serous drainage is on the dressing. There are no signs or symptoms of infections. The dressing was last dated and changed on the night shift, and was therefore reapplied.

Auscultation of the patient's lungs is clear in the upper lobes anteriorly and posteriorly with diminished and faint coarse breath sounds in the bases anteriorly and posteriorly. Respirations are nonlabored on the mechanical ventilator. A moderate amount of yellow sputum is suctioned from the #6 Shiley tracheostomy. There is 1+ edema of the bilateral lower extremities. Radial pulses are 2+ bilaterally and pedal pulses are 1+ bilaterally. The patient shakes his head "no" when asked if he has pain. No facial grimacing or restlessness is observed. Pupils are equal, round, and reactive to light. The patient's Foley catheter output is clear yellow. Vital signs are: blood pressure 149/89 mm Hg; heart rate 87/min, sinus rhythm; respirations 20/min; temperature 37.9° C (100.2° F); pulse oximeter reading is 93% on 2 liters of oxygen via nasal cannula.

1. Identify the top three priority patient problems from the list below.
   - Altered skin integrity
   - Inability to sustain spontaneous ventilation
   - Impaired Swallowing
   - Impaired Physical Mobility
   - Potential for infection
2. Chart the clinical findings in a nursing note for the patient in a body systems format. Include any Additional Notes pertinent for documentation.

CASE STUDY: THE PATIENT WITH A TUNNELED DIALYSIS CATHETER

Use a separate sheet of paper to answer the questions in this Case Study, or go to the "Prepare for Class" folder on your Evolve website at http://evolve.elsevier.com/Iggy/ to download and complete as a word processing file. Answer guidelines for this Case Study are also available on your Evolve website.

A patient who has end-stage kidney disease is hospitalized for a potassium level of 6.3 mEq/L. The patient has a tunneled dialysis catheter in place for hemodialysis, which is done three times a week. On assessment, the patient states that he is anuric. His blood pressure is 107/59 mm Hg, heart rate is 69/min, respirations on room air are 22/min, and his temperature is 37.5° C (99.5° F). His pulse oximeter reading is 93% at rest. The patient's lungs are auscultated clear in the bilateral upper lobes anteriorly and posteriorly, and diminished in the bilateral lower lobes anteriorly and posteriorly. A bio-occlusive dressing is in place over the tunneled catheter that is clean, dry, and intact. There are no signs or symptoms of infection at the insertion site of the catheter. The patient denies any shortness of breath or chest pain. Peaked T waves are noted on ECG and physician has been notified. Current labs indicate a blood urea nitrogen level of 62 mg/dL and a creatinine level of 3.7 mg/dL.

Upon admission to the room, the patient is oriented to the use of the call light that was placed within reach, his side rails are placed in the up position on both sides, and all surrounding floor space is clear. The patient is instructed to call the nurse for assistance when he desired to sit in the chair or requires bathroom assistance. He states understanding and is able to demonstrate the correct use of the call light.

The physician has prescribed one ampule of bicarbonate IV and 4 units of regular insulin IV.

1. Identify the top three patient problems to document in a nursing note. Chart the clinical findings using these three patient problems, and include any Additional Notes pertinent for documentation.
   - Potential for potassium imbalance
   - Potential for infection
   - Altered urinary elimination
   - Potential for fluid volume imbalance
2. What action will the nurse take to carry out the medication order?

CASE STUDY: THE PATIENT RECEIVING INTRAVENOUS THERAPY

Use a separate sheet of paper to answer the questions in this Case Study, or go to the "Prepare for Class" folder on your Evolve website at http://evolve.elsevier.com/Iggy/ to download and complete as a word processing file. Answer guidelines for this Case Study are also available on your Evolve website.

The patient is an older adult resident at a skilled nursing facility. She needs to receive IV antibiotics and fluids for pneumonia via a peripheral catheter. She is alert and cooperative and understands the need for therapy.

1. What considerations does the nurse have in establishing a peripheral IV site in an older patient?

2. What should be included in the documentation for initiating IV therapy for this patient?

3. The patient reports that her arm hurts where she is receiving the IV, especially when the antibiotic is given. What is the nurse's best action at this time?

4. What possible complications may explain her discomfort?

5. After examining the site, the nurse decides to discontinue the IV. It is restarted in her other arm, and the infusion set at 50 mL/hr as ordered. When the nurse rechecks her in an hour, the entire 1000 mL bag of normal saline has infused. The patient reports shortness of breath and she has puffiness around her eyes and engorged neck veins. Assessment of breath sounds reveals crackles over both lower lobes, and her blood pressure is 154/96 mm Hg. Another nurse says that the patient is experiencing speed shock because the saline went in too fast. Is the nurse correct? Explain your answer.

6. What should the nurse do at this time?

16
CHAPTER

Care of Preoperative Patients

STUDY/REVIEW QUESTIONS

1. Which statements best describe the preoperative period? *(Select all that apply.)*
    a. It begins when the patient makes the appointment with the surgeon to discuss the need for surgery.
    b. It ends at the time of transfer to the surgical suite.
    c. It is a time during which the patient's need for surgery is established.
    d. It begins when the patient is scheduled for surgery.
    e. It is a time during which the patient receives testing and education related to impending surgery.

2. A female patient is having a biopsy of a nodule found in the right breast. Which classification identifies this surgery?
    a. Urgent
    b. Minor
    c. Cosmetic
    d. Diagnostic

3. A patient who can barely ambulate with a walker at home is having a left total knee replacement. What is the most appropriate category for this surgery?
    a. Urgent
    b. Restorative
    c. Simple
    d. Palliative

4. A colostomy is scheduled to be done on a patient who has severe Crohn's disease. What is the correct classification for this surgery?
    a. Palliative
    b. Minor
    c. Restorative
    d. Curative

5. A male patient has a facial scar on his forehead from a third-degree burn. What is the correct classification for this surgery?
    a. Major
    b. Restorative
    c. Cosmetic
    d. Curative

6. An appendectomy is being performed on a patient with appendicitis. What is the correct classification for this surgery?
    a. Curative
    b. Diagnostic
    c. Urgent
    d. Radical

7. A patient with an abdominal aortic aneurysm is having surgical repair. What is the correct classification for this surgery?
    a. Restorative
    b. Emergent
    c. Urgent
    d. Minor

8. A 76-year-old patient is having a bilateral cataract removal. What is the correct classification for this surgery?
    a. Major
    b. Cosmetic
    c. Elective
    d. Emergent

9. A 47-year-old patient is having surgery to remove kidney stones. What is the correct classification for this surgery?
    a. Restorative
    b. Emergent
    c. Palliative
    d. Urgent

10. The nurse screens a preoperative patient for conditions that may increase the risk for complications during the perioperative period. Which conditions are possible risk factors? *(Select all that apply.)*
    a. Emotionally stable
    b. 67 years old
    c. Obesity
    d. Marathon runner
    e. Pulmonary disease

11. A 75-year-old patient is having an exploratory laparotomy tomorrow. The wife tells the nurse that at night the patient gets up and walks around his room. What does the nurse do next after hearing this information?
    a. Notifies the physician
    b. Develops a plan to keep the patient safe
    c. Obtains an order for sleep medication
    d. Tells the patient not to get out of bed at night

12. Discharge planning is done for patients who have had which types of surgery? *(Select all that apply.)*
    a. Minor
    b. Urgent
    c. Palliative
    d. Curative
    e. Emergent

13. The nurse has received a patient in the holding area who is scheduled for a left femoral-popliteal bypass. What are the priority safety measures for this patient before surgery? *(Select all that apply.)*
    a. The operative limb is marked by the surgeon.
    b. The patient is positively identified by checking the name and date of birth.
    c. The patient is asked to confirm the marked operative limb.
    d. The patient is identified by checking the name and room number.
    e. The patient is instructed to verify any family members waiting.

14. In the preoperative setting, the nurse functions as a patient advocate when which factors are assessed in the discharge planning process? *(Select all that apply.)*
    a. Support systems
    b. Any known allergies
    c. Self-care capabilities
    d. Preference for route of administration of analgesics
    e. Home environment

15. The nurse is preparing the patient for surgery. Which common laboratory tests does the nurse anticipate to be ordered? *(Select all that apply.)*
    a. Total cholesterol
    b. Electrolyte levels
    c. Uric acid
    d. Clotting studies
    e. Serum creatinine

16. Which statement is true regarding the patient who has given consent for a surgical procedure?
    a. Information necessary to understand the nature of and reason for the surgery has been provided.
    b. The length of stay in the hospital has been preapproved by the managed care provider.
    c. Information about the surgeon's experience has been provided.
    d. The nurse has provided detailed information about the surgical procedure.

17. Which statement best describes the collaborative roles of the nurse and surgeon when obtaining the informed consent?
    a. The nurse is responsible for having the informed consent form on the chart for the physician to witness.
    b. The nurse may serve as a witness that the patient has been informed by the physician before surgery is performed.
    c. The nurse may serve as witness to the patient's signature after the physician has the consent form signed before preoperative sedation is given and before surgery is performed.
    d. The nurse has no duties regarding the consent form if the patient has signed the informed consent form for the physician, even if the patient then asks additional questions about the surgery.

18. A patient with diabetes is scheduled for surgery at 0700. What are the actions, in order of priority, that the nurse will perform preoperatively? *(Select based on priority order.)*

    _____ a. Modify the dose of insulin given based on the patient's blood glucose.

    _____ b. Complete the preoperative checklist before 0700.

    _____ c. Have non-licensed personnel obtain the patient's Accucheck and vital signs.

    _____ d. Check if the patient has any jewelry on and call security to secure valuables.

19. Which postoperative interventions will the nurse typically teach a patient to prevent complications following surgery? *(Select all that apply.)*
    a. Range of motion exercises
    b. Massaging of lower extremities
    c. Taking pain medication only when experiencing severe pain
    d. Incision splinting
    e. Deep-breathing exercises

CASE STUDY: THE PREOPERATIVE PATIENT (1)

Use a separate sheet of paper to answer the questions in this Case Study, or go to the "Prepare for Class" folder on your Evolve website at http://evolve.elsevier.com/Iggy/ to download and complete as a word processing file. Answer guidelines for this Case Study are also available on your Evolve website.

A 37-year-old Chinese-American man who was rock climbing fell 20 feet onto his left side and sustained a closed fracture to his left radius. It is immobilized in a splint. Prior to this incident, the patient had a history of tonsillectomy at 5 years old, usual childhood diseases, and otherwise negative medical history. The patient is scheduled for surgery this morning under general anesthesia. Present assessment of the patient since admission to the unit 2 hours ago reveals the patient reporting pain in his left arm and slight shortness of breath. When the nurse asks him to rate his pain on a scale of 0 to 10 (with 0 being no pain and 10 being the worst pain imaginable), he rates the pain in his left arm a 7. He is alert and oriented to date, place, and name.

Vital signs are: blood pressure 139/72 mm Hg; heart rate 92; respirations 28/min; temperature 37.1° C (98.7° F); pulse oximetry 89% on room air. Respirations are regular and slightly shallow. Oxygen is applied at 2 L via nasal cannula. A pulse oximetry reading of 93% was retaken after 5 minutes on oxygen. The nurse calls the surgeon to report her concerns about the patient's report of feeling short of breath. Auscultated lung sounds are clear but diminished in the left base posteriorly and anteriorly. The patient has a nonproductive, dry cough. His left hand is warm to the touch, and his nail beds blanch in 2 seconds. He denies any numbness or tingling in his left hand or fingers, and can move all fingers and grasp the nurse's hand. His palpated radial pulses are 2+ bilaterally. He reports that he has no known drug allergies and no known reaction to general anesthesia.

1. Document a nursing note for this patient using a body systems format. Include any Additional Notes that may be pertinent for documentation.

2. What might be the medical problem the patient is experiencing, causing the feeling of shortness of breath?

3. What would the ethnic considerations be for this Chinese-American patient?

CASE STUDY: THE PREOPERATIVE PATIENT (2)

Use a separate sheet of paper to answer the questions in this Case Study, or go to the "Prepare for Class" folder on your Evolve website at http://evolve.elsevier.com/Iggy/ to download and complete as a word processing file. Answer guidelines for this Case Study are also available on your Evolve website.

The patient is a 42-year-old woman who is scheduled for a total hysterectomy under general anesthesia this morning. She is admitted to the preoperative area in the same-day surgery admitting area. During the admission assessment, the patient mentions to the nurse that her last menses was 2 months ago and that the bleeding was heavier than usual, which she assumes is why her surgeon is recommending the surgery. When asking her about medications that she takes, the patient denies taking any prescription medicines but does mention taking a baby aspirin a day and assorted herbal medicines for the bleeding.

1. What assessment should the nurse make to determine this patient's nutritional status and potential risk from the preoperative preparation and surgery?
2. Which laboratory results should the nurse review? State the rationales for doing so.
3. Prioritize teaching needs for this patient before surgery.
4. Develop a teaching-learning plan for this patient's postoperative care.
5. Identify any patient conditions or information that is to be shared with the surgeon or anesthesiologist.
6. The patient states that she doesn't know whether her hysterectomy will be done vaginally or abdominally. Recognizing that the patient is in need of more information, what would the nurse do?
7. The patient asks if she will lose a lot of blood in surgery and, if so, can her daughter donate blood that she can receive if needed. What teaching would you give the patient concerning blood donations?
8. Identify which category of surgery is related to each aspect of this patient's impending surgery.
   a. Reason:
   b. Urgency:
   c. Degree of risk of surgery:
   d. Extent of surgery:
9. While this patient is waiting in the preoperative area, she begins to cry, saying she is fearful of the surgery and "going under." What interventions could be used to reduce the patient's anxiety?
10. The patient is about to be sent to the operating room. What items on a final checklist should be evaluated before leaving the preoperative area?

17
CHAPTER

Care of Intraoperative Patients

STUDY/REVIEW QUESTIONS

1. Which nursing intervention can reduce a preoperative patient's anxiety?
   a. Provide a climate of privacy, comfort, and confidentiality when caring for the patient.
   b. Instruct the patient that after the preoperative medication has taken effect, the anxiety will go away.
   c. Avoid discussing the activities taking place around the patient while in the holding area.
   d. Assist members of the surgical team readying the operating room suite.

2. A patient is hospitalized for acute cholelithiasis. On the intake admission, which information does the nurse include? *(Select all that apply.)*
   a. Any spiritual or cultural considerations of the patient
   b. History of the patient or family
   c. When the patient plans to return to work
   d. What food preferences the patient has postsurgery
   e. The patient's medical history

3. A patient with left breast cancer is scheduled for a left mastectomy. The patient has informed the surgeon and nurse that she is a Jehovah's Witness and does not want any blood transfusions. In preparation for intraoperative care of this patient, what measures does the nurse take? *(Select all that apply.)*
   a. Obtain 2 units of packed red blood cells, typed and crossmatched.
   b. Make physician aware of patient's request for no blood transfusions.
   c. Ensure autotransfusion device is in place intraoperatively.
   d. Ensure patient has a medical necessity order for emergency blood transfusion.
   e. Inform the patient of potential risks if blood transfusion is not given.

4. To reduce the incidence of patients with a known history or risk of malignant hyperthermia (MH), what best practices are put in place in the operating room? *(Select all that apply.)*
   a. List of medications available for emergency treatment of MH
   b. Dedicated MH cart with treatment medications
   c. Treatment before, during, and after surgery if the patient has a known history or risk
   d. Additional nursing support on call if MH develops
   e. Available MH hotline number

5. A patient has a malignant hyperthermia (MH) incident during surgery. To whom does the nurse report this incident?
   a. North American Malignant Hyperthermia Registry
   b. The Joint Commission
   c. Centers for Disease Control
   d. Occupational Safety and Health Administration

Matching. Match the perioperative personnel with the descriptions of duties in the perioperative area.

Personnel
a. Surgeon
b. Holding area nurse
c. Anesthesiologist
d. Circulating nurse
e. Scrub nurse
f. Specialty nurse

Duties

_____ 6. Coordinates, oversees, and participates in the patient's nursing care while the patient is in the operating room

_____ 7. Assumes responsibility for the surgical procedure and any surgical judgments about the patient

_____ 8. Manages the patient's care while the patient is in this area and initiates documentation on a perioperative nursing record

_____ 9. Educated in a particular type of surgery and responsible for intraoperative nursing care specific to patients needing that type of surgery

_____ 10. Sets up the sterile field, assists with the draping of the patient, and hands sterile supplies, sterile equipment, and instruments to the surgeon

_____ 11. Physician who specializes in the administration of anesthetic agents

12. During surgery, what things do anesthesia personnel monitor, measure, and assess? *(Select all that apply.)*
    a. Intake and output
    b. Vital signs
    c. Cardiopulmonary function
    d. Level of anesthesia
    e. Family concerns
    f. Room temperature

Matching. *Match the nursing interventions with their stages of general anesthesia.*

Stages of Anesthesia
a.   Stage 1
b.   Stage 2
c.   Stage 3
d.   Stage 4

Nursing Interventions

_____ 13.   Prepare for and assist in treatment of cardiovascular and/or pulmonary arrest. Document in record.

_____ 14.   Shield patient from extra noise and physical stimuli. Protect the patient's extremities. Assist anesthesia personnel as needed. Stay with patient.

_____ 15.   Close operating room doors and control traffic in and out of room. Position patient securely with safety belts. Maintain minimal discussion in operating room.

_____ 16.   Assist anesthesia personnel with intubation of patient. Place the patient in position for surgery. Prep the patient's skin in area of operative site.

17.   The acute, life-threatening complication of malignant hyperthermia (MH) results from the use of which agents?
   a.   Hypnotics and neuromuscular blocking agents
   b.   Succinylcholine and inhalation agents
   c.   Nitrous oxide and pancuronium for muscle relaxation
   d.   Fentanyl and regional anesthesia for spinal block

18.   Which clinical features are found in an MH crisis? *(Select all that apply.)*
   a.   Sinus tachycardia
   b.   Tightness and rigidity of the patient's jaw area
   c.   Lowering of the blood pressure
   d.   A decrease in the end-tidal carbon dioxide level
   e.   Skin mottling and cyanosis
   f.   An extremely elevated temperature at onset
   g.   Tachypnea

19.   The surgical team understands that time is crucial in recognizing and treating an MH crisis. Once recognized, what is the treatment of choice?
   a.   Danazol gluconate
   b.   Dilantin sodium
   c.   Diazepam sulfate
   d.   Dantrolene sodium

20.   Which factors may lead to an anesthetic overdose in a patient? *(Select all that apply.)*
   a.   Amount of anesthesia retained by fat cells
   b.   Patient who is older
   c.   Slowed metabolism and drug elimination
   d.   An uncooperative patient
   e.   Liver or kidney disease

21.   A patient experiences MH immediately after induction of anesthesia. What interventions, in order of priority, does the nurse carry out? *(Select based on priority order.)*

   _____   a.   Administer IV dantrolene sodium (Dantrium) 2 to 3 mg/kg.

   _____   b.   Apply a cooling blanket over the torso.

   _____   c.   Assess ABGs and serum chemistries.

   _____   d.   Stop all inhalation anesthetic agents and succinylcholine.

   _____   e.   Monitor cardiac rhythm by electrocardiography to assess for dysrhythmias.

22. What techniques are essential to performing a proper surgical scrub of the hands by the surgeon, assistants, and scrub nurse? *(Select all that apply.)*
    a. Use a broad-spectrum, surgical antimicrobial solution.
    b. Scrub for 2 minutes, followed by a rinse with water.
    c. Use an alcohol-based antimicrobial solution.
    d. Hold hands higher than the elbows during the scrub and rinse.
    e. Scrub for 3 to 5 minutes, followed by a rinse with water.
    f. Hold hands below the elbows during the scrub and rinse.

Matching. *Match the nursing interventions with the potential complications, which can be prevented with appropriate patient positioning and monitoring.*

Anatomic Area/Complications
a. Brachial plexus/paralysis; loss of sensation
b. Radial nerve/wrist drop
c. Medial or ulnar nerves (hand deformities)/peroneal nerve (foot drop)
d. Tibial nerve/loss of sensation on the plantar surface of the foot
e. Joints/stiffness, pain, inflammation

Interventions
_____ 23. Support the wrist with padding; do not overtighten wrist straps.

_____ 24. Place pillow or foam padding under bony prominences; maintain good body alignment; slightly flex joints and support with pillows, trochanter rolls, and pads.

_____ 25. Place a safety strap above the ankle; do not place equipment on lower extremities.

_____ 26. Pad the elbow, avoid excessive abduction, secure the arm firmly on an arm board positioned at shoulder level.

_____ 27. Place a safety strap above or below the area. Place a pillow or padding under the knees.

28. In which situations is regional anesthesia used instead of general anesthesia? *(Select all that apply.)*
    a. For an endoscopy or cardiac catheterization
    b. In patients who have had an adverse reaction to general anesthesia
    c. In some cases when pain management after surgery is enhanced by regional anesthesia
    d. In patients with serious medical problems
    e. When the patient has a preference and a choice is possible

Matching. Match the anesthetic agent with its characteristic.

Agents
a. Halothane
b. Nitrous oxide
c. Desflurane
d. Thiopental sodium
e. Ketamine HCl
f. Propofol
g. Fentanyl
h. Midazolam

Characteristics
_____ 29. Induces amnesia around the event
_____ 30. Can depress respiratory and cardiac functions
_____ 31. Dissociative emergence reactions; can induce nausea and vomiting
_____ 32. Excellent postoperative analgesia and epidural anesthesia
_____ 33. Short-acting; patient becomes responsive quickly postoperatively
_____ 34. Less irritating to respiratory tract than other inhalation agents
_____ 35. May increase heart rate and lower BP during induction
_____ 36. Needs addition of other agents for longer procedures

37. To avoid electrical safety problems during surgery, what does the nurse do?
    a. Observes for breaks in sterile technique
    b. Continuously assists the anesthesia provider
    c. Ensures proper placement of the grounding pads
    d. Monitors the operating room with available cameras

38. Which medical condition increases a patient's risk for surgical wound infection?
    a. Anxiety
    b. Hiatal hernia
    c. Diabetes mellitus
    d. Amnesia

Matching. Match the type of anesthesia with its appropriate definition.

Type of Anesthesia
a. Topical anesthesia
b. Local infiltration
c. Nerve block
d. Spinal anesthesia
e. Epidural anesthesia

Definitions

_____ 39. Injection of the anesthetic agent into the epidural space; the spinal cord areas are never entered. Used for lower extremity surgeries, as well as anorectal, vaginal, perineal, and hip surgeries.

_____ 40. Injection of anesthetic agent into or around a nerve or group of nerves, resulting in blocked sensation and motor impulse transmission. Used to prevent pain during a procedure or to identify the cause of pain. A type of regional anesthesia.

_____ 41. Agents applied directly to the area of skin or mucous membrane to be anesthetized. Onset is within 1 minute; duration is up to 30 minutes.

_____ 42. Injection of an anesthetic agent directly into the tissue around an incision, wound, or lesion. Blocks peripheral nerve function at its origin.

_____ 43. Also called *intrathecal block*; injection of anesthetic agent into the cerebrospinal fluid in the subarachnoid space. Used for lower abdominal and pelvic surgery.

44. Which patient would be a candidate for moderate sedation? *(Select all that apply.)*
    a. Endoscopy
    b. Cesarean section delivery
    c. Closed fracture reduction
    d. Cardiac catheterization
    e. Suturing a laceration
    f. Abdominal surgery
    g. Cardioversion

45. A patient is requesting moderate sedation for repair of a torn meniscus and has no medical contraindications. How does the nurse respond to this patient's request?
    a. "Your surgeon will decide if you will receive moderate sedation or general anesthesia."
    b. "You can discuss your request for moderate sedation with your surgeon and anesthesiologist."
    c. "Most patients prefer general anesthesia. Can you tell me why you want moderate sedation?"
    d. "It can be frightening to see surgery done on yourself. You need to think about that."

46. Which medical condition influences whether a patient is to have moderate sedation for a laparoscopic cholecysectomy?
    a. Hypertension
    b. Osteoporosis
    c. Hypothyroidism
    d. Chronic obstructive pulmonary disease

CASE STUDY: THE INTRAOPERATIVE PATIENT (1)

Use a separate sheet of paper to answer the questions in this Case Study, or go to the "Prepare for Class" folder on your Evolve website at http://evolve.elsevier.com/Iggy/ to download and complete as a word processing file. Answer guidelines for this Case Study are also available on your Evolve website.

A 67-year-old man is wheeled into the surgical suite to repair a thoracic ascending aortic aneurysm. The patient has a right subclavian central line with a bio-occlusive dressing over the insertion site of the catheter. Intravenous fluid of $D_5 0.45$ normal saline is infusing at 70 mL/hr. A Foley catheter #18 F is placed, resulting in 175 mL of clear yellow urine output. There is bilateral pedal edema 2+ and ankle edema 1+ bilateral. The heart monitor shows a sinus rhythm of 93 beats/min with occasional premature ventricular contractions. Auscultation of the lungs reveals faint crackles in bilateral posterior bases, but all other lung fields are clear. The surgeon and anesthesiologist have agreed on general anesthesia. The nail beds are pink with a capillary refill of less than 2 seconds. Radial pulses are 2+ bilaterally and pedal pulses are 1+ bilaterally. Vital signs are: temp 99.2° F, respirations 26, blood pressure 132/73 mm Hg right upper extremity.

A time-out was done prior to placing the patient on the surgical table. The patient was correctly identified and the correct procedure was verified. The nurse from the unit reported that the wife and family were in the waiting room. Prior to administering general anesthesia, the patient was alert and oriented to person, place, time, and situation. In addition, the surgical nurse noted that the patient was able to answer simple questions and follow simple commands. He was able to move all extremities and denied any numbness or tingling. The nurse reported from the unit that patient ambulated independently without assistance. The patient's skin is warm, dry, and intact.

1. Document the patient's case using the following categories:
   - Vital signs
   - Cardiac
   - Respiratory
   - Neurologic
   - Integumentary
   - Genitourinary/gastrointestinal
   - Psychological support
   - Additional notes
2. What was done to verify that surgery was being performed on the correct patient?
3. Why is it important for the nurse to include the patient's neurologic assessment when he is having surgery for a thoracic aortic aneurysm?

CASE STUDY: THE INTRAOPERATIVE PATIENT (2)

Use a separate sheet of paper to answer the questions in this Case Study, or go to the "Prepare for Class" folder on your Evolve website at http://evolve.elsevier.com/Iggy/ to download and complete as a word processing file. Answer guidelines for this Case Study are also available on your Evolve website.

A 71-year-old man is scheduled to receive orthopedic surgery in 3 hours. The nurse in the holding area has assessed the patient and begins to prepare him for the surgical procedure.

1. While this patient is in the holding area, members of the surgical team are preparing the surgical suite. Identify factors related to physical safety in the surgical suite and give the rationale for each.

2. Identify three factors related to what the surgical team does to minimize risk of surgical infection for the patient; also identify the rationale for each.

3. The patient sees the surgical team scrubbing their hands and arms and states, "Oh, it makes me feel good to know that their hands are going to be sterile for my surgery." Evaluate this statement.

4. The surgeon, nurse, and anesthesiologist have discussed anesthesia options with the patient, who agrees that an epidural anesthetic will be a good choice for him. What are potential complications the surgical team should be aware of with this choice? What are the symptoms of these potential complications?

5. Identify the circulating nurse's responsibilities for this patient during the intraoperative period.

6. As the surgical team closes the operative wound, what type of skin closures would you expect to see?

18 CHAPTER

Care of Postoperative Patients

STUDY/REVIEW QUESTIONS

1. Which description illustrates the beginning of the postoperative period?
   a. Completion of the surgical procedure and arousal of the patient from anesthesia
   b. Discharge planning initiated in the preoperative setting
   c. Closure of the patient's surgical incision
   d. Completion of the surgical procedure and transfer of the patient to the postanesthesia care unit (PACU) or intensive care unit

2. What is the primary purpose of a PACU?
   a. Follow-through on the surgeon's postoperative orders
   b. Ongoing critical evaluation and stabilization of the patient
   c. Prevention of lengthened hospital stay
   d. Arousal of patient following the use of conscious sedation

3. A patient develops respiratory distress after having a left total hip replacement. The patient develops labored breathing and a pulse oximetry reading is 83% on 2 L nasal cannula. Which intervention is appropriate for unlicensed personnel to perform?
   a. Assess change in patient's respiratory status.
   b. Order necessary medications to be administered.
   c. Intubate the patient for maintenance of airway and assisted breathing.
   d. Take vital signs.

4. Which signs/symptoms are considered postoperative complications? *(Select all that apply.)*
   a. Sedation
   b. Pain at the surgical site
   c. Pulmonary embolism
   d. Hypothermia
   e. Wound evisceration

5. If a patient experiences a wound dehiscence, which description illustrates what is happening with the wound?
   a. Purulent drainage is present at incision site because of infection.
   b. Extreme pain is present at incision site.
   c. A partial or complete separation of outer layers is present at incision site.
   d. The inner and outer layers of the incision are separated.

6. A patient who is 2 days postoperative for abdominal surgery states, "I coughed and heard something pop." The nurse's immediate assessment reveals an opened incision with a portion of large intestine protruding. Which statements apply to this clinical situation? *(Select all that apply.)*
   a. Incision dehiscence has occurred.
   b. This is an emergency situation.
   c. The wound must be kept moist with normal saline-soaked sterile dressings.
   d. This is an urgent situation.
   e. Incision evisceration has occurred.

7. In the PACU, the nurse assesses that a patient is bleeding profusely from an abdominal incision. What actions, in order of priority, does the nurse perform? *(Select in order of priority.)*
    _____ a. The surgeon is paged.
    _____ b. The nurse applies pressure to the dressing.
    _____ c. Unlicensed assistive personnel (UAP) are asked to get additional dressing supplies.
    _____ d. A complete blood count is ordered.

Short Answer.

8. The nurse transfers a patient to the PACU who had an incision and drainage of an abscess in the right groin with general anesthesia. Blood pressure is 80/47 mm Hg, heart rate 117/min in sinus tachycardia, respiratory rate 28/min, pulse oximeter reading 93% on oxygen at 3 L nasal cannula, temp is 38.5° C. The Jackson-Pratt drain has 70 mL of a cream-colored output. Normal saline is infusing at 150 mL/hr.
    The surgeon sends orders to bolus the patient with 500 mL IV over 1 hour of normal saline, draw two sets of blood cultures, and culture drainage from the Jackson-Pratt drain. The patient has a history of vulvar cancer and had a needle biopsy of the right groin 1 week ago. In addition, the patient has a history of hypertension and is taking lisinopril 5 mg PO daily. The patient has no known drug allergies. The patient is a full code.
    Using the SBAR reporting method, indicate the appropriate responses for this case.
    a. Situation:

    b. Background:

    c. Assessment:

    d. Recommendation:

9. Clinical Note: A postoperative patient in the PACU has had an open reduction internal fixation of a left fractured femur. Vital signs are blood pressure 87/49 mm Hg, heart rate 100/min sinus rhythm, respirations 22/min, temp 98.3° F. The Foley catheter has a total amount of 110 mL of clear, yellow urine in the last 4 hours. Which body systems have been assessed by the nurse? *(Select all that apply.)*
    a. Respiratory
    b. Cardiovascular
    c. Neurovascular
    d. Integumentary
    e. Renal/urinary

10. Clinical Note: A patient cared for in the PACU has had a colostomy placed for treatment of Crohn's disease. The nurse assesses that an abdominal dressing is 25% saturated with serosanguineous drainage and notes that the incision is intact. An IV is infusing with D_5/lactated Ringer's at 100 mL/hr through a 20-g peripheral IV access. Auscultation of abdomen reveals hypoactive bowel sounds in all 4 quadrants, abdomen soft, and no distension. Foley catheter is in place and draining yellow urine with sediment, 375 mL output in Foley bag. Which body systems have been assessed by the nurse? *(Select all that apply.)*
    a. Renal/urinary
    b. Gastrointestinal
    c. Respiratory
    d. Musculoskeletal
    e. Integumentary

11. Clinical Note: A 49-year-old patient is in the PACU following a frontal craniotomy for repair of a ruptured cerebral aneurysm. The nurse assesses that the patient's eyes open on verbal stimulation. Pupils are equal, reactive to light, and prompt 3 mm. The patient's hand grasps are equal and strong. When the nurse asks the patient to state name, the patient states name correctly. The patient has had one episode of nausea and vomiting. Incision edges are dry and approximated with sutures. Lungs are slightly diminished per auscultation and the nurse observes the patient is using abdominal accessory muscles to breathe. Which body systems has the nurse assessed? *(Select in order of assessment.)*
    _____ a. Cardiovascular
    _____ b. Gastrointestinal
    _____ c. Neurologic
    _____ d. Integumentary
    _____ e. Respiratory

Matching. *Identify the assessment findings that may be noted for patients in the PACU with their corresponding body systems. Answers may be used more than once. More than one body system may be involved in an assessment finding.*

Body Systems

a.   Respiratory
b.   Cardiovascular
c.   Fluid and electrolyte balance
d.   Neurologic
e.   Renal/urinary
f.   Gastrointestinal
g.   Integumentary

Assessment Findings

_____ 12.   Eyes open on command

_____ 13.   Symmetrical chest wall expansion

_____ 14.   Foley catheter to facilitate drainage

_____ 15.   Absent dorsalis pedis pulsations

_____ 16.   Use of accessory muscles

_____ 17.   Large amount of sanguineous drainage

_____ 18.   Negative Homans' sign

_____ 19.   IV infusion of dextrose 5% Ringer's lactate

_____ 20.   States name when asked

_____ 21.   Rounded, firm abdomen

_____ 22.   Exhalation felt from nose or mouth

_____ 23.   Decreased blood pressure

_____ 24.   Wound edges approximated

_____ 25.   Dry mucous membranes

_____ 26.   Vomiting

_____ 27.   Pupils constrict equally

_____ 28.   Sternal retraction

_____ 29.   Nasogastric tube in place

_____ 30.   Evisceration

_____ 31.   Dullness over symphysis pubis

_____ 32.   Tenting

_____ 33.   Faint heart sounds

_____ 34.   Wound dressing dry

_____ 35.   Absent bowel sounds

_____ 36.   Vesicular crackles

_____ 37.   Hand grips equal

_____ 38.   Simultaneous apical and radial pulsations

_____ 39.   Dehiscence

_____ 40.   Snoring

41. A patient arrives in the PACU. Which action does the nurse perform first?
    a. Assess for a patent airway and adequate gas exchange.
    b. Rate the patient's pain using the 0-10 pain assessment scale.
    c. Position the patient in a supine position to prevent aspiration.
    d. Calculate the PCA pump maximum dose per hour to avoid an overdose.

42. A patient arrives at the PACU and the nurse notes a respiratory rate of 10 with sternal retractions. The report from anesthesia personnel indicates that the patient had received fentanyl during surgery. Place in sequential order, using the numbers 1 to 7, the nursing interventions to be performed.

    _____ a. Monitor the patient for effects of anesthetic for at least 1 hour.

    _____ b. Have suction available appropriate to the patient's available airway.

    _____ c. Closely monitor vital signs and pulse oximetry readings until the patient responds.

    _____ d. Do not leave the patient unattended until he or she is able to respond fully.

    _____ e. Observe for significant reversal of anesthesia.

    _____ f. Administer oxygen as ordered, monitoring pulse oximetry.

    _____ g. Maintain an open airway through positioning and suction as needed.

43. The nurse is teaching incisional care to a patient who has been discharged after abdominal surgery. Which instructions does the nurse include?
    a. Do not rub or touch the incision site.
    b. Practice proper handwashing.
    c. Clean the incision site two times a day with soap and water.
    d. Splint the incisional site as often as needed for comfort.

44. The health care team determines a patient's readiness for discharge from the PACU by noting a postanesthesia recovery score of at least 10. After determining that all criteria have been met, the patient is discharged to the hospital unit or home. Review the patient profiles after 1 hour in the PACU listed below. Number the patients in order of anticipated discharge from the PACU area.

    _____ a. 10-year-old girl, tonsillectomy, general anesthesia. Duration of surgery 30 minutes. Immediate response to voice. Alert to place and person. Able to move all extremities. Respirations even, deep, rate of 20. VS are within normal limits. IV solution is D_5RL. Has voided on bedpan. Eating ice chips. Complaining of sore throat.

    _____ b. 35-year-old woman, cesarean section, epidural anesthesia. Duration of surgery 27 minutes. Awake and alert. Able to bend knees and lift lower extremities. Respirations 16 breaths/min and unlabored. Foley draining 300 mL urine. IV of RL infusing. VS are within normal limits.

    _____ c. 55-year-old man, repair of fractured lower left leg. General anesthesia. Duration of surgery 1 hour, 30 minutes. Drowsy, but responds to voice. Nausea and vomiting twice in PACU. No urge to void at this time. IV infusing D_5NS. Pedal pulses noted in both lower extremities. VS: T 98.6° F; P 130; R 24; BP 124/76.

    _____ d. 24-year-old man, reconstruction of facial scar. General anesthesia. Duration of surgery 2 hours. Sleeping, groans to voice command. VS are within normal limits. Respirations 10 breaths/min. No urge to void. IV of D_5RL infusing. Complains of pain in surgical area.

    _____ e. 42-year-old woman, colonoscopy. IV conscious sedation. Awake and alert. Up to bathroom to void. IV discontinued. Resting quietly in chair. VS are within normal limits.

45. The nurse is caring for a patient who has had abdominal surgery. After a hard sneeze, the patient reports pain in the surgical area, and the nurse immediately sees that the patient has a wound evisceration. What should the nurse do? Include in your answer the timing of the interventions.

46. Which intervention for postsurgical care of a patient is correct?
    a. When positioning the patient, use the knee gatch of the bed to bend the knees and relieve pressure.
    b. Gentle massage on the lower legs and calves helps promote venous blood return to the heart.
    c. Encourage bedrest for 3 days after surgery to prevent complications.
    d. The patient should splint the surgical wound for support and comfort when getting out of bed.

47. The morning after a patient's lower leg surgery, the nurse notes that the dressing is wet from drainage. The surgeon has not yet been in to see the patient on rounds. What does the nurse do about the dressing?
    a. Removes the dressing and puts on a dry, sterile dressing
    b. Reinforces the dressing by adding dry, sterile dressing material on top of the existing dressing
    c. Applies dry, sterile dressing material directly to the wound, then retapes the original dressing
    d. Does nothing to the dressing but calls the surgeon to evaluate the patient immediately

48. The health care provider removed a patient's original surgical dressing 2 days after surgery and is discharging the patient home on daily dressing changes. Which actions does the nurse take for this patient's discharge teaching? *(Select all that apply.)*
    a. Ask the patient's family or significant other to observe the dressing change.
    b. Ask the UAP to get dressing supplies for the patient.
    c. Instruct that the drainage will appear serosanguinous.
    d. Instruct the patient to go to the ED for problems related to dressing changes.
    e. Have the case manager arrange for a home health nurse to ensure that dressing changes are done and there are no complications of infection.

CASE STUDY: THE POSTOPERATIVE PATIENT (1)

Use a separate sheet of paper to answer the questions in this Case Study, or go to the "Prepare for Class" folder on your Evolve website at http://evolve.elsevier.com/Iggy/ to download and complete as a word processing file. Answer guidelines for this Case Study are also available on your Evolve website.

A patient has arrived in the PACU 15 minutes postoperatively after having a right thoracotomy for lobectomy for lung cancer. Right anterior chest tube is set at -20 cm of suction. There is 275 mL serosanguinous drainage output in the atrium. No subcutaneous air is around the chest tube insertion site or elsewhere. There is no air leak noted in the atrium when the patient coughs. Respirations are regular and nonlabored, 20/min. Lungs are clear in the anterior and posterior upper lobes with diminished breath sounds auscultated in the anterior and posterior lower lobes, and a few crackles around the site of the chest tube insertion. Note that the patient has a dry, nonproductive cough occasionally. Nails beds are pink, with capillary refill less than 2 seconds. Pulse oximeter reading is 95% on 3 L oxygen via nasal cannula. Bilateral ankles and feet have edema 1+, nonpitting. Peripheral IV access 18 g in place with 0.45 NS with 20 mEq KCL infusing at 100 mL/hr. No redness or edema is noted at the IV insertion site.

The patient reports pain at the surgical chest site and rates the pain a 7 on a scale of 0 to 10 with 10 being the worst pain experienced. The nurse medicated the patient with fentanyl IV push 50 mcq. A Foley catheter is in place with 400 mL clear yellow urine output. Dressing is placed over the right thoracic posterior chest site of surgery and the chest tube dressing is clean, dry, and intact. A Jackson-Pratt drain is placed distal to the posterior chest incision with 40 mL bloody drainage. The patient is drowsy but arousable to verbal stimuli, then is alert and oriented to person, name, and place. The patient moves all extremities on command.

1. From the following list, identify the **top three** priority patient problems for which to document.
   - Altered skin integrity related to surgical incision
   - Potential for infection related to the incision site for bacterial invasion
   - Potential for impaired respiratory function
   - Alteration in immune system, lung cancer
   - Acute Pain related to incision and immobility

2. What measures will reduce the potential for respiratory complications?

3. What measures can reduce the risk of a postoperative patient from developing deep vein thrombosis?

4. List at least three risk factors for the development of DVT.

CASE STUDY: THE POSTOPERATIVE PATIENT (2)

Use a separate sheet of paper to answer the questions in this Case Study, or go to the "Prepare for Class" folder on your Evolve website at http://evolve.elsevier.com/Iggy/ to download and complete as a word processing file. Answer guidelines for this Case Study are also available on your Evolve website.

A 30-year-old woman is admitted to the recovery area following a laparoscopy for an ovarian cyst removal. She is a small woman: 5 feet 1 inch and 103 pounds. Her surgery lasted 1 hour and 45 minutes, and the circulating nurse reported that she had a severe hemorrhage from the surgical site during that time. Upon admission to the PACU, the patient's blood pressure is 112/62, pulse range is 84 to 92, and respirations are 20 and shallow. She is groggy but answers when asked questions. An IV infusion of 1000 mL of D_5 Ringer's lactate is infusing at a rate of 200 mL per hour, and 800 mL remains in the bottle. During surgery, 100 mL of D_5 Ringer's lactate and 500 mL of normal saline were infused. An endotracheal tube (ET) is in place.

1. What assessments should the nurse perform before removing the ET?

2. How often should the nurse monitor the patient's vital signs?

A very slight amount of drainage is present on her dressing. Her blood pressure has been rising slowly and is now 20 mm Hg higher than the time recorded during surgery. She is restless and her respirations are 24 per minute.

3. After reviewing the above data, the nurse performs further assessment. What additional parameters should be assessed and why?

4. The nurse contacts the surgeon who orders the IV rate be reduced to 100 mL per hour. What is the reason for this order?

5. The patient's condition stabilizes and she is transferred to the postsurgical nursing unit. Discuss the information that the PACU nurse should report to the unit nurse.

19 CHAPTER

Inflammation and the Immune Response

STUDY/REVIEW QUESTIONS

1. Which statements about the purpose of the immune system are true? *(Select all that apply.)*
   a. The immune system provides protection from and eliminates or destroys microorganisms.
   b. The immune system is able to identify non-self proteins and cells.
   c. The immune system removes foreign proteins and other substances.
   d. The immune system protects against allergic/anaphylactic reactions.
   e. The immune system is able to prevent healthy body cells from being destroyed.

2. Which factors may affect the function of the immune system? *(Select all that apply.)*
   a. Nutritional status
   b. Environmental conditions
   c. Drugs
   d. Previous/current disease
   e. Age

3. The immune system responsible for self-tolerance has the ability to do what? *(Select all that apply.)*
   a. Recognize self versus non-self.
   b. Be recognized by T-lymphocyte helper/inducer T cells.
   c. Recognize different proteins on cell membranes.
   d. Recognize self versus the inflammatory response.
   e. Identify non-self which includes all invading cells and organisms.

4. From where do most immune cells originate?
   a. Thymus
   b. Spleen
   c. Liver
   d. Bone marrow

5. How does the body determine self from non-self cells?
   a. Red blood cells use T-lymphocyte helper cells.
   b. Leukocytes use human leukocyte antigens.
   c. Leukocytes use the macrophages.
   d. White blood cells use the stem cells.

6. A patient has sustained a severe right ankle sprain, and the nurse is explaining the process of inflammation to the patient and family. Which information does the nurse include? *(Select all that apply.)*
   a. The presence of inflammation does not always indicate that an infection is present.
   b. It occurs in response to tissue injury.
   c. It provides long-term protection.
   d. It is a specific body defense to invasion or injury.
   e. How widespread the symptoms are depends on the intensity and severity of the initiating injury.

7. The nurse is instructing a patient with an immune system disease about what the major functions of immunity are. Which information does the nurse include? *(Select all that apply.)*
   a. Immunity requires three immunity processes.
   b. Inflammation process is natural immunity.
   c. The gastrointestinal system is part of natural immunity.
   d. Antibody-mediated immunity produces new red blood cells.
   e. Cell-mediated immunity circulates T-lymphocytes.

8. The actions of leukocytes provide the body protection against invading organisms. Which is *not* one of those actions?
   a. Phagocytic destruction of foreign invaders and unhealthy or abnormal self cells
   b. Lytic destruction of foreign invaders and unhealthy self cells
   c. Production of antibodies directed against invaders
   d. Production of cytokines that decrease specific leukocyte growth and activity

9. Which statement about the inflammatory response is true?
   a. Response is different with each incident.
   b. Response is the same whether the insult to the body is a burn or otitis media.
   c. Response depends on the location in the body.
   d. Response is specific to the cell type invaded or injured.

10. The inflammatory response is present in which conditions? *(Select all that apply.)*
    a. Sprain injuries to joints
    b. Surgical wounds
    c. Poison ivy
    d. Scalding burn injury
    e. Appendicitis

11. Which cell types associated with the inflammatory response participate in phagocytosis?
    a. Neutrophils and eosinophils
    b. Macrophages and neutrophils
    c. Macrophages and eosinophils
    d. Eosinophils and basophils

12. The body produces the most of which type of white blood cell?
    a. Macrophages
    b. Eosinophils
    c. Neutrophils
    d. Band neutrophils

Matching. *Match the cell characteristics with the types of cells. Answers may be used more than once.*

Cell Types
a. Neutrophil
b. Macrophage
c. Basophil
d. Eosinophil

Characteristics

_____ 13. 12- to 18-hour life span

_____ 14. 1% to 2% of total WBCs

_____ 15. Contains chemicals such as histamine

_____ 16. Can participate in multiple episodes of phagocytosis

_____ 17. When mature, capable of phagocytosis

_____ 18. Clinical sign of left shift indicates not enough mature cells being produced

_____ 19. Liver and spleen have greatest concentration

_____ 20. Vascular leak syndrome

_____ 21. The number in circulation increases during an allergic response

22. Which statements about phagocytosis are true? *(Select all that apply.)*
    a. It is a process that engulfs invaders and destroys them by enzymatic degradation.
    b. It rids the body of debris and destroys foreign invaders.
    c. It is done in a predictable manner.
    d. It is a function of all leukocytes.
    e. Phagocytosis involves six very important steps.

23. When an injury or invasion occurs, which functions will the phagocytic cell perform? *(Select all that apply.)*
    a. Release chemotaxins or leukotaxins
    b. Initiate repair of damaged tissue
    c. Generate specific antibodies
    d. Gain direct contact with the antigen or invader
    e. Recognize "non-self"

24. Complement activation and fixation is a mechanism of opsonization. When stimulated, phagocytic adherence includes 20 different inactive protein components that will:
    a. Cause individual complement proteins to activate, join together, surround the antigen, and adhere.
    b. Join together, cause individual complement proteins to activate, surround the antigen, and adhere.
    c. Cause individual phagocytic cells to clump together, forming a barrier to an invader.
    d. Stimulate the bone marrow to increase production of macrophages.

25. What are phagocytes capable of doing?
    a. Making antibodies
    b. Ingesting cells
    c. Secreting complement
    d. Producing insulin

26. A patient is seen in the emergency department for a scalding burn to the left dorsal surface of the hands and fingers from one day ago. The nurse assesses the injury to have redness, swelling, warmth to touch, and the patient reports pain in the hand. The nurse observes that the patient has limited ability to hold a pen and limited range of motion. What do these findings indicate? *(Select all that apply.)*
    a. Stage II of inflammation
    b. The result of an antigen-antibody interaction
    c. Cardinal signs of inflammation
    d. A vascular response
    e. Stage I of inflammation

27. In which stage are all the signs of inflammation present?
    a. I
    b. II
    c. III
    d. IV

28. At the time of inflammation, a colony-stimulating factor stimulates bone marrow to perform which action?
    a. Produce leukocytes in less time
    b. Produce immature leukocytes
    c. Release immature leukocytes
    d. Synthesize immunoglobulins

29. The substance commonly called "pus" is produced by exudate in which stage of inflammation?
    a. I
    b. II
    c. III
    d. IV

30. Which statements correctly describe characteristics of the phagocytosis process? *(Select all that apply.)*
    a. Neutrophils are a functional part of phagocytosis.
    b. Platelets are a functional part of phagocytosis.
    c. During phagocytosis, invading microorganisms are attacked and destroyed.
    d. During phagocytosis, dead tissue is removed.
    e. Immunoglobulins are critical to the defense of the host against pathogenic bacteria and fungi.

31. When B-lymphocytes, part of the antibody-mediated immunity (AMI) response, become sensitized to an antigen, what do they do next?
    a. Release colony-stimulating factors
    b. Cause leukocytes to aggregate
    c. Generate specific antibodies
    d. Suppress phagocytosis

32. When a person is exposed to an antigen, seven special actions take place in sequence. In which step do antibodies bind to the antigen and form an immune complex?
    a. 2
    b. 4
    c. 5
    d. 7

33. Which cells interact in the presence of an antigen to start antibody production? *(Select all that apply.)*
    a. B-lymphocytes
    b. Macrophages
    c. Neutrophils
    d. T-helper/inducer cells
    e. T-suppressor cells

34. Which statement about B-lymphocytes sensitizing to one antigen is true?
    a. Once sensitized, B-lymphocytes are always sensitized to that antigen.
    b. Plasma cells produce the antigen.
    c. The plasma cell lies dormant until the next exposure.
    d. Memory cells prevent plasma cells from oversecreting antibodies.

35. In what way is AMI different from cell-mediated immunity (CMI)?
    a. AMI is more powerful than CMI.
    b. AMI can be transferred from one person to another; CMI cannot.
    c. CMI requires constant re-exposure for "boosting;" AMI does not.
    d. CMI requires inflammatory actions for best function; AMI function is independent of inflammatory actions.

Matching. *Match the actions with the antibody-binding reactions.*

Antibody-Binding Reactions
a. Agglutination
b. Lysis
c. Precipitation
d. Inactivation (neutralization)
e. Complement fixation

Actions
_____ 36. Cell membrane destruction

_____ 37. Large, insoluble antibody molecules

_____ 38. Clumping-like antibody action

_____ 39. Activated by IgG and IgM

_____ 40. Covers antigen's active site

41. Which statement is true about innate-native immunity?
    a. It is genetically determined, nonspecific, and cannot be transferred.
    b. It adapts to individual exposure and invasion.
    c. It can be altered by environmental or physiologic changes.
    d. It requires a special interaction with antibody-mediated immunity for activation.

Matching. *Match the type of immunity with its correct definition.*

Immunity Types
a. Natural active
b. Artificial active
c. Innate-native
d. Passive
e. Active

Definitions
_____ 42. Immunity that occurs when antibodies are created in another person or animal

_____ 43. Immunity which is a naturally occurring feature of a person

_____ 44. Protections developed by vaccination or immunization

_____ 45. Antigens enter the body and the body makes antibodies against the antigen

_____ 46. Antigen enters the body without human assistance; antibodies are made against the antigen

47. Which cells are the T-lymphocyte subsets that are critically important to CMI? *(Select all that apply.)*
    a. Helper/inducer T-cell
    b. Suppressor T-cell
    c. Cytotoxic/cytolytic T-cell
    d. Natural killer cells
    e. Cytokines

48. Which statement best describes the function of CD4+ (cluster of differentiation 4, or T4+) cells?
    a. They participate in specialized episodes of phagocytosis directed against cancer cells.
    b. They provide a frame or lattice for tissue repair and regeneration after inflammatory events.
    c. They secrete lymphokines that can enhance the activity of other WBCs.
    d. They deliver a "lethal hit" of lytic substance to a target cell in response to antibody-dependent lysis.

Matching. *Match each type of cell with its function. Answers may be used more than once.*

Cell Type
a. Suppressor cell
b. Natural killer cell
c. Helper/inducer T-cell
d. Cytotoxic/cytolytic T-cell

Function
_____ 49. Prevents overreaction

_____ 50. Binds with infected cell's antigen that results in death of affected cell

_____ 51. Secretes lymphokines that stimulate activities of other cells of the immune system

_____ 52. Exerts cytotoxic effect without first undergoing period of sensitization

_____ 53. Regulates variety of inflammatory and immune responses

54. A patient who is in good health is naturally assisted in cancer prevention by which type of immunity?
   a. Cell-mediated
   b. Innate
   c. Lymphokine
   d. Humoral

55. The action of which cell types must be suppressed to prevent acute rejection of transplanted organs? *(Select all that apply.)*
   a. Eosinophils
   b. Suppressor T-cells
   c. Natural killer cells
   d. Cytotoxic/cytolytic T-cells
   e. Helper/inducer T-cells

56. During surgery, a patient who had a heart transplant is experiencing rejection of the organ. What type of rejection is this?
   a. Acute
   b. Chronic
   c. Hyperacute
   d. Transplant

57. Which type of organ transplant rejection does not always mean immediate loss of the organ?
   a. Rejection of suppressor T-cells
   b. Chronic
   c. Acute
   d. Hyperacute

58. A patient who had an organ transplant 2 months ago is experiencing rejection of the organ. What type of rejection is this?
   a. Acute
   b. Hyperacute
   c. Delayed
   d. Chronic

Matching. Match the types of rejection with their descriptors. Answers may be used more than once.

Types of Rejection
a.   Hyperacute
b.   Acute
c.   Chronic

Descriptors

_____ 59.   Immediate

_____ 60.   Includes both cellular and antibody-mediated mechanisms

_____ 61.   Rejection cannot be stopped

_____ 62.   Occurs within 1 week to 3 months

_____ 63.   Leads to organ destruction

_____ 64.   Does not mean loss of transplant

_____ 65.   Accelerated graft atherosclerosis

_____ 66.   Triggers blood clotting cascade

_____ 67.   Fibrotic and scarlike tissue

_____ 68.   Major cause of death in heart transplant patients

_____ 69.   Is antibody-mediated

70.   A patient was admitted to the hospital for acute rejection after a kidney transplant that occurred 2 months ago. What are the appropriate interventions for this patient? *(Select all that apply.)*
   a.   Immunosuppressant therapy to limit damage and save the organ
   b.   Counseling for the patient and family about the inability to save the organ
   c.   Intravenous fluids and a low-sodium diet
   d.   Cardiac catheterization
   e.   Organ biopsy to diagnose impaired function

71.   How does the immune system respond to a graft when a transplant rejection occurs? *(Select all that apply.)*
   a.   Anticoagulation causes damage to the graft cells.
   b.   Natural killer cells cause lysis of the organ cells.
   c.   Interleukin-1 causes clotting and leads to necrosis.
   d.   Cytotoxic/cytolytic T-cells destroy and eliminate non-self cells.
   e.   The host's immune system starts inflammation and immunologic actions to destroy non-self cells.

72.   What precaution or intervention has the highest priority for a patient going home on maintenance drugs after receiving a kidney transplant?
   a.   Monitoring for bacterial and fungal infections
   b.   Avoiding the use of table salt
   c.   Measuring abdominal girth daily
   d.   Avoiding blood donation

Matching. Match each antibody characteristic with its correct antibody type.

Antibody Types
a. IgA
b. IgE
c. IgG
d. IgM

Characteristics

_____ 73. Mediates ABO incompatibility reactions in blood transfusions

_____ 74. Mediates many types of allergic reactions

_____ 75. Present in body secretions such as tears, mucus, saliva

_____ 76. Has the highest percentage in the blood

77. The nurse is instructing a patient who has undergone an organ transplant about immunosuppressant medications. What information does the nurse include? *(Select all that apply.)*
   a. All immunosuppressive medications increase the risk of infection and cancer.
   b. These medications are used for maintenance therapy of the graft.
   c. These medications will be gradually discontinued.
   d. These medications are essential to preventing transplant rejection.
   e. Some immunosuppressive medications may stimulate hyperglycemia.

78. In order to combat rejection of a transplanted kidney, what medication given before and after the transplant surgery and that uses monoclonal antibodies is administered to the patient?
   a. Daclizumab (Zenapax)
   b. Tacrolimus FK 506 (Prograf)
   c. Cyclosporin
   d. Muromonab-CD3 (OKT3)

79. Muromonab-CD3 (OKT3) is another essential drug given to patients who are having an organ transplant. Which characteristics apply to taking this medication? *(Select all that apply.)*
   a. There is a high incidence of flu-like symptoms.
   b. Induction of capillary leak syndrome is common.
   c. An antibody is also used to prevent T-cell activities.
   d. It mediates many types of immunosuppression.
   e. Premedication with corticosteroids may be required.

80. A patient is admitted with pneumonia and has developed sepsis. What can the findings from a differential WBC count reveal about this patient? *(Select all that apply.)*
   a. If an infection is present
   b. Whether an infection is bacterial or viral
   c. The tissue type from the human leukocyte antigen
   d. Whether the patient has active immunity
   e. The type of antibody response occurring

81. Which statements correctly pertain to the drug sirolimus (Rapamune)? *(Select all that apply.)*
   a. It is an autoimmune agent.
   b. It is used for prophylaxis of organ rejection.
   c. It is an immunosuppressive agent.
   d. It requires that trough levels be monitored regularly.
   e. Grapefruit juice inhibits CYP3A4-mediated metabolism of this medication.

CASE STUDY: THE PATIENT WITH A HEART TRANSPLANT

Use a separate sheet of paper to answer the questions in this Case Study, or go to the "Prepare for Class" folder on your Evolve website at http://evolve.elsevier.com/Iggy/ to download and complete as a word processing file. Answer guidelines for this Case Study are also available on your Evolve website.

A 38-year-old man who had a heart transplant 7 weeks ago is admitted to the hospital for dyspnea and 3+ bilateral edema in the lower extremities. Auscultation of the lungs reveals crackles in the bilateral posterior bases; otherwise breath sounds are clear in the anterior and posterior upper lobes. Pulse oximeter is at 88% on room air. Further nursing assessment reveals that the patient takes cyclosporine, prednisone, and tacrolimus as prescribed. In addition, the patient states he has not adhered 100% of the time to the 2-gram sodium diet he was instructed on prior to discharge home. He is alert and oriented to person, place, and time. He follows simple commands and ambulates with a steady gait with no assistive devices.

Vital signs are: blood pressure 110/63 mm Hg; heart rate 69/min in sinus arrhythmia; respiratory rate 30/min; temp 38.7° C (101.6° F). The patient states that he has gained 3 lbs in the last day and 7 lbs total over the past 7 days.

Oxygen is administered immediately at 2 L per nasal cannula and a pulse oximeter reading is retaken showing 93%. The physician orders laboratory tests and a biopsy.

1. From the following list, select the **top two** priority problems for this patient. Also include any Additional Notes pertinent for documentation.
   - Behavior modification
   - Decreased Cardiac Output
   - Noncompliance
   - Deficient Knowledge
   - Impaired oxygenation
2. What factors place a patient at high risk for hyperacute rejection?
3. What does maintenance therapy for a transplant patient entail?
4. Prepare a teaching plan for the patient that focuses on the importance of compliance with diet and lifestyle modification.

20
CHAPTER

Care of Patients with Arthritis and Other Connective Tissue Diseases

STUDY/REVIEW QUESTIONS

1. Identify these abbreviations commonly used in relation to connective tissue disease.

   a. CTD _____

   b. DJD _____

   c. OA _____

   d. ESR _____

   e. TJR _____

   f. TJA _____

   g. DVT _____

   h. CPM _____

   i. RA _____

   j. TMJ _____

   k. SLE _____

2. A rheumatic disease is any condition or disease of which body system?
   a. Cardiovascular
   b. Hematopoietic
   c. Integumentary
   d. Musculoskeletal

3. Connective tissue diseases are characterized by which features? *(Select all that apply.)*
   a. Chronic pain
   b. Dry skin
   c. Decreased function
   d. Joint deterioration
   e. Autoimmune disorder

4. What are the known causes of osteoarthritis? *(Select all that apply.)*
   a. Smoking
   b. Aging
   c. Decrease in the production of synovial fluid
   d. Decrease in proteoglycans
   e. Obesity

5. Which are features of osteoarthritis? *(Select all that apply.)*
   a. Excessive formation of scar tissue
   b. Narrowing of the joint space, formation of bone spurs
   c. Nerve degeneration resulting in joint paresthesias
   d. Bone cyst formation and joint subluxation
   e. Progressive deterioration of the loss of cartilage in one or more joints
   f. Thinning cartilage

6. In what way does obesity influence the development of osteoarthritis?
   a. The obese person has a reduced inflammatory response with less joint swelling.
   b. The high body fat levels of the obese patient lubricate joints and improve mobility.
   c. The extra weight of obesity increases the degeneration rate of hip and knee joints.
   d. Obesity has no positive or negative influence on development of osteoarthritis.

7. Which patients are more likely to develop osteoarthritis? *(Select all that apply.)*
   a. Obese older woman living alone
   b. Slender, nonsmoking, middle-aged man
   c. Muscular, young construction worker
   d. Young woman with family history of rheumatoid arthritis
   e. Middle-aged adult with multiple knee injuries from playing soccer in high school

8. Which terms might a patient use to describe crepitus? *(Select all that apply.)*
   a. Spasms of surrounding muscles
   b. Increasing joint pain and stiffness
   c. A continuous grating sensation
   d. Protruding bony lumps
   e. Limited movement

9. The nurse is preparing an educational session for a group of patients newly diagnosed with osteoarthritis. What lifestyle changes that may slow joint degeneration does the nurse suggest? *(Select all that apply.)*
   a. Keep body weight within normal limits.
   b. Quit smoking.
   c. Do not participate in any strenuous activity.
   d. Avoid risk-taking behaviors that may result in trauma.
   e. Avoid high-intensity repetitive movement of knee joints whenever possible.

10. The presence of fluid in the knees may be diagnosed as which condition?
    a. Subcutaneous swelling
    b. Joint nodules
    c. Joint effusions
    d. Joint deformities

11. Osteoarthritis affecting the spine may present as what kind of pain?
    a. Localized pain at L3-4, bone spurs, stiffness, and muscle spasm
    b. Radiating pain at L3-4, C4-6, stiffness, muscle spasms, and bone spurs
    c. Localized pain at T6 to T12, stiffness, and muscle atrophy
    d. Radiating pain throughout the spine, stiffness, and muscle spasms

12. Which responses from a patient with advanced osteoarthritis alerts the nurse to a problem coping with the image and role changes necessitated by disease progression? *(Select all that apply.)*
    a. "I used to be a playground assistant; now I work with children who need help with reading."
    b. "I must be getting younger. I used to tie my shoes; now I am using Velcro closures just like my kids."
    c. "I find it easier to do my ironing sitting down rather than standing up."
    d. "I try to avoid public places so no one will see my ugly hands."
    e. "My joints are so stiff all the time, I can't be bothered to go outside."

13. To determine an alteration in a patient's body image and self-esteem, what does the nurse assess as priorities? *(Select all that apply.)*
    a. Church affiliation
    b. Personal care of self
    c. Demeanor as happy or sad
    d. Expression of feeling of reacting to change
    e. Number of years the patient has been married

14. The nurse is teaching a patient with osteoarthritis about taking prescribed ibuprofen (Motrin). Which statements by the patient indicate a correct understanding of the medication? *(Select all that apply.)*
    a. "I'll take the medication between meals."
    b. "The medication will affect my appetite."
    c. "The medication will help my pain and swelling."
    d. "I should stop the medication if my joints swell."
    e. "I should contact my health care provider if I have frequent upset stomach or notice dark tarry stools."

15. Which treatment modalities might the nurse expect for a patient who is undergoing nonsurgical management of chronic joint pain? *(Select all that apply.)*
    a. Immobilization to promote rest
    b. Weight control
    c. Analgesics
    d. Exercise balanced with rest
    e. Thermal modalities

16. When educating a patient about total joint arthroplasty (TJA), what does the nurse do first?
    a. Asks whether the patient has insurance
    b. Reviews instructions and ask the patient to repeat them back
    c. Assesses the patient's knowledge and begins education if needed
    d. Asks if the doctor has explained the procedure

17. For preoperative care of a patient scheduled for total joint arthroplasty (TJA), what does the nurse plan to do? *(Select all that apply.)*
    a. Provide written or videotaped information about the procedure.
    b. Assess the patient's understanding of the procedure.
    c. Assess and include the patient's support people or family.
    d. Include interdisciplinary providers, if possible.
    e. Assist in scheduling needed dental procedures after the surgery.

18. Which items are contraindications for total joint arthroplasty? *(Select all that apply.)*
    a. Infection
    b. Severe pain
    c. Advanced osteoporosis
    d. Severe inflammation
    e. Open wound

19. The nurse is preparing an educational session for a patient who is preparing to undergo hip replacement. Which potential complications does the nurse make the patient aware of? *(Select all that apply.)*
    a. Venous thromboembolism
    b. Hip dislocation
    c. Overgrowth of bone
    d. Neurovascular compromise
    e. Infection

20. The nurse is preparing an educational program for student nurses on the orthopedic unit. Which three signs of hip dislocation would be included in this offering?

    a. _____

    b. _____

    c. _____

21. Which interventions can the nurse use to prevent or manage infections in patients who have undergone TJR? *(Select all that apply.)*
    a. Use aseptic technique for wound care and emptying of drains.
    b. Wash hands thoroughly when caring for patients.
    c. Culture drainage fluid if a change is observed.
    d. Monitor temperature.
    e. Report excessive inflammation or drainage to the provider.

True or False? Read each statement and write T for true or F for false in the blanks provided.

_____ 22. The most potentially life-threatening complication following TJA is venous thromboembolism (VTE).

_____ 23. The TJA patient's erythrocyte sedimentation rate (ESR) is elevated, which may indicate infection at the site.

_____ 24. Early ambulation is an effective method of preventing VTE.

25. Which preoperative tests are performed for a patient scheduled to undergo a total hip arthroplasty (THA)? *(Select all that apply.)*
    a. Review of risk factors for clotting disturbance
    b. X-ray of operative hip
    c. CT of operative hip
    d. Biopsy of operative hip
    e. MRI of operative hip

26. A patient is reluctant to consider hip surgery because of a fear of blood transfusion reaction. What is the nurse's best response?
    a. "No one will force you to receive blood if you don't want it."
    b. "You could donate your own blood for several weeks before the surgery."
    c. "Why do you think you are going to have a blood transfusion reaction?"
    d. "Blood products are very safe these days and there are numerous safety protocols."

27. A patient is receiving LMWH therapy to prevent postoperative DVT. Which routine assessments are most important for this patient during anticoagulation therapy? *(Select all that apply.)*
    a. Ensure that antiembolic stockings or sequential compression devices are in use.
    b. Monitor CBC and platelet counts.
    c. Monitor aPTT levels.
    d. Check stools for occult blood.
    e. Monitor the surgical site for bleeding.

28. How does a continuous peripheral nerve blockade (CPNB) device work?
    a. Infuses intravenous opioids.
    b. Infuses a local anesthetic into the surgical site.
    c. Circulates cold liquids within a wrap around the incision site.
    d. Stimulates vibration-sensitive receptors in the incision area to "close the gate" on pain.

29. Adlea is a refined capsaicin product. If infused directly into the surgical joint, how is its mechanism of action described?
    a. Numbness results from calcium flooding the nerve cells, which then shut down.
    b. Capsaicin shuts down C fiber receptors.
    c. Depletes calcium stores in nerve cells and blocks pain transmission.
    d. Local anesthetic numbs nerves in the operative region.

30. Postoperative total hip replacement patients can develop numerous complications. Which interventions are most important in preventing complications? *(Select all that apply.)*
    a. Bedrest with pillow between the legs
    b. Adequate diet and fluid intake
    c. Getting out of bed on the first postoperative day
    d. Sitting on the side of the bed
    e. Frequent assessment of the patient's pain

31. Which postoperative complication occurs more frequently among patients who have total hip replacements than among patients who have total knee replacements?
    a. Deep vein thrombosis
    b. Joint dislocation
    c. Acute pain
    d. Infection

32. For patients who have TJAs, the risk of deep vein thrombosis (DVT) is high. Which statements are true? *(Select all that apply.)*
    a. Older adults are at high risk for DVT and compromised circulation.
    b. Thinner patients are more at risk than obese patients.
    c. Patients with a history of DVT are at high risk for recurrence.
    d. Leg exercises must be started in the immediate postoperative period.
    e. Use of an abduction splint will decrease the risk of DVT.

33. A patient had a total hip arthroplasty. Which interventions does the nurse perform to prevent a DVT from occurring? *(Select all that apply.)*
    a. Instruct to delay ambulation postoperatively.
    b. Apply thigh-high stockings.
    c. Administer an anticoagulant such as aspirin.
    d. Use the foot sole pumps as needed.
    e. Apply sequential compression devices (SCDs).

34. To prevent a DVT, several types of anticoagulant medications can be ordered. Which is the most commonly used drug during hospitalization?
    a. Oral or parenteral aspirin
    b. Warfarin
    c. Intravenous tPA
    d. Subcutaneous low-molecular–weight (LMW) heparin

35. It is important to monitor which laboratory test for patients on anticoagulant therapy with LMW heparin after total joint arthroplasty? *(Select all that apply.)*
    a. Prothrombin time and international normalized ratio (INR)
    b. Oxygen saturation
    c. Complete blood count
    d. Activated partial thromboplastin time
    e. Platelet count

36. Postoperative care for total knee replacement may include which techniques? *(Select all that apply.)*
    a. Hot compresses to the incisional area
    b. Continuous passive motion (CPM) used immediately or several days postoperatively
    c. Ice packs or cold packs to the incisional area
    d. The use of a CPM machine in the daytime and an immobilizer at night
    e. Maintaining abduction

37. Postoperative care following finger and wrist replacements includes which techniques? *(Select all that apply.)*
    a. Traction
    b. Joint wrapped in a bulky dressing
    c. Splint, brace, or cast
    d. Abduction pillow
    e. Elevation of the arm to prevent edema
    f. CPM machine

38. Which interventions does the nurse implement to improve mobility for a patient who has undergone a THR? *(Select all that apply.)*
    a. Encourage use of assistive devices such as a walker when ambulating.
    b. Recommend to quickly decrease rest periods between activities.
    c. Instruct to flex the hips 90 degrees or greater.
    d. Instruct to sit on a soft chair with a raised back.
    e. Instruct in the use of a raised toilet seat.

39. What is an important health teaching point for a patient with TJA?
    a. "Do as much as you can as often as you can."
    b. "Reach beyond the physical therapist's instructions."
    c. "Protect the joint."
    d. "No pain, no gain."

40. Although arthritis is not curable, many "cures" are marketed to patients with the disease. What does the nurse encourage the patient to do?
    a. Take advantage of clinical trials or experimental therapy.
    b. Check with the Arthritis Foundation for appropriate modalities.
    c. Buy special liniments and creams.
    d. Take herbals and vitamins.

41. When evaluating a patient with arthritis and TJA, the nurse assesses for which expected outcome?
    a. Perform ADLs with one person assisting.
    b. Verbally express comfort and pain relief.
    c. Ambulate with crutches or a walker.
    d. Perform passive range of motion (ROM) exercises three times a shift.

42. Which statements regarding rheumatoid arthritis (RA) are true? *(Select all that apply.)*
    a. It is a chronic, progressive, systemic inflammatory process.
    b. It primarily affects the synovial joints.
    c. It is known to have periods of remission.
    d. It occurs most often in older men and women.
    e. It often involves an inflamed, red rash.

43. Because of the inflammatory process in RA, a pannus forms in the joint. What is a pannus?
    a. Scar tissue restricting the joint
    b. Vascular granulation tissue in the joint
    c. Necrotic tissue sloughing into the joint
    d. Fluid encapsulated in the joint

44. What common musculoskeletal health problem is often associated with RA?
    a. Paget's disease
    b. Fibromyalgia
    c. Marfan syndrome
    d. Osteoporosis

45. Although the etiology of RA is unknown for certain, it is considered to be what type of disorder?
    a. An autoimmune disease
    b. Associated with aging
    c. Genetic
    d. The result of joint misuse

46. For the following manifestations of RA, specify whether they are early (E) or late (L) manifestations.

    _____ a. Joint deformities

    _____ b. Joint inflammation

    _____ c. Osteoporosis

    _____ d. Vasculitis

    _____ e. Subcutaneous nodules

    _____ f. Paresthesias

    _____ g. Low-grade fever

    _____ h. Anemia

47. Which patient-reported symptoms are typical of RA? *(Select all that apply.)*
    a. "My hands are stiff, swollen, and tender."
    b. "My right hand is weak."
    c. "My pain and stiffness is worse in the morning."
    d. "My knees are swollen and stiff."
    e. "I am weak and fatigued."

48. When a patient has RA of the temporomandibular joint, what is the major complaint?
    a. Pain on chewing and opening the mouth
    b. Headache at the temple
    c. Toothache
    d. Earache

49. What is the most common area of involvement of RA in the spine?
    a. Lumbar spine
    b. Sacral spine
    c. Cervical spine
    d. Thoracic spine

50. Complications of spinal involvement in RA may be seen as which signs/symptoms? *(Select all that apply.)*
    a. Compression of the phrenic nerve that controls the diaphragm
    b. Resulting subluxation of the first and second vertebrae
    c. Becoming quadriplegic or quadriparetic
    d. Bilateral sciatic pain in the legs
    e. Numbness of the hands and feet

51. In patients with RA, where might Baker's cysts be located?
    a. Ankles
    b. Wrists
    c. Popliteal bursae
    d. Achilles tendon

52. In late RA, the patient may have systemic involvement called "flareups." How are these characterized? *(Select all that apply.)*
    a. Moderate to severe weight loss
    b. Fever and fatigue
    c. Muscle atrophy
    d. Joint contractures
    e. Complete loss of mobility

53. Which condition is *not* consistent with the patient with RA?
    a. Ischemia
    b. Deformed joints
    c. Weight loss
    d. Subcutaneous nodules

54. What are the manifestations of Sjögren's syndrome in patients with advanced RA? *(Select all that apply.)*
    a. Dry eyes
    b. Dry mouth
    c. Nodules in the lungs
    d. Enlarged spleen and liver
    e. Vaginal dryness

55. What might a psychosocial examination of a patient with advanced RA reveal? *(Select all that apply.)*
    a. Role changes
    b. Poor self-esteem and body image
    c. Grieving and depression
    d. Loss of control and independence
    e. Inability to perform relaxation techniques

56. In RA, autoantibodies (rheumatoid factors [RFs]) are formed that attack healthy tissue, especially synovium, causing which condition?
    a. Nerve pain
    b. Bone porosity
    c. Ischemia
    d. Inflammation

57. In which conditions will the elevation of an ESR be seen? *(Select all that apply.)*
    a. Inflammation or infection in the body
    b. Pregnancy
    c. Inflammatory autoimmune disease
    d. Anemia
    e. Muscular dystrophy

58. What CBC laboratory values does the nurse expect for a patient with RA? *(Circle "high" or "low" for each value.)*
    a. Hemoglobin: High   Low
    b. Hematocrit: High   Low
    c. RBC: High   Low
    d. WBC: High   Low
    e. Platelets: High   Low

59. Arthrocentesis done on the patient with RA may reveal which elements in the synovial fluid of the joint? *(Select all that apply.)*
    a. Glucose and glycogen
    b. Inflammatory cells and immune complexes
    c. Protein, such as albumin
    d. Platelet aggregation
    e. Increased WBCs

60. The nurse is teaching a patient about the common side effects of chronic salicylate and NSAID therapy. Which body system side effects does the nurse focus on in the teaching plan?
    a. Central nervous system
    b. Skin
    c. Gastrointestinal
    d. Cardiovascular

Matching. *Match each drug with the possible side effect of which the nurse should be aware in patients with RA.*

Drugs
a. NSAIDs
b. Steroids
c. Plaquenil (Antimalarial)
d. Methotrexate (Rheumatrex)
e. Minocycline
f. Analgesics
g. Etanercept (Enbrel)
h. Gold salts
i. Leflunomide (Arava)

Side Effects
_____ 61. Headache, dizziness, drowsiness

_____ 62. Diabetes, infection, hypertension

_____ 63. Gastrointestinal problems

_____ 64. Bone marrow suppression, mouth sores

_____ 65. Rash, blood dyscrasias, renal involvement

_____ 66. Red, itchy rash at injection site

_____ 67. Retinal toxicity

_____ 68. Low incidence of adverse effects and resistance

_____ 69. Hair loss, diarrhea, decreased WBCs and platelets

70. The nurse is performing an assessment of a patient with RA. Which findings does the nurse expect?
    a. Head and neck pain
    b. Early morning joint pain
    c. Increased ROM in the hands
    d. Absence of joint swelling

71. The nurse's plan of care for a patient with RA includes which interventions? *(Select all that apply.)*
    a. Ensure optimal pain relief.
    b. Utilize the prone position.
    c. Encourage frequent rest periods.
    d. Decrease exercise to every other day.
    e. Recommend liberal use of arthritic creams.

Matching. *Match the drugs to their correct descriptions.*

Drugs
a. NSAIDs
b. Methotrexate
c. Biologic response modifiers

Descriptions

_____ 72. The first choice for the treatment of mild RA

_____ 73. The first choice for the treatment of moderate to severe RA

_____ 74. Requires a purified protein derivative (PPD) test be performed to rule out the presence of tuberculosis

75. Which statement best describes discoid lupus?
    a. It is the most frequently diagnosed type of lupus.
    b. It results in an increase in immune complexes within the joint cavity.
    c. It is not a systemic condition and is limited to involvement of the skin.
    d. It is a lupus-like syndrome that occurs in patients taking certain medications.

76. What can be expected for a patient with recently diagnosed systemic lupus erythematosus (SLE)?
    a. An acute inflammatory disorder
    b. Spontaneous remission and exacerbations
    c. Symptoms limited to arthritis
    d. Symptoms limited to skin lesions

77. What is the most common cause of death in patients with SLE?
    a. Cardiac failure
    b. Skin involvement
    c. Central nervous system involvement
    d. Renal failure

78. Which laboratory test is the only significant test for diagnosing a patient with discoid lupus?
    a. Antinuclear antibody
    b. Serum complement
    c. Complete blood count
    d. Skin biopsy

79. Which finding does the nurse expect to see in a patient admitted with limited systemic sclerosis?
    a. Multiple joint deformities
    b. Chronic use of immunosuppressant therapy
    c. Rash and discoid lesions
    d. CREST syndrome

80. A patient with scleroderma may have which problems? *(Select all that apply.)*
    a. Dysphagia, esophageal reflux
    b. Smooth tongue
    c. Malabsorption problems causing malodorous diarrhea stools
    d. Butterfly lesions on the face and nose
    e. Spiderlike hemangiomas

81. Raynaud's phenomenon in a patient with scleroderma may present as which signs/symptoms? *(Select all that apply.)*
    a. Digit necrosis
    b. Excruciating pain
    c. Autoamputations of digits
    d. Periungual lesions
    e. Peripheral neuropathy

82. What are characteristics of primary gout? *(Select all that apply.)*
    a. Results from medications such as diuretics
    b. Sodium urate deposited in the synovium
    c. Affects large joints most commonly
    d. Affects middle-aged and older men
    e. Peak time of onset after age 50

83. What part of the body is first affected by gout?
    a. Fingers
    b. Knees
    c. Great toe
    d. Shoulder

True or False? *Read each statement and write T for true or F for false in the blanks provided. If the statement is false, correct the statement to make it true.*

_____ 84. The patient with acute gout cannot tolerate having the joint touched or moved.

_____ 85. The patient with chronic gout may have tophi on the outer ear.

86. A patient was prescribed the combination drug of probenicid and colchicine for the treatment of gout. How does the health care team evaluate the effectiveness of the therapy?
    a. Monitor the serum uric acid level.
    b. Check the results of urinalysis.
    c. Review the patient's compliance with a low-purine diet.
    d. Assess the mobility of affected joints.

87. Polymyalgia rheumatica and temporal arteritis present with which symptoms? *(Select all that apply.)*
    a. Stiffness
    b. Low-grade fever
    c. Arthralgias
    d. Decreased ESR
    e. Polycythemia

88. Patients with ankylosing spondylitis have the threat of which condition?
    a. Compromised respiratory function
    b. Cardiac involvement
    c. Hip pain
    d. Dysphagia

89. Which are common findings in a patient with Reiter's syndrome? *(Select all that apply.)*
    a. Conjunctivitis
    b. Erythema and psoriasis
    c. Arthritis
    d. Paresthesias and fatigue
    e. Urethritis

90. Which manifestations are expected in a patient with Marfan syndrome? *(Select all that apply.)*
    a. Obesity
    b. Shortened hands and feet
    c. Short, swollen fingers
    d. Excessive height
    e. Elongated hands and feet

91. Lyme disease is identified early by which signs/symptoms? *(Select all that apply.)*
    a. Known bite from deer tick
    b. Bull's-eye rash at onset
    c. Facial paralysis
    d. Dysphagia
    e. Generalized erythema

True or False? *Read each statement and write T for true or F for false in the blanks provided. If the statement is false, correct the statement to make it true.*

_____ 92. Lyme disease is treated with antibiotics over an extended period of time (10 to 21 days).

_____ 93. Pseudogout is a mimic of gout depositing uric acid crystals in the joints.

94. The nurse assessing a patient with fibromyalgia identifies the trigger points by palpation. In which specific areas does the nurse expect to elicit pain and tenderness? *(Select all that apply.)*
   a. Neck
   b. Lips
   c. Trunk
   d. Lower back
   e. Upper back

95. A patient is prescribed amitriptyline (Elavil) for the diagnosis of fibromyalgia. What kind of drug is this medication?
   a. Anti-inflammatory
   b. Antirheumatic
   c. Antidepressant
   d. Antipsychotic

Matching. *Match the disease or condition with its definition.*

Diseases/Conditions
a. Polyarthralgia
b. Polymyositis
c. Polymyalgia rheumatica
d. Giant cell arteritis
e. Ankylosing spondylitis
f. Sjögren's syndrome
g. Lyme disease

Definitions

_____ 96. Systemic infectious disease that is caused by the spirochete *Borrelia burgdorferi*

_____ 97. Affects the vertebral column and causes spinal deformities

_____ 98. Diffuse, inflammatory disease of skeletal (striated) muscle

_____ 99. Systemic vasculitis that affects large and midsized arteries

_____ 100. Aching around multiple joints

_____ 101. Clinical syndrome characterized by stiffness, weakness, and aching of the proximal musculature

_____ 102. Inflammatory condition in which secretory ducts and glands are obstructed

CASE STUDY: THE PATIENT WITH RHEUMATOID ARTHRITIS

Use a separate sheet of paper to answer the questions in this Case Study, or go to the "Prepare for Class" folder on your Evolve website at http://evolve.elsevier.com/Iggy/ to download and complete as a word processing file. Answer guidelines for this Case Study are also available on your Evolve website.

The patient comes to the clinic with symptoms of fatigue and hand and wrist pain for 3 months. The patient reports the fatigue has started to interfere with sleep, and NSAIDs have provided minimal pain relief. The nurse assesses that the proximal interphalangeal (PCP) and metacarpophalangeal (MCP) joints of both hands are warm, swollen, and painful to touch with limited ROM. Diagnostic tests reveal a positive rheumatoid factor, elevated antinuclear antibody (ANA), and ESR of 32 mm/hr. The patient is diagnosed with RA, and the health care provider prescribes a regimen of prednisone 10 mg orally daily, methotrexate (Rheumatrex) 15 mg orally weekly, and folate once per day.

1. What clinical manifestations of RA did the patient exhibit? Explain the pathophysiologic basis for these clinical manifestations.

2. Document the discharge teaching instructions provided to the patient for prednisone, methotrexate (Rheumatrex), and folate therapy.

3. What are four minimum interventions the nurse can suggest to manage the patient's fatigue?

Care of Patients with HIV Disease and Other Immune Deficiencies

STUDY/REVIEW QUESTIONS

1. Which statements about immunodeficiency are true? *(Select all that apply.)*
   a. It causes a decrease in the patient's risk for infection.
   b. It may be acquired or congenital.
   c. It occurs when a person's body cannot recognize antigens.
   d. It is the same as autoimmunity.
   e. It may cause varied reactions from mild, localized health problems to total immune system failure.

Matching. Match the descriptions with the types of immunodeficiencies.

Immunodeficiencies
a. Primary
b. Secondary
c. Human immunodeficiency virus (HIV)
d. Acquired immunodeficiency syndrome (AIDS)
e. Immunodeficiency

Descriptions

_____ 2. Last and most serious stage of HIV infection

_____ 3. Disease/deficiency present since birth

_____ 4. Chronic infection with immunodeficiency virus

_____ 5. Disease/deficiency acquired as a result of viral infection, contact with a toxin, or medical therapy

_____ 6. Deficient immune response as a result of impaired or missing immune components

Short Answer: *Define the following terms.*

7.   Retrovirus:

8.   HIV protease:

9.   HIV:

10.   AIDS:

11.   Which immune function abnormalities are a result of HIV infection? *(Select all that apply.)*
      a.   Lymphocytosis
      b.   CD4+ cell depletion
      c.   Increased CD8+ cell activity
      d.   Long macrophage life span
      e.   Lymphocytopenia

12.   Which groups are experiencing increased numbers of HIV infections? *(Select all that apply.)*
      a.   Men having sex with other men
      b.   Intravenous drug users
      c.   Women having sex with men
      d.   African Americans
      e.   Hispanics

13.   Which descriptions are characteristic of a non-progressor? *(Select all that apply.)*
      a.   Has been infected for 10 years
      b.   Is asymptomatic
      c.   Has no CD4+ or T-lymphocytes
      d.   Is immunocompetent
      e.   Are functional antibodies

14.   Which statements about the transmission of HIV are true? *(Select all that apply.)*
      a.   HIV may only be transmitted during the end stages of the disease.
      b.   Those with recent HIV infection and high viral load are very infectious.
      c.   Those with end-stage HIV and no drug therapy are very infectious.
      d.   HIV is only transmitted with sexual contact with an infected person.
      e.   All people infected with HIV will quickly progress to AIDS.

15.   Which conditions may be the first signs of HIV in women? *(Select all that apply.)*
      a.   Vaginal candidiasis
      b.   Bladder infections
      c.   Cervical neoplasia
      d.   Pelvic inflammatory disease (PID)
      e.   Mononucleosis

16.   Which statements regarding HIV/AIDS among older adults are true? *(Select all that apply.)*
      a.   The risk for HIV infection after exposure is minimal for older adults.
      b.   Older men are more susceptible to HIV infection than are older women.
      c.   It is not necessary to assess an older adult for a history of drug abuse.
      d.   Older adults who participate in high-risk behaviors are susceptible to HIV infection.
      e.   Cognitive deficit associated with the disease may appear earlier in older adults with HIV.

17.   What is the most important means of preventing HIV spread or transmission?
      a.   Engineering
      b.   Education
      c.   Isolation
      d.   Counseling

18.   HIV can be transmitted by which routes? *(Select all that apply.)*
      a.   Viral
      b.   Sexual
      c.   Parenteral
      d.   Airborne
      e.   Perinatal

19. Highly activated antiretroviral therapy (HAART) causes what effect?
    a. Reversal of a patient's antibody status
    b. Decrease of the viral load
    c. Increase of the viral load
    d. More detectable HIV

20. A patient is an IV drug user who regularly shares needles and syringes with friends. What information does the nurse provide to decrease the patient's risk of HIV through shared needles and syringes after each use?
    a. Fill and flush the syringe with clear water, then fill the syringe with bleach, shake approximately 30-60 seconds, and rinse with clear water.
    b. Fill and flush the syringe with water, then fill the syringe with soap and hot water, shake 2 minutes, and rinse with cold water.
    c. Rinse needles after each use with a bleach and water solution, then allow to air dry.
    d. Rinse needles after each use with rubbing alcohol and water solution, then rinse with water.

21. Which practices are recommended by the CDC to prevent sexual transmission of HIV? *(Select all that apply.)*
    a. Use of latex or polyurethane condoms for genital and anal intercourse
    b. Use of natural membrane condoms for genital and anal intercourse
    c. Use of topical contraceptives
    d. Use of antiviral medications
    e. Use of a latex barrier for genital and anal intercourse

22. What is the difference between a pathogenic infection and an opportunistic infection?

23. Which opportunistic infections can be observed in AIDS? *(Select all that apply.)*
    a. Protozoan
    b. Viral
    c. Bacterial
    d. Fungal
    e. Gastroenteritis

24. A patient with *Pneumocystis jiroveci* pneumonia (PCP) usually presents with which symptoms? *(Select all that apply.)*
    a. Dyspnea, tachypnea, persistent dry cough, and fever
    b. Cough with copious thick sputum, fever, and dyspnea
    c. Chest pain and difficulty swallowing
    d. Fever, persistent cough, and vomiting
    e. Fatigue and weight loss

25. A patient presenting with toxoplasmosis may have which signs and symptoms? *(Select all that apply.)*
    a. Speech difficulty
    b. Shortness of breath
    c. Visual changes
    d. Impaired gait
    e. Mental status changes

26. Cryptosporidiosis is a form of intestinal infection in which diarrhea can amount to a loss of how many liters of fluid per day?
    a. 1 to 2
    b. 3 to 5
    c. 5 to 8
    d. 15 to 20

27. Where can candidiasis occur in the body? *(Select all that apply.)*
    a. Mouth
    b. Esophagus
    c. Vagina
    d. Nose
    e. Ears

True or False? *Read each statement and write T for true or F for false in the blanks provided. If the statement is false, correct the statement to make it true.*

_____ 28. Cryptococcosis is a type of meningitis.

_____ 29. Histoplasmosis is a localized respiratory infection.

_____ 30. *Mycobacterium avium-intracellulare* complex (MAC) is the most common bacterial infection among people with HIV/AIDS.

31. Where in the body can cytomegalovirus (CMV) present with symptoms? *(Select all that apply.)*
    a. Eyes, causing visual impairment
    b. The kidneys as glomerulonephritis
    c. Respiratory tract, causing pneumonitis
    d. Gastrointestinal tract, causing colitis
    e. The heart as cardiomyopathy

32. How does the herpes simplex virus (HSV) manifest itself in patients with HIV and AIDS? *(Select all that apply.)*
    a. Maculopapular lesions that can spread
    b. A chronic ulceration after vesicles rupture
    c. Vesicles located in the perirectal, oral, and genital areas
    d. Numbness and tingling occurring before the vesicle forms
    e. Itching localized in the perianal area

33. Shingles results from varicella zoster virus (VZV) leaving the nerve ganglia and entering the body by which route?
    a. Mucous membranes
    b. Pulmonary spaces
    c. Body fluids and other tissue areas
    d. Bone marrow

34. Lymphomas associated with AIDS include which types? *(Select all that apply.)*
    a. Non-Hodgkin's B cell
    b. Immunoblastic
    c. Hodgkin's
    d. Burkitt's
    e. Primary brain

35. Which treatments are intended to boost the immune system? *(Select all that apply.)*
    a. Radiation therapy
    b. Hematopoietic growth factors
    c. Lymphocyte transfusion
    d. Administration of interleukin-2
    e. Infusion of lymphokines

36. Which conditions cause severe pain in HIV disease and AIDS? *(Select all that apply.)*
    a. Enlarged organs
    b. Peripheral neuropathy
    c. Tumors
    d. High fevers
    e. Dry skin

37. What methods or agents are used to treat Kaposi's sarcoma? *(Select all that apply.)*
    a. Radiotherapy
    b. Chemotherapy
    c. Antibiotics
    d. Cryotherapy
    e. Surgery

38. Which actions are useful in helping orient a patient? *(Select all that apply.)*
    a. Repeating person, place, and time
    b. Using clocks and calendars
    c. Giving the Mini-Mental State Examination (MMSE) screening test
    d. Having familiar items present
    e. Providing uninterrupted time

39. The nurse assesses a patient diagnosed with advanced AIDS for malnutrition. Which findings does the nurse most likely assess? *(Select all that apply.)*
    a. Pain
    b. Anorexia
    c. Urinary incontinence
    d. Diarrhea
    e. Vomiting

40. Corticosteroids perform which actions? *(Select all that apply.)*
    a. Block the movement of neutrophils and monocytes through cell membranes.
    b. Increase cell production in the bone marrow.
    c. Reduce the number of circulating T cells, resulting in suppressed cell-mediated immunity.
    d. Decrease intracranial pressure.
    e. Constrict blood vessels.

True or False? Read each statement and write T for true or F for false in the blanks provided. If the statement is false, correct the statement to make it true.

_____ 41. The person with HIV infection can transmit the virus to others at all stages of disease.

_____ 42. Lesions resulting from Kaposi's sarcoma are painful and have purulent drainage.

_____ 43. AIDS dementia complex (ADC) is caused by infection of the cells in the central nervous system by HIV.

_____ 44. Patients with HIV should know that as CD4+ counts lower, clinical manifestations decrease.

_____ 45. The viral load test measures the presence of HIV genetic material in the patient's blood and helps with monitoring the disease progression.

_____ 46. Antiretroviral drug therapy kills the virus before it is able to replicate.

_____ 47. HIV is more easily transmitted from infected female to uninfected male than from infected male to uninfected female.

48. Which methods or items are means of transmitting HIV? *(Select all that apply.)*
    a. Sexual intercourse
    b. Household utensils
    c. Breast milk
    d. Toilet facilities
    e. Mosquitoes

49. The nurse is teaching a patient about preventing HIV infection through sexual contact. Which statement made by the patient indicates effective teaching?
    a. "A latex condom with spermicide provides the best protection against getting infected with HIV."
    b. "Mutually monogamous sex with a noninfected partner will best prevent HIV infection."
    c. "Contraceptive methods like implants and injections are recommended to prevent HIV transmission."
    d. "If my partner and I are both HIV-positive, unprotected sex is permitted."

50. For each laboratory test, indicate whether the presence of HIV will increase (I), decrease (D), or cause no change (NC) in the levels.

    _____ a. CD4+

    _____ b. CD8+

    _____ c. WBC

    _____ d. Lymphocytes

51. A patient diagnosed with HIV is receiving medications to reduce the viral load and improve CD4+ lymphocyte counts. Which term accurately describes this HIV/AIDS drug regimen?
    a. Interferon treatment
    b. Antiviremia
    c. ELISA administration
    d. HAART therapy

CASE STUDY: THE PATIENT WITH HIV

Use a separate sheet of paper to answer the questions in this Case Study, or go to the "Prepare for Class" folder on your Evolve website at http://evolve.elsevier.com/Iggy/ to download and complete as a word processing file. Answer guidelines for this Case Study are also available on your Evolve website.

A 42-year-old man who was diagnosed as HIV-positive 10 years ago is admitted to the hospital with AIDS. He has been on antiretroviral therapy since his diagnosis, and his CD4+ count has consistently been above 500 for the past 10 years. He now reports increased dyspnea for 3 days and "being very cold." The nurse assesses a dry nonproductive cough and crackles in the right and lower lung bases. Vital signs are BP 156/90 mm Hg, HR 110 BPM, RR 28-30 breaths/min and regular, and an oral temperature of 102.4° F. Diagnostic tests reveal a WBC count of 4000/μL, lymphocytes 13%, CD4+ T cell count of 300/mm^3, CD4+ count of 160 mm^3, and decreased RBC and thrombocyte levels. The patient is currently receiving HAART and tells the nurse that he is having difficulty remembering to take his medications.

1. What is the significance of the patient's CD4+ cell count?

2. What nursing interventions will be most helpful for this patient?

3. The patient asks for an explanation of HAART and asks why one drug cannot be prescribed. Document the teaching regarding HAART the nurse would give.

4. What nursing considerations are necessary to ensure the patient is compliant with his antiretroviral medication therapy?

22

CHAPTER

Care of Patients with Immune Function Excess: Hypersensitivity (Allergy) and Autoimmunity

STUDY/REVIEW QUESTIONS

1. Which type I hypersensitivity reaction requires immediate intervention by the nurse?
   a. PPD test result of 10 mm
   b. Anaphylaxis
   c. Vasculitis
   d. Fever

2. "Overreactions" to invaders or foreign antigens can be the result of what? *(Select all that apply.)*
   a. Hypersensitivity
   b. Allergic response
   c. Autoimmune response
   d. Phagocytosis
   e. Increased cardiac output

3. Which statement best describes allergy or hypersensitivity?
   a. Excessive response to the presence of an antigen
   b. Excessive response against self-cells and cell products
   c. Failure of the immune system to recognize self cells as normal
   d. Failure of the immune system to recognize foreign cells and microbial invaders

Matching. Match the type of hypersensitivity to a clinical example. Types may be used more than once.

Hypersensitivities
a. Type I: immediate
b. Type II: cytotoxic
c. Type III: immune complex-mediated
d. Type IV: delayed
e. Type V: stimulated

Clinical Examples
_____ 4. Autoimmune hemolytic anemia
_____ 5. Poison ivy
_____ 6. Hay fever
_____ 7. Graves' disease
_____ 8. Serum sickness
_____ 9. Anaphylaxis
_____ 10. Myasthenia gravis
_____ 11. Graft rejection
_____ 12. Allergic asthma
_____ 13. Vasculitis

14. Which type of therapy for allergy management administers small increasing amounts of identified allergens subcutaneously?
    a. Alternative
    b. Progressive
    c. Symptomatic
    d. Desensitization

Short Answer.

15. What is an allergen?

16. What is leukotriene's rule in the secondary phase of an allergic reaction?

17. What is histamine and what kind of symptoms occur with a histamine reaction?

18. What are the symptoms of rhinorrhea?

19. Which techniques are used for allergy management? *(Select all that apply.)*
    a. Avoidance
    b. Desensitization
    c. Conization
    d. Antibiotics
    e. Injections

20. Which methods are used for testing for allergies? *(Select all that apply.)*
    a. Topical serums
    b. Scratch test
    c. Intravenous
    d. Intradermal
    e. Skin biopsy

Matching. *Match the drug types with their corresponding actions.*

Drug Types
a. Decongestant
b. Antihistamine
c. Corticosteroids
d. Mast cell stabilizers
e. Leukotriene antagonist

Actions

_____ 21. Competes for histamine at histamine receptor sites

_____ 22. Causes vasoconstriction, reducing edema; may be combined with anticholinergics

_____ 23. Decreases inflammation and immune response in a short time

_____ 24. Prevents mast cells from opening when allergen binds with IgE

_____ 25. Prevents leukotriene synthesis and blocks leukotriene receptors

26. The nurse is reviewing the health history of a patient who reports allergic rhinitis, and who has been taking OTC decongestants for these symptoms. Which chronic health problems cause the nurse to recommend that the patient stop taking the OTC medication immediately? *(Select all that apply.)*
    a. Osteoarthritis
    b. Hypertension
    c. Diabetes mellitus
    d. Glaucoma
    e. Pancreatitis

27. For a patient who is having an anaphylactic reaction, which common symptoms will manifest almost immediately after being exposed to an allergen? *(Select all that apply.)*
    a. Angioedema
    b. Apprehension
    c. Chills
    d. Fever
    e. Urticaria

28. A patient in anaphylaxis who is going into respiratory failure will demonstrate which symptoms? *(Select all that apply.)*
    a. Laryngeal edema
    b. Hypoxemia
    c. Hypocapnia
    d. Dehydration
    e. Crackles
    f. Wheezing
    g. Dry mouth

29. For the patient with anaphylaxis described above, which priority treatment does the nurse expect to administer?
    a. Education regarding the use of the EpiPen
    b. Epinephrine injection
    c. Intravenous 0.9% normal saline
    d. Intravenous corticosteroids

True or False? *Read each statement and write T for true or F for false in the blanks provided. If the statement is false, correct the statement to make it true.*

_____ 30. Rhinitis may or may not be an allergic response.

_____ 31. After the proper dose of epinephrine is administered to a patient having an anaphylactic reaction, the nurse must wait 60 minutes before repeating the dose.

_____ 32. Latex allergies are manifested only in dermatitis, so latex-free gloves are the only necessary precaution for those with a latex allergy.

_____ 33. A patient who is allergic to bananas could possibly develop a latex allergy.

_____ 34. Patients with a history of anaphylaxis should carry a prescription for injectable epinephrine at all times.

35. The nurse is assessing a patient experiencing a cytotoxic reaction to IV drugs. What does the nurse do first?
    a. Discontinue drug administration.
    b. Decrease the infusion rate.
    c. Call the health care provider.
    d. Increase the IV fluid rate.
    e. Notify the Rapid Response Team.

36. What are the clinical manifestations of systemic lupus erythematosus that are caused by immune complex reaction? *(Select all that apply.)*
    a. Vasculitis, nephritis
    b. Hypertension, anemia
    c. Destruction of mucus-producing glands
    d. Increased urinary output
    e. Arthritis

37. Serum sickness occurs less frequently than in the past for what reason?
    a. Vaccines are no longer made from horse and rabbit serum.
    b. Patients have become less sensitive to allergens.
    c. Penicillin and related drugs and some animal serums are antitoxins.
    d. Manufacturing techniques produce vaccines that contain fewer impurities.

38. Which responses are characterized as type IV delayed hypersensitivity reactions? *(Select all that apply.)*
    a. Positive PPD test for tuberculosis
    b. Anaphylaxis after insect sting
    c. Thrombocytopenic purpura
    d. Contact dermatitis
    e. Graft rejection

39. What is the most important aspect of treating type V stimulating reactions?
    a. Medication management and observation for adverse effects
    b. Removing stimulated tissue to return the organ to normal functioning
    c. Monitoring for other organ involvement
    d. Surgical removal of secondary immune tissue

40. Which descriptions best characterize autoimmunity? *(Select all that apply.)*
    a. Cell-mediated immune response that does not cause an antibody-mediated response
    b. The synthetic substances used to stimulate or suppress the response of the immune system
    c. Inappropriate immune response to one's own healthy cells and tissues
    d. An altered immune response that results in an immediate hypersensitivity reaction
    e. Immune system failing to recognize certain body cells or tissues as self, triggering immune reactions

41. Which disorders are types of autoimmune diseases? *(Select all that apply.)*
    a. Polyarteritis nodosa
    b. Systemic lupus erythematosus
    c. Hypothyroidism
    d. Rheumatic fever
    e. Hashimoto's thyroiditis

42. Autoimmune diseases occur mostly in which group of women?
    a. African American
    b. Asian American
    c. White
    d. Hispanic

43. What is the most common cause of Sjögren's syndrome thought to be?
    a. A bacterial infection
    b. A viral infection
    c. Inflammation
    d. An allergic reaction

44. The nurse suspects Sjögren's syndrome because the patient reports which common symptoms? *(Select all that apply.)*
    a. Increased tooth decay
    b. Burning and itching of the eyes
    c. Painful intercourse
    d. Nosebleeds
    e. Shortness of breath

45. The nurse expects the lab values on a patient with Sjögren's syndrome to include which results? *(Select all that apply.)*
    a. Increased presence of general antinuclear antibodies
    b. Elevated levels of IgM rheumatoid factor
    c. Decreased presence of anti-SS-A or anti-SS-B antibodies
    d. Decreased erythrocyte sedimentation rate
    e. Increased circulating platelets

46. Which symptomatic treatments does the nurse expect to implement for a patient with Sjögren's syndrome? *(Select all that apply.)*
    a. Water-soluble lubricants
    b. Artificial tears
    c. Room humidifiers
    d. Beta-blockers
    e. Nonsteroidal anti-inflammatory drugs (NSAIDs)

47. Goodpasture's syndrome is a disorder of autoantibodies against which two body components?

48. What do the symptoms of Goodpasture's syndrome include? *(Select all that apply.)*
    a. Hemoptysis
    b. Increased urine output
    c. Bradycardia
    d. Shortness of breath
    e. Weight loss
    f. Generalized edema

49. Which organs are often damaged which can cause death in Goodpasture's syndrome? *(Select all that apply.)*
    a. Heart
    b. Liver
    c. Lungs
    d. Thyroid
    e. Kidney

50. A patient has been diagnosed with Goodpasture's syndrome. Which drug therapies does the nurse expect to administer? *(Select all that apply.)*
    a. Corticosteroids
    b. Low-dose chemotherapy
    c. Vasopressors
    d. Antibiotics
    e. Muscle relaxants

51. Plasmapheresis may be used to treat immune complex responses such as Goodpasture's syndrome. Which statement best describes this treatment?
    a. Blood is circulated through a machine that removes excess fluids.
    b. 300 to 500 mL of blood is intermittently removed to decrease immune complexes.
    c. Autoantibodies are removed from blood plasma.
    d. IV immunoglobulins (IVIGs) are infused.

52. Which nursing intervention is most important for the nurse to do before administering any drug or therapeutic agent to a patient?
    a. Ask the patient about allergies to drugs or other substances.
    b. Compare the wristband name with the drug administration record.
    c. Verify the order with the prescriber.
    d. Calculate the prescribed drug dosage twice.

53. A patient who had a PPD test has redness and a 9 mm induration at the injection site. The nurse suspects which type of hypersensitivity reaction?
    a. Type I, immediate
    b. Type II, cytotoxic
    c. Type III, immune complex-mediated
    d. Type IV, delayed

54. A patient reports a runny nose with clear drainage, watery eyes, and a scratchy throat. The nurse determines the patient has been in close contact with several cats. Which hypersensitivity reaction does the nurse suspect the patient is experiencing?
    a. Type I, immediate
    b. Type II, cytotoxic
    c. Type III, immune complex-mediated
    d. Type IV, delayed

55. The nurse is assessing a patient with shortness of breath, hemoptysis, tachycardia, and generalized edema. Which autoimmune disorder does the nurse suspect this patient is experiencing?
    a. Goodpasture's syndrome
    b. Transplant reaction
    c. Glomerulonephritis
    d. Hemolytic reaction

CASE STUDY: THE PATIENT WITH HYPERSENSITIVITY

Use a separate sheet of paper to answer the questions in this Case Study, or go to the "Prepare for Class" folder on your Evolve website at http://evolve.elsevier.com/Iggy/ to download and complete as a word processing file. Answer guidelines for this Case Study are also available on your Evolve website.

A 62-year-old woman is admitted for total knee replacement surgery. Following surgery, cefazolin sodium (Ancef), 2 g, was ordered to be given intravenous piggyback (IVPB) every 8 hours for 24 hours. She received her first dose when she arrived at the orthopedic unit after surgery. Vital signs upon arrival: BP 136/84, P 88, R 12, T 98.8° F.

1. Before administering the cefazolin sodium (Ancef), the nurse asks the patient about drug allergies. Which drug allergy causes the nurse to question the administration of the cefazolin sodium and why?

Thirty minutes after the medication was started, the patient calls the nurse and reports "itching all over" and difficulty breathing. The nurse notes facial edema and audible wheezing. The patient's skin is red with large, swollen blotches over her arms, trunk, and back. Her systolic blood pressure is 118/78, pulse 108, and respirations 24. The IVPB antibiotic bag has infused about three-fourths of the dose.

2. What should the nurse's *first* action be?

3. What medications and by what route should the nurse expect the physician to prescribe? Explain the rationale for the medications used in this situation. What other interventions should follow?

4. Below is the documentation of the patient incident recorded by the nurse. What documentation should entry #3 contain?

   Initial Entry: VS on arrival to unit BP 136/84, P 88, R 12, T 98.8° F. Patient medication allergies reviewed prior to administration of Ancef 2 g IVPB. IV site clear, without redness or swelling. Ancef IVPB infusing without difficulty.

   Entry #2: VS BP 118/78, P 108, R 24. Patient c/o "itching all over." Patient SOB, with audible wheezing noted, skin reddened with blotches on arms, trunk, and back. IVPB stopped. Dr. X notified. Medications administered as ordered by Dr. X.

   Entry #3:

23 CHAPTER

Cancer Development

STUDY/REVIEW QUESTIONS

1. Nurses have an important role in which components of cancer care? *(Select all that apply.)*
   a. Disclosing the initial diagnosis of cancer
   b. Education of the public regarding cancer prevention
   c. Education of the public regarding early detection
   d. Advising the patient about the various cancer treatment options
   e. Determining the best treatment modalities for the patient's cancer

2. Which statement is true about hypertrophy and hyperplasia?
   a. Hypertrophy and hyperplasia are the same, except that one is in an organ and the other is in tissue.
   b. Hypertrophy is the expansion of cells; hyperplasia is an increased number of cells.
   c. Hypertrophy is an increase in the number of cells; hyperplasia is the expansion of cells.
   d. Hypertrophy is a decrease in the number of cells; hyperplasia is the shrinkage of cells.

3. Which are characteristics of neoplasia? *(Select all that apply.)*
   a. New or continued cell growth that is not needed for tissue replacement
   b. Is always malignant
   c. Has a parent cell that was normal
   d. Typically leads to death
   e. Is always abnormal
   f. Some cause no harm

4. Which statements about cell mitosis are true? *(Select all that apply.)*
   a. It is a term for cell division.
   b. Mitosis occurs to develop normal tissue.
   c. Mitosis occurs to replace damaged or lost tissue.
   d. Mitosis occurs randomly throughout the life cycle.
   e. *Apoptosis* is another term for mitosis.
   f. Mitosis occurs only when body conditions and nutrition are appropriate.

5. Which areas of the body contain cells which grow throughout the life span? *(Select all that apply.)*
   a. Heart
   b. Hair
   c. Brain
   d. Bone marrow
   e. Skin

Matching. *Match the terms with the correct definitions.*

Terms

a. Differentiated function
b. Mitosis
c. Apoptosis
d. Euploidy
e Hypertrophy
f. Hyperplasia
g. Aneuploidy

Definitions

_____ 6. Growth that causes tissue to increase in size by enlarging each cell

_____ 7. Cell division

_____ 8. The special function of a normal cell which contributes to homeostasis

_____ 9. Programmed cell death

_____ 10. Normal number of chromosomes within the cells

_____ 11. Growth that causes tissue to increase in size by increasing the number of cells

_____ 12. Abnormal number of chromosomes in a cell

13. How is a gene that is "turned on" described?
    a. Repressed
    b. Suppressed
    c. Expressed
    d. Depressed

14. Benign cells have which characteristics? *(Select all that apply.)*
    a. Tissue unnecessary for normal function
    b. Resemble the parent tissue
    c. Have a small nucleus
    d. Perform their differentiated function
    e. Invade other tissues
    f. Nonmigratory
    g. Aneuploid

15. Which statements are true of cancer cells? *(Select all that apply.)*
    a. They are slow-growing.
    b. Cancer cells divide nearly continuously.
    c. They are harmful to the body.
    d. They are abnormal.
    e. Cancer cells contain a small nucleus.
    f. They have an unlimited life span.

16. Why do cancer cells spread throughout the body? *(Select all that apply.)*
    a. They make little fibronectin.
    b. They are able to metastasize.
    c. They are persistent in their growth.
    d. Cell division occurs under adverse conditions.
    e. They have only one enzyme on their surface.

17. Which are actions of carcinogens? *(Select all that apply.)*
    a. Damage the DNA
    b. Change the activity of a cell
    c. Turn off proto-oncogenes
    d. Create allergic reactions
    e. Begin the initiation step of carcinogenesis

True or False? *Read each statement and write T for true or F for false in the blanks provided. If the statement is false, correct the statement to make it true.*

_____ 18. If growth conditions are right, widespread metastatic disease can develop from just one cancer cell.

_____ 19. In carcinogenesis and oncogenesis, a normal cell undergoes malignant transformation.

_____ 20. Initiators start irreversible mutations in a normal cell.

_____ 21. Once a cell has been initiated, it is a recognizable tumor.

_____ 22. As the tumor cells grow, there are changes within the tumor cells themselves allowing for "selection advantages."

23. Which characteristics describe the initiated cell's responses to the promoter? *(Select all that apply.)*
    a. Promoted or enhanced cell growth
    b. Shortened latency period
    c. Lengthened latency period
    d. Metastasis
    e. Irreversible changes in the cell

24. Promoters may include which factors? *(Select all that apply.)*
    a. Chemicals
    b. Hormones
    c. Drugs
    d. Antibodies
    e. Viruses

25. If a primary tumor is located in a vital organ, what happens?
    a. The organ's rate of cell division is increased.
    b. The organ's response to injury is decreased.
    c. There is interference with the organ's functioning.
    d. Function of the organ is initially increased.

26. Which statement correctly describes metastatic tumors?
    a. They are caused by cells breaking off from the primary tumor.
    b. They become less malignant over time.
    c. They are usually less harmful than a primary tumor.
    d. They become the tissue of the organ where they spread.

27. During metastasis, which actions take place? *(Select all that apply.)*
    a. Tumor vascularization results in blood supply to the tumor.
    b. Enzymes open up pores in the patient's blood vessels.
    c. Clumps of the cells break off for transport.
    d. Cells stop circulating and then invade.
    e. Increased tumor size causes invasion of surrounding tissues.

28. Which characteristics describe a "high-grade" tumor? *(Select all that apply.)*
    a. Barely resembles the parent cell
    b. Slow-growing
    c. Rapidly metastasizes
    d. Easiest to cure
    e. Very aggressive

29. Which information can be obtained from grading a tumor? *(Select all that apply.)*
    a. Cause of the cancer
    b. Location of metastasis
    c. Evaluating prognosis and appropriate therapy
    d. How long the cancer has been present
    e. Cell differentiation

30. What information can be obtained by surgical staging?
    a. Assessment of tumor size
    b. Number of tumors
    c. Sites of tumors
    d. Pattern of spread of tumors
    e. Pain related to tumors

31. What are the primary factors influencing the development of cancer? *(Select all that apply.)*
    a. Environmental exposure to carcinogens
    b. Gender of the patient
    c. Genetic predisposition
    d. Immune function
    e. Health history

32. What factors influence cancer development in a patient?

33. Which statements are true regarding tobacco use and cancer risk? *(Select all that apply.)*
    a. Tobacco is considered an initiator of cancer.
    b. Tobacco is considered a promoter of cancer.
    c. A person's risk for cancer depends on the amount of tobacco use.
    d. A person's risk for cancer depends on the type of tobacco use.
    e. Those who receive secondhand tobacco smoke have the same risk for cancer as those in direct contact with tobacco smoke.

34. Ionizing radiation is found in which elements? *(Select all that apply.)*
    a. Radon
    b. Uranium
    c. Soil
    d. Water
    e. Medical x-rays

35. Which factors are forms of UV radiation? *(Select all that apply.)*
    a. Sun (solar)
    b. Tanning beds
    c. Medical x-rays
    d. Radon
    e. Germicidal lights

36. A few viruses are known as *oncoviruses* because they perform which actions? *(Select all that apply.)*
    a. Infect the cell
    b. Break the DNA chain
    c. Insert their own genetic material
    d. Mutate the cell's DNA
    e. Grow slowly

37. How does the immune system protect the body from cancer? *(Select all that apply.)*
    a. By using cell-mediated immunity
    b. By using natural killer cells
    c. By using antibody-mediated immunity
    d. By using helper T-cells
    e. Identifying cancer cells as "non-self" cells

38. Which people are considered to be at greater risk for developing cancer? *(Select all that apply.)*
    a. Organ transplant recipients
    b. Adults over the age of 60
    c. People with AIDS
    d. African Americans
    e. People who are immunocompromised

39. For which types of cancer is risk modifiable? *(Select all that apply.)*
    a. Breast
    b. Colon
    c. Ovarian
    d. Prostate
    e. Cervical
    f. Lymphatic

40. Which are cancers that have genetic predisposition? *(Select all that apply.)*
    a. Breast
    b. Colorectal
    c. Melanoma
    d. Bladder
    e. Lung

41. Which groups have the highest rate of incidence, death rate, and largest increase in incidence of cancer? *(Select all that apply.)*
    a. Whites
    b. Hispanics
    c. African Americans
    d. Asian Americans
    e. Lower socioeconomic people

42. Which patient would have the best prognosis for survival based on the TNM staging classification listed?
    a. $T_{IS}N_0M_0$
    b. $T_xN_xM_x$
    c. $T_2N_1M_0$
    d. $T_2N_3M_1$

43. The American Cancer Society reports that the cancer incidence and survival rate are related to which factors? *(Select all that apply.)*
    a. Gender
    b. Availability of health care services
    c. Early health care
    d. Age
    e. Race

44. Which are included in the seven warning signs of cancer? *(Select all that apply.)*
    a. Hoarseness
    b. A thickening lump
    c. Obvious change in a mole
    d. Inability of a sore to heal
    e. Difficulty swallowing

45. Which are dietary practices that may help reduce the risk of cancer? *(Select all that apply.)*
    a. Low-fat diet
    b. Avoidance of nitrates
    c. Eating foods high in vitamins A and C
    d. Maximize intake of red meat
    e. Increase fiber intake

46. Which measures are considered secondary prevention for cancer? *(Select all that apply.)*
    a. Yearly mammography for women over age 40
    b. Avoidance of tobacco
    c. Yearly fecal occult blood testing in adults
    d. Removing colon polyps
    e. Using sunscreen when outdoors
    f. Colonoscopy at age 50 and then every 10 years
    g. Chemoprevention with vitamin therapy

24 CHAPTER

Care of Patients with Cancer

STUDY/REVIEW QUESTIONS

1. Which type of cancer puts patients at greatest risk for infection?
   a. Breast cancer
   b. Leukemia
   c. Lung cancer
   d. Prostate cancer

2. Cancer invading the bone marrow can cause which effects? *(Select all that apply.)*
   a. Hypokalemia
   b. Decreased RBCs
   c. Pathologic fractures
   d. Degenerative joint disease
   e. Thrombocytopenia

3. Which statements about gastrointestinal function and cancer are true? *(Select all that apply.)*
   a. Only cancers within the gastrointestinal system alter gastrointestinal function.
   b. Tumors may increase the metabolic rate.
   c. A low-fat diet improves survival rates for people with cancer.
   d. The liver is a common site of cancer metastasis.
   e. Gaining weight during cancer therapy indicates successful treatment.

4. Which common hematologic conditions result from cancer invading the bone marrow? *(Select all that apply.)*
   a. Cachexia
   b. Anemia
   c. Bruising
   d. Thrombocytopenia
   e. Bleeding

True or False? *Read each statement and write T for true or F for false in the blanks provided. If the statement is false, correct the statement to make it true.*

_____ 5. Pain is present with all cancers.

_____ 6. Patients with lung cancer can develop pulmonary edema and dyspnea.

_____ 7. The primary goal of cancer treatment is to cure the patient.

_____ 8. Surgery for a cancer patient may be a part of diagnosis or treatment.

9. A patient asks the nurse why untreated cancers cause gastrointestinal problems. Which responses are appropriate? *(Select all that apply.)*
   a. "A tumor in the bowel can decrease your ability to absorb necessary nutrients."
   b. "The tumor makes you not feel hungry or thirsty and affects your urinary output."
   c. "It stops the absorption of necessary fat and protein enzymes."
   d. "Cancers in the GI tract are known to cause related bowel problems."
   e. "Tumors may increase metabolic needs which you are unable to meet."

10. Which factors determine the type of therapy for cancer? *(Select all that apply.)*
    a. Type and location of cancer
    b. Overall health of the patient
    c. Whether the cancer has metastasized
    d. Family history and genetics
    e. Previous lymph node biopsy

11. Which examples illustrate appropriate prophylactic cancer surgery? *(Select all that apply.)*
    a. Excision of lesions shown on biopsy to be "precancerous"
    b. Removal of tissue which may be predisposed to cancer development due to family history
    c. Removal of a mole that is often irritated by the patient's waistband
    d. Breast reconstruction after a mastectomy
    e. Removing part of a tumor to provide pain relief

12. What is the purpose of cytoreductive surgery for cancer?
    a. Cancer prevention by removal of "at-risk" tissue
    b. Cancer control by reducing the size of the tumor
    c. Cancer cure by removing all gross and microscopic tumor tissue
    d. Improving the function or appearance of a previously treated body area

13. Palliative surgery may be performed for which reasons? *(Select all that apply.)*
    a. Relieving pain
    b. Relieving an obstruction
    c. Curing the cancer
    d. Diagnostic staging
    e. Destroying the tumor

14. For what purposes may cancer survivors need reconstructive surgery? *(Select all that apply.)*
    a. Breast reconstruction
    b. Revision of scars and release of contractures
    c. Bowel reconstruction
    d. Pain relief
    e. Increase organ function

True or False? *Read each statement about radiation therapy and write T for true or F for false in the blanks provided. If the statement is false, correct the statement to make it true.*

_____ 15. Cell damage occurs with any exposure to radiation, which may cause the cell to die or lose the ability to divide.

_____ 16. The dosage of radiation is commonly determined by cell cycle.

_____ 17. Normal cells are not damaged during radiation therapy.

_____ 18. Each cell has its own response to radiation, such as dying, becoming sterile, or repairing itself.

_____ 19. The goal of radiation therapy is to administer enough treatment to kill all of the cancer cells.

_____ 20. Brachytherapy involves the use of isotopes placed on or near the cancer tissue, making the patient hazardous to others.

_____ 21. Unsealed radiation sources can be given orally, intravenously, or as an instillation in a body cavity, making patients and their excrement radioactive for 48 hours.

_____ 22. Needles and seeds for sealed radiation sources make the patient and his or her excrement radioactive.

_____ 23. Teletherapy is also called *beam therapy*.

24. What is the meaning of the "inverse square law" for radiation exposure?
   a. The further away a person is from a radiation source, the less radiation is absorbed.
   b. When chemotherapy is added to the treatment regimen, less radiation is needed.
   c. As the distance from the radiation source increases, more tumor cells are killed.
   d. Less radiation is needed if natural sources are used.

25. Which factors are used to determine a cancer patient's absorbed radiation dose? *(Select all that apply.)*
   a. Intensity of radiation exposure
   b. Proximity of radiation source to the cells
   c. Duration of exposure
   d. Age of the patient
   e. Previous radiation therapy

26. Which statements about stereotactic body radiotherapy are true? *(Select all that apply.)*
   a. The radiation beam is broken into thousands of smaller beams.
   b. A greater number of normal cells are "spared."
   c. Three-dimensional tumor imaging is used.
   d. Higher radiation doses may be used.
   e. Radiation is implanted in the patient's tissue.

27. Why is the therapeutic dose of radiation fractionated for cancer treatment?
   a. To reduce total treatment cost
   b. To ensure a higher cancer cell kill with less damage to normal cells
   c. To prevent profound bone marrow suppression with resulting anemia
   d. To allow time for chemotherapy to first reduce the tumor size

28. At what point is a patient radioactive when receiving radiation treatment by teletherapy and therefore a potential danger to other people?
   a. The patient is never radioactive
   b. When the linear accelerator is turned on
   c. For the first 24 to 48 hours after treatment
   d. Until the radiation source has decayed by at least one half-life

29. What are the side effects of radiation? *(Select all that apply.)*
   a. Altered taste sensation
   b. Skin changes and permanent local hair loss
   c. Diarrhea and tooth loss
   d. Immunosuppression and weight gain
   e. Fatigue

30. For a patient undergoing external radiation therapy, what do the nurse's instructions include? *(Select all that apply.)*
   a. Do not remove the markings.
   b. Do not use lotions or ointments.
   c. Avoid direct skin exposure to sunlight for up to a year.
   d. Use soap and water on the affected skin.
   e. Do not rub treated areas.

31. Why does the nurse wear a dosimeter when providing care to a patient receiving brachytherapy?
   a. Indicate special expertise in radiation therapy.
   b. Protect the nurse from absorbing radiation.
   c. Determine the amount of radiation exposure experienced.
   d. Ensure that the radiation source remains active.

32. What are the rationales for chemotherapy as a cancer treatment? *(Select all that apply.)*
   a. Increases survival time for the patient
   b. Decreases the patient's risk for life-threatening complications
   c. Systemic treatment for cancer cells that may have escaped from the primary tumor
   d. Concentrates in secondary lymphoid tissues and prevents widespread metastasis
   e. Less expensive and safer than radiation therapy

Matching. *Match each type of chemotherapy with the corresponding action.*

Chemotherapy
a.   Antimitotic agents
b.   Topoisomerase inhibitor
c.   Antimetabolites
d.   Anti-tumor antibiotics

Type of Action

_____ 33.   "Counterfeit" chemicals that fool cancer cells into using them, but prevent cell division

_____ 34.   Causes major damage to DNA and RNA synthesis

_____ 35.   Cross-links DNA; prevents RNA synthesis

_____ 36.   A plant source that interferes with formation of microtubules

37.   What is the lowest level of bone marrow activity and WBCs called?
a.   Anemia
b.   Nadir
c.   Leukopenia
d.   Immunosuppression

38.   Each chemotherapeutic agent has a specific nadir. What is important to do when giving combination therapy?
a.   Give two agents with like nadirs.
b.   Avoid giving agents with like nadirs at the same time.
c.   Allow for one agent's nadir to recover before giving another agent.
d.   Give two agents from the same drug class.

39.   Chemotherapy drug dosage is based on total body surface area (TBSA); therefore, what is it important for the nurse to do?
a.   Ask the patient's height and weight.
b.   Weigh and measure the patient's height.
c.   Assess body mass index.
d.   Measure abdominal girth.

40.   What does a course of chemotherapy normally include? *(Select all that apply.)*
a.   Rounds every week for a total of 6 weeks
b.   Variance with patient's responses to therapy
c.   Timed dosing of the therapy to minimize normal cell damage
d.   A concurrent dose of radiation
e.   The administration of one specific anticancer drug

41.   Most chemotherapy is administered intravenously. Which are major potential complications? *(Select all that apply.)*
a.   Electrolyte imbalance
b.   Tissue damage
c.   Extravasation
d.   Thrombus formation
e.   Bruising

42.   What is the major side effect that limits the dose of chemotherapy?
a.   Nausea and vomiting
b.   Peripheral neuropathy
c.   Bone marrow suppression
d.   Dry desquamation of the skin

43.   The nurse administering a vesicant must be prepared for complications and must have knowledge of which information? *(Select all that apply.)*
a.   The antidote
b.   The pH of the vesicant
c.   The correct method of documentation for extravasation
d.   Type of available dressings
e.   How to use hot or cold packs

44.   Indicate which chemotherapeutic agents are vesicants (V) and which are irritants (I).
_____ a.   Daunorubicin
_____ b.   Mitomycin C
_____ c.   Bleomycin
_____ d.   Vincristine
_____ e.   Paclitaxel

45. When thinning or loss of hair is a known side effect of a drug being administered, what does the nurse do? *(Select all that apply.)*
    a. Have the patient use gentle hair shampoo.
    b. Help the patient select wigs, turbans, or scarves.
    c. Instruct the patient that hair loss is permanent.
    d. Remind the patient to avoid washing the hair.
    e. Suggest complementary and alternative therapies to the patient.

46. Which statements are true regarding nausea and vomiting related to chemotherapy administration? *(Select all that apply.)*
    a. It is a common side effect of emetogenic agents.
    b. It usually lasts for 1 to 2 days after administration.
    c. It lasts as long as 3 weeks after administration.
    d. It is purely psychosomatic.
    e. Most chemotherapy drugs do not induce vomiting.

47. Which phrase best describes stomatitis?
    a. Lesions located in the GI tract
    b. An infection within the stomach lining
    c. A generalized infection within the bowel lining
    d. Sores located in the mouth

48. Because of the rapid cell division in the gastrointestinal tract, what is the effect of chemotherapy?
    a. Kills off the cells immediately
    b. Prevents the body from replacing cells
    c. Causes cells to be killed more rapidly than they can be produced
    d. Helps to increase cell division

49. What techniques are included in oral care for a patient with stomatitis? *(Select all that apply.)*
    a. Observation
    b. Hard-bristled toothbrush
    c. Saline mouthwash
    d. Glycerin swabs
    e. Commercial mouthwashes
    f. Petrolatum jelly to lips after each mouth care

50. Bone marrow suppression causes a decrease in which bodily components to occur? *(Select all that apply.)*
    a. Leukocytes
    b. Parenchyma
    c. Erythrocytes
    d. Platelets
    e. Blood

51. What clinical manifestations does the nurse expect in a patient who has chemotherapy-induced bone marrow suppression? *(Select all that apply.)*
    a. Alopecia
    b. Fatigue
    c. Bleeding gums
    d. Dry skin
    e. Diarrhea
    f. Pallor

True or False? Read each statement about biological response modifiers and write T for true or F for false in the blanks provided. If the statement is false, correct the statement to make it true.

_____ 52. Biological response modifier drugs stimulate the immune system to recognize cancer cells and take action to eliminate or destroy them.

_____ 53. Some BRMs stimulate recovery of bone marrow function after treatment-induced suppression.

54. The nurse is responsible for teaching both the immunosuppressed patient and the family about health promoting activities. Which are the most important activities to teach? *(Select all that apply.)*
    a. Handwashing
    b. Isolation
    c. Boiling dishes
    d. Wearing masks
    e. Eliminating fresh fruit from the patient's diet

Short Answer. *Discuss the use of the following biological response modifiers (BRMs) and their role in cancer treatment.*

55.   Interleukin:

56.   Interferon:

57.   The biological response modifiers have which positive effects on patients receiving chemotherapy? *(Select all that apply.)*
a.   Less risk of life-threatening infections
b.   Reduced incidence of alopecia
c.   Reduced severity of nausea
d.   Able to tolerate higher doses of chemotherapy
e.   Euphoria and increased libido

58.   Side effects of interleukin therapy can be dramatic. The patient may need to be treated in a critical care unit for which side effects? *(Select all that apply.)*
a.   Fluid shifts
b.   Severe inflammatory reaction
c.   Capillary leak
d.   Nausea and vomiting
e.   Tissue swelling

59.   What are common immediate reactions to biological response modifier therapy?
a.   Fever, chills, nausea and vomiting, malaise
b.   Fever, chills, rigor, malaise
c.   Hypertension, constipation
d.   Hives, diarrhea, low back pain

60.   A patient with cancer tells the nurse she has numbness and weakness in her legs. What is the nurse's best response?
a.   "Are you having any back pain?"
b.   "Have you been exercising vigorously?"
c.   "When was your last dose of pain medication?"
d.   "Don't worry. This is a normal response to chemotherapy."

61.   Which interventions does the nurse implement for a patient receiving chemotherapy to prevent the serious side effects of sepsis and disseminated intravascular coagulation? *(Select all that apply.)*
a.   Strict handwashing
b.   Monitoring of WBCs and clotting factors
c.   Education of the patient and family
d.   Isolation of the patient
e.   Frequent thorough patient assessment

Matching. *Match the colony stimulating factor (CSF) agent with the type of cell affected.*

CSF Agents
a.   Sargramostim (Leukine)
b.   Epoietin alfa (Epogen, Procrit)
c.   Filgrastim (Neupogen)
d.   Oprelvekin (Neumega)

Cell Types
_____ 62.   Erythrocytes

_____ 63.   Neutrophils

_____ 64.   Platelets

_____ 65.   Monocytes and macrophages

66. A patient with lymphoma reports severe facial swelling, tightness of the gown collar, and epistaxis. Which complication does the nurse suspect?
    a. Tumor lysis syndrome
    b. Cancer-induced hypercalcemia
    c. Superior vena cava syndrome
    d. Congestive heart failure

67. Which severe side effects of chemotherapy may cause a patient's death? *(Select all that apply.)*
    a. Myeloid leukemia
    b. Sepsis
    c. Allergic reactions
    d. Blood transfusions
    e. Disseminated intravascular coagulation

68. A patient has a diagnosis of cancer with a gram-negative infection. The nurse assesses bleeding from many sites throughout the body. For which condition does the nurse expect to perform nursing interventions?
    a. Sepsis
    b. Anemia
    c. Disseminated intravascular coagulation
    d. SIADH

69. A patient diagnosed with bone cancer reports fatigue, loss of appetite, and constipation. Which laboratory result does the nurse report immediately?
    a. Potassium level of 4.2 mEq/L
    b. Magnesium level of 2.0 mg/dL
    c. Sodium level of 140 mEq/L
    d. Calcium level of 10.5 mEq/dL

70. A patient with advanced breast cancer reports severe back pain and leg weakness. Based on these symptoms, what does the nurse suspect?
    a. Isolated limb perfusion
    b. Lower back cancer
    c. Spinal cord compression
    d. Bladder tumor

CASE STUDY: THE PATIENT RECEIVING CHEMOTHERAPY

Use a separate sheet of paper to answer the questions in this Case Study, or go to the "Prepare for Class" folder on your Evolve website at http://evolve.elsevier.com/Iggy/ to download and complete as a word processing file. Answer guidelines for this Case Study are also available on your Evolve website.

A 63-year-old woman is seen in the cancer therapy unit for her first round of chemotherapy for breast cancer. She had a lumpectomy 2 months ago and a double-lumen peripherally inserted central catheter (PICC) line inserted at that time. She is going to be taking the oral chemotherapy agent capecitabine (Xeloda); and will receive only her first dose while hospitalized today. She will return at a later date for continuation of therapy with an IV chemotherapy agent. She will also be taking ondansetron (Zofran) for nausea.

1. What instructions should the nurse give the patient about taking capecitabine (Xeloda)?

2. Before giving chemotherapy, the nurse prepares to give the ondansetron. The patient asks why she is getting that medication "when I'm not even nauseated." How should the nurse answer the patient?

3. After 10 days, the patient comes to the office for follow-up laboratory work. The results are as follows:
   - Sodium: 135 mEq/L
   - Potassium: 3.7 mEq/L
   - Hemoglobin: 8.5 g/dL
   - Hematocrit: 25%
   - Red blood cells: 2.3 million/mm^3
   - White blood cells: 2.8 mm^3
   - Platelets: 45,000 mm^3/mL

   Which laboratory values are expected at this time? What is the cause of these altered laboratory values?

4. What, if anything, can be done to protect this patient during this period? What other drugs may be ordered at this time?

CHAPTER 25

Care of Patients with Infection

STUDY/REVIEW QUESTIONS

Matching. Match the terms related to infection to their correct definitions.

Terms

a. Communicable
b. Reservoirs
c. Pathogen
d. Pathogenicity
e. Colonization
f. Susceptible host
g. Virulence
h. Normal flora

Definitions

_____ 1. Causative agent

_____ 2. Infection recipient

_____ 3. Ability to cause disease

_____ 4. Degree of communicability

_____ 5. Characteristic bacteria

_____ 6. Pathogenic microbes present but no symptoms

_____ 7. Sources of infectious agents

_____ 8. Transmitted from person to person

9. Transmissions of infection require a reservoir. Which is an example of an animate reservoir?
   a. People
   b. Water
   c. Soil
   d. IV solution

Matching. Match each type of pathogen with its description.

Pathogens

a. Toxin
b. Exotoxin
c. Endotoxin

Descriptions

_____ 10. Substances produced and released by certain bacteria, such as tetanus and diphtheria, into the surrounding environment

_____ 11. Substances produced in cell walls of certain bacteria, such as typhoid, and released by cell lysis

_____ 12. Protein molecules released by bacteria to affect host cells at distant sites

13. Which factors increase a patient's susceptibility to infection? *(Select all that apply.)*
    a. Alcohol consumption
    b. Steroid use
    c. Diabetes mellitus
    d. Nicotine use
    e. Oral contraceptives
    f. High-protein diet
    g. Advanced age

14. Which nursing intervention best decreases a patient's susceptibility to infection?
    a. Using standard precautions
    b. Removing soiled linens
    c. Restricting all visitors
    d. Avoiding direct contact

Matching. *Match the portal of entry with its method of transmission. Answers may be used more than once.*

Portals of Entry
a. Bloodstream
b. Skin/mucous membrane
c. Genitourinary tract
d. Gastrointestinal tract
e. Respiratory tract

Methods of Transmission
_____ 15. Droplet
_____ 16. Ingestion
_____ 17. Intravascular device
_____ 18. Insect bite
_____ 19. Catheterization
_____ 20. Laceration

Matching. *Match the contact site for infection to its mode of transmission. Answers may be used more than once.*

Modes of Transmission
a. Airborne
b. Droplet
c. Vector
d. Direct
e. Indirect

Contact Sites
_____ 21. Skin-to-skin
_____ 22. Contaminated needle
_____ 23. Sneezing
_____ 24. Contaminated food
_____ 25. Lyme disease

26. A patient admitted with a postoperative abdominal wound infection is diagnosed with methicillin-resistant *Staphylococcus aureus* (MRSA). While performing a physical examination on this patient, which personal protective equipment must the nurse wear? *(Select all that apply.)*
    a. Gown
    b. Gloves
    c. Mask
    d. Shoe covers
    e. Goggles

27. The nurse is preparing to hang an IV of 1 g vancomycin in 250 mL of normal saline for a patient diagnosed with MRSA infection. The medication is to infuse over 1.5 hours. The nurse sets the pump at what rate? (Record your answer using a whole number.) _____ mL/hr

28. The new nurse is discussing planned interventions to reduce the risk of a patient feeling isolated while on airborne precautions. Which statement by the new nurse requires follow-up from the preceptor?
    a. "I have arranged to have the newspaper delivered to the room daily."
    b. "I will leave the door propped open to increase auditory and visual stimuli."
    c. "I have demonstrated the use of television and radio controls for the patient."
    d. "I will bundle my activities in order to have more time to talk to the patient while in the room."

29. Handwashing, rather than using alcohol-based hand rub, must be performed during which situation?
    a. After contact with a patient who has a temperature of 101° F
    b. Before having direct contact with patients
    c. Before donning and after removing sterile gloves
    d. After contact with a patient who has had diarrhea for 3 days

30. Appropriate methods of infection control include which precautions? *(Select all that apply.)*
    a. Utilizing effective hand hygiene
    b. Using appropriate personal protective equipment
    c. Limiting time spent with patients
    d. Using standard precautions
    e. Administering prophylactic antibiotics

31. During the shift-to-shift hand-off, the nurse is informed that a patient is experiencing urticaria. What question does the nurse ask to clarify the condition of urticaria?
    a. "Were isolation precautions initiated?"
    b. "Did the patient receive an antibiotic before the onset?"
    c. "Was a culture specimen obtained from the site?"
    d. "Does the patient have a history of MRSA?"

32. The nurse is observing a new graduate nurse perform hand hygiene. Which observation indicates a need for further instruction?
    a. Wetting hands before applying soap
    b. Holding hands higher than the elbows
    c. Using friction under running water
    d. Washing for at least 15 seconds

33. Which situation requires using soap and water for handwashing?
    a. Before a sterile dressing change
    b. After removing sterile gloves
    c. Dry skin
    d. Hands feeling sticky

Matching. *Match each precaution with the example of its use.*

Precautions
a. Contact precautions
b. Droplet precautions
c. Standard precautions
d. Airborne precautions

Uses
_____ 34. All body secretions and excretions, most membranes and tissue, excluding perspiration, are potentially infectious.

_____ 35. Uses negative airflow rooms, high-efficiency particulate air (HEPA) filters, or ultraviolet (UV) lights.

_____ 36. Infection transmitted by droplet; an example is meningitis.

_____ 37. Transmission by touch of patient or environment; examples are methicillin-resistant *Staphylococcus aureus* (MRSA) and vancomycin-resistant *Enterococcus* (VRE).

38. How are complications of infection usually caused? *(Select all that apply.)*
    a. Incorrect choice of antibiotic
    b. Poor patient compliance
    c. Patient unable to afford medication
    d. The patient's overall health condition
    e. The patient taking too much of the prescribed medication

39. A localized infection may include which symptoms? *(Select all that apply.)*
    a. Chills
    b. Cool and clammy skin
    c. Fever
    d. Pain
    e. Pus
    f. Redness
    g. Swelling

Matching. *Match each diagnostic test with its description.*

Tests
a. Biopsy
b. Scanning
c. Ultrasonography
d. Radiographic studies
e. Erythrocyte sedimentation rate
f. Complete blood count
g. Culture
h. Sensitivity

Descriptions

_____ 40. Pathogen is isolated for identification.

_____ 41. Pathogen is tested for antibiotic reactions.

_____ 42. Checks WBC, neutrophils, lymphocytes, monocytes, eosinophils, and basophils.

_____ 43. Measures rate of RBC fall through plasma; increased rate indicates infection or inflammation.

_____ 44. X-ray films used to monitor infection.

_____ 45. Noninvasive procedure: used particularly for diagnosing heart valve problems.

_____ 46. Use of radioactive agents to determine presence of inflammation.

_____ 47. Tissue specimen obtained for tissue culture.

48. A patient has had a bacterial infection for 3 days and laboratory results show the percentage of immature neutrophils has increased at a greater rate than mature neutrophils. How does the nurse interpret these findings?
    a. The patient is very sick and immunocompromised.
    b. There is a unilateral shift to the right in the differential.
    c. The infection was caused by antimicrobial agents.
    d. There is a shift to the left in the differential.

True or False? *Read each statement about infection and write T for true or F for false in the blanks provided. If the statement is false, correct the statement to make it true.*

_____ 49. Antibiotic therapy should not begin until after the culture specimen is obtained.

_____ 50. Patients with a temperature greater than 100° F are considered to have a systemic infection.

_____ 51. Older adult patients may have a severe infection with no fever.

_____ 52. A superinfection is an infection with an extremely resistant microbe.

53. In a patient with an infection, which common interventions may be used to reduce fever? *(Select all that apply.)*
   a. Antipyretic drugs such as aspirin or acetaminophen
   b. External cooling, cooling blankets, cool compresses
   c. Fluid administration, oral and IV
   d. Antimicrobial therapy with antibiotic, antiviral, or antifungal agents
   e. Opening the windows and door to the patient's room

54. Name the antimicrobials that correspond to each drug action listed below.
   a. Inhibits reproduction

   b. Injures the cytoplasmic membrane

   c. Inhibits nucleic acid synthesis

   d. Inhibits cell wall synthesis

55. A patient has been prescribed gentamicin drug therapy. Which nursing intervention ensures effective antimicrobial therapy?
   a. Avoid the use of acetaminophen while on this medication.
   b. Deliver a sufficient dosage and duration of therapy.
   c. Take the medication with food.
   d. Closely monitor the patient's temperature.

Matching. *Match the organism to its disease manifestation.*

Organisms
a. *Escherichia coli*
b. *Plasmodium* sp.
c. Pinworm
d. *Streptococcus* sp.
e. *Pneumocystis jiroveci*
f. *Entamoeba histolytica*
g. Rickettsiae
h. Rhinovirus
i. *Candida albicans*

Disease Manifestations
_____ 56. Rocky Mountain spotted fever
_____ 57. Thrush
_____ 58. Diarrhea
_____ 59. Common cold
_____ 60. Malaria
_____ 61. Urinary tract infection
_____ 62. Anal pruritus
_____ 63. Pharyngitis
_____ 64. Pneumonia

65. A patient is diagnosed with mycobacterium tuberculosis. Which nursing intervention does the nurse implement for this patient?
    a. Wash hands before and after entering the room.
    b. Ensure the patient has a private room with negative airflow.
    c. Use contact and droplet precautions.
    d. Place contaminated gloves outside the room.

66. Which individual is at greatest risk for exposure to a blood-borne pathogen?
    a. Nursing assistant who is helping a patient to ambulate
    b. Nurse who is changing the tubing on a patient's IV infusion
    c. Physician who is injecting a patient with a local anesthetic
    d. Janitorial worker who is mopping an area where a patient vomited

67. A patient reports fever, chills, headache, and swollen glands in the groin and axillary areas. When the nurse assesses multiple reddened areas on both lower extremities, the patient states, "Those are flea bites from the refugee camp mission that I went to." What does the nurse suspect?
    a. Plague *(Yersinia pestis)*
    b. Erythema multiforme (Stevens-Johnson syndrome)
    c. Smallpox (variola virus)
    d. Measles (rubeola)

68. A patient who had previously reported flu-like symptoms which seemed to be improving woke up today with severe dyspnea, tachycardia, fever, and diaphoresis. What does the nurse suspect?
    a. Meningitis
    b. Influenza
    c. Inhalation anthrax *(Bacillus anthracis)*
    d. Respiratory syncytial virus

69. A patient who has returned from a camping trip reports severe vomiting and diarrhea and is experiencing symmetrical flaccid paralysis. The patient reports eating mostly canned foods during the trip. What does the nurse suspect?
    a. Meningitis
    b. Botulism
    c. Variola virus
    d. Inhalation anthrax

70. The nurse is caring for multiple patients in a temporary hospital after severe flooding in the area. Several patients have high fever, headache, and a papular rash over the face and extremities, including the palms of the hands. Some of the skin lesions are vesicular and pustular. What does the nurse suspect?
    a. Pandemic infection
    b. Superinfection
    c. Plague *(Yersinia pestis)*
    d. Smallpox (variola virus)

26
CHAPTER

Assessment of the Skin, Hair, and Nails

STUDY/REVIEW QUESTIONS

Matching. *Match each property with its appropriate layer of skin.*

Layer of Skin
a. Fat
b. Dermis
c. Epidermis

Property

_____ 1. Contains elastin

_____ 2. Serves as insulator

_____ 3. Contains no cells

_____ 4. Collagen is main component

_____ 5. Does not have a separate blood supply

_____ 6. Provides padding

_____ 7. Innermost layer of skin

_____ 8. Rich in sensory nerves

_____ 9. Synthesis of vitamin D

_____ 10. Melanin production

11. A dark-skinned patient is admitted for pneumonia. What is the most accurate method to assess for cyanosis in this patient?
    a. Observe for shallow and rapid respirations.
    b. Check the tongue and lips for a gray color.
    c. Auscultate for decreased breath sounds throughout lung fields.
    d. Inspect the palms and soles for a yellow-tinged color.

12. A patient is at risk for hypovolemia. The nurse assesses this patient's skin using which assessment technique?
    a. Brush the skin surface and observe for flaking.
    b. Push on the skin and observe for blanching.
    c. Gently pinch the skin on the chest and observe for tenting.
    d. Push on the skin over the tibia and observe for depth of indentation.

13. A patient with a history of congestive heart failure goes to the outpatient clinic for a follow-up appointment. How does the nurse assess for dependent edema in this patient?
    a. Palpate the dorsum of the foot or the medial ankle.
    b. Weigh the patient and compare to the baseline weight.
    c. Check the patient's buttocks or lower back.
    d. Ask the patient about intake and output.

14. The nurse is assessing the skin of an older adult patient who is at risk for dehydration due to excessive vomiting. The skin appears dry and loose. Where is the best site for the nurse to check skin turgor on this patient?
    a. Facial cheek
    b. Upper arm
    c. Anterior chest
    d. Mid-thigh

15. The nurse is preparing patient education material about healthy skin. What is the single most important preventive health behavior the nurse promotes?
    a. Limit continuous sun exposure.
    b. Drink plenty of water.
    c. Practice good skin hygiene.
    d. Eat a well-balanced diet.

16. A thin and malnourished patient requires emergency abdominal surgery. After the operation, in order to promote wound healing, what does the nurse encourage?
    a. High-calorie diet
    b. Low-sodium and low-carbohydrate diet
    c. High-quality protein diet
    d. Low-fat diet with vitamin supplements

Matching. Match the definition or characteristic of the integumentary system with the correct term.

Terms
a. Elastin
b. Sebum
c. Lichenified
d. Pruritus
e. Petechiae
f. Ecchymoses
g. Macular
h. Papular
i. Turgor
j. Hirsutism

Defining Characteristics
_____ 17. Itching

_____ 18. Small, reddish-purple lesions that do not fade or blanch when pressure is applied

_____ 19. Raised rash

_____ 20. Skin becomes thickened

_____ 21. Lubricates the skin and reduces water loss from the skin surface

_____ 22. Indicates amount of skin elasticity

_____ 23. Excessive growth of body hair or hair growth in abnormal body areas

_____ 24. Large bruised areas of hemorrhage; vary in size

_____ 25. Fine, flat rash

_____ 26. Major component of the elastic fiber

27. The nursing student must perform a skin assessment on an older adult patient and observe for signs of skin breakdown. What does the student do to meet the clinical objective and demonstrate good time-management skills?
    a. Examine the skin while bathing or assist the patient with hygiene.
    b. Complete the assessment before the end of the clinical experience.
    c. Check to see if the primary nurse has already completed the assessment.
    d. Perform the examination when the patient willingly consents and agrees.

28. The nurse is caring for a patient who sustained trauma and blood loss. The patient is alert and anxious, blood pressure is low, and the heart rate is high. Which skin characteristics are most likely to manifest during impending shock?
    a. Dry, flushed appearance
    b. Cool, pale, moist skin
    c. Bluish color that blanches with pressure
    d. Poor turgor with a rough texture

29. A patient is being referred to a dermatologist for evaluation of a rash of unknown origin. The patient has trouble articulating specific information because of "nervousness." Which questions does the nurse use to help the patient practice for the specialist appointment? *(Select all that apply.)*
    a. "Why do you have the rash?"
    b. "When did you first notice the rash?"
    c. "Where on the body did the rash first start?"
    d. "How do you feel about the skin rash?"
    e. "Are you having an itching or burning sensation?"
    f. "What makes the problem better or worse?"
    g. "Have you been having fever or sore throat?"

30. In regulating body temperature, how much evaporative water loss can occur during hot weather or exercise?
    a. 600 mL/day
    b. 900 mL/day
    c. 2 L/day
    d. 10 to 12 L/day

31. The nurse is caring for a very dark-skinned patient who has high risk for thrombocytopenia. Which area of the patient's body is the best place to check for petechiae?
    a. Anterior chest
    b. Oral mucosa
    c. Palmar surface
    d. Periorbital area

32. The nurse is performing a skin assessment on a patient and notes an area on the forearm that feels hard or "woody." What does the nurse interpret this physical finding as?
    a. Inflammation
    b. Subcutaneous fat
    c. Psoriasis
    d. Skin cancer

33. Age-related changes in the integumentary system include a decrease in which factors? *(Select all that apply.)*
    a. Vitamin D production
    b. Thickness of epidermis
    c. Thickness of dermis
    d. Epidermal permeability
    e. Dermal blood flow

34. During a patient hand-off, the nurse is informed that the patient has xerosis of the bilateral lower extremities. Based on this information, the nurse expects to assess which clinical finding on the lower extremities?
    a. Loss of hair
    b. Liver spots
    c. Dry skin
    d. Paper-thin skin

35. A decreased number of active melanocytes in an older adult leads to which result?
    a. Decreased wound healing
    b. Decreased skin tone and elasticity
    c. Increased skin transparency
    d. Increased sensitivity to sun exposure

36. It is important for the nurse to avoid taping the skin of an older adult patient due to a decrease in which integumentary factor?
    a. Vitamin D production
    b. Thickness of epidermis
    c. Dermal blood flow
    d. Epidermal permeability

37. In an older adult, decreased vitamin D production increases the patient's susceptibility to which condition?
    a. Osteomalacia
    b. Osteodystrophy
    c. Hypothermia
    d. Dry skin

38. In caring for an older adult patient, the room may need to be kept warmer because of a decrease in which integumentary factor?
    a. Sebum production
    b. Subcutaneous fat layer
    c. Thickness of epidermis
    d. Number of active melanocytes

39. While obtaining a health history on a patient with a chronic skin condition, the nurse observes that the patient does not make eye contact and keeps the affected area covered with a scarf. What is the most appropriate nursing action?
    a. Explain all actions and procedures to the patient.
    b. Explain to the patient that it is normal to be embarrassed.
    c. Discuss the patient's behavior with another nurse for validation.
    d. Explore the patient's feelings about the condition.

40. The nurse is assessing the skin of an older patient. Which assessment finding needs follow-up?
    a. Multiple liver spots on the arms
    b. Xerosis on the lower extremities
    c. Presence of cherry hemangiomas
    d. One light brown macule (6.5 cm) on the right scapula

41. A patient reports a rash that itches, but denies fever, shortness of breath, or other symptoms. Which questions does the nurse ask to help determine if the patient is having an allergic reaction? *(Select all that apply.)*
    a. "Are you taking any new medications?"
    b. "Have you been using any different soaps or lotions?"
    c. "Is your skin unusually dry or flaky?"
    d. "Have you been exposed to any new cleaning solutions?"
    e. "Have you noticed any new bruises or brownish discolorations?"
    f. "Have you had any changes in your diet?"

42. The nurse is performing a physical exam on a patient and observes a dark asymmetrical lesion on the patient's back. The patient states, "I can't see back there and I don't know how long it has been there." What is the most important intervention for this patient?
    a. Encourage the patient to make an appointment with a dermatologist.
    b. Teach the patient how to do a total skin self-evaluation.
    c. Instruct the patient on self-care measures, such as use of sunscreen.
    d. Obtain an order for a fungal culture and take a fungal specimen.

43. To differentiate between color changes in the nail bed related to vascular supply and those from pigment disposition, what does the nurse do?
    a. Examine the nail plate under a Wood's light.
    b. Assess for thickness.
    c. Blanch the nail bed.
    d. Evaluate for lesions.

44. The nurse is taking a medication history of a patient and performing a physical assessment on the skin. During the assessment the nurse notes that the skin is thin, fragile, and papery. The nurse specifically asks if the patient takes which type of medication?
    a. Anticoagulants
    b. Oral hypoglycemics
    c. Steroids
    d. Herbal preparations

45. A young female patient reports an unusual increase in facial hair. Which question helps the nurse to identify the need for a genital examination?
    a. "Have you noticed any bruising or unusual bleeding?"
    b. "Have you noticed any deepening of your voice quality?"
    c. "Are you having any trouble urinating?"
    d. "Does your skin seem unusually dry and flaky?"

46. Which statement about dandruff is true?
    a. Dandruff flakes are caused by a dry scalp.
    b. Dandruff is merely a cosmetic problem.
    c. Severe dandruff could cause hair loss.
    d. Brushing your hair every day prevents dandruff.

47. The nurse is caring for several older adult patients in a long-term care facility. The patient with which disorder has the greatest risk to develop a staphylococcal infection secondary to an ingrown toenail?
    a. Chronic obstructive pulmonary disease
    b. Hypertension
    c. Osteoarthritis
    d. Diabetes mellitus

Matching. *Match each alteration in color to its underlying cause or condition.*

Alteration in Color
a. Blue
b. Yellow-orange
c. Red (erythema)
d. Brown
e. White (pallor)

Underlying Cause or Condition

_____ 48. Pregnancy (melasma), Addison's disease

_____ 49. Bleeding from vessels into tissue

_____ 50. Liver disorders, chronic renal failure, or increased hemolysis of red blood cells

_____ 51. Vasoconstriction, sudden emotional upset

_____ 52. Fever, cellulitis

53. The nurse is assessing a patient who is African American with very dark skin. Which technique does the nurse use to assess the health of the nail?
    a. Gently squeeze the end of the finger, exert downward pressure, then release the pressure.
    b. Obtain a color chart to identify the normal color of nails for the dark-skinned patient.
    c. Observe the nail bed for a pale pink color and a shiny, smooth surface.
    d. Soak the fingertips in warm water, then gently push back the cuticle.

54. A patient reports a subjective sensation of pain and tenderness "because my arthritis is flaring up." In order to assess for inflammation, what does the nurse do?
    a. Place the hand just above the area and feel for radiant warmth.
    b. Use fingertips to gently depress tissue area and then release and observe.
    c. Use the back of the hand to palpate the area for warmth.
    d. Using the palmar surface of the hand, make a circular motion over the area.

55. A patient has a history of mild congestive heart failure. The nurse is assessing the patient's lower extremities; the skin is tight and shiny, but the patient currently denies pain or distress, saying "Oh, my legs just get like that." How does the nurse interpret these findings?
    a. Fluid retention and edema
    b. Early signs of poor circulation
    c. Early stage of infection
    d. Normal for this patient

56. The nurse is caring for a patient who is several days postoperative. The nursing assistant reports that the patient's linens were changed, but are wet again. The nurse notes that the patient's skin is excessively warm and moist. What is the nurse's priority action?
    a. Initiate intake and output
    b. Take the patient's temperature
    c. Direct the nursing assistant to change the linens
    d. Help the patient with hygiene

Matching. *Identify the probable causes for each skin manifestation identified below.*

Causes
a. Dehydration, sudden severe weight loss, or normal aging
b. Fungal infection
c. Hormone imbalance
d. Prolonged hypoxia or lung cancer

Manifestations
_____ 57. Increased body hair growth on the face in the female patient

_____ 58. Drumstick appearance of nail shape

_____ 59. Decreased skin turgor

_____ 60. "Heaped up" appearance of the older adult's toenail

61. The nurse is assessing a patient's skin and notes a slightly darkened area over the left ankle. The patient denies pain, but reports a recent problem with the area. Based on the skin appearance and the patient's report, what does the nurse do next?
    a. Ask the patient if there was a serious and deep burn to the area.
    b. Observe the area for scar tissue.
    c. Ask the patient if there was an inflammation to the area.
    d. Take a scraping of the skin for culture.

62. The nurse is caring for an older adult patient with very dark skin. The patient has a low hemoglobin and hematocrit. How does the nurse assess for pallor in this patient?
    a. Observe the mucous membranes for an ash-gray color.
    b. Use indirect and low fluorescent lighting.
    c. Gently push on the skin and watch for blanching.
    d. Inspect the conjunctivae for a yellowish color.

63. The nurse is interviewing a patient who has come to the walk-in clinic and observes the patient has matted hair, body odor, and soiled clothes. Which conditions does the nurse assess for that could be contributing to the patient's overall hygiene? *(Select all that apply.)*
    a. Range of motion and strength to perform self-care
    b. Access to shower facilities and a laundry
    c. Financial ability to pay water and heating bills
    d. Patient's perception of how he or she appears to others
    e. Diabetes mellitus or hypertension
    f. Intactness of sensory functions (i.e., sight, smell)
    g. Patient's knowledge (or memory) of how to perform hygiene care

64. The health care provider has ordered diagnostic testing to determine whether a patient has a fungal infection of the skin. Which test does the nurse prepare the patient for?
    a. Shave biopsy
    b. Punch biopsy
    c. Wood's light examination
    d. KOH test

65. A patient reports a history of chronic liver problems; liver enzyme tests and bilirubin results are pending. In order to assess for jaundice, where is the best place for the nurse to look for a yellowish discoloration?
    a. Hard palate
    b. Sclera
    c. Palms
    d. Conjunctivae

Matching. Match the terms to the description of the skin lesion configurations.

Terms
a. Annular
b. Universal
c. Serpiginous
d. Coalesced
e. Clustered
f. Diffuse
g. Linear
h. Circumscribed
i. Circinate

Description
_____ 66. Ringlike with raised borders around flat, clear centers of normal skin

_____ 67. Circular

_____ 68. Well-defined with sharp borders

_____ 69. Several lesions grouped together

_____ 70. Lesions that merge with one another and appear confluent

_____ 71. Widespread, involving most of the body with intervening areas of normal skin

_____ 72. Occurring in a straight line

_____ 73. With wavy borders, resembling a snake

_____ 74. All areas of the body involved, with no areas of normal-appearing skin

75. The nurse is collecting a superficial specimen for a suspected fungal infection from a patient's groin area. What is the correct technique to obtain this specimen?
    a. Obtain a small sample of tissue by using a biopsy needle.
    b. Express exudate from a lesion and use a sterile swab to collect the fluid.
    c. Gently scrape scales with a tongue blade into a clean container.
    d. Aspirate fluid from the lesion using sterile technique.

76. The nurse has collected several specimens from patients who have skin conditions. Which specimen must be immediately placed on ice?
    a. Punch biopsy performed with sterile technique for collection of a tissue piece.
    b. Exudate taken by sterile technique and swabbed on a bacterial culture medium.
    c. Aspirate taken by sterile technique, placed in a bacterial culture tube.
    d. Vesicle fluid taken by sterile technique and placed in a viral culture tube.

77. A patient is scheduled to have a punch biopsy for a lesion on the mid-back. What does the nurse tell the patient about the procedure?
    a. There will be a small scar similar to any surgical procedure.
    b. The surgeon uses a scalpel to punch through the lesion.
    c. A local anesthetic is used and it causes a temporary burning sensation.
    d. The physician uses a lens that punches the skin to reveal the shape of the lesion.

78. The nurse is caring for a patient who had an excisional biopsy for a skin lesion. What does the post-procedural care for this patient include? *(Select all that apply.)*
    a. Monitor the biopsy site for bleeding.
    b. Instruct the patient to keep the site clean and dry for at least 24 hours.
    c. Teach the patient to clean the site daily after the dressing is removed.
    d. Remove dried blood or crusts with diluted hydrogen peroxide.
    e. Instruct the patient to report any redness or excessive drainage.
    f. Advise the patient that the sutures will be removed in 7 to 10 days.

79. The health care provider instructs the nurse to prepare a light-skinned patient for examination, which includes evaluation of skin pigment changes. Which piece of equipment does the nurse obtain to assist the provider with this examination?
    a. Wood's light
    b. Glass slide
    c. Biopsy tray
    d. Non-fluorescent light

Matching. *Match each primary lesion with its description.*

Primary Skin Lesion
a. Macule
b. Papule
c. Patch
d. Plaques
e. Nodule
f. Vesicle
g. Pustule
h. Wheals
i. Fissure
j. Cyst

Descriptions
_____ 80. Nodule filled with liquid or semisolid material that can't be expressed

_____ 81. Flat lesion <1 cm in diameter

_____ 82. Macules >1 cm in diameter

_____ 83. Elevated, marble-like lesions >1 cm wide and deep

_____ 84. Elevated, irregular, and transient areas of dermal edema

_____ 85. Linear cracks in the skin

_____ 86. Elevated lesions <1 cm in diameter

_____ 87. Elevated patches >1 cm in diameter

_____ 88. Blister <1 cm in diameter filled with clear fluid

_____ 89. Vesicle filled with cloudy fluid

CASE STUDY: THE OLDER ADULT WITH SKIN CHANGES

Use a separate sheet of paper to answer the questions in this Case Study, or go to the "Prepare for Class" folder on your Evolve website at http://evolve.elsevier.com/Iggy/ to download and complete as a word processing file. Answer guidelines for this Case Study are also available on your Evolve website.

The older adult patient comes to the clinic for an annual health checkup. The patient reports good general health, but reports that her skin feels very dry and would like recommendations for "a nice skin cream." The patient also expresses some concern about "these ugly age spots" and "a lot of moles and warts as I get older." The patient's friend was recently diagnosed with skin cancer, and asks "Would you look at these moles for me?"

Assessment of the integumentary system reveals dry skin of the bilateral lower extremities, multiple reddish cherry angiomas on the upper extremities, four flat, brown lesions less than 1 cm in diameter on the upper back area, and a bruise (2 cm in diameter) on the right forearm.

1. What questions may the nurse ask to obtain a thorough health history from the patient?

2. Explain what the ABCDE features are that are associated with skin cancer.

3. What type of information and reassurance should be given to this patient about normal changes associated with aging?

4. What additional information would be appropriate to include in the teaching plan for this patient?

5. Using narrative charting, document the findings of the above integumentary assessment.

Care of Patients with Skin Problems

STUDY/REVIEW QUESTIONS

Matching. *Match the terms with their correct descriptions.*

Terms

a. Xerosis
b. Pruritus
c. Lichenification
d. Erythema
e. Urticaria
f. Debris
g. Débride
h. Re-epithelialization
i. Granulation
j. Contraction
k. Cellulitis
l. Eschar
m. Maceration

Descriptions

_____ 1. Mushiness

_____ 2. Inflammation of the skin cells

_____ 3. Scar tissue

_____ 4. Redness

_____ 5. Itching

_____ 6. Dead cells and tissues

_____ 7. Black, gray, or brown nonviable, denatured collagen

_____ 8. Pull the wound edges inward along the path of least resistance

_____ 9. Thickening

_____ 10. Dry skin

_____ 11. Hives

_____ 12. Production of new skin cells by undamaged epidermal cells

_____ 13. Remove exudate and dead tissue

14. The nurse is directing the home health aide in the care of an older adult patient. The patient reports dry skin and wants help in applying an emollient cream. What does the nurse direct the aide to do?
    a. Assist the patient to soak for 20 minutes in a warm bath and then apply the cream to slightly damp skin within 2 to 3 minutes after bathing.
    b. Generously apply the cream and leave it on for 15 to 20 minutes, then bathe the patient, especially the genital and axillary areas.
    c. Use an antimicrobial skin soap and wash the patient carefully, then apply the emollient cream, especially to the leg area.
    d. Use extra-warm water with added bath oil, then gently pat the patient dry and apply more oil and cream to the skin.

15. Which patients are at risk for pressure ulcers? *(Select all that apply.)*
    a. A confused patient who likes to wander through the halls
    b. A middle-aged quadriplegic patient who is alert and conversant
    c. A bedridden patient who is in the late stage of Alzheimer's
    d. A very heavy patient who must be assisted to move in the bed
    e. An ambulatory patient who has occasional urinary incontinence
    f. A thin patient who sits for long periods and refuses meals

16. The nurse is caring for an obese patient who has been on bedrest for several days. The nurse observes that the patient is beginning to develop redness on the sacral area. What intervention is used to decrease the shearing force?
    a. Place the patient in a high Fowler's position.
    b. Instruct the patient to use arms and legs to push when moving self in bed.
    c. Obtain an order for the patient to be up 3 to 4 times per day in a recliner chair.
    d. Place the patient in a side-lying position.

17. The nurse is reviewing the results of a pressure mapping on a patient at high risk for pressure ulcers. The map shows a red area over the hips. How does the nurse interpret this evidence?
    a. Normal finding because there is always pressure on the hip area
    b. Greater heat production associated with greater pressure
    c. Cooler skin associated with lower pressure
    d. Validation of observable skin redness and breakdown

18. The nurse is assessing the nutritional status of a patient at risk for skin breakdown who has been refusing to eat the hospital food. Which indicator is the most sensitive in identifying inadequate nutrition for this patient?
    a. Serum albumin level of 3.0 mg/dL
    b. Prealbumin level of 17.5 mg/dL
    c. Lymphocyte count of 1700/mm^3
    d. Weight loss of 10% of total body weight

19. Seeing a reddened area on a patient's skin, the nurse presses firmly with fingers at the center of the area and sees that the area blanches with pressure. The nurse interprets this finding as changes related to which factor?
    a. Inflammation
    b. Infection
    c. Blood vessel dilation
    d. Tissue damage

20. The nurse is assessing a wound on a patient's abdomen. What is the correct technique?
    a. Stand on the right side of the bed and lay a sterile cotton swab across the width and the length of the wound.
    b. Read the previous nursing documentation and follow the same pattern that other nurses are using for standardization.
    c. Assess the wound as a clock face with 12 o'clock in the direction of the patient's head and 6 o'clock in the direction of the patient's feet.
    d. Observe the wound after the dressing is removed and estimate the shape and record the appearance.

21. The nurse is assessing a patient's wound every day for signs of healing or infection. Which finding is a positive indication that healing is progressing as expected?
    a. Eschar starts to lift and separate from the tissue beneath which appears dry and pale.
    b. Area appears pale pink, progressing to a spongy texture with a beefy red color.
    c. Tissue is softer and more yellow and wound exudate increases substantially.
    d. Ulcer surface is excessively moist with a deep reddish-purple color.

22. The student nurse is irrigating a large pressure ulcer on a patient's hip, and notes a small opening in the skin with purulent drainage. Which technique does the student use to check for tunneling?
    a. Ask the primary nurse if the physician will order an ultrasound.
    b. Palpate the surface of the wound to identify spongy areas.
    c. Continue to flush the wound and watch the flow of the fluid.
    d. Use a sterile cotton-tipped applicator to probe gently for a tunnel.

23. The nurse is assessing a patient's skin and notes a 2" × 2" purplish-colored area on the coccyx with skin intact. These findings suggest which stage of a pressure ulcer?
    a. Suspected deep tissue injury
    b. Stage I pressure ulcer
    c. Stage II pressure ulcer
    d. Unstageable

24. When developing a plan of care for a patient who is at high risk for skin breakdown, what does the nurse include in the plan of care? *(Select all that apply.)*
    a. Applying a pressure reduction overlay to the mattress
    b. Frequent repositioning of the patient
    c. Instructing UAP to assess the patient's skin daily
    d. Instructing UAP to massage reddened areas
    e. Using positioning devices to keep heels pressure-free

25. Which expected outcome is most appropriate for a patient with a 1" × 1" stage II sacral decubitus?
    a. Patient will consume >75% of meals.
    b. Patient will sit up in chair three times a day.
    c. Wound will show granulation and decrease in size.
    d. Patient will rate pain at an acceptable level.

26. A patient receiving negative pressure wound therapy (NPWT) should be monitored closely for which potential complication?
    a. Bleeding
    b. Infection
    c. Pain
    d. Nausea

27. Which class of medication would exclude a patient from participating in negative pressure wound therapy (NPWT)?
    a. Antihypertensives
    b. Anticoagulants
    c. Nonsteroidal anti-inflammatory drugs
    d. Antidepressants

28. A patient on the unit has herpes zoster. Which staff members would be best to assign for the care of this patient?
    a. Any staff member, as long as PPE is utilized
    b. Staff members who have had chickenpox
    c. Staff members who have completed training on herpes zoster
    d. Staff members with no small children at home

29. The ED nurse is giving discharge instructions to the parents of a child who has been diagnosed with bedbug bites. What instructions does the nurse give to the parents? *(Select all that apply.)*
    a. Wash linens and clothing in hot water and dry on high heat.
    b. Use a topical insecticide as needed.
    c. Discard deeply infested furniture or mattresses.
    d. Place items that cannot be washed in the sunlight to be heated.
    e. Steam-clean all carpets and curtains.

30. A patient diagnosed with bedbug bites says to the nurse "I am so embarrassed. I shower daily and do not live in an unclean environment." Which response by the nurse is most appropriate?
    a. "You don't need to give me any explanations."
    b. "Showering will not kill bedbugs."
    c. "Can you tell me what you understand about bedbugs?"
    d. "Bedbugs are too small to be seen by the human eye."

31. Which statement about palmoplantar pustulosis (PPP) is true?
    a. It is easily treated with UV light therapy and corticosteroids.
    b. It is often associated with social and physical disabilities.
    c. It is an extremely rare form of psoriasis.
    d. It causes patchy scaling on the hands and feet.

32. A mother reports that her child has dry skin with itching that seems to worsen at night. What nonpharmacologic interventions does the nurse teach to the mother? *(Select all that apply.)*
    a. Keep the child's fingernails trimmed short and filed, to reduce skin damage.
    b. Place mittens or splints on the child's hands at night if the scratching is causing skin tears during sleep.
    c. Ensure a warm and moderately humid sleeping environment.
    d. Read the child a relaxing and familiar story to reduce stress.
    e. Colloidal oatmeal bath may give temporary relief.

33. After eating a food that triggered an allergic reaction, a patient developed hives. In addition to over-the-counter diphenhydramine (Benadryl), what does the nurse suggest to the patient for self-care?
    a. Avoid alcohol consumption which can potentiate the sedative effect of Benadryl.
    b. Warm environments and warm showers will accelerate metabolism and recovery.
    c. Use an emollient cream or lotion after bathing to reduce the itching.
    d. Apply a topical antibiotic cream after bathing in the evening.

34. The nurse is examining a patient's skin and sees large, sore-looking, raised bumps with pustular heads. Which method does the nurse use to obtain a specimen to test for a bacterial infection?
    a. Take a culture swab of the purulent material.
    b. Take cells from the base of a lesion for a Tzanck's smear.
    c. Scrape scales from the lesions and prepare a slide with KOH.
    c. Assist the physician with a skin biopsy.

35. The nurse is teaching a patient about self-care for a minor bacterial skin infection. What is the most important aspect the nurse emphasizes?
    a. Apply warm compresses twice a day.
    b. Do not squeeze any pustules or crusts.
    c. Apply astringent compresses.
    d. Bathe daily with an antibacterial soap.

36. A patient is diagnosed with psoriasis vulgaris. Which description of the characteristic lesions of psoriasis would the nurse expect to see in the patient's documentation?
    a. Plaques surmounted by silvery-white scales
    b. Circular areas of redness
    c. Multiple blisters with a yellowish crust
    d. Patches of tender, raised areas limited to extremities

37. What does the treatment for psoriasis include? *(Select all that apply.)*
    a. UV light therapy
    b. Calcipotriene (Dovonex) topical cream
    c. Topical methotrexate
    d. Oral ciprofloxacin
    e. Corticosteroids

38. What is the most common symptom of pruritus?
    a. Blisters
    b. Itching
    c. Flaking
    d. Tenderness

39. The nurse is teaching an older adult about how to deal with and prevent dry skin. What information does the nurse include? *(Select all that apply.)*
    a. Use a room humidifier during the winter months or whenever the furnace is in use.
    b. Take a complete bath or shower every day.
    c. Maintain a daily fluid intake of 1000 mL unless contraindicated.
    d. Use a superfatted, nonalkaline soap instead of deodorant soap.
    e. Rinse the soap thoroughly from the skin.
    f. Vigorously rub the skin until it is free of moisture.
    g. Avoid clothing that continuously rubs the skin, such as tight belts or pantyhose.

Matching. Match each tinea infection with its corresponding location.

Infection
a. Tinea capitis
b. Tinea manus
c. Tinea cruris
d. Tinea pedis
e. Tinea corporis

Location
_____ 40. Feet

_____ 41. Hands

_____ 42. Groin (jock itch)

_____ 43. Scalp

_____ 44. Smooth skin surfaces

45. The nurse is teaching a patient about treatment of pediculosis. What information does the nurse include? *(Select all that apply.)*
    a. Proper use of topical sprays or creams, such as permethrin or lindane
    b. Abstinence of sexual intercourse with the infected person
    c. Treatment of the patient's social contacts
    d. Side effects of ciprofloxacin (Cipro) or doxycycline (Doryx, Vibramycin)
    e. Washing clothing and bedding in hot water with detergent

46. The school nurse is examining a child and observes linear ridges in the skin. The child reports intense itching, especially at night. The nurse scrapes the lesion and examines it under a microscope. For which condition should the child be treated?
    a. Head lice
    b. Scabies
    c. Body lice
    d. Dermatitis

47. The school nurse discovers a child has tinea capitis. What does the nurse instruct the parents to do?
    a. Treat the family pet and temporarily isolate the pet.
    b. Refrain from sharing items like combs or hats.
    c. Scrub the shower area and keep the feet dry.
    d. Ensure all family members carefully wash their hands.

48. The nurse is assessing the pedicle flap that has been used to cover a patient's wound, and observes a pale flap with delayed capillary filling when blanched. How does the nurse interpret this finding?
    a. Inadequate venous drainage
    b. Inadequate lymphatic drainage
    c. Inadequate arterial perfusion
    d. Expected flap condition

49. A patient returns from surgery with a large graft site on the sacral area. Which task is delegated to unlicensed assistive personnel?
    a. Turn the patient every 2 hours.
    b. Explain to the patient that he will be in a side-lying or prone position for 7 to 10 days.
    c. Give the patient a backrub.
    d. Trim the gauze close to the skin surface to prevent accidental removal of the dressing.

50. The nurse is giving discharge instructions to a patient and family who must continue dressing changes and wound care at home. Which point does the nurse emphasize to help the family prevent infection and minimize cost?
    a. Scrupulous handwashing before and after wound care
    b. Use of sterile water for flushing and sterile dressing materials
    c. Use of clean gloves for performing dressing changes
    d. Careful disposal of contaminated dressings in a biohazard bag

51. The nurse is caring for a 25-year-old patient who recently had a rhinoplasty as part of reconstruction after cancer treatment. The patient is swallowing repeatedly and belching. What does the nurse suspect?
    a. Postnasal bleeding
    b. Respiratory distress
    c. Edema and swelling
    d. Anxiety

52. A patient has been prescribed isotretinoin (Accutane) for a skin condition. What information does the nurse tell the patient about this drug? *(Select all that apply.)*
    a. It may cause dry, chapped lips.
    b. It is the first choice for acne treatment.
    c. Strict birth control measures are necessary.
    d. Liver function studies should be monitored while on this therapy.
    e. It is used for superficial lesions.

53. The nurse is caring for a patient with toxic epidermal necrolysis (TEN). Which nursing action is included in the nursing care plan?
    a. Assessing input and output
    b. Administering antibiotics as prescribed
    c. Monitoring for hyperthermia
    d. Managing inflammation with steroid creams

54. A patient is prescribed a topical steroid for treatment of contact dermatitis. Which instruction does the nurse provide to the patient about this drug?
    a. Moisten dressings with warm tap water; place over topical steroids for short periods.
    b. Apply topical steroids then cover with an occlusive dressing.
    c. Apply a topical corticosteroid sparingly on the face.
    d. Discontinue the use of topical steroids when symptoms subside.

55. Which statement is true about the application and use of topical preparations?
    a. A stiff paste should be applied to large areas such as the trunk or legs.
    b. Using a water-soluble cream in the groin area could cause maceration.
    c. Using an oil-based ointment in the axillary area could cause folliculitis.
    d. An oil-based gel should be massaged into hairy areas.

Matching. *Match the disorders with their descriptions. Disorders may be used more than once.*

Disorders
a. Toxic epidermal necrolysis
b. Stevens-Johnson syndrome
c. Contact dermatitis
d. Lichen planus
e. Hansen's disease
f. Acne
g. Pemphigus vulgaris
h. Cutaneous anthrax
i. Seborrheic keratoses
j. Pilonidal cyst
k. Keloid
l. Nevus

Descriptions

_____ 56. A rash caused by toxic injury to the skin as a result of contact with an irritant substance

_____ 57. A chronic, contagious, systemic mycobacterial infection of the peripheral nervous system with skin involvement

_____ 58. A drug-induced skin reaction that may include a mix of vesicles, erosions, and crusts

_____ 59. Painless boil-like lesions and eschar that form regardless of treatment used

_____ 60. A rare, chronic blistering disease with high morbidity and mortality

_____ 61. A rare, acute drug reaction of the skin that gradually heals in 2 to 3 weeks with widespread peeling of the epidermis

_____ 62. Purple, flat-topped, itchy papules over the wrists and inner surfaces of the forearms

_____ 63. Also known as leprosy

_____ 64. Comedone lesions

_____ 65. Removed for cosmetic reasons or if a lesion becomes irritated from friction

_____ 66. A lesion of the sacral area that often has a sinus tract extending into deeper tissue structures

_____ 67. Overgrowth of a scar with excessive accumulation of collagen and ground substance

_____ 68. Mole, a benign growth of the pigment-forming cells

69. A patient has a partial-thickness wound. How long does the nurse anticipate the healing by epithelialization will take?
    a. 24 hours
    b. 2 to 3 days
    c. 5 to 7 days
    d. 12 to 14 days

70. A toddler is miserable with itching from chickenpox. Which type of bath is the best to help relieve the toddler's discomfort?
    a. Milk
    b. Emollient
    c. Tar with Polytar formula
    d. Aveeno colloidal oatmeal

71. The nurse is performing daily wound care and dressing changes on a patient with a full-thickness wound. The patient protests when the nurse attempts to débride the wound. What is the nurse's best response?
    a. "Re-epithelialization, granulation, and contraction are natural body processes that will occur if this tissue is removed."
    b. "I know this is uncomfortable, but don't you want your wound to heal as fast as possible? This treatment allows the body to heal itself."
    c. "Harmful bacteria can grow in the dead tissue and it also interferes with the body's attempt to fill in the wound with new cells and collagen."
    d. "I would never force a patient to do anything, but this really is the best treatment for the wound that you have."

72. A patient has a stage III pressure ulcer over the left trochanter area that has a thick exudate. The wound bed is visible and beefy red, and the edges are surrounded with swollen pink tissue. The exudate has an odor. Which dressing is best for this wound?
    a. Transparent
    b. Alginate
    c. Continuous dry gauze
    d. Pigskin or cadaver skin

73. The nurse is caring for a patient with arterial insufficiency in the lower right leg. In order to prevent leg ulcers, what does the nurse do?
    a. Elevates the leg frequently.
    b. Places the leg in a dependent position.
    c. Places a heel protector on the right foot.
    d. Encourages the patient to walk briskly.

74. The nurse is caring for a patient who had surgical débridement with a skin graft on the leg. The patient returns from the operating room with the graft site immobilized and a bulky cotton pressure dressing in place. What does the nurse do next?
    a. Encourages elevation and complete rest of the grafted area.
    b. Removes the dressing and cleans the wound every shift.
    c. Encourages the patient to get up and ambulate as soon as he is awake and alert.
    d. Monitors the dressing for a small amount of bleeding which is expected.

75. Place the physiologic steps of healing of partial-thickness wounds in the correct order using the numbers 1 through 8.

    _____ a. Skin injury is followed immediately by local inflammation.

    _____ b. The protective barrier is re-established.

    _____ c. The cell layer thickens and stratifies to resemble normal skin.

    _____ d. New skin cells move into open spaces on the wound surface.

    _____ e. Regrowth across the opening area is only one cell layer thick at first.

    _____ f. Fibrin clot acts as a frame or scaffold to guide cell movement.

    _____ g. Growth factors are released to stimulate epidermal cell division.

    _____ h. There is formation of a fibrin clot.

76. The nurse is caring for several patients who are incontinent of stool and urine. Which task is delegated to unlicensed assistive personnel?
    a. Inspect the skin daily for any areas of redness.
    b. Massage the reddened areas after cleaning.
    c. Wash the skin with a pH-balanced soap to maintain normal acidity.
    d. Change the absorbent pads or garments every 4 hours.

77. The nurse is caring for a patient in a prolonged coma after a serious head injury. The nurse uses which interventions to prevent the development of pressure ulcers for this patient? *(Select all that apply.)*
    a. Use pillows or padding devices to keep heels pressure-free.
    b. Assess heel positioning every 8 hours.
    c. Delegate turning and positioning every 2 hours.
    d. Obtain an order for a pressure-relief device.
    e. Give special attention to fleshy or muscular areas.

78. The nurse is assessing a patient's skin and observes a superficial infection with a raised, red rash with small pustules. How does the nurse interpret this finding?
    a. Minor skin trauma
    b. Folliculitis
    c. Furuncles
    d. Cellulitis

79. A patient has a painful and unsightly herpes simplex blister on her lip, and would like to have her school photo delayed until after the lesion has resolved. How long does the nurse tell the patient the outbreak may last?
    a. 2 to 3 days
    b. 3 to 5 days
    c. 3 to 10 days
    d. Up to 2 weeks

80. The nurse is caring for a patient who needs frequent oral hygiene and endotracheal suctioning. In this particular circumstance, the nurse wears gloves to prevent contracting and spreading which organism?
    a. Herpetic whitlow
    b. Herpes zoster
    c. Methicillin-resistant *Staphylococcus aureus*
    d. Streptococcus

81. The nurse hears in report that a patient admitted for an elective surgery also has herpes zoster. Which factor causes contact isolation to be initiated for this patient?
    a. Fever and malaise are present as accompanying symptoms.
    b. Other patients or staff members have never had chickenpox.
    c. Lesions are present as fluid-filled blisters.
    d. Lesions are present and crusted over.

82. A patient is diagnosed with a primary herpetic infection. The nurse questions an order for which drug?
    a. Acyclovir (Zovirax)
    b. Valacyclovir (Valtrex)
    c. Ketoconazole (Nizoral)
    d. Famciclovir (Famvir)

83. The public health nurse is reviewing case files of people who were exposed and treated for cutaneous anthrax. Which patient who develops the disease warrants further investigation as a possible bioterrorism exposure?
    a. Farmer
    b. Veterinarian
    c. Tannery worker
    d. Construction worker

84. A patient reported painless raised vesicles that itched. Within a few days, there was bleeding in the center and then it sank inwards. Now it looks black and leathery. Which question does the nurse ask in order to elicit more information about this patient's condition?
    a. "Do you remember being bitten by an insect?"
    b. "Do you work with or around animals?"
    c. "Have you noticed any mite or lice infestations?"
    d. "Have you had exposure to new soaps, lotions, or foods?"

85. A patient underwent cryosurgery for removal of a small lesion. The nurse teaches the patient to clean the area to prevent infection. What does the patient use for cleaning?
    a. Soap and water
    b. Hydrogen peroxide
    c. Alcohol
    d. Betadine

86. A patient is diagnosed with chronic psoriasis and is prescribed a topical therapy of anthralin (Lasan). What does the nurse teach the patient about proper use of this drug?
    a. Apply the paste every night before going to bed.
    b. Check for local tissue reaction.
    c. Apply the drug generously to the lesion and surrounding skin.
    d. Use two forms of contraception.

87. What does the nurse teach a patient about ultraviolet (UV) therapy for psoriasis?
    a. Use a commercial tanning bed service but limit exposure to 2 to 3 times per week.
    b. Use the sun as an inexpensive source of UV; inspect skin daily for overexposure.
    c. Wear dark glasses during and after treatment if psoralen is prescribed.
    d. Expect generalized redness with edema and tenderness after the treatment.

Matching. Match the skin disorder with its description.

Skin Disorder
a. Melanoma
b. Basal cell carcinoma
c. Actinic keratosis
d. Squamous cell carcinoma

88. Which are examples of benign skin tumors? *(Select all that apply.)*
    a. Pilonidal cyst
    b. Nevus
    c. Hemangioma
    d. Actinic keratoses
    e. Keloid
    f. Seborrheic keratoses
    g. Melanoma

Description
_____ 89. Most common cause: ultraviolet exposure; metastasis is rare.

_____ 90. Invades locally and is potentially metastatic; arises from epidermis.

_____ 91. Pigmented skin cancer that is highly metastatic.

_____ 92. Premalignant lesions of the cells of the epidermis.

93. The nurse is examining the nevi on a patient's back and neck. Because about 50% of malignant melanomas arise from moles, which finding is a concern to warrant further investigation?
    a. Regular, well-defined borders
    b. Uniform dark brown color
    c. Rough surface
    d. Sudden report of itching

94. *Koebner's phenomenon* is known as a greater risk for which disorder/condition?
    a. Skin cancer
    b. Psoriasis
    c. Nevus
    d. Keloids

95. Which statement is true about Mohs' surgery used to treat squamous cell carcinoma?
    a. Cure rates are high and there is less removal of healthy tissue compared with other surgical methods.
    b. The surgeon places an electric probe on the wound, and remnants of the tumor are destroyed by thermal energy.
    c. Local anesthesia is seldom needed because most patients have only minor discomfort during the procedure.
    d. Wounds created by this treatment heal by second intention, and scarring is usually minimal.

96. The nurse is talking to a patient who is planning to have cosmetic plastic surgery. Which patient statement prompts the nurse to report concerns to the surgeon?
    a. "Having this surgery is going to help increase my self-confidence."
    b. "I know this surgery is going to solve my marital problems."
    c. "I have been thinking about having this surgery for a long time."
    d. "I am nervous about having the surgery, but I can't wait to see the outcome."

97. The nurse is doing preoperative teaching for a patient who is scheduled to have cosmetic plastic surgery. The nurse decides the surgeon must be notified when the patient adamantly refuses to comply with which instruction?
    a. Take NSAIDs for pain associated with the procedure.
    b. Stop drinking an evening alcoholic cocktail prior to the procedure.
    c. Maintain a moderate calorie, low-fat diet after the procedure.
    d. Stop smoking cigarettes either before or after the procedure.

98. The nurse is caring for a patient who had facial reconstruction surgery. In order to decrease pressure in the head region, what does the nurse instruct the patient to do?
    a. Rest in bed in a supine position and log-roll to change position.
    b. Chew, talk, and smile to normally use and exercise the facial muscles.
    c. Avoid bending over, blowing the nose, sneezing with the mouth closed.
    d. Take small and frequent sips of fluid through a straw.

99. An older patient who is receiving chemotherapy is diagnosed with toxic epidermal necrolysis. In addition to identifying the causative agent, what does the nurse monitor for?
    a. Fluid and electrolyte imbalance, caloric intake, and hypothermia
    b. Shortness of breath, hypertension, and cardiac dysrhythmias
    c. Nausea, vomiting, diarrhea, and severe abdominal pain
    d. Severe itching with tenderness and edema of the skin

100. The nurse is caring for a patient with localized leprosy who recently immigrated to the U.S. The patient is fearful because she has seen others with leprosy deformity. What is the nurse's best response?
    a. "The progression of the disease is limited to the current area of skin involvement."
    b. "Widespread, faintly red macules suggest that your body is limiting the disease."
    c. "One or two isolated red plaques suggest that your body has high immunity."
    d. "There are drugs that can reverse the physical deformities and cure the disease."

CASE STUDY: THE PATIENT WITH MALIGNANT MELANOMA

Use a separate sheet of paper to answer the questions in this Case Study, or go to the "Prepare for Class" folder on your Evolve website at http://evolve.elsevier.com/Iggy/ to download and complete as a word processing file. Answer guidelines for this Case Study are also available on your Evolve website.

A 44-year-old Caucasian woman is admitted for local wide excision of a large mole that has been diagnosed as malignant melanoma on her upper thigh. Her past history is negative for serious illness. She was hospitalized for the birth of her three children. She admits to being an "avid sun worshipper" and is noted to have very dark brown skin and some premature aging of the facial skin.

1. Considering the possible etiology of melanoma, what effect does the exposure to sunlight have on this form of cancer?

2. During her preoperative instructions, the patient asks why she is going to have a 4-inch circle of skin and tissue removed to get rid of a "mole." What information should the nurse consider before responding to her question?

3. The patient has a wide excision of the melanoma, and the surgical site is closed with a split-thickness skin graft from the opposite thigh. Following surgery, the wound is dressed with a bulky dressing, and the donor site is covered with a pressure dressing. When the nurse is assessing the dressings, the patient asks to "peek" at the surgical site so that she can see where the mole had been. How should the nurse respond?

4. On the following morning, the patient reports that the donor site "hurts worse than the cancer site." What should the nurse say and what interventions are appropriate?

5. On the third day after surgery, the bulky dressing is removed. The wound appears wet with cloudy fluid oozing from it, and the skin graft is unattached to the wound. The surrounding tissues are red and swollen. The patient's vital signs are within normal limits with the exception of a low-grade temperature of 99.6° F and WBCs from yesterday are normal at 8.6. What is the likely cause of these features in the graft site?

6. Using the ISBARR format, how would the nurse communicate these findings to the appropriate health care provider?

Care of Patients with Burns

STUDY/REVIEW QUESTIONS

Matching. *Match each term with its corresponding definition.*

Terms
a. Dermal appendages
b. Anesthetic
c. Avascular
d. Eschar
e. Desquamation
f. Fasciotomy
g. Viable
h. Hyperkalemia
i. Hyponatremia
j. Hemoconcentration
k. Catabolism

Definitions
_____ 1. Decreased sodium levels

_____ 2. Peeling of dead skin

_____ 3. Living

_____ 4. Sweat and oil glands and hair follicles

_____ 5. Burn crust

_____ 6. Elevated potassium levels

_____ 7. Without a blood supply

_____ 8. Incision through the eschar and fascia

_____ 9. Reduces pain

_____ 10. Fat and protein breakdown

_____ 11. Elevated blood osmolarity, hemoglobin, and hematocrit

12. A patient was burned on the forearm after tripping and falling against a wood-burning stove. There are currently several small blisters over the burn area. What does the nurse advise the patient to do about the blisters?
    a. Leave the blisters intact because they protect the wound from infection
    b. Use a sterile needle to open a tiny hole in each blister to drain the fluid
    c. Allow blisters to increase in size; then open them to prevent immunosuppression
    d. Leave the blisters intact unless the pain and pressure increase

13. The nurse is caring for a patient who has 30% total body surface area (TBSA) burn. During the first 12 to 36 hours, the nurse carefully monitors the patient for which status changes related to capillary leak syndrome?
    a. Bradycardia and pitting edema
    b. Hypertension and decreased urine output
    c. Tachycardia and hypotension
    d. Respiratory depression and lung crackles

14. The home health nurse is visiting an older couple for the initial visit. In observing the household, the nurse identifies several behaviors and environmental factors to address. Which identified factors increase the risk for burns and/or household fires? *(Select all that apply.)*
    a. Several potholders hanging within easy reach from the stove
    b. Ashtray with old cigarette butts on the bedside table
    c. Space heater very close to the bed
    d. Single smoke detector in the kitchen
    e. Back exit hall of the house used as a storage space

15. The nurse is caring for several patients on the burn unit who have sustained extensive tissue damage. The nurse should monitor for which electrolyte imbalance that is typically associated with the initial third-spacing fluid shift?
    a. Hypercalcemia
    b. Hypernatremia
    c. Hypokalemia
    d. Hyperkalemia

16. The nurse is reviewing the hemoglobin and hematocrit results for a patient recently admitted for a severe burn. Which result is most likely related to vascular dehydration?
    a. Hematocrit of 58%
    b. Hemoglobin of 14 g/dL
    c. Hematocrit of 42%
    d. Hemoglobin of 10 g/dL

17. The nurse is performing a morning assessment on a patient admitted for serious burns to the extremities. For what reason does the nurse assess the patient's abdomen?
    a. To perform a daily full head-to-toe assessment
    b. To assess for nausea and vomiting related to pain medication
    c. To assess for a paralytic ileus secondary to reduced blood flow
    d. To monitor increased motility that may result in cramps and diarrhea

18. The nurse is interviewing and assessing an electrician who was brought to the emergency department (ED) after being "electrocuted." Bystanders report that he was holding onto the electrical source "for a long time." The patient is currently alert with no respiratory distress. During the interview, what does the nurse assess for?
    a. Knowledge of electrical safety
    b. Burn marks on the dominant hand
    c. Injuries based on reports of pain
    d. Entrance and exit wounds

19. A patient was involved in a house fire and suffered extensive full-thickness burns. In the long-term, what issue may this patient have trouble with?
    a. Intolerance for vitamin C
    b. Metabolism of vitamin K
    c. Activation of vitamin D
    d. Absorption of vitamin A

20. During shift report, the nurse learns that a new patient was admitted for an inhalation injury. The auscultation of the lungs has revealed wheezing over the mainstream bronchi since admission. During the nurse's assessment of the patient, the wheezing sounds are absent. What does the nurse do next?
    a. Document these findings because they indicate that the patient is improving.
    b. Assess for respiratory distress because of potential airway obstruction.
    c. Obtain an order to discontinue oxygen therapy because it is no longer needed.
    d. Encourage use of incentive spirometry to prevent atelectasis.

21. What is the maximum temperature that the skin can tolerate without injury?
    a. 102° F
    b. 104° F
    c. 110° F
    d. 120° F

22. The nurse is caring for several patients who have sustained burns. The patient with which initial injury is the *least* likely to experience severe pain when a sharp stimulus is applied?
    a. Severe sunburn after lying in the sun for several hours
    b. Deep full-thickness burn from an electrical accident
    c. Partial-thickness burn from picking up a hot pan
    d. Deep partial-thickness burn after a motorcycle accident

23. The nurse is reviewing arterial blood gas (ABG) results for a patient with 35% TBSA burn in the emergent phase: pH is 7.26; Pco_2 is 36 mm Hg; and HCO_3^- is 19 mEq/L. What condition does the nurse suspect the patient has?
    a. Metabolic alkalosis
    b. Metabolic acidosis
    c. Respiratory acidosis
    d. Respiratory alkalosis

24. A patient comes to the clinic to be treated for burns from a barbeque fire. Although the patient does not appear to be in any respiratory distress, the nurse suspects an inhalation injury after observing which findings? *(Select all that apply.)*
    a. Burns to the face
    b. Bright cherry-red color to lips
    c. Singed nose hairs
    d. Edema of the nasal septum
    e. Black carbon particles around the mouth
    f. Sweet, sugary smell to the breath

25. The nurse is caring for a burn patient who received rigorous fluid resuscitation in the ED for hypotension and hypovolemic shock. In assessing renal function for the first 24 hours, what finding does the nurse anticipate?
    a. Output will be approximately equal to fluid intake.
    b. Output will be decreased compared to fluid intake.
    c. Urine will have a very low specific gravity and a pale-yellow color.
    d. Output will be managed with diuretics.

26. A patient sustained a superficial-thickness burn over a large area of the body. The patient is crying with discomfort and is very concerned about the long-term effects. What does the nurse tell the patient to expect?
    a. "Healing should occur in 3 to 6 days with no scarring or complications."
    b. "The pain should be less because more of the nerve endings were destroyed."
    c. "The wound will appear red and dry with some white areas."
    d. "The leathery eschar will have to be removed before healing can occur."

27. The nurse is caring for a patient brought to the ED after bending over the engine of his car when it exploded in his face. What is the priority for this patient?
    a. Initiate fluid resuscitation
    b. Secure the airway
    c. Manage pain and discomfort
    d. Prevent infection

28. The nurse is caring for a patient who sustained carbon monoxide poisoning while working on his car engine in an enclosed space. What assessment finding does the nurse anticipate?
    a. Patient will be cyanotic because of hypoxia.
    b. Blood gas value of Pao_2 will be very low.
    c. Patient will report a headache.
    d. Patient will report a dry and irritated throat.

29. For which patient would the rule of nines method of calculating burn size be most appropriate?
    a. Child who weighs at least 50 pounds
    b. Adult whose weight is proportionate to height
    c. Adult who weighs under 300 pounds
    d. Child whose weight is proportionate to height

30. Which criterion describes a full-thickness burn wound? *(Select all that apply.)*
    a. The wound is red and moist and blanches easily.
    b. There is destruction to the epidermis and dermis.
    c. There are no skin cells for regrowth.
    d. The burned tissue is avascular.
    e. The burn wound will not be painful.

31. The nurse is assessing a patient with a burn wound to the back and chest area. Which assessment findings are consistent with a superficial-thickness burn wound? *(Select all that apply.)*
    a. Redness
    b. Pain
    c. Mild edema
    d. Moisture
    e. Eschar

32. The nurse observes peeling of dead skin on the legs of a patient with a superficial-thickness burn wound. What is the most accurate description of this assessment finding?
    a. Blanching
    b. Desquamation
    c. Slough
    d. Fluid shift

33. The epidermis can grow back after a burn injury due to which component in this layer of skin?
    a. Blood vessels
    b. Dermal appendages
    c. Subcutaneous tissue
    d. Lymph vessels

34. Which type of burn wound damages the epidermis, dermis, fascia, and tissues?
    a. Superficial
    b. Partial thickness
    c. Full-thickness
    d. Deep full-thickness

35. Which type of burn destroys the sweat glands, resulting in decreased excretory ability?
    a. Superficial
    b. Partial-thickness
    c. Full-thickness
    d. Deep full-thickness

36. During the early phase of a burn injury, there is a drastic increase in capillary permeability. What does this physiologic change place the patient at risk for?
    a. Acute kidney injury
    b. Fluid overload
    c. Increased cardiac output
    d. Hypovolemic shock

37. An adult patient is admitted to the burn unit after being burned in a house fire. Assessment reveals burns to the entire face, back of the head, anterior torso, and circumferential burns to both arms. Using the rule of nines, what is the extent of the burn injury?
    a. 18%
    b. 24%
    c. 45%
    d. 54%

38. What is the most effective intervention for preventing transmission of infection to a burn patient?
    a. Use of PPE for anyone entering the patient's room
    b. Maintaining reverse isolation during the resuscitation phase
    c. Use of designated equipment for patient use
    d. Performing hand hygiene correctly and when appropriate

39. Which vaccine is routinely administered when a burn patient is admitted to the hospital?
    a. Hepatitis B
    b. Tetanus
    c. Influenza
    d. Pneumonia

40. A patient has severe burns to the anterior surface of the body from a short exposure to high temperatures at a worksite furnace. Which area of the body is most vulnerable to a deep burn injury?
    a. Anterior chest
    b. Upper arms
    c. Palmar surface of hands
    d. Eyelids

41. A patient has sustained a burn which appears red and moist. The nurse gently applies pressure to the area to assess for what sign/symptom?
    a. Intensity of pain
    b. Blanching
    c. Pitting edema
    d. Fluid-filled blisters

42. What is the primary reason to avoid infection with burn injuries?
    a. Prevent extensive scar formation
    b. Prevent sepsis
    c. Avert worsening of pain
    d. Avoid fever and inflammation

43. The nurse is caring for several patients on the burn unit. Which patients have the greatest risk for developing respiratory problems? *(Select all that apply.)*
    a. Patient who was in a storage room where chemicals caught fire
    b. Patient who was working in an area where steam escaped from a pipe
    c. Patient who sustained a circumferential burn to the chest area
    d. Patient who was burned when a firecracker exploded prematurely
    e. Patient who was found unconscious in a slow-burning house fire

44. The nurse is caring for a firefighter who was trapped for a prolonged period of time by burning debris. During the shift, the nurse notes a progressive hoarseness, a brassy cough, and the patient reports increased difficulty with swallowing. How does the nurse interpret these changes?
    a. Temporary discomfort that can be treated with sips of cool fluids
    b. Signs and symptoms of probable carbon monoxide poisoning
    c. Signs indicating a pulmonary injury and possible airway obstruction
    d. Expected findings considering the mechanism of injury

45. The nurse has just received report on a patient admitted for steam inhalation burns. The patient is alert and conversant, but reports that his throat feels raw. His wife says that he sounds hoarse compared to usual. Considering these findings, which order does the nurse question?
    a. Continuous pulse oximetry
    b. Vital signs and airway assessment every shift
    c. Intubation equipment at the bedside
    d. Oxygen 2 L via nasal cannula to maintain saturation of greater than 90%

46. The nurse is caring for a burn patient who was stabilized by and transferred from a small rural hospital. The patient develops a new complaint of shortness of breath. On auscultation, the nurse hears crackles throughout the lung fields. What does the nurse suspect is causing this patient's symptoms?
    a. Pulmonary fluid overload due to fluid resuscitation
    b. Exposure to carbon monoxide that was undiagnosed
    c. Fat emboli secondary to extensive injury
    d. Excessive oxygen therapy at the first facility

47. The nurse is caring for several patients on the burn unit. Which of these patients has the most acute need for cardiac monitoring?
    a. Older adult woman who spilled hot water over her legs while boiling noodles
    b. Teenager with facial burns that occurred when he threw gasoline on a campfire
    c. Young woman who was struck by lightning while jogging on the beach
    d. Middle-aged man who fell asleep while smoking and sustained burns to the chest

48. A patient is transported to the ED for severe and extensive burns that occurred while he was trapped in a burning building. The patient is severely injured with respiratory distress and the resuscitation team must immediately begin multiple interventions. Which task is delegated to unlicensed assistive personnel (UAP)?
a. Position the patient's head to open the airway and assist with intubation.
b. Assist the respiratory therapist to maintain a seal during bag-valve-mask ventilation.
c. Prepare the intubation equipment and set up the oxygen flowmeter.
d. Elevate the head of the bed to achieve a high-Fowler's position.

49. The nursing student notes on the care plan that the burn patient she is caring for is at risk for organ ischemia. Based on the student's knowledge of the pathophysiology of burns, which etiology does the nursing student select?
a. Related to hypovolemia and myoglobin release
b. Related to fluid overload and peripheral edema
c. Related to prolonged resuscitation and hypoxia
d. Related to direct blunt trauma to the kidneys

50. The student nurse is caring for a patient who has been in the burn unit for several weeks. The patient needs assistance with the bedpan to have a bowel movement, and the student nurse notes that the stool is black with a tarry appearance. What does the student nurse do next?
a. Report this finding to the primary nurse or the instructor.
b. Obtain a stool specimen to be sent to the laboratory for analysis.
c. Test for the presence of occult blood with a hemoccult card and reagent.
d. Perform a dietary assessment to determine if the stool color is related to food.

51. A patient who lives in a rural community sustained severe burns during a house fire at 10 AM. The rural EMS started a peripheral IV at 11:00 AM at a keep vein open (KVO) rate. The patient was admitted to the hospital at 1:00 PM. In calculating the fluid replacement, at what time is the fluid for the first 8-hour period completed?
a. 6:00 PM
b. 7:00 PM
c. 8:00 PM
d. 9:00 PM

52. A patient in the burn intensive care unit weighed 80 kg (preburn weight). The physician orders titration of IV fluid to achieve 0.5 mL/kg/hr urine output. What is the minimal hourly urine output for this patient?
_____ mL/hr

53. A burn patient with which condition is most likely to have mannitol (Osmitrol) ordered as part of the drug therapy?
a. Peripheral edema associated with burns on the lower extremities
b. Inhalation burns around the mouth causing mucosal swelling
c. Electrical burn and myoglobin in the urine
d. Smoke inhalation and superficial burns to the forearms

54. A patient was admitted to the burn unit approximately 6 hours ago after being rescued from a burning building. In the ED, he reported a dry, irritated throat "from breathing in the fumes," but otherwise had no airway complaints. During the shift, the nurse notes that the patient has suddenly developed marked stridor. The nurse anticipates preparing the patient for which emergency procedure?
a. Bronchoscopy
b. Intubation
c. Needle thoracotomy
d. Escharotomy

55. A patient was admitted for burns to the upper extremities after being trapped in a burning structure. The patient is also at risk for inadequate oxygenation related to inhalation of smoke and superheated fumes. Which diagnostic test best monitors this patient's gas exchange?
    a. Complete blood count
    b. Myoglobin level
    c. Carboxyhemoglobin level
    d. Chest x-ray

56. A patient in the burn intensive care unit is receiving vecuronium (Norcuron). What is the priority nursing intervention for this patient?
    a. Have emergency intubation equipment at the bedside.
    b. Ensure that all the equipment alarms are on and functional.
    c. Closely monitor the patient's urinary output every hour.
    d. Ensure that daily drug levels and electrolyte values are obtained.

57. The priority expected outcome during the resuscitation phase of a burn injury is to maintain which factor?
    a. The airway
    b. Cardiac output
    c. Fluid replacement
    d. Patient comfort

58. Which statement about the resuscitation phase of a burn injury is accurate?
    a. It occurs in the prehospital timeframe.
    b. It continues for about 4 hours after the burn.
    c. It continues for about 48 hours after the burn.
    d. It continues until the patient is stable.

59. The release of myoglobin from damaged muscle in patients with major burns can result in which potential complication?
    a. Paralytic ileus
    b. Acute kidney injury
    c. Limited mobility
    d. Hypovolemia

60. A burn patient in the fluid resuscitation phase is experiencing dyspnea. What are the priority interventions for this patient? *(Select all that apply.)*
    a. Elevate the head of bed to 45 degrees.
    b. Maintain patient in the supine position.
    c. Notify the Rapid Response Team.
    d. Administer an analgesic to calm the patient.
    e. Apply humidified oxygen.

61. The vasodilating effects of carbon monoxide in patients with carbon monoxide poisoning cause what clinical manifestation?
    a. Cyanosis around the lips
    b. Generalized pallor
    c. Cherry-red skin color
    d. Mottled skin color

62. The nurse is caring for a burn patient about to undergo hydrotherapy. Which complementary therapies are appropriate for pain management in this patient? *(Select all that apply.)*
    a. Administration of IV opioid analgesics
    b. Allowing the patient to make decisions regarding pain control
    c. Playing music in the background
    d. Use of meditative breathing
    e. Use of guided imagery

63. A burn patient refuses to eat. The potential problem of weight loss related to increased metabolic rate and reduced calorie intake is identified for this patient. What method does the nurse use to correctly weigh this patient?
    a. Weigh once a week after morning hygiene and compare to previous weight.
    b. Weigh daily at the same time of day and compare to preburn weight.
    c. Use a bed scale and subtract the estimated weight of linens.
    d. Weigh daily without dressings or splints and compare to preburn weight.

64. The student nurse is preparing to assist with hydrotherapy for a burn patient. The supervising nurse instructs the student to obtain the necessary equipment before beginning the procedure. What equipment does the student nurse obtain? *(Select all that apply.)*
    a. Scissors and forceps
    b. Hydrogen peroxide
    c. Mild soap or detergent
    d. Pressure dressings
    e. Washcloths and gauze sponges
    f. Chlorhexidine sponges

65. The nurse is applying a dressing to cover a burn on a patient's left leg. What technique does the nurse use?
    a. Consider the depth of the injury and amount of drainage, and work distal to proximal.
    b. Change the dressing every 4 hours or when the drainage leaks through the dressing.
    c. Consider the patient's mobility and the area of injury, and work proximal to distal.
    d. Use multiple gauze layers and roller gauze to pad and protect the joint areas.

66. The nurse has just received a phone report on a burn patient being transferred from the burn intensive care unit to the step-down burn unit. Which task is appropriate to delegate to unlicensed assistive personnel (UAP) in order to prepare the room?
    a. Place sterile sheets and a sterile pillowcase on the bed.
    b. Place a new disposable stethoscope in the room.
    c. Clear a space in the corner for the patient's flowers.
    d. Hang a sign on the door to prohibit entry of visitors.

67. The nurse is monitoring the nutritional status of a burn patient. Which indicators does the nurse use? *(Select all that apply.)*
    a. Amount of food the patient eats
    b. Weight to height ratio
    c. Serum albumin
    d. Amount of water the patient drinks
    e. Blood glucose
    f. Serum potassium

68. The nurse is educating a patient who has sustained burns to the dominant hand. What kind of active range of motion exercises does the nurse instruct the patient to perform?
    a. Exercise the hand, thumb, and fingers every hour while awake.
    b. Exercise the fingers and thumb at least three times a day.
    c. Use the hands to perform activities of daily living.
    d. Squeeze a soft rubber ball several times a day.

69. A burn patient must have pressure dressings applied to prevent contractures and reduce scarring. For maximum effectiveness, what procedure pertaining to the pressure garments is implemented?
    a. Changed every 24 to 48 hours to prevent infection
    b. Worn at least 23 hours a day until the scar tissue matures
    c. Removed for hygiene and during sleeping
    d. Applied with aseptic technique

70. The family reports that the burn patient is unable to perform self-care measures, so someone has been "doing everything for her." The nurse finds that the patient has the knowledge and the physical capacity to independently perform self-care. What is the nurse's best response?
    a. "What can your family do to help you feel better and stronger?"
    b. "You should be doing these things for yourself to increase your self-esteem."
    c. "What has been happening since you were discharged from the hospital?"
    d. "Let's review the principles of self-care that you learned in the hospital."

71. A patient who sustained severe burns to the face with significant scarring and disfigurement will soon be discharged from the hospital. Which intervention is best to help the patient make the transition into the community?
    a. Discuss cosmetic surgery that could occur over the next several years.
    b. Focus on the positive aspects of going home and being with family.
    c. Teach the family to perform all aspects of care for the patient.
    d. Encourage visits from friends and short public appearances before discharge.

72. What does the process of full-thickness wound healing include? *(Select all that apply.)*
    a. Healing occurs by wound contraction.
    b. Eschar must be removed.
    c. Large blisters are protective and left undisturbed.
    d. Skin grafting may be necessary.
    e. Fasciotomy may be needed to relieve pressure and allow normal blood flow.

73. Which statement about the third-spacing or capillary leak syndrome in a patient with severe burns is accurate?
    a. It usually happens in the first 36 to 48 hours.
    b. It is a leak of plasma fluids into the interstitial space.
    c. It is present only in the burned tissues.
    d. It can usually be prevented with diuretics.

74. As a result of third-spacing, during the acute phase, which electrolyte imbalances may occur? *(Select all that apply.)*
    a. Hyperkalemia
    b. Hypokalemia
    c. Hypernatremia
    d. Hyponatremia
    e. Hypokalemia
    f. Hypercalcemia

75. Because of the fluid shifts in burn patients, what effects on cardiac output does the nurse expect to see?
    a. An initial increase, then normalized in 24 to 48 hours
    b. Depressed up to 36 hours after the burn
    c. Improved with fluid restriction
    d. Responsive to diuretics as evidenced by urinary output

76. A patient with burn injuries is being discharged from the hospital. What important points does the nurse include in the discharge teaching? *(Select all that apply.)*
    a. Signs and symptoms of infection
    b. Drug regimens and potential medication side effects
    c. Definition of full-thickness burns
    d. Correct application and care of pressure garments
    e. Comfort measures to reduce scarring
    f. Dates for follow-up appointments

77. A patient has sustained significant burns which have created a hypermetabolic state. In planning care for this patient, what does the nurse consider?
    a. Increased retention of sodium
    b. Decreased secretion of catecholamines
    c. Increased caloric needs
    d. The decrease in core temperature

78. The nurse is reviewing the laboratory results for several burn patients who are approximately 24 to 36 hours postinjury. What laboratory results related to the fluid remobilization in these patients does the nurse expect to see?
    a. Anemia
    b. Metabolic alkalosis
    c. Hypernatremia
    d. Hyperkalemia

79. Local tissue resistance to electricity varies in different parts of the body. Which tissue has the *most* resistance?
    a. Skin epidermis
    b. Tendons and muscle
    c. Fatty tissue
    d. Nerve tissue and blood vessels

80. A patient was rescued from a burning house and treated with oxygen. Initially, the patient had audible wheezing and wheezing on auscultation, but after approximately 30 minutes the wheezing stopped. The patient now demonstrates substernal retractions and anxiety. What action does the nurse take at this time?
    a. Recognize an impending airway obstruction and prepare for immediate intubation.
    b. Continue to monitor the patient's respiratory status and initiate pulse oximetry.
    c. Document this finding as evidence of improvement and continue to observe.
    d. Stay with and encourage the patient to remain calm and breathe deeply.

81. The nurse is caring for a young woman who sustained burns on the upper extremities and anterior chest while attempting to put out a kitchen grease fire. Which laboratory results does the nurse expect to see during the resuscitation phase? *(Select all that apply.)*
    a. Potassium level of 3.2 mEq/L
    b. Glucose level of 180 mg/dL
    c. Hematocrit of 49%
    d. pH of 7.20
    e. Sodium level of 139 mEq/L

True or False? *Read each statement about the correct procedure for débridement and write T for true or F for false in the blanks provided.*

_____ 82. Eschar and other cellular debris are removed from the wound.

_____ 83. Nonviable tissue is removed during hydrotherapy.

_____ 84. Sterile saline is used during débridement.

_____ 85. Small blisters are usually opened.

_____ 86. Includes both mechanical and enzymatic actions.

87. A patient has sustained a burn to the right ankle. The physician has applied the initial dressing to the ankle, and the nurse assists the patient into bed and positions the ankle to prevent contracture. What is the correct position the nurse uses?
    a. Dorsiflexion
    b. Adduction
    c. External rotation
    d. Hyperextension

88. A patient has sustained a severe burn greater than 30% TBSA. What is the best way to assess renal function in this patient?
    a. Measure urine output and compare this value with fluid intake.
    b. Weigh the patient every day and compare that to the dry weight.
    c. Note the amount of edema and measure abdominal girth.
    d. Assist the patient with a urinal or bedpan every 2 hours.

89. The nurse is caring for an African-American patient with a burn injury. The patient appears to be having severe pain and discomfort that are unrelated to the burned areas. The nurse advocates that the physician order which additional test?
    a. Sickle cell for trait
    b. Drug screen for opiate abuse
    c. X-rays to identify bone injuries
    d. ECG to identify cardiac dysrhythmias

90. The physician has ordered an escharotomy for a patient because of constriction around the patient's chest. The nurse is teaching the patient and family about the procedure. Which statement by the family indicates a need for additional teaching?
    a. "He doesn't do well under general anesthesia."
    b. "He'll be awake for the procedure."
    c. "He will receive medication for sedation and pain."
    d. "We could stay with him at the bedside during the procedure."

91. The nurse is caring for a firefighter who was brought in for burns around the face and upper chest. Airway maintenance for this patient with respiratory involvement includes what action?
    a. Monitoring for signs and symptoms of upper airway edema during fluid resuscitation
    b. Inserting a nasopharyngeal or oropharyngeal airway when the patient's airway is completely obstructed
    c. Obtaining an order for PRN oxygen per nasal cannula
    d. Frequently suctioning the mouth with a Yankauer suction

92. At what point does fluid mobilization occur in patients with burns?
    a. After the scar tissue is formed and fluids are no longer being lost.
    b. Within the first 4 hours after the burns were sustained.
    c. After 36 hours when the fluid is reabsorbed from the interstitial tissue.
    d. Immediately after the burns occur.

93. The nurse is caring for a patient with chronic pain associated with an old burn injury. Which nonpharmacologic intervention does the nurse use to help relieve the patient's pain?
    a. Nitrous oxide
    b. Cool room temperature to reduce discomfort
    c. Massaging nonburned areas
    d. Intravenous narcotics due to delayed tissue absorption

Matching. *Match the different types of dressing materials with their descriptions.*

Dressing Materials
a. Artificial skin
b. Xenograft
c. Allograft
d. Biobrane
e. Cultured skin
f. Amniotic membrane
g. Synthetic dressing

Descriptions
_____ 94. Biologic dressing from a cadaver provided by a skin bank

_____ 95. Membrane obtained from an animal donor

_____ 96. Does not develop a blood supply; it disintegrates in about 48 hours

_____ 97. Cells are grown in a laboratory to produce cell sheets

_____ 98. Silastic epidermis and a porous dermis made from beef collagen and shark cartilage

_____ 99. Made up of a nylon fabric that is partially embedded into a silicone film

_____ 100. Made of solid silicone and plastic membranes

101. A patient with a burn injury had an autograft. The nurse learns in report that the donor site is on the upper thigh. What type of wound does the nurse expect to find at donor site?
    a. Stage 1
    b. Partial-thickness
    c. Full-thickness
    d. Stage 4

102. To prevent the complication of Curling's ulcer, what does the nurse anticipate the physician will order?
    a. Nasogastric tube insertion
    b. H_2 histamine blockers
    c. Abdominal assessment every 4 hours
    d. Systemic antibiotic

103. Several patients are transported from an industrial fire to a local ED. Which factors increase the risk of death for these patients? *(Select all that apply.)*
    a. Male gender
    b. Age greater than 60 years
    c. Burn greater than 40% TBSA
    d. Presence of an inhalation injury
    e. Presence of contact burns

104. What is the most essential patient data needed for calculating the fluid rates, energy requirements, and drug doses for the burn patient?
    a. Age
    b. Previous health history
    c. Preburn weight
    d. Current weight

105. Which drug therapy reduces the risk of wound infection for burn patients?
    a. Large doses of oral antifungal medications every 4 hours
    b. Silver nitrate solution covered by dry dressings applied every 4 hours
    c. Silver sulfadiazine (Silvadene) on full-thickness injuries every 4 hours
    d. Broad-spectrum antibiotics given intravenously

106. A patient has sustained a relatively large burn. The nurse anticipates that the patient's nutritional requirements may exceed how many kcal/day?
    a. 1500
    b. 2000
    c. 3000
    d. 5000

107. Which feelings are most typically expressed by the burn patient? *(Select all that apply.)*
    a. Suspicion
    b. Regression
    c. Apathy
    d. Denial
    e. Suicidal ideations
    f. Anger

108. A patient has been depressed and withdrawn since her injury and has expressed that "life will never be the same." Which nursing intervention best promotes a positive image for this burn patient?
    a. Discussing the possibility of reconstructive surgery with the patient
    b. Allowing the patient to choose a colorful scarf to cover the burned area
    c. Playing cards or board games with the patient
    d. Encouraging the patient to consider how fortunate she is to be alive

109. A 28-year-old male patient sustained second- and third-degree burns on his legs (30%) when his clothing caught fire while he was burning leaves. He was hosed down by his neighbor and has arrived at the ED in severe discomfort. What is the priority problem for this patient at this time?
    a. Acute pain related to damaged or exposed nerve endings
    b. Decreased fluid volume related to electrolyte imbalance
    c. Potential for inadequate oxygenation
    d. Diminished self-image related to the appearance of legs

110. Which patient has the highest risk for a fatal burn injury?
    a. 4-year-old child
    b. 32-year-old man
    c. 45-year-old woman
    d. 77-year-old man

111. **Crossword Puzzle.** Complete the crossword puzzle by answering the questions below.

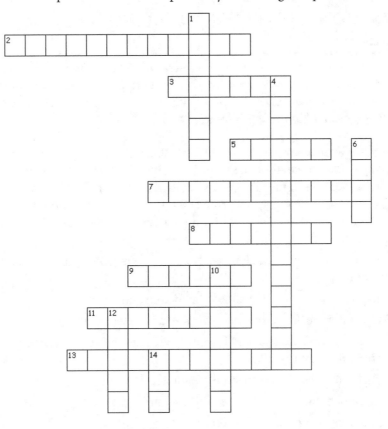

Across

2. A patient has noticed that the skin is peeling off 3 days after a severe sunburn. What is this called?

3. Also known as "burn crust."

5. The nurse monitors for this severe complication of a full-thickness burn by watching for tachycardia, decreased blood pressure, decreased peripheral pulses, and other signs of decreased cardiac output.

7. After spending the day at the beach, a teenage girl has a severe sunburn. This is an example of a _____-thickness burn.

8. _____-thickness burn involves the entire epidermis and varying parts of the dermis.

9. To assess whether a superficial partial-thickness wound is present, the nurse notes that the wound is red, moist, and _____ when pressure is applied.

11. A patient is admitted to a burn trauma unit after suffering a severe electrical shock. He is in the _____ phase of burn injury.

13. The patient in Question 11 has severe edema. This is due to a fluid shift, known as _____ _____ (two words).

Down

1. A patient who was admitted with a severe burn after spilling hot liquid on his legs will be receiving a heterograft. The most common heterograft, which is compatible with human skin, is made from _____.

4. After 48 hours, the patient in Question 11 begins to produce large amounts of urine. This is known as fluid _____.

6. A patient is admitted after a house fire with severe burns across her body. The burns have destroyed the entire epidermis and dermis layers. This is known as a _____-thickness wound.

10. A camper spills bacon grease on his foot while cooking breakfast. This type of burn is a ____ burn.

12. An older adult man tips over a tea kettle with boiling water and burns the skin of his abdomen and thighs. This type of heat injury is a _____ burn, or a scald.

14. A patient suffers burns on her arms after the sleeves of her robe catch fire while she is cooking breakfast. This type of burn injury is known as a _____ heat injury.

CASE STUDY: THE OLDER ADULT WITH SEVERE BURNS

Use a separate sheet of paper to answer the questions in this Case Study, or go to the "Prepare for Class" folder on your Evolve website at http://evolve.elsevier.com/Iggy/ to download and complete as a word processing file. Answer guidelines for this Case Study are also available on your Evolve website.

An older adult woman arrives in the ED at 11:00 AM. According to her family, she was cooking and accidentally spilled a pot of boiling liquids while trying to move the pan from the stove to the table. She sustained severe burns on her arms, anterior trunk, and legs. The injury occurred at 9:00 AM, but she was home alone and tried to administer first aid before notifying her family. She weighs 70 kg and the burns are estimated at 50% TBSA.

1. Identify the age-related changes that increase morbidity and mortality in the older adult.

2. Identify information that should be included in a history.

3. Why is it important to evaluate the size and extent of the burn?

4. Using the Parkland (Baxter) formula, calculate the fluids needed for the first 8 hours after injury.

5. What time does the first 8-hour period end?

6. How much fluid is required for the 24 hours?

7. Hourly urine output is adjusted to _____ mL/kg.

8. Tissue destruction caused by a burn injury causes local and systemic problems. Identify six of these potential problems.

9. Early detection of wound infection is important. The wound should be examined for which six signs of infection?

10. Identify priority problems for patients with burn injuries in the resuscitation phase who have sustained a burn injury greater than 25% TBSA.

11. The patient reported severe pain in the areas of the burn, rated as an 8 on the 0-10 pain scale. The nurse administered 1 mg IV dilaudid. Use the focus charting method (also known as the DAR method—data, action, response) to document this.

29 CHAPTER

Assessment of the Respiratory System

STUDY/REVIEW QUESTIONS

Matching. Match each function/description of the airway with its corresponding location.

Locations
a. Upper airway
b. Lower airway

Functions/Descriptions

_____ 1. Traps particles not filtered by nares

_____ 2. Traps organisms entering nose and mouth

_____ 3. Trachea

_____ 4. Contains cilia to move mucus to trachea

_____ 5. Composed of alveoli for gas exchange

_____ 6. Pharynx, or throat

_____ 7. Place where the trachea divides into the right and left bronchi

_____ 8. Larynx

_____ 9. Dividing point where solid foods and fluids are separated from air

_____ 10. Epiglottis

_____ 11. Pleura

_____ 12. Alveoli

13. A patient comes to the health care provider's office for an annual physical. The patient reports having a persistent nagging cough. Which question does the nurse ask first about this symptom?
    a. "When did the cough start?"
    b. "Do you have a family history of lung cancer?"
    c. "Have you been running a fever"
    d. "Do you have sneezing and congestion?"

14. When blood passes through the lungs, oxygen _____ from the alveoli into the red blood cells.

15. A patient reports smoking a pack of cigarettes a day for 9 years. He then quit for 2 years, then smoked 2 packs a day for the last 30 years. What are the pack-years for this patient?
    a. 39 years
    b. 69 years
    c. 19.5 years
    d. 41 years

16. Pulmonary function tests are scheduled for a patient with a history of smoking who reports dyspnea and chronic cough. What will patient teaching information about this procedure include?

    a. Do not smoke for at least 2 weeks before the test.
    b. Bronchodilator drugs may be withheld 2 days before the test.
    c. The patient will breathe through the mouth and wear a nose clip during the test.
    d. The patient will be expected to walk on a treadmill during the test.

17. A patient is scheduled to have a pulmonary function test (PFT). Which type of information does the nurse include in the nursing history so that PFT results can be appropriately determined?

    a. Age, gender, race, height, weight, and smoking status
    b. Occupational status, activity tolerance for activities of daily living
    c. Medication history and history of allergies to contrast media
    d. History of chronic medical conditions and surgical procedures

Matching. *Match each PFT with its description.*

PFTs
a. Forced expiratory volume (FEV)
b. Functional residual capacity (FRC)
c. Forced vital capacity (FVC)
d. Residual volume (RV)
e. Total lung capacity (TLC)

Descriptions

_____ 18. Maximal amount of forced air that can be exhaled after maximal inspiration

_____ 19. Amount of air in lungs at the end of maximal inhalation

_____ 20. Amount of air remaining in lungs after normal exhalation

_____ 21. Maximal amount of air that can be exhaled over a specific time

_____ 22. Amount of air remaining in lungs at the end of full, forced exhalation

23. The nurse is caring for an older adult who uses a wheelchair and spends over half of each day in bed. Which intervention is important in promoting pulmonary hygiene related to age and decreased mobility?

    a. Obtain an order for PRN oxygen via nasal cannula.
    b. Encourage the patient to turn, cough, and deep-breathe.
    c. Reassure the patient that immobility is temporary.
    d. Monitor the respiratory rate and check pulse oximetry readings.

24. The nurse is assessing a middle-aged patient who reports a decreased tolerance for exercise and that she must work harder to breathe. Which questions assist the nurse in determining what these changes are related to? *(Select all that apply.)*

    a. "Do you have anemia?"
    b. "When did you first notice these symptoms?"
    c. "Do you or have you ever smoked cigarettes?"
    d. "How often do you exercise?"
    e. "Are you coughing up any colored sputum?"

25. A patient has had a bronchoscopy and was NPO for several hours before the test. Now a few hours after the test, the patient is hungry and would like to eat a meal. What does the nurse do?
    a. Order a meal because the patient is now alert and oriented.
    b. Check pulse oximetry to be sure oxygen saturation has returned to normal.
    c. Check for a gag reflex before allowing the patient to eat.
    d. Assess for nausea from the medications given for the test.

26. After a bronchoscopy procedure, the patient coughs up sputum which contains blood. What is the best nursing intervention for this patient?
    a. Assess vital signs and respiratory status and notify the physician of the findings.
    b. Monitor the patient for 24 hours to see if blood continues in the sputum.
    c. Send the sputum to the lab for cytology for possible lung cancer.
    d. Reassure the patient this is a normal response after a bronchoscopy.

27. Before a bronchoscopy procedure, the patient received benzocaine spray as a topical anesthetic to numb the oropharynx. The nurse is assessing the patient after the procedure. Which finding suggests that the patient is developing methemoglobinemia?
    a. The patient has a decreased hematocrit level.
    b. The patient does not respond to supplemental oxygen.
    c. The blood sample is a bright cherry-red color.
    d. The patient experiences sedation and amnesia.

28. The nurse is caring for several patients who had diagnostic testing for respiratory disorders. Which diagnostic test has the highest risk for the postprocedure complication of pneumothorax?
    a. Bronchoscopy
    b. Laryngoscopy
    c. Computed tomography of lungs
    d. Percutaneous lung biopsy

29. A patient's pulse oximetry reading is 89%. What is the nurse's priority action?
    a. Recheck the reading with a different oximeter.
    b. Apply supplemental oxygen and recheck the oximeter reading in 15 minutes.
    c. Assess the patient for respiratory distress and recheck the oximeter reading.
    d. Place the patient in the recovery position and monitor frequently.

30. A patient demonstrates labored shallow respirations and a respiratory rate of 32/min with a pulse oximetry reading of 85%. What is the priority nursing intervention?
    a. Notify respiratory therapy to give the patient a breathing treatment.
    b. Start oxygen via nasal cannula at 2 L/min.
    c. Obtain an order for a stat arterial blood gas (ABG).
    d. Encourage coughing and deep-breathing exercises.

31. Which factors or conditions cause a decreased (below normal) $PETCO_2$ level due to abnormal ventilation? *(Select all that apply.)*
    a. Hyperthermia
    b. Hypotension
    c. Apnea
    d. Hyperventilation
    e. Hypothermia

32. The nurse is reviewing ABG results from an 86-year-old patient. Which results would be considered normal findings for a patient of this age?
    a. Normal pH, normal Pao_2, normal $Paco_2$
    b. Normal pH, decreased Pao_2, normal $Paco_2$
    c. Decreased pH, decreased Pao_2, normal $Paco_2$
    d. Decreased pH, decreased Pao_2, decreased $Paco_2$

33. Upon performing a lung sound assessment of the anterior chest, the nurse hears moderately loud sounds on inspiration that are equal in length with expiration. In what area is this lung sound considered normal?
    a. Trachea
    b. Primary bronchi
    c. Lung fields
    d. Larynx

34. Which sounds in the smaller bronchioles and the alveoli indicate normal lung sounds?
    a. Harsh, hollow, and tubular blowing
    b. Nothing; normally no sounds are heard
    c. Soft, low rustling; like wind in the trees
    d. Flat and dull tones with a moderate pitch

35. What is the characteristic of normal lung sounds that should be heard throughout the lung fields?
    a. Short inspiration, long expiration, loud, harsh
    b. Soft sound, long inspiration, short quiet expiration
    c. Mixed sounds of harsh and soft, long inspiration and long expiration
    d. Loud, long inspiration and short, loud expiration

36. Upon assessing the lungs, the nurse hears short, discrete popping sounds "like hair being rolled between fingers near the ear" in the bilateral lower lobes. How is this assessment documented?
    a. Rhonchi
    b. Wheezes
    c. Fine crackles
    d. Coarse crackles

37. The nurse is taking a history on a patient who reports sleeping in a recliner chair at night because lying on the bed causes shortness of breath. How is this documented?
    a. Orthopnea
    b. Paroxysmal nocturnal dyspnea
    c. Orthostatic nocturnal dyspnea
    d. Tachypnea

38. On the diagram below, indicate the correct sequence (1 through 26) for percussion and auscultation for the anteroposterior assessment of the lungs.

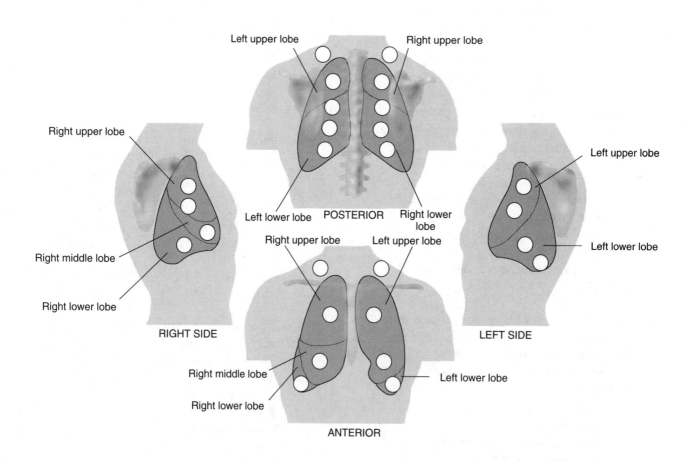

39. What conditions shift the curve to the right, meaning hemoglobin will dissociate oxygen? *(Select all that apply.)*
    a. Increased carbon dioxide concentration
    b. Decreased tissue concentration of glucose breakdown products
    c. Increased tissue pH (alkalosis)
    d. Decreased tissue temperature
    e. Decreased tissue pH (acidosis)

40. What observations does the nurse make when performing a general assessment of a patient's lungs and thorax? *(Select all that apply.)*
    a. Symmetry of chest movement
    b. Rate, rhythm, and depth of respirations
    c. Use of accessory muscles for breathing
    d. Comparison of the anteroposterior diameter with the lateral diameter
    e. Measurement of the length of the chest cavity
    f. Assessment of chest expansion and respiratory excursion

41. Which assessment finding is an objective sign of chronic oxygen deprivation?
    a. Continuous cough productive of clear sputum
    b. Audible inspiratory and expiratory wheeze
    c. Chest pain that increases with deep inspiration
    d. Clubbing of fingernails and a barrel-shaped chest

42. The nurse is palpating a patient's chest and identifies an increased tactile fremitus or vibration of the chest wall produced when the patient speaks. What does the nurse do next?
    a. Observe for other findings associated with subcutaneous emphysema.
    b. Document the observation as an expected normal finding.
    c. Observe the patient for other findings associated with a pneumothorax.
    d. Document the observation as a pleural friction rub.

43. The nurse reviews the complete blood count results for the patient who has chronic obstructive pulmonary disease (COPD) and lives in a high mountain area. What lab results does the nurse expect to see for this patient?
    a. Increased red blood cells
    b. Decreased neutrophils
    c. Decreased eosinophils
    d. Increased lymphocytes

44. The nurse is inspecting a patient's chest and observes an increase in anteroposterior diameter of the chest. When is this an expected finding?
    a. With a pulmonary mass
    b. Upon deep inhalation
    c. In older adult patients
    d. With chest trauma

45. While percussing a patient's chest and lung fields, the nurse notes a high, loud, musical, drumlike sound similar to tapping a cheek that is puffed out with air. What is the nurse's priority action?
    a. Document this expected finding using words like, "high," "loud," and "hollow."
    b. Immediately notify the physician because the patient has an airway obstruction.
    c. Assess the patient for air hunger or pain at the end of inhalation and exhalation.
    d. Palpate for crackling sensation underneath the skin or for localized tenderness.

46. What is the best position for a patient to assume for a thoracentesis?
    a. Side-lying, affected side exposed, head slightly raised
    b. Lying flat with arm on affected side across the chest
    c. Sitting up, leaning forward on the overbed table
    d. Prone position with arms above the head

47. Which procedure has a risk for the complication of pneumothorax?
    a. Thoracentesis
    b. Bronchoscopy
    c. PFT
    d. Ventilation-perfusion scan

48. A patient has undergone a percutaneous lung biopsy. After the procedure, what tests are done to confirm that there is no pneumothorax? *(Select all that apply.)*
    a. Computed tomography
    b. Pulmonary function test
    c. Magnetic resonance imaging
    d. Digital chest radiography
    e. Chest x-ray

49. The respiratory therapist consults with and reports to the nurse on the sputum production of several respiratory patients. The patient producing which kind of sputum needs priority attention?
    a. Thick and yellow
    b. Watery mucoid
    c. Pink and frothy
    d. Rust-colored

50. A patient who had a thoracentesis is now experiencing the following clinical manifestations: rapid shallow respirations, rapid heart rate, and pain on the affected side that is worse at the end of inhalation. The nurse assesses that this patient has developed a

    _____.

51. For what reasons would a patient have a bronchoscopy? *(Select all that apply.)*
    a. Obtain samples for cultures
    b. Diagnose pulmonary disease
    c. View upper airway structures
    d. Administer medications
    e. Obtain samples for biopsy

52. The nurse has just received a patient from the recovery room who is somewhat drowsy, but is capable of following instructions. Pulse oximetry has dropped from 95% to 90%. What is the priority nursing intervention?
    a. Administer oxygen at 2 L/min by nasal cannula, then reassess.
    b. Have the patient perform coughing and deep-breathing exercises, then reassess.
    c. Administer Narcan to reverse narcotic sedation effect.
    d. Withhold narcotic pain medication to reduce sedation effect.

Matching. *Match the pulmonary function capacities and functions with the correct corresponding assessment findings. One answer will not be used.*

Capacities and Functions
a. Forced vital capacity (FVC)
b. Forced expiratory volume in 1 sec (FEV_1)
c. Forced expiratory flow (FEF)
d. Functional residual capacity (FRC)
e. Diffusion capacity of carbon monoxide (DLCO)

Assessment Findings

_____ 53. Reduced in patients with obstructive disease and increased with exercise or congestive heart failure

_____ 54. After a maximum deep breath, amount of air quickly exhaled

_____ 55. Not used to measure larger airway obstructions

_____ 56. After a maximum deep breath, the maximum amount of air exhaled in the first 1 second

57. What is a pulse oximeter used to measure?
    a. Oxygen perfusion in the extremities
    b. Pulse and perfusion in the extremities
    c. Generalized tissue perfusion
    d. Oxygen saturation in the red blood cells

58. Which aspect of PFTs would be considered a normal result in the older adult?
    a. Increased forced vital capacity
    b. Decline in forced expiratory volume in 1 second
    c. Decrease in diffusion capacity of carbon monoxide
    d. Increased functional residual capacity

59. In the older adult, there is a loss of elastic recoiling of the lung and decreased chest wall compliance. What is the result of this occurrence?
    a. The thoracic area becomes shorter.
    b. The patient has an increased activity tolerance.
    c. There is an increase in anteroposterior ratio.
    d. The patient has severe shortness of breath.

60. In the older adult, there is a decreased number of functional alveoli. To assist the patient to compensate for this change related to aging, what does the nurse do?
    a. Encourage the patient to ambulate and change positions.
    b. Allow the patient to rest and sleep frequently.
    c. Have face-to-face conversations when possible.
    d. Obtain an order for supplemental oxygen.

61. The nurse teaches a patient about the impact of cigarette smoking on the lower respiratory tract. Which statement by the patient indicates an understanding of the information?
    a. "Smoking increases my susceptibility to respiratory infections."
    b. "If I stop smoking the damage to my lungs will be reversed."
    c. "Cigarette smoke affects my ability to cough out secretions from the lungs."
    d. "Smoking makes the large and small airways get bigger."

62. A patient reports fatigue and shortness of breath when getting up to walk to the bathroom; however, the pulse oximetry reading is 99%. The nurse identifies a diagnosis of Activity intolerance. Which laboratory value is consistent with the patient's subjective symptoms?
    a. BUN of 15 mg/dL
    b. WBC count of 8000/mm^3
    c. Hemoglobin of 9 g/dL
    d. Glucose 160 mg/dL

63. The nurse is performing a respiratory assessment including pulse oximetry on several patients. Which conditions or situations may cause an artificially low reading? *(Select all that apply.)*
    a. Fever
    b. Anemia
    c. Receiving narcotic pain medications
    d. Peripheral artery disease
    e. History of respiratory disease such as cystic fibrosis or tuberculosis

64. A patient who had neck surgery for removal of a tumor reports "not being able to breathe very well." The nurse observes that the patient has decreased chest movement and an elevated pulse. A bronchoscopy is ordered. For what reason did the physician order a bronchoscopy for this patient?
    a. Reverse and relieve any obstruction caused during the neck surgery
    b. Assess the function of vocal cords or remove foreign bodies from the larynx
    c. Aspirate pleural fluid or air from the pleural space
    d. Visualize the larynx (airway structures) to use as a guide for intubation

65. A patient returns to the unit after bronchoscopy. In addition to respiratory status assessment, which assessment does the nurse make in order to prevent aspiration?
    a. Presence of pain or soreness in throat
    b. Time and amount of last oral fluid intake
    c. Type and location of chest pain
    d. Presence or absence of gag reflex

66. The nurse hears fine crackles during a lung assessment of the patient who is in the initial postoperative period. Which nursing intervention helps relieve this respiratory problem?
    a. Monitor the patient with a pulse oximeter.
    b. Encourage coughing and deep-breathing.
    c. Obtain an order for a chest x-ray.
    d. Obtain an order for high-flow oxygen.

67. In performing a respiratory assessment, which finding is considered the principal or main sign of respiratory disease?
    a. Sputum production
    b. Continuous cough
    c. Fever with congestion
    d. Increased respiratory rate

68. When assessing the distance between the ribs (intercostal space) on a patient with emphysema, the distance is (increased or decreased).

69. A patient with a pH of 7.48 and respiratory difficulties indicates respiratory _____.

70. The nurse is performing a respiratory assessment on an older adult patient. Which question is not appropriate to ask when using the Gordon's Functional Health Pattern Assessment approach?
    a. "How has your general health been?"
    b. "Have you had any colds this past year?"
    c. "Do you have sufficient energy to do what you like to do?"
    d. "When was the last time you were hospitalized?"

71. Tissue oxygen delivery through dissociation from hemoglobin is based on which factor?
    a. Saturation
    b. Oxygen tension
    c. Unloading from hemoglobin
    d. Tissues' need for oxygen

72. The nurse makes observations about several respiratory patients' abilities to perform activities of daily living in order to quantify the level of dyspnea. Which patient is considered to have Class V dyspnea?
    a. Experiences subjective shortness of breath when walking up a flight of stairs
    b. Limited to bed or chair and experiences shortness of breath at rest
    c. Can independently shower and dress, but cannot keep pace with similarly aged people
    d. Experiences shortness of breath during aerobic exercise such as jogging

73. The nurse is reviewing the arterial blood gas results for a 25-year-old trauma patient who has new onset of shortness of breath and demonstrates shallow and irregular respirations. The arterial blood gas results are: pH, 7.26; P_{CO_2}, 47%; P_{O_2}, 89%; HCO_3, 24. What imbalance does the nurse suspect this patient has?
    a. Respiratory acidosis
    b. Respiratory alkalosis
    c. Metabolic acidosis
    d. Metabolic alkalosis

CASE STUDY: RESPIRATORY TRACT ASSESSMENT

Use a separate sheet of paper to answer the questions in this Case Study, or go to the "Prepare for Class" folder on your Evolve website at http://evolve.elsevier.com/Iggy/ to download and complete as a word processing file. Answer guidelines for this Case Study are also available on your Evolve website.

The adult patient reports to the pulmonary clinic reporting a productive cough that "won't go away." She is a 62-year-old married housewife whose children are grown. She smoked two packs of cigarettes per day for 20 years, but she has not smoked for the past 10 years. She contracted a "virus" 4 weeks ago, which "settled in her chest." Her usual remedies have not resulted in improvement in her status.

1. What additional subjective data should the nurse elicit from this patient?

2. What physical assessments should the nurse perform on this patient?

3. What effect does this patient's 10 years of not smoking have on the condition of her lungs?

4. The physician orders a chest x-ray and a sputum specimen. What should the nurse tell this patient about these tests?

5. Document a nursing note for the patient using the following format:
   • Chief complaint:
   • Nursing note:

After 1 week, this patient reports no improvement, and the chest x-ray results also indicate that there is no change. A bronchoscopy is scheduled to be done in the outpatient surgical unit the following day. (The physician would prefer to do an MRI scan, but the patient has an inner-ear implant.)

6. Prepare a teaching-learning plan for this patient regarding the bronchoscopy. Consider restrictions related to breathing during the procedure.

7. When the patient reports to the outpatient surgical unit the next morning, what assessments should the nurse make?

8. Both the patient and her husband are very anxious. Describe interventions that the nurse should implement to assist the patient and her spouse.

9. A topical anesthetic agent is applied to the pharynx immediately before the bronchoscopy is to begin. What is the purpose of this agent?

10. What special actions must the nurse take after the procedure is completed and the patient is taken to the PACU?

11. What equipment should be available when she arrives?

12. What are the reasons for having this equipment available?

30 CHAPTER

Care of Patients Requiring Oxygen Therapy or Tracheostomy

STUDY/REVIEW QUESTIONS

1. At what times is oxygen therapy needed for a patient? *(Select all that apply.)*
   a. To treat hypoxia
   b. To treat hypothermia
   c. To treat hypoxemia
   d. When the normal 35% oxygen level in the air is inadequate
   e. When the normal 21% oxygen level in the air is inadequate

2. Which conditions can increase the body's need for more oxygen? *(Select all that apply.)*
   a. Hypothyroid
   b. Sickle cell disease
   c. Infection in the blood
   d. Body temperature of 101° F
   e. Hemoglobin level of 8.7 g/dL

3. To improve a patient's oxygenation to a normal level, the amount of oxygen administered is based on which factors? *(Select all that apply.)*
   a. Symptom management only
   b. Pulse oximetry reading
   c. Respiratory assessment
   d. The patient's subjective complaints
   e. Arterial blood gas results

4. _____ is the result of constant pressure exerted by a tracheostomy cuff causing tracheal dilation and erosion of cartilage.

5. What are the hazards of administering oxygen therapy? *(Select all that apply.)*
   a. Oxygen supports and enhances combustion.
   b. Oxygen itself can burn.
   c. Each electrical outlet in the room must be covered if not in use.
   d. All electrical equipment in the room must be grounded.
   e. Solutions with high concentrations of alcohol or oil cannot be used in the room.

6. A patient requires home oxygen therapy. When the home health nurse enters the patient's home for the initial visit, he observes several issues that are safety hazards related to the patient's oxygen therapy. What hazards do these include? *(Select all that apply.)*
   a. Bottle of wine in the kitchen area
   b. Package of cigarettes on the coffee table
   c. Several decorative candles on the mantelpiece
   d. Grounded outlet with a green dot on the plate
   e. Electric fan with a frayed cord in the bathroom
   f. Computer with a three-pronged plug

7. Before completing the morning assessment, the nurse concludes that a patient is experiencing inadequate oxygenation and tissue perfusion as a result of respiratory problems. Which assessment findings support the nurse's conclusion? *(Select all that apply.)*
   a. Inspiratory and expiratory effort is shallow, even, and quiet.
   b. Patient must take a breath after every third or fourth word.
   c. Skin is pale, pink, and dry.
   d. Patient appears strained and fatigued.
   e. Pulse of 95 beats/min, respiratory rate of 30/min.
   f. Patient does not want to eat.

8. The home health nurse has been caring for a patient with a chronic respiratory disorder. Today the patient seems confused when she is normally alert and oriented x 3. What is the priority nursing action?
   a. Notify the physician about the mental status change.
   b. Take vital signs and check the pulse oximeter readings.
   c. Ask the patient's family when this behavior started.
   d. Perform a mental status examination.

9. The nurse is caring for several patients on a general medical-surgical unit. The nurse would question the necessity of oxygen therapy for a patient with which condition?
   a. Pulmonary edema with decreased arterial Po_2 levels
   b. Valve replacement with increased cardiac output
   c. Anemia with a decreased hemoglobin and hematocrit
   d. Sustained fever with an increased metabolic demand

10. When a patient is requiring oxygen therapy, what is important for the nurse to know?
   a. Patients require 1 to 10 L/min by nasal cannula in order for oxygen to be effective.
   b. Oxygen-induced hypoventilation is the priority when the $Paco_2$ levels are unknown.
   c. Why the patient is receiving oxygen, expected outcomes, and complications.
   d. The goal is the highest Fio_2 possible for the particular device being used.

11. A patient with chronic obstructive pulmonary disease (COPD) is admitted to the hospital with oxygen-induced hypoventilation. What is the respiratory stimulus to breathe for this patient?
   a. High carbon dioxide (60 to 65 mm Hg) level in the blood that rose over time
   b. Low level of carbon dioxide concentration in the blood, as sensed by the chemoreceptors in the brain
   c. Low level of oxygen concentration in the blood, as sensed by the peripheral chemoreceptors
   d. Oxygen narcosis which stimulates central chemoreceptors in the brain

12. The nurse is administering oxygen to a patient who is hypoxic and has chronic high levels of carbon dioxide. Which oxygen therapy prevents a respiratory complication for this patient?
   a. Fio_2 higher than the usual 2 to 4 L/min per nasal cannula
   b. Venturi mask of 40% for the delivery of oxygen
   c. Lower concentration of oxygen (1 to 2 L/min) per nasal cannula
   d. Variable Fio_2 via partial rebreather mask

13. A patient is at high risk or unknown risk for oxygen-induced hypoventilation. What must the nurse monitor for?
   a. Signs of nonproductive cough, chest pain, crackles, and hypoxemia
   b. Change of skin tone from pink to gray color after several minutes of oxygen therapy
   c. Signs and symptoms of hypoventilation rather than hypoxemia
   d. Changes in level of consciousness, apnea, and respiratory pattern

14. A patient is receiving a high concentration of oxygen as a temporary emergency measure. Which nursing action is the most appropriate to prevent complications associated with high-flow oxygen?
    a. Auscultate the lungs every 4 hours for oxygen toxicity.
    b. Increase the oxygen if the Pao$_2$ level is less than 93 mm Hg.
    c. Monitor the prescribed oxygen level and length of therapy.
    d. Decrease the oxygen if the patient's condition does not respond.

15. Increased risk for oxygen toxicity is related to which factors? *(Select all that apply.)*
    a. Continuous delivery of oxygen at greater than 50% concentration
    b. Delivery of a high concentration of oxygen over 24 to 48 hours
    c. The severity and extent of lung disease
    d. Neglecting to monitor the patient's status and reducing oxygen concentration as soon as possible
    e. Excluding measures such as continuous positive airway pressure (CPAP) or positive end-expiratory pressure (PEEP)

16. The patient is receiving humidified oxygen which places the patient at high risk for which problem?
    a. Injury related to the moisture in the tube
    b. Infection related to the condensation in the tubing
    c. Limited mobility related to reliance on equipment
    d. Impaired skin integrity related to the mask

17. A patient is receiving warmed and humidified oxygen. The respiratory therapist informs the nurse that several other patients on other units have developed hospital-acquired infections and *Pseudomonas aeruginosa* has been identified as the organism. What does the nurse do?
    a. Place the patient in respiratory isolation.
    b. Obtain an order for a sputum culture.
    c. Change the humidifier every 24 hours.
    d. Obtain an order to discontinue the humidifier.

18. Nursing interventions to prevent infection in patients with humidified oxygen include which actions?
    a. Use sterile normal saline to provide moisture.
    b. Drain condensation into the humidifier.
    c. Drain condensation from the water trap.
    d. Maintain a sterile closed system at all times.

19. Which factors are considered hazards associated with oxygen therapy? *(Select all that apply.)*
    a. Increased combustion
    b. Oxygen narcosis
    c. Oxygen toxicity
    d. Absorption atelectasis
    e. Oxygen-induced hypoventilation

20. A patient is receiving warmed and humidified oxygen. In discarding the moisture formed by condensation, why does the nurse minimize the time that the tubing is disconnected?
    a. To prevent the patient from desaturating
    b. To reduce the patient's risk of infection
    c. To minimize the disturbance to the patient
    d. To facilitate overall time management

21. What is the best description of the nurse's role in the delivery of oxygen therapy?
    a. Receiving the therapy report from the respiratory therapist
    b. Evaluating the response to oxygen therapy
    c. Contacting respiratory therapy for the devices
    d. Being familiar with the devices and techniques used in order to provide proper care

22. A patient with an oxygen delivery device would like to ambulate to the bathroom but the tubing is too short. Extension tubing is added. What is the maximum length of the tubing that can be added in order to deliver the amount of oxygen needed for that device?
    a. 25 feet
    b. 35 feet
    c. 45 feet
    d. 50 feet

23. A patient is being discharged and requires home oxygen therapy with a reservoir-type nasal cannula. He asks the nurse, "Why can't I just take this nasal cannula that I have been using in the hospital?" What is the nurse's best response?
    a. "The doctor ordered the cannula, so your insurance company should cover the cost."
    b. "With the used cannula there is a risk of a hospital-acquired infection."
    c. "This special nasal cannula allows you to decrease the oxygen flow by 50%."
    d. "This nasal cannula is much better. It is more flexible and comfortable to wear."

24. A patient is receiving oxygen therapy through a non-rebreather mask. What is the correct nursing intervention?
    a. Maintain liter flow so that the reservoir bag is up to one-half full.
    b. Maintain 60% to 75% Fio_2 at 6 to 11 L/min.
    c. Ensure that valves and rubber flaps are patent, functional, and not stuck.
    d. Assess for effectiveness and switch to partial rebreather for more precise Fio_2.

25. A patient with a facemask at 5 L/min is able to eat. Which nursing intervention is performed at mealtimes?
    a. Change the mask to a nasal cannula of 6 L/min or more.
    b. Have the patient work around the face mask as best as possible.
    c. Obtain a physician order for a nasal cannula at 5 L/min.
    d. Obtain a physician order to remove the mask at meals.

26. The physician orders transtracheal oxygen therapy for a patient with respiratory difficulty. What does the nurse tell the patient's family is the purpose of this type of oxygen delivery system?
    a. Delivers oxygen directly into the lungs.
    b. Keeps the small air sacs open to improve gas exchange.
    c. Prevents the need for an endotracheal tube.
    d. Provides high humidity with oxygen delivery.

27. A patient has an inflated cuffed #8 Shiley tracheostomy and is on a ventilator. The tracheostomy tube is pulsating in synchrony with the patient's heartbeat. What does the nurse do first?
    a. Apply direct pressure to the innominate artery at the stoma site.
    b. Prepare the patient for immediate surgical repair.
    c. Notify the physician of the pulsating tube.
    d. No immediate management is needed unless there is bleeding.

28. A patient requires long-term airway maintenance following surgery for cancer of the neck. The nurse is using a piece of equipment to explain the procedure and mechanism that are associated with this long-term therapy. Which piece of equipment does the nurse most likely use for this patient teaching session?
    a. Tracheostomy tube
    b. Nasal trumpet
    c. Endotracheal tube
    d. Nasal cannula

29. A patient is receiving preoperative teaching for a partial laryngectomy and will have a tracheostomy postoperatively. How does the nurse define a tracheostomy to the patient?
    a. Opening in the trachea that enables breathing
    b. Temporary procedure that will be reversed at a later date
    c. Technique using positive pressure to improve gas exchange
    d. Procedure that holds open the upper airways

30. A patient returns from the operating room and the nurse assesses for subcutaneous emphysema which is a potential complication associated with tracheostomy. How does the nurse assess for this complication?
    a. Checking the volume of the pilot balloon
    b. Listening for airflow through the tube
    c. Inspecting and palpating for air under the skin
    d. Assessing the tube for patency

31. A patient with a tracheostomy without a tube in place develops increased coughing, inability to expectorate secretions, and difficulty breathing. What are these assessment findings related to?
    a. Overinflation of the pilot balloon
    b. Tracheoesophageal fistula
    c. Cuff leak and rupture
    d. Tracheal stenosis

32. A patient returns from the operating room after having a tracheostomy. While assessing the patient, which observations made by the nurse warrant immediate notification of the physician?
    a. Patient is alert but unable to speak and has difficulty communicating his needs.
    b. Small amount of bleeding present at the incision.
    c. Skin is puffy at the neck area with a crackling sensation.
    d. Respirations are audible and noisy with an increased respiratory rate.

33. A patient was intubated for acute respiratory failure, and there is an endotracheal tube in place. Which nursing intervention is *not* appropriate for this patient?
    a. Ensure that the oxygen is warmed and humidified.
    b. Suction the airway, then the mouth, and give oral care.
    c. Suction the airway with the oral suction equipment.
    d. Position the tubing so it does not pull on the airway.

34. To prevent accidental decannulation of a tracheostomy tube, what does the nurse do?
    a. Obtain an order for continuous upper extremity restraints.
    b. Secure the tube in place using ties or fabric fasteners.
    c. Allow some flexibility in motion of the tube while coughing.
    d. Instruct the patient to hold the tube with a tissue while coughing.

35. A patient has a recent tracheostomy. What necessary equipment does the nurse ensure is kept at the bedside? *(Select all that apply.)*
    a. Ambu bag
    b. Pair of wire cutters
    c. Oxygen tubing
    d. Suction equipment
    e. Tracheostomy tube with obturator

36. Which statement by the nursing student indicates an understanding of the deflation of the tracheostomy cuff?
    a. "The cuff is deflated to allow the patient to speak."
    b. "The cuff is deflated to permit suctioning more easily."
    c. "The cuff should never be deflated because the patient will choke."
    d. "The cuff should be deflated to facilitate access for tracheostomy care."

37. A patient has a temporary tracheostomy following surgery to the neck area to remove a benign tumor. Which nursing intervention is performed to prevent obstruction of the tracheostomy tube?
    a. Provide tracheal suctioning when there are noisy respirations.
    b. Provide oxygenation to maintain pulse oximeter readings.
    c. Inflate the cuff to maximum pressure and check it once per shift.
    d. Suction regularly and PRN with a Yankauer suction.

38. A patient sustained a serious crush injury to the neck and had a tracheostomy tube placed yesterday. As the nurse is performing tracheostomy care, the patient suddenly sneezes very forcefully and the tracheostomy tube falls out onto the bed linens. What does the nurse do?
    a. Ventilate the patient with 100% oxygen and notify the physician.
    b. Quickly and gently replace the tube with a clean cannula kept at the bedside.
    c. Quickly rinse the tube with sterile solution and gently replace it.
    d. Give the patient oxygen; call for assistance and a new tracheostomy kit.

39. A patient with a tracheostomy or endotracheal tube has inline suctioning. Which nursing interventions apply to proper suctioning technique? *(Select all that apply.)*
    a. Oxygenate the patient before suctioning.
    b. Instruct the patient that he or she is going to be suctioned.
    c. Suctioning time is the same for a tracheostomy and an endotracheal tube.
    d. The suction line is unlocked after suctioning is completed.
    e. The suction tubing is locked after suctioning is completed.

40. What are possible complications that can occur with suctioning from an artificial airway? *(Select all that apply.)*
    a. Infection
    b. Coughing
    c. Hypoxia
    d. Tissue (mucosa) trauma
    e. Vagal stimulation
    f. Bronchospasm
    g. Cardiac dysrhythmias

41. A patient required emergency intubation and currently has an artificial airway in place. Oxygen is being administered directly from the wall source. Why would warmed and humidified oxygen be a more appropriate choice for this patient?
    a. Helps prevent tracheal damage
    b. Promotes thick secretions
    c. Is more comfortable for the patient
    d. Is less likely to cause oxygen toxicity

42. A patient has an endotracheal tube and requires frequent suctioning for copious secretions. What is a complication of tracheal suctioning?
    a. Atelectasis
    b. Hypoxia
    c. Hypercarbia
    d. Bronchodilation

43. The nurse has explained the endotracheal suctioning procedure to a patient, gathered equipment, washed hands, and set low wall suction. Indicate the correct steps of completing the suctioning procedure in order using 1 through 9.
    _____ a. Open the suction kit.
    _____ b. Pour sterile saline into sterile container.
    _____ c. Preoxygenate the patient.
    _____ d. Discard supplies, wash hands, and document.
    _____ e. Put on sterile gloves.
    _____ f. Keep catheter sterile; attach to suction.
    _____ g. Withdraw catheter, applying suction and twirling catheter.
    _____ h. Insert catheter into trachea without suctioning.
    _____ i. Lubricate catheter tip in sterile saline solution.

44. The nurse has explained the tracheostomy care procedure to a patient, gathered equipment, and washed hands. Indicate the correct steps of completing the tracheostomy care procedure in order using 1 through 10.
    _____ a. Remove old dressing and excess secretions.
    _____ b. Wash hands, dispose of equipment, and document.
    _____ c. Suction tracheostomy tube if necessary.
    _____ d. Put on sterile gloves.
    _____ e. Reinsert inner cannula into outer cannula.
    _____ f. Open tracheostomy kit and pour peroxide into one side of container and saline into another.
    _____ g. Clean stoma site and plate.
    _____ h. Rinse inner cannula in sterile saline.
    _____ i. Remove inner cannula; place it in peroxide solution use brush to clean.
    _____ j. Change tracheostomy ties if needed and place new tracheostomy dressing.

45. While the nursing student changes a patient's tracheostomy dressing, the nurse observes the student using a pair of scissors to cut a 4 x 4 gauze pad to make a split dressing that will fit around the tracheostomy tube. What is the nurse's best action?
    a. Give the student positive reinforcement for use of materials and technique.
    b. Report the student to the instructor for remediation of the skill.
    c. Change the dressing immediately after the student has left the room.
    d. Direct the student in the correct use of materials and explain the rationale.

46. The nurse is caring for a patient with a tracheostomy who has recently been transferred from the ICU, but he has had no unusual occurrences related to the tracheostomy or his oxygenation status. What does the routine care for this patient include?
    a. Thorough respiratory assessment at least every 2 hours
    b. Maintaining the cuff pressure between 50 and 100 mm Hg
    c. Suctioning as needed; maximum suction time of 20 seconds
    d. Changing the tracheostomy dressing once a day

47. A patient with a tracheostomy is being discharged to home. In patient teaching, what does the nurse instruct the patient to do?
    a. Use sterile technique when suctioning.
    b. Instill tap water into the artificial airway.
    c. Clean the tracheostomy tube with soap and water.
    d. Increase the humidity in the home.

48. A patient with a permanent tracheostomy is interested in developing an exercise regimen. Which activity does the nurse advise the patient to avoid?
    a. Aerobics
    b. Tennis
    c. Golf
    d. Swimming

49. A patient with an endotracheal tube in place has dry mucous membranes and lips related to the tube and the partial open mouth position. What techniques does the nurse use to provide this patient with frequent oral care?
    a. Cleanses the mouth with glycerin swabs.
    b. Provides alcohol-based mouth rinse and oral suction.
    c. Cleanses with a mixture of hydrogen peroxide and water.
    d. Uses toothettes or a soft-bristled brush moistened in water.

50. A patient with a tracheostomy who receives unnecessary suctioning can experience which complications? *(Select all that apply.)*
    a. Bronchospasm
    b. Mucosal damage
    c. Impaired gag reflex
    d. Bronchodilation
    e. Bleeding

51. A patient with a tracheostomy tube is able to speak and is no longer on mechanical ventilation. Which type of tracheostomy tube does this patient have? *(Select all that apply.)*
    a. Cuffless tube
    b. Fenestrated tube with inner cannula removed and the red stopper locked in place
    c. Standard inflated cuffed tube
    d. Size #6 Shiley inflated cuffed with a Passy-Muir valve
    e. Size #6 Shiley deflated cuffed that is capped

Matching. *Match each type of tracheostomy tube with its description.*

Tracheostomy Tubes
a. Double-lumen tube
b. Single-lumen tube
c. Cuffed tube
d. Cuffless tube
e. Fenestrated tube
f. Cuffed fenestrated tube
g. Metal tracheostomy tube
h. Talking tracheostomy tube

Descriptions
_____ 52. Used with patients who can speak while on a ventilator for a long-term basis

_____ 53. Has a cuff that seals airway when inflated

_____ 54. Used for long-term management of patients not on mechanical ventilation or at high risk for aspiration

_____ 55. Has three parts—outer cannula, inner cannula, and obturator

_____ 56. Used for permanent tracheostomy

_____ 57. Used often with patients with spinal cord paralysis or muscular disease who do not require a ventilator all the time

_____ 58. Has no inner cannula and is used for patients with long or extra-thick necks

_____ 59. Used when weaning a patient from a ventilator; allows the patient to speak

60. A patient has a cuffed tracheostomy tube without a pressure relief valve. To prevent tissue damage of the tracheal mucosa, what does the nurse do?
    a. Deflate the cuff every 2 to 4 hours and maintain as needed.
    b. Change the tracheostomy tube every 3 days or per hospital policy.
    c. Assess and record cuff pressures each shift using the occlusive technique.
    d. Assess and record cuff pressures each shift using minimal leak technique.

61. An older adult patient is at risk for aspirating food or fluids. Which are the most appropriate nursing actions to prevent this problem? *(Select all that apply.)*
    a. Provide close supervision if the patient is self-feeding.
    b. Instruct the patient to tilt the head back when swallowing.
    c. Obtain an order for a clear liquid diet and offer small but frequent amounts.
    d. Instruct the patient to tuck the chin down when swallowing.
    e. Place the patient in an upright position.

62. An older adult patient sustained a stroke several weeks ago and is having difficulty swallowing. To prevent aspiration during mealtimes, what does the nurse do?
    a. Hyperextend the head to allow food to enter the stomach and not the lungs.
    b. Give thin liquids after each bite of food to help "wash the food down."
    c. Encourage "dry swallowing" after each bite to clear residue from the throat.
    d. Maintain a low-Fowler's position during eating and for 2 hours afterwards.

63. A patient with a tracheostomy tube is currently alert and cooperative but seems to be coughing more frequently and producing more secretions than usual. The nurse determines that there is a need for suctioning. Which nursing intervention does the nurse use to prevent hypoxia for this patient?
    a. Allow the patient to breathe room air prior to suctioning.
    b. Avoid prolonged suctioning time.
    c. Suction frequently when the patient is coughing.
    d. Use the largest available catheter.

64. The nurse is suctioning the secretions from a patient's endotracheal tube. The patient demonstrates a vagal response by a drop in heart rate to 54 and a drop in blood pressure to 90/50. After stopping suctioning, what is the nurse's priority action?
    a. Allow the patient to rest for at least 10 minutes.
    b. Monitor the patient and call the Rapid Response Team.
    c. Oxygenate with 100% oxygen and monitor the patient.
    d. Administer atropine according to standing orders.

65. A patient with a tracheostomy is unable to speak. He is not in acute distress, but is gesturing and trying to communicate with the nurse. Which nursing intervention is the best approach in this situation?
    a. Rely on the family to interpret for the patient.
    b. Ask questions that can be answered with a "yes" or "no" response.
    c. Obtain an immediate consult with the speech therapist.
    d. Encourage the patient to rest rather than struggle with communication.

66. Which clinical finding in a patient with a recent tracheostomy is the most serious and requires immediate intervention?
    a. Increased cough and difficulty expectorating secretions
    b. Food particles in the tracheal secretions
    c. Pulsating tracheostomy tube in synchrony with the heartbeat
    d. Set tidal volume on the ventilator not being received by the patient

67. The nurse is providing discharge instructions for a patient who must perform self-care of a tracheostomy. The patient has been cheerful and cooperative during the hospital stay and has demonstrated interest and capability in performing self-care. But now the patient begins crying and refuses to leave the hospital. What is the nurse's best response?
    a. "You have done so well with your self-care. I am sure that you will be okay."
    b. "Let me call your family. They can help you to get home and get settled."
    c. "You have been brave and cheerful, but there is something that is worrying you."
    d. "We'll delay this teaching until later. Let's choose a scarf for you to wear home."

CASE STUDY: THE PATIENT WITH A TRACHEOSTOMY

Use a separate sheet of paper to answer the questions in this Case Study, or go to the "Prepare for Class" folder on your Evolve website at http://evolve.elsevier.com/Iggy/ to download and complete as a word processing file. Answer guidelines for this Case Study are also available on your Evolve website.

The nurse is caring for a 75-year-old man who was admitted for laryngeal cancer and surgery. The patient was transferred from the ICU several days ago. He has a tracheostomy and the tracheostomy collar is in place. He is receiving high-flow oxygen at 8 L/min. In shift report, the nurse learns that the patient is alert and oriented to person, place, and time. He is able to feed himself and independently perform most basic ADLs. He appears to be anxious and is having difficulty coping with the tracheostomy. He has a large amount of yellow mucus secretions from the tracheostomy and a specimen has been sent for culture and sensitivity. He is increasingly resistant to tracheostomy care and suctioning, although the need to deal with the excessive secretions has been explained to him. He expresses in written notes how frustrated he is by his inability to communicate verbally. His pulse is 85 beats/min; blood pressure is 135/60; respirations 20/min; temperature 100° F; pulse oximetry reading 95%.

1. List six complications associated with tracheostomy.
2. What assessment findings would accompany an airway obstruction related to the patient's excessive secretions?
3. List interventions to prevent obstruction.
4. Explain the prevention of tissue damage that could occur because the patient has a tracheostomy.
5. What assessment findings indicate that the patient should be suctioned?
6. Write a dialogue to enlist the patient's cooperation for the suctioning procedure. Include an explanation of the purpose, the procedure, and the patient's role. (Role play this with a classmate.)
7. Discuss special considerations for this older patient who has a tracheostomy.
8. Describe nursing interventions and several alternative communication methods to try with this patient.
9. Document a nursing note for the patient using these categories:
   - Respiratory
   - Communication
   - Neurologic
   - Additional notes

31 CHAPTER

Care of Patients with Noninfectious Upper Respiratory Problems

STUDY/REVIEW QUESTIONS

1. The nurse is caring for several patients who are at risk because of problems related to the upper airway. What is the priority assessment for these patients?
   a. Thickness of oral secretions; encourage ingestion of oral fluids
   b. Anxiety and pain; provide reassurance and NSAIDs
   c. Adequacy of oxygenation; ensure an unobstructed air passageway
   d. Evidence of spinal cord injuries; obtain order for x-rays

2. Which factors contribute to sleep apnea? (Select all that apply.)
   a. Smoking
   b. A short neck
   c. Athletic lifestyle
   d. Small uvula
   e. Enlarged tonsils or adenoids
   f. Underweight for height and gender

3. The nurse is instructing a patient about a scheduled polysomnograph. Which patient statement indicates understanding of the procedure?
   a. "The test can be done in the doctor's office and will take 2 to 3 hours."
   b. "I shouldn't eat anything after midnight the night before, and someone must accompany me."
   c. "The test determines the depth and type of sleep and muscle movement."
   d. "The test determines the amount of sleep I need for adequate rest."

4. A patient has been diagnosed with sleep apnea. Which assessment findings indicate that the patient is having complications associated with sleep apnea?
   a. Side effects of hypoxemia, hypercapnia, and sleep deprivation
   b. Decrease in arterial carbon dioxide levels and sleep deprivation
   c. Respiratory alkalosis with retention of carbon dioxide
   d. Irritability, obesity, and enlarged tonsils or adenoids

5. A patient has been diagnosed with airway obstruction during sleep. The nurse most likely includes patient education about which device for home use?
   a. CPAP to deliver a positive airway pressure
   b. Oxygen via facemask to prevent hypoxia
   c. Neck brace to support the head and facilitate breathing
   d. Nebulizer treatments with bronchodilators

6. A patient is at risk for aspiration related to open vocal cord paralysis. What does the nurse teach the patient to do? (Select all that apply.)
   a. Raise the chin while swallowing
   b. Breathe slowly through an open mouth immediately after swallowing
   c. Hold the breath during swallowing
   d. Tilt the head backward during and immediately after swallowing
   e. Tuck the chin down and tilt the head forward during swallowing

7. A patient has been diagnosed with vocal nodules. The health care provider recommends conservative treatment that includes lifestyle modifications. What does the nurse teach the patient to do? *(Select all that apply.)*
   a. Give the voice a rest from speaking, including no whispering
   b. Avoid humid climate conditions
   c. Use stool softeners to decrease straining
   d. Limit intake of caffeinated beverages
   e. Avoid heavy lifting

8. The nurse is assessing a patient who reports being struck in the face and head several times. During the assessment, a pink-tinged drainage from the nares is observed. Which nursing action provides relevant assessment data?
   a. Have the patient gently blow the nose and observe for bloody mucus.
   b. Test the drainage with a reagent to check the pH.
   c. Ask the patient to describe the appearance of the face before the incident.
   d. Place a drop of the drainage on a filter paper and look for a yellow ring.

9. While playing football at school, a patient injured his nose resulting in a possible simple fracture. The patient's parents call the nurse seeking advice. What does the nurse tell the parents to do?
   a. Ask the school nurse to insert a nasal airway to ensure patency.
   b. Apply an ice pack and allow the patient to rest in a supine position.
   c. Seek medical attention within 24 hours to minimize further complications.
   d. Monitor the symptoms for 24 hours and contact the physician if there is bleeding.

10. A patient had a rhinoplasty and is preparing for discharge home. A family member is instructed by the nurse to monitor the patient for postnasal drip by using a flashlight to look in the back of the throat. If bleeding is noted, what does the nurse tell the family member to do?
    a. Place ice packs on the back of the neck and apply pressure to the nose.
    b. Hyperextend the neck and apply pressure and ice packs as needed.
    c. Seek immediate medical attention for the bleeding.
    d. Monitor for 24 hours if the bleeding appears to be a small amount.

11. The nurse is teaching a patient about post-rhinoplasty care. Which patient statement indicates an understanding of the instruction?
    a. "I will have a very large dressing on my nose."
    b. "I will have bruising around my eyes, nose, and face."
    c. "There will be swelling that will cause a loss of sense of smell."
    d. "My nose will be three times its normal size for 3 weeks."

12. A patient with an active nosebleed is admitted to the emergency department. What interventions, in priority order, does the nurse use to attempt to stop the nosebleed? *(Select in order of priority.)*

    _____ a. Apply an ice pack to the nose.

    _____ b. Have the patient sit upright with the head forward.

    _____ c. Monitor the color and amount of blood.

    _____ d. Apply direct lateral pressure to the nose.

    _____ e. If bleeding continues, place nasal packing.

13. The nurse is caring for an older adult patient with a history of noncompliance with prescribed metoprolol (Toprol XL) and recurrent nosebleeds. Which assessment finding is the most significant in relation to this patient's risk for repeated nosebleeds?
    a. Irregular apical pulse of 58 beats/min
    b. Open-mouth breathing with respiratory rate of 28/min
    c. Asymptomatic blood pressure of 180/110 mm Hg
    d. Subjective chills and oral temperature of 97.2° F

14. After being treated in the emergency department for posterior nosebleed, the patient is admitted to the hospital. The nasal packing is in place and vital signs are stable. The patient has an IV of normal saline at 125 mL/hr. What is the priority for nursing care?
    a. Airway management
    b. Managing potential dehydration
    c. Managing potential decreased cardiac output
    d. Monitoring for potential infection

15. A patient is admitted for a posterior nosebleed. Posterior packing is in place and, in addition, the patient is on oxygen therapy, antibiotics, and opioid analgesics. What is the priority assessment?
    a. Tolerance of packing or tubes
    b. Gag and cough reflexes
    c. Mouth breathing
    d. Skin breakdown around the nares

16. A patient reports noticing a change in the character of nasal discharge and speech quality, and a subjective feeling of blockage in the nasal passages. To gather additional relevant information, which question is the most appropriate to ask this patient?
    a. "Are you experiencing any soreness or tightness in your throat?"
    b. "Do you have a history of nasal polyps?"
    c. "Do you take over-the-counter medications on a regular basis?"
    d. "Do you have a history of frequent nosebleeds?"

17. The nurse is caring for a patient who has just returned from rhinoplasty surgery. Which assessment finding warrants additional assessment and concern?
    a. Bilateral packing of both nares in place
    b. Moustache pad in place
    c. Demonstrated repeated swallowing
    d. Traces of bruising around the eyes

18. A patient returns from surgery following a rhinoplasty. The nursing assistant places the patient in a supine position to encourage rest and sleep. Which action should the nurse take first?
    a. Teach the patient how to use the bed controls to position herself.
    b. Explain the purpose of the semi-Fowler's position to the nursing assistant.
    c. Place the patient in a semi-Fowler's position and assess for aspiration.
    d. Post a notice at the head of the bed to remind personnel about positioning.

19. The nurse is caring for a patient who had a nasoseptoplasty. Which action is the best to delegate to the licensed practical nurse?
    a. Administer a stool softener to ease bowel movements.
    b. Assess the patient's airway and breathing after general anesthesia.
    c. Evaluate the patient's emotional reaction to the facial edema and bruising.
    d. Take vital signs every 4 hours as ordered by the physician.

20. To assess for potential vocal cord paralysis in a patient, what does the nurse ask the patient about? *(Select all that apply.)*
    a. "Do you yell and scream at sporting events frequently?"
    b. "Have you experienced any trauma to your vocal cords recently?"
    c. "Do you have gastroesophageal reflux disease?"
    d. "Do you have any diseases of the vagus nerve?"
    e. "Were you recently intubated for a prolonged time period with an endotracheal tube?"

21. The nurse is providing postoperative nursing care for a patient with surgical correction of a deviated septum. Which intervention is part of the standard care for this patient?
    a. Apply ice to the nasal area and eyes to decrease swelling and pain.
    b. Encourage deep coughing to prevent atelectasis and clear secretions.
    c. Administer NSAIDs or Tylenol every 4 to 6 hours for pain relief.
    d. Apply moist heat and humidity to the nasal area for comfort and circulation.

22. The nurse is monitoring a child who has been admitted for a fever of unknown origin. The child also reports a sore throat and demonstrates reluctance to eat and drink. Which assessment finding indicates an upper airway obstruction which requires immediate intervention?
    a. Stridor
    b. Crepitus
    c. Weak cough
    d. Subcutaneous emphysema

23. A patient arrives in the emergency department with a severe crush injury to the face with blood gurgling from the mouth and nose and obvious respiratory distress. The nurse prepares to assist the physician with which procedure to manage the airway?
    a. Performing a needle thoracotomy
    b. Inserting an endotracheal tube
    c. Performing a tracheotomy
    d. Inserting a nasal airway and giving oxygen

24. A patient with facial trauma has undergone surgical intervention to wire the jaw shut. In performing discharge teaching with this patient, which topics does the nurse cover? *(Select all that apply.)*
    a. Oral care
    b. Activity
    c. Use of wire cutters
    d. Communication
    e. Aspiration prevention

25. The nurse is assessing a patient with significant and obvious facial trauma after being struck repeatedly in the face. Which finding is the priority and requires immediate intervention?
    a. Asymmetry of the mandible
    b. Restlessness and gurgling respirations
    c. Nonparallel extraocular movements
    d. Pain upon palpation over the nasal bridge

26. The nurse enters the room and the patient is crying. When the nurse asks the patient what happened, the patient says, "The doctor told me I have a LeFort I fracture of my face." What is the nurse's best response?
    a. "Don't worry; a LeFort I fracture is much less serious than a LeFort III."
    b. "You have an excellent doctor who will take good care of you."
    c. "Let me get you a mirror and you will see that it's not so bad."
    d. "What is your main concern about the LeFort I fracture?"

27. A patient has an inner maxillary fixation. The nurse encourages the patient to eat which kind of food?
    a. Milkshakes
    b. Cottage cheese
    c. Tea and toast
    d. Tuna and noodle casserole

28. A patient enters the emergency department after being punched in the throat. What does the nurse monitor for?
    a. Aphonia
    b. Dry cough
    c. Crepitus
    d. Loss of gag reflex

29. A patient has sustained a mandible fracture and the surgeon has explained that the repair will be made using a resorbable plate. The patient discloses to the nurse that he has not told the surgeon about his substance abuse and illicit drug dependence. What is the nurse's best response?
    a. "Why didn't you talk to your surgeon about this issue?"
    b. "You should tell the surgeon, but it is your choice."
    c. "It is important for your surgeon to know about this information."
    d. "You shouldn't be ashamed; your surgeon will still repair your fracture."

30. A patient has had an inner maxillary fixation for a mandibular fracture. Which piece of equipment should be kept at the bedside at all times?
    a. Water Pik
    b. Wire cutters
    c. Pair of hemostats
    d. Emesis basin

31. A patient who was in a motor vehicle accident and sustained laryngeal trauma is being treated in the emergency department with humidified oxygen and is being monitored every 15 to 30 minutes for respiratory distress. Which assessment finding may indicate the need for further intervention?
    a. Respiratory rate 24, Pao_2 80 to 100, no difficulty with communication
    b. Pulse oximetry 96%, anxious, fatigued, blood in sputum, abdominal breathing
    c. Confused and disoriented, difficulty producing sounds, pulse oximetry 80%
    d. Anxious, respiratory rate 30, talking rapidly about the accident, warm to touch

32. A patient in the emergency department with laryngeal trauma has developed shortness of breath with stridor and decreased oxygen saturation. What is the priority action?
    a. Insert an oral or nasal airway.
    b. Assess for tachypnea, anxiety, and nasal flaring.
    c. Obtain the equipment for a tracheostomy.
    d. Apply oxygen and stay with the patient.

33. An older adult patient who is talking and laughing while eating begins to choke on a piece of meat. What is the initial emergency management for this patient?
    a. Several sharp blows between the scapulae
    b. Call the Rapid Response Team
    c. Nasotracheal suctioning
    d. Abdominal thrusts (Heimlich maneuver)

True or False? Read each statement about head and neck cancers and write T for true or F for false in the blanks provided. If the statement is false, correct the statement to make it true.

_____ 34. Head and neck cancers are usually squamous cell carcinomas.

_____ 35. Diagnosis is usually not made until the disease is advanced.

_____ 36. Signs and symptoms of the disease are related to the location of the cancer.

_____ 37. Red velvety patches are called *leukoplakia*.

_____ 38. Many diagnostic tests are performed. CT scan aids in finding the exact location of a tumor, whereas MRI defines soft tissue invasion.

_____ 39. Discharge teaching for all partial or total laryngectomy patients includes tracheostomy care.

_____ 40. Patients may have tubes removed before they are discharged from the hospital.

_____ 41. Discharge teaching for a total laryngectomy patient includes stoma care, which combines wound and airway care.

42. Following radiation therapy for head and neck cancer, the nurse instructs the patient about which potential side effects? *(Select all that apply.)*
   a. Skin redness and tenderness
   b. Numbness of the mouth, lips, or face
   c. Dysphagia
   d. Hoarseness
   e. Xerostomia

43. What type of treatment has the highest cure rate for small cancers of the head and neck?
   a. Surgery
   b. Chemotherapy
   c. Laser surgery
   d. Radiation therapy

44. The nursing student is preparing patient teaching materials about head and neck cancer. Which statement is accurate and included in the patient teaching information?
   a. It metastasizes often to the brain.
   b. It usually develops over a short time.
   c. It is often seen as red edematous areas.
   d. It is often seen as white patchy mucosal lesions.

45. The nurse is interviewing a patient to assess for risk factors related to head and neck cancer. Which questions are appropriate to include? *(Select all that apply.)*
   a. "How many servings per day of alcohol would you typically drink?"
   b. "Have you had frequent episodes of acute or chronic visual problems?"
   c. "Have you had a problem with sores in your mouth?"
   d. "When was the last time you saw your dentist?"
   e. "Do you have recurrent laryngitis or frequent episodes of sore throat?"
   f. "How many packs per day do you smoke and for how many years?"

46. Which patient has the highest risk for developing cancer of the larynx and should be alerted about relevant lifestyle modifications to decrease this risk?
   a. 57-year-old male with alcoholism
   b. 18-year-old marijuana smoker
   c. 28-year-old female with diabetes
   d. 34-year-old male who snorts cocaine

47. The nurse is caring for a patient with a laryngeal tumor. In order to facilitate comfort and breathing for the patient, which type of position does the nurse use?
   a. Sims'
   b. Supine
   c. Fowler's
   d. Prone

48. A patient suffers from chronic xerostomia related to past radiation therapy treatments. Which intervention does the nurse use to assist the patient with this symptom?
   a. Offer small frequent meals.
   b. Suggest a moisturizing spray.
   c. Explain fluid restrictions.
   d. Teach to wash with mild soap and water.

49. The nurse is assessing a patient's skin at the site of radiation therapy to the neck. Which skin condition is expected in relation to the radiation treatments?
   a. Red, tender, and peeling
   b. Shiny, pale, and tight
   c. Puffy and edematous
   d. Pale, dry, and cool

50. Which surgical procedure of the neck area poses no risk postoperatively for aspiration?
    a. Total laryngectomy
    b. Transoral cordectomy
    c. Hemilaryngectomy
    d. Partial laryngectomy

51. The nurse is caring for a postoperative patient who had a neck dissection. Which assessment finding is expected?
    a. Bulky gauze dressing is present that is dry and intact over the site.
    b. The patient can speak normally, but reports a sore throat.
    c. Permanent gastrostomy tube is present with continuous tube feedings.
    d. The patient has shoulder muscle weakness and limited range of motion.

52. The nursing student is caring for an older adult patient who sustained a stroke and is confused and having trouble swallowing. Which statement by the nursing student indicates an understanding of aspiration precautions for this patient?
    a. "I will administer pills as whole tablets; they are easier to swallow."
    b. "If the patient coughs, I will discontinue feeding and contact the physician."
    c. "I will keep the head of bed elevated during and after feeding."
    d. "I will encourage small amounts of fluids such as water, tea, or juices."

53. The nurse observes that a patient is having difficulty swallowing and has initiated aspiration precautions. Which procedure does the nurse expect the physician to order for this patient?
    a. Chest x-ray of the neck and chest
    b. CT scan of the head and neck
    c. Barium swallow under fluoroscopy
    d. Direct and indirect laryngoscopy

54. A patient has had neck dissection surgery with a reconstructive flap over the carotid artery. Which intervention is appropriate for the flap care?
    a. Evaluate the flap every hour for the first 72 hours.
    b. Monitor the flap by gently placing a Doppler on the flap.
    c. Position the patient so that the flap is in the dependent position.
    d. Apply a wet-to-dry dressing to the flap.

55. The nurse is caring for several patients who require treatment for laryngeal cancer. Which treatment/procedure requires patient education about aspiration precautions?
    a. Total laryngectomy
    b. Laser surgery
    c. Radiation therapy
    d. Supraglottic laryngectomy

56. Which statement by the patient indicates understanding about radiation therapy for neck cancer?
    a. "My voice will initially be hoarse but should improve over time."
    b. "There are no side effects other than a hoarse voice."
    c. "Dry mouth after radiation therapy is temporary and short-term."
    d. "My throat is not directly affected by radiation."

57. What does the nurse include in the teaching session for a patient who is scheduled to have a partial laryngectomy?
    a. Supraglottic method of swallowing
    b. Presence of a tracheostomy tube and nasogastric tube for feeding due to postoperative swelling
    c. Not being able to eat solid foods
    d. Permanence of the tracheostomy, referred to as a *laryngectomy stoma*

58. A patient has been transferred from the intensive care unit to the medical-surgical unit after a laryngectomy. What does the nurse suggest to encourage the patient to participate in self-care?
    a. Changing the tracheostomy collar
    b. Suctioning the mouth with a Yankauer suction
    c. Checking the stoma with a flashlight
    d. Observing the color of the reconstructive flap

59. The nurse is caring for a patient who had reconstructive neck surgery and observes bright red blood spurting from the tissue flap that is covering the carotid artery. What is the priority action?
    a. Call the surgeon and alert the operating room.
    b. Call the Rapid Response Team.
    c. Apply immediate, direct pressure to the site.
    d. Apply a bulky sterile dressing and secure the airway.

60. A patient is experiencing acute anxiety related to hospitalization stress and an inability to accept changes related to laryngeal cancer. The patient wants to leave the hospital, but agrees to try a medication to "help me calm down." For which medication does the nurse obtain a PRN order?
    a. Amitriptyline (Elavil)
    b. Modafinil (Provigil)
    c. Morphine sulfate (Statex)
    d. Lorazepam (Ativan)

61. A patient with a recent diagnosis of sinus cancer states that he wants another course of antibiotics because he believes he simply has another sinus infection. What is the nurse's best response?
    a. "I'll call the physician for the antibiotic prescription."
    b. "Why are you doubting your doctor's diagnosis?"
    c. "Let me bring you some information about sinus cancer."
    d. "What did the doctor say to you about your condition?"

62. The nurse identifies the priority problem of reduced self-concept related to perceived disfigurement created by tracheostomy for a young female patient. What does the nurse recommend for this patient? *(Select all that apply.)*
    a. Encourage the family to bring several attractive scarves.
    b. Assist the patient to identify realistic goals.
    c. Redirect conversation topics away from body image.
    d. Obtain an order for a psychiatric social services consult.
    e. Have the patient talk with someone who has adapted to having a tracheostomy.

63. A patient is unable to speak following a cordectomy. Which action is delegated to the nursing assistant to assist the patient in dealing with communication issues?
    a. Politely tell the patient not to communicate.
    b. Teach the patient how to use hand signals.
    c. Allow extra time to accomplish ADLs because of communication limitations.
    d. Give step-by-step instructions during the ADLs and discourage two-way communication.

64. The nurse is assessing a patient who has had a neck dissection with removal of muscle tissue, lymph nodes, and the eleventh cranial nerve. Which assessment finding is anticipated because of the surgical procedure?
    a. Shoulder drop with an increased limitation of movement
    b. Asymmetrical eye movements and a change of visual acuity
    c. Blood and serous fluid under the reconstructive flap
    d. Facial swelling with discoloration and bruising around the eyes

65. A patient is having radiation therapy to the neck and reports a sore throat and difficulty swallowing. Which statement by the nursing student indicates a correct understanding of symptom relief for this patient?
    a. "The patient should not swallow anything too cold or too hot."
    b. "I will give the patient a mouthwash with an alcohol base."
    c. "I will help the patient with a saline gargle."
    d. "The patient should be reassured that the sore throat is temporary."

66. The physician orders the discontinuation of the nasogastric tube for a patient with a total laryngectomy. Before discontinuing the tube, which action is performed?
    a. The physician and the nurse will assess the patient's ability to swallow.
    b. Reassure the patient that eating and swallowing will be painless and natural.
    c. The nutritionist will evaluate the patient's nutritional status.
    d. The patient will be offered a PRN analgesic or an anxiolytic medication.

67. A patient is learning esophageal speech and reports that he feels bloated after a practice session. To assist the patient with this issue, what does the nurse do?
    a. Refer the patient to the American Cancer Society Visitor Program.
    b. Obtain an order for PRN antacids.
    c. Reassure the patient that the discomfort is worth the long-term benefit.
    d. Notify the speech therapist about the symptom.

68. A patient has had surgery for cancer of the neck. Which behavior indicates that the patient understands how to perform self-care to prevent aspiration?
    a. Chooses thin liquids that cause coughing, but knows to take small sips.
    b. Eats small frequent meals that include a variety of textures and nutrients.
    c. Asks for small frequent sips of nutrition supplement as a bedtime snack.
    d. Positions self upright before eating or drinking anything.

69. A patient is receiving enteral feedings and a nasogastric tube is in place. In order to prevent aspiration, which precautions are used? *(Select all that apply.)*
    a. No bolus feedings are given at night.
    b. Hold the feeding if the residual volume exceeds 20 mL.
    c. Vary the time of feedings according to the patient's preference.
    d. Check the pH of the secretions.
    e. Elevate the head of bed during and after feedings.
    f. Evaluate the patient's tolerance of the feedings.

70. A patient has demonstrated anxiety since a diagnosis of neck cancer. The surgery and radiation therapy are completed. Which behavior indicates that the patient's anxiety is decreasing?
    a. Repeatedly asks the same questions and seeks to revalidate all information.
    b. States that he is less anxious, but is irritable and tense whenever questioned.
    c. Makes a plan to contact the American Cancer Society Visitor Program.
    d. Makes a plan to share personal belongings with friends and family.

71. Which side effects would a patient with obstructive sleep apnea report? *(Select all that apply.)*
    a. Excessive daytime sleepiness
    b. Excessive daytime hyperactivity
    c. Inability to concentrate
    d. Excessive production of sputum
    e. Irritability

CASE STUDY: THE PATIENT WITH AN ORAL LESION

Use a separate sheet of paper to answer the questions in this Case Study, or go to the "Prepare for Class" folder on your Evolve website at http://evolve.elsevier.com/Iggy/ to download and complete as a word processing file. Answer guidelines for this Case Study are also available on your Evolve website.

A patient is admitted with a report of left ear pain for 3 1/2 weeks. On assessment the patient is noted to have slight difficulty articulating his words. A sore is noted on the left lateral aspect of the tongue. The patient reports that he has had a "cold" for a several weeks.

Oral cavity reveals poor dentition and odorous breath. History reveals the patient has smoked 1 1/2 packs/day for 20 years. He drinks 1-2 beers a day. Weight is 67 kg (147 lbs) and records from 8 months ago indicate his weight was 89 kg (195 lbs). The patient states that he has found himself eating smaller portions and softer foods. He ambulates without assistance, gait is slow and steady. No peripheral edema of lower or upper extremities. Pulses palpated 2+ bilateral radial and 2+ bilateral pedal. Vital signs: Temp 37.2° C (98.9° F), heart rate 87/min sinus rhythm, respirations 22/min, and blood pressure 138/72 mm Hg. Patient reports mild pain from left ear ache and sore on tongue. He rates his pain 3-4 on a scale of 0 to 10 (0 being no pain and 10 being the worst pain imaginable).

1. What are the warning signs of head and neck cancer found in the patient?
2. What are the risk factors of head and neck cancer for this patient?
3. Document a nursing note for this patient using these categories:
   - Communication/oral cavity
   - Pain management
   - Nutritional intake
   - Additional notes
4. What imaging assessment will likely be ordered for this patient?

CASE STUDY: THE PATIENT WITH AN UPPER RESPIRATORY CONDITION

Use a separate sheet of paper to answer the questions in this Case Study, or go to the "Prepare for Class" folder on your Evolve website at http://evolve.elsevier.com/Iggy/ to download and complete as a word processing file. Answer guidelines for this Case Study are also available on your Evolve website.

The patient is a 45-year-old man whose chief complaint is hoarseness and a sensation of a lump in his throat when swallowing. He reports that he can swallow, but it feels like some foods are getting stuck in the back of his throat. There is no bleeding and he denies any trauma or recent illness, although he does note that he wakes in the morning with a vague sore throat which has been going on for several months. The patient expresses guilt and fear related to lifestyle choices. He is fearful that he has cancer.

1. What additional questions should the nurse ask?

The physician determines that the patient may be at risk for cancer. The nurse must explain that the patient will have several kinds of diagnostic testing.

2. What laboratory tests are most likely to be ordered for this patient?

In addition to the laboratory tests, the patient is scheduled to have a bronchoscopy.

3. Explain the purpose and the procedure in terms that the patient will understand.

The patient is diagnosed with vocal cord polyps. The doctor informs him that the condition is not cancerous and that it will be managed conservatively.

4. Prepare a teaching plan for this patient.

32 CHAPTER

Care of Patients with Noninfectious Lower Respiratory Problems

STUDY/REVIEW QUESTIONS

Matching: *Match each characteristic of disease that is associated with chronic airflow limitation (CAL). Answers will be used more than once.*

Types of Diseases
a. Asthma
b. Chronic bronchitis
c. Pulmonary emphysema

Characteristics of CAL Diseases

_____ 1. Affects smaller airways

_____ 2. Chronic thickening of bronchial walls

_____ 3. Decreased surface area of alveoli

_____ 4. Destruction of alveolar walls

_____ 5. Hypercapnia

_____ 6. Impaired mucociliary clearance

_____ 7. Increased airway resistance

_____ 8. Increased eosinophils

_____ 9. Increased secretions

_____ 10. Affects work of breathing

_____ 11. Intermittent bronchospasm

_____ 12. Intermittent mucosal edema

_____ 13. Intermittent excess mucus production

_____ 14. Loss of elastic recoil

_____ 15. Mast cell destabilization

_____ 16. Elastin broken down by proteases

_____ 17. Stimulation of disease process by allergies

_____ 18. Possibly results in respiratory acidosis

_____ 19. Narrowed airway lumen due to inflammation

_____ 20. Narrowing of airway from smooth muscle constriction

_____ 21. Disease triggered by anti-inflammatory drugs used to treat disease

22. The nurse is caring for an older adult patient with a chronic respiratory disorder. Which interventions are best to use in caring for this patient? *(Select all that apply.)*
    a. Provide rest periods between activities such as bathing, meals, and ambulation.
    b. Place the patient in a supine position after meals to allow for rest.
    c. Schedule drug administration around routine activities to increase adherence to drug therapy.
    d. Arrange chairs in strategic locations to allow the patient to walk and rest.
    e. Teach the patient to avoid getting the pneumococcal vaccine.
    f. Encourage the patient to have an annual flu vaccination.

23. The nurse is caring for an older adult patient with a history of chronic asthma. Which problem related to aging can influence the care and treatment of this patient?
    a. Asthma usually resolves with age, so the condition is less severe in older adult patients.
    b. It is more difficult to teach older adult patients about asthma than to teach younger patients.
    c. With aging, the beta-adrenergic drugs do not work as quickly or strongly.
    d. Older adult patients have difficulty manipulating handheld inhalers.

24. The nurse is presenting a community education lecture about respiratory disorders. Which statement by a participant indicates a correct understanding of the information?
    a. "Bronchitis is a genetic disease that affects many organs."
    b. "In bronchial asthma, an airway obstruction can be caused by inflammation."
    c. "In chronic bronchitis, the tissue damage is only temporary and is reversible."
    d. "Smoking cessation reverses the tissue damage caused by emphysema."

25. A patient with chronic obstructive pulmonary disease (COPD) is likely to have which findings on assessment? *(Select all that apply.)*
    a. Body odor and unkempt hair
    b. Sitting in a chair leaning forward with elbows on knees
    c. Unintentional weight gain
    d. Decreased appetite
    e. Unexplained weight loss

26. A patient with COPD has dyspnea and mucus production that usually results in poor _____ intake and decreased _____.

27. The nurse is helping a patient learn about managing her asthma. What does the nurse instruct the patient to do?
    a. Keep a symptom diary to identify what triggers the asthma attacks.
    b. Make an appointment with an allergist for allergy therapy.
    c. Take a low dose of aspirin every day for the anti-inflammatory action.
    d. Drink large amounts of clear fluid to keep mucus thin and watery.

28. The nurse is taking a medical history on a new patient who has come to the office for a checkup. The patient states that he was supposed to take a medication called Singulair (montelukast), but that he never got the prescription filled. What is the best response by the nurse?
    a. "When did you first get diagnosed with a respiratory disorder?"
    b. "Why didn't you get the prescription filled?"
    c. "Tell me how you feel about your decision to not fill the prescription."
    d. "Are you having any problems with your asthma?"

29. The nurse teaches a patient with asthma to monitor for which problem while exercising?
    a. Increased peak expiratory flow rates
    b. Wheezing from bronchospasm
    c. Swelling in the feet and ankles
    d. Respiratory muscle fatigue

30. A patient with asthma is repeatedly not compliant with the medication regimen, which has resulted in the patient being hospitalized for a severe asthma attack. Which interventions does the nurse suggest to help the patient manage asthma on a daily basis? *(Select all that apply.)*
   a. Encourage active participation in the plan of care.
   b. Help the patient develop a flexible plan of care.
   c. Have the pharmacist establish a plan of care.
   d. Teach the patient about asthma and its treatment plan.
   e. Assess symptom severity using a peak flowmeter 1-2 times per week.

31. A child attending day camp has asthma, and her parent packed and sent with her all of her medicine in a small carry bag. The child has an asthma attack that is severe enough to warrant a rescue drug. Which medication from the child's bag is best to use for the acute symptoms?
   a. Omalizumab (Xolair)
   b. Fluticasone (Flovent)
   c. Salmeterol (Serevent)
   d. Albuterol (Proventil)

32. What are the three main goals of asthma treatment?
   a. _____
   b. _____
   c. _____

33. For a patient who is a nonsmoker, which classic assessment finding of chronic airflow limitation is particularly important in diagnosing asthma?
   a. Cough
   b. Dyspnea
   c. Audible wheezing
   d. Tachypnea

34. A patient who is allergic to dogs experiences a sudden "asthma attack." Which assessment findings does the nurse expect for this patient?
   a. Slow, deep, pursed-lip respirations
   b. Breathlessness and difficulty completing sentences
   c. Clubbing of the fingers and cyanosis of the nail beds
   d. Bradycardia and irregular pulse

35. A patient is experiencing an asthma attack and shows an increased respiratory effort. Which arterial blood gas value is more associated with the early phase of the attack?
   a. $Paco_2$ of 60 mm Hg
   b. $Paco_2$ of 30 mm Hg
   c. pH of 7.40
   d. Pao_2 of 98 mm Hg

36. A patient who has well-controlled asthma has what kind of airway changes?
   a. Chronic, leading to hyperplasia
   b. Temporary and reversible
   c. Open alveoli
   d. Permanent and irreversible

37. What are the goals for drug therapy in the treatment of asthma? *(Select all that apply.)*
   a. Drugs are used to stop an attack once it has started.
   b. Weekly drugs are used to reduce the asthma response.
   c. Combination drugs are avoided in the treatment of asthma.
   d. Some patients only require drug therapy during an asthma episode.
   e. Drugs are used to change airway responsiveness.

38. The nurse is teaching a patient how to interpret peak expiratory flow readings and to use this information to manage drug therapy at home. Which statement by the patient indicates a need for additional teaching?
    a. "If the reading is in the green zone, there is no need to increase the drug therapy."
    b. "Red is 50% below my 'personal best'; I should try a rescue drug and seek help."
    c. "If the reading is in the yellow zone, I should increase my use of my inhalers."
    d. "If frequent yellow readings occur, I should see my doctor for a change in medications."

39. A patient with chronic bronchitis often shows signs of hypoxia. Which clinical manifestation is the priority to look out for in this patient?
    a. Chronic, nonproductive, dry cough
    b. Clubbing of fingers
    c. Large amounts of thick mucus
    d. Barrel chest

40. The nurse is taking a history for a patient with chronic pulmonary disease. The patient reports often sleeping in a chair that allows his head to be elevated rather than going to bed. The patient's behavior is a strategy to deal with which condition?
    a. Paroxysmal nocturnal dyspnea
    b. Orthopnea
    c. Tachypnea
    d. Cheyne-Stokes

41. A patient has chronic bronchitis. The nurse plans interventions for inadequate oxygenation based on which set of clinical manifestations?
    a. Chronic cough, thin secretions, and chronic infection
    b. Respiratory alkalosis, decreased $Paco_2$, and increased Pao_2
    c. Areas of chest tenderness and sputum production (often with hemoptysis)
    d. Large amounts of thick secretions and repeated infections

42. A patient has COPD with chronic difficult breathing. In planning this patient's care, what condition must the nurse acknowledge is present in this patient?
    a. Decreased need for calories and protein requirements since dyspnea causes activity intolerance
    b. COPD has no effect on calorie and protein needs, meal tolerance, satiety, appetite, and weight
    c. Increased metabolism and the need for additional calories and protein supplements
    d. Anabolic state, which creates conditions for building body strength and muscle mass

43. In obtaining a history for a patient with chronic airflow limitation, which risk factor is not related to potentially causing or triggering the disease process?
    a. Cigarette smoking
    b. Occupational and air pollution
    c. Genetic tendencies
    d. Smokeless tobacco

44. Which statement is true about the relationship of smoking cessation to the pathophysiology of COPD?
    a. Smoking cessation completely reverses the damage to the lungs.
    b. Smoking cessation slows the rate of disease progression.
    c. Smoking cessation is an important therapy for asthma but not for COPD.
    d. Smoking cessation reverses the effects on the airways but not the lungs.

45. A patient has a history of COPD but is admitted for a surgical procedure that is unrelated to the respiratory system. Nevertheless, to prevent any complications related to the patient's COPD, what does the nurse do?
    a. Assess the patient's respiratory system every 8 hours.
    b. Monitor for signs and symptoms of pneumonia.
    c. Give high-flow oxygen to maintain pulse oximetry readings.
    d. Instruct the patient to use a tissue if coughing or sneezing.

46. The nurse is instructing a patient regarding complications of COPD. Which statement by the patient indicates the need for additional teaching?
   a. "I have to be careful because I am susceptible to respiratory infections."
   b. "I could develop heart failure, which could be fatal if untreated."
   c. "My COPD is serious, but it can be reversed if I follow my doctor's orders."
   d. "The lack of oxygen could cause my heart to beat in an irregular pattern."

47. What is the purpose of pulmonary function testing?
   a. Determines the oxygen liter flow rates required by the patient
   b. Measures blood gas levels before bronchodilators are administered
   c. Evaluates the movement of oxygenated blood from the lung to the heart
   d. Distinguishes airway disease from restrictive lung disease

48. A patient with respiratory difficulty has completed a pulmonary function test before starting any treatment. The peak expiratory flow (PEF) is 15% to 20% below what is expected for this adult patient's age, gender, and size. The nurse anticipates this patient will need additional information about which topic?
   a. Further diagnostic tests to confirm pulmonary hypertension
   b. How to manage asthma medications and identify triggers
   c. Smoking cessation and its relationship to COPD
   d. How to manage the acute episode of respiratory infection

49. Patients with asthma are taught self-care activities and treatment modalities according to the "step method." Which symptoms and medication routines relate to step III?
   a. Symptoms occur daily; daily use of inhaled corticosteroid, add a long-acting beta agonist
   b. Symptoms occur more than once per week; daily use of anti-inflammatory inhaler
   c. Symptoms occur less than once per week; use of rescue inhalers once per week
   d. Frequent exacerbations with limited physical activity; increased use of rescue inhalers

50. Why is a high-liter flow of oxygen contraindicated in a patient with COPD?
   a. The patient depends on a hypercapnic drive to breathe.
   b. The patient depends on a hypoxic drive to breathe.
   c. Receiving too much oxygen over a short time results in headache.
   d. Tolerance develops; therefore high doses needed later will be ineffective.

51. In assisting a patient with chronic airflow limitation to relieve dyspnea, which sitting position offers the patient no benefit?
   a. On edge of chair, leaning forward with arms folded and resting on a small table
   b. In a low semi-reclining position with the shoulders back and knees apart
   c. Forward in a chair with feet spread apart and elbows placed on the knees
   d. Head slightly flexed, with feet spread apart and shoulders relaxed

52. The nurse is developing a teaching plan for a patient with chronic airflow limitation using the priority patient problem of insufficient knowledge related to energy conservation. What does the nurse advise the patient to avoid?
   a. Performing activities at a relaxed pace throughout the day with rest periods
   b. Working on activities that require using arms at chest level or lower
   c. Eating three large meals per day
   d. Talking and performing activities separately

53. A patient with COPD has meal-related dyspnea. To address this issue, which drug does the nurse offer the patient 30 minutes before the meal?
    a. Albuterol (Ventolin)
    b. Guaifenesin (Organidin)
    c. Fluticasone (Flovent)
    d. Pantoprazole sodium (Protonix)

54. The laboratory result for a patient's theophylline level is 18 mcg/mL. What action does the nurse take?
    a. Place the results in the patient's chart because the value is within therapeutic range.
    b. Immediately alert the physician because the value indicates that the dose is too high.
    c. Contact the physician during AM rounds to get a prescription to increase the dose.
    d. Immediately assess the patient for adverse reactions related to a toxic level.

55. A patient is receiving ipratropium (Atrovent) and reports nausea, blurred vision, headache, and inability to sleep. What action does the nurse take?
    a. Administer a PRN medication for nausea and a mild PRN sedative.
    b. Report these symptoms to the physician as signs of overdose.
    c. Obtain a physician's request for an ipratropium level.
    d. Tell the patient that these side effects are normal and not to worry.

56. A patient with asthma has been prescribed a Flovent inhaler. What is the purpose of this drug for the patient?
    a. Relaxes the smooth muscles of the airway
    b. Acts as a bronchodilator in severe episodes
    c. Reduces obstruction of airways by decreasing inflammation
    d. Reduces the histamine effect of the triggering agent

57. What is the advantage of using the aerosol route for administering short-acting beta$_2$ agonists?
    a. Achieves a rapid and effective anti-inflammatory action
    b. Reduces the risk for fungal infections
    c. Increases patient compliance because it is easy to use
    d. Provides rapid therapy with fewer systemic side effects

58. The nurse is teaching a patient with chronic airflow limitation about his medications. What is the correct sequence for administering aerosol treatments?
    a. Bronchodilator should be taken 5 to 10 minutes after the steroid.
    b. Bronchodilator should be taken at least 5 minutes before other inhaled drugs.
    c. Bronchodilator should be taken immediately after the steroid.
    d. Bronchodilator and steroid are two different classes of drugs, so sequence is irrelevant.

59. A patient has been prescribed cromolyn sodium (Intal) for the treatment of asthma. Which statement by the patient indicates a correct understanding of this drug?
    a. "It opens my airways and provides short-term relief."
    b. "It is the medication that should be used 30 minutes before exercise."
    c. "It is not intended for use during acute episodes of asthma attacks."
    d. "It is a steroid medication, so there are severe side effects."

60. After the nurse has instructed a patient with COPD in the proper coughing technique, which action the next day by the patient indicates the need for additional teaching or intervention?
    a. Coughing upon rising in the morning
    b. Coughing before meals
    c. Coughing after meals
    d. Coughing at bedtime

61. A family member of a patient with COPD asks the nurse, "What is the purpose of making him cough on a routine basis?" What is the nurse's best response?
    a. "We have to check the color and consistency of his sputum."
    b. "We don't want him to feel embarrassed when coughing in public, so we actively encourage it."
    c. "It improves air exchange by increasing airflow in the larger airways."
    d. "If he cannot cough, the physician may elect to do a tracheostomy."

62. The nurse is teaching and assisting a patient with controlled coughing. Place the steps for the "controlled coughing" in the correct order using the numbers 1 through 7.

    _____ a. Turns shoulders inward, bends head downward, and hugs pillow to stomach

    _____ b. Repeats the procedure at least twice

    _____ c. Returns to a sitting position and then takes a comfortable deep breath

    _____ d. Takes three to five deep breaths

    _____ e. Bends forward slowly while coughing two or three times from the same breath

    _____ f. Rests and performs mouth care

    _____ g. Sits in a chair or on the side of a bed with feet placed firmly on the floor

63. A patient with a history of bronchitis for greater than 20 years is hospitalized. With this patient's history, what is a potential complication?
    a. Right-sided heart failure
    b. Left-sided heart failure
    c. Renal disease
    d. Stroke

64. The nurse notes these clinical findings in the patient from the previous question: fatigue, dependent edema, distended neck veins, and cyanotic lips. What condition is the patient exhibiting?
    a. COPD
    b. Cor pulmonale
    c. Asthma
    d. Lung cancer

65. A patient is admitted with asthma. Which assessment findings are most likely to indicate that the patient's asthma condition is deteriorating and progressing toward respiratory failure?
    a. Rales, rhonchi, and productive cough with yellow sputum
    b. Tachypnea; thick, tenacious sputum; and hemoptysis
    c. Audible breath sounds, wheezing, and use of accessory muscles
    d. Respiratory alkalosis; slow, shallow respiratory rate

66. A patient has returned several times to the clinic for treatment of respiratory problems. Which action does the nurse perform first?
    a. Obtain a history of the patient's previous respiratory problems and response to therapy.
    b. Ask the patient to describe his compliance to the prescribed therapies.
    c. Obtain a request for diagnostic testing, including a tuberculosis and human immune deficiency virus (HIV) evaluation.
    d. Listen to the patient's lungs, obtain a pulse oximetry reading, and count the respiratory rate.

67. A patient is undergoing diagnostic testing for possible cystic fibrosis (CF). Which nonpulmonary assessment findings does the nurse expect to observe in a patient with CF? *(Select all that apply.)*
    a. Peripheral edema
    b. Abdominal distention
    c. Steatorrhea
    d. Constipation
    e. Gastroesophageal reflux

68. The nurse is caring for a patient who has cystic fibrosis. Which assessment findings indicate the need for exacerbation therapy? *(Select all that apply.)*
    a. New-onset crackles
    b. Increased activity tolerance
    c. Increased frequency of coughing
    d. Increased chest congestion
    e. Increased Sao$_2$
    f. At least a 10% decrease in FEV$_1$

69. A patient with cystic fibrosis (CF) is admitted to the medical-surgical unit for an elective surgery. Which infection control measure is best for this patient?
    a. It is best to put two patients with CF in the same room.
    b. Standard Precautions including handwashing are sufficient.
    c. The patient is to be placed on Contact Isolation.
    d. Measures that limit close contact between people with CF are needed.

70. The nurse is working for a manufacturing company and is responsible for routine employee health issues. Which primary prevention is most important for those employees at high risk for occupational pulmonary disease?
    a. Screen all employees by use of chest x-ray films twice a year.
    b. Advise employees not to smoke and to use masks and ventilation equipment.
    c. Perform pulmonary function tests once a year on all employees.
    d. Refer at-risk employees to a social worker for information about pensions.

71. A patient had prolonged occupational exposure to petroleum distillates and subsequently developed a chronic lung disease. This patient is advised to seek frequent health examinations because there is a high risk for developing which respiratory disease condition?
    a. Tuberculosis
    b. Cystic fibrosis
    c. Lung cancer
    d. Pulmonary hypertension

72. The nurse has completed a community presentation about lung cancer. Which statement from a participant demonstrates an understanding of the information presented?
    a. "The primary prevention for reducing the risk of lung cancer is to stop smoking and avoid secondhand smoke."
    b. "The overall 5-year survival rate for all patients with lung cancer is 85%."
    c. "The death rate for lung cancer is less than prostate, breast, and colon cancer combined."
    d. "Cures are most likely for patients who undergo treatment for stage III disease."

73. A patient with lung cancer has been readmitted for periodic confusion and reports of lower back pain. These symptoms could be a manifestation of _____ and _____ metastasis.

74. Which sites are commonly affected by lung cancer metastasis? *(Select all that apply.)*
    a. Heart
    b. Bone
    c. Liver
    d. Colon
    e. Brain

True or False? *Read each statement about lung cancer and write T for true or F for false in the blanks provided. If the statement is false, correct the statement to make it true.*

_____ 75. There are two primary classifications of lung cancer—small cell and non–small cell.

_____ 76. Non–small cell lung cancer is further divided into three types—squamous, adenocarcinoma, and large cell.

_____ 77. Hypoglycemia could be one manifestation of paraneoplastic syndrome.

_____ 78. Wearing a specialized mask can decrease the risk of developing occupation-related lung cancer.

_____ 79. Onset of symptoms is a positive sign of early disease.

_____ 80. A chest x-ray film is a good screening tool for lung cancer.

_____ 81. Surgical intervention for non–small cell cancer is the goal for curing the patient.

_____ 82. A wedge resection is a form of surgical intervention that removes a small localized section of the diseased lung.

83. A patient who smokes is assessed for which warning signs associated with cancer? *(Select all that apply.)*
    a. Dyspnea
    b. Dark yellow-colored sputum
    c. Persistent cough or change in cough
    d. Abdominal pain and frequent stools
    e. Recurring episodes of pleural effusion

84. Which statement is true about radiation therapy for lung cancer patients?
    a. It is given daily in "cycles" over the course of several months.
    b. It causes hair loss, nausea, and vomiting for the duration of treatment.
    c. It causes dry skin at the radiation site, fatigue, and changes in appetite with nausea.
    d. It is the best method of treatment for systemic metastatic disease.

85. The nurse is taking a report on a patient who had a pneumonectomy 4 days ago. Which question is the best to ask during the shift report?
    a. "Does the physician want us to continue encouraging use of the spirometer?"
    b. "How much drainage did you see in the Pleur-Evac during your shift?"
    c. "Do we have a request to 'milk' the patient's chest tube?"
    d. "Does the surgeon want the patient placed on the nonoperative side?"

86. The nurse is caring for a patient with a chest tube. What is the correct nursing intervention for this patient?
    a. The patient is encouraged to cough and do deep-breathing exercises frequently.
    b. "Stripping" of the chest tubes is done routinely to prevent obstruction by blood clots.
    c. Water level in the suction chamber need not be monitored, just the collection chamber.
    d. Drainage containers are positioned upright or on the bed next to the patient.

87. Upon observation of a chest tube setup, the nurse reports to the physician that there is a leak in the chest tube and system. How has the nurse identified this problem?
    a. Drainage in the collection chamber has decreased.
    b. The bubbling in the suction chamber has suddenly increased.
    c. Fluctuation in the water seal chamber has stopped.
    d. There was onset of vigorous bubbling in the water seal chamber.

88. The physician's prescriptions indicate an increase in the suction to –20 cm for a patient with a chest tube. To implement this, the nurse performs which intervention?
    a. Increases the wall suction to the medium setting, and observes gentle bubbling in the suction chamber
    b. Adds water to the suction and drainage chambers to the level of –20 cm
    c. Stops the suction, adds sterile water to level of –20 cm to the water seal chamber, and resumes the wall suction
    d. Has the patient cough and deep-breathe, and monitors level of fluctuation to achieve –20 cm

89. A patient is fearful that she might develop lung cancer because her father and grandfather died of cancer. She seeks advice about how to modify lifestyle factors that contribute to cancer. How does the nurse advise this patient?
    a. Not to worry about air pollution unless there is hydrocarbon exposure
    b. Quit her job if she has continuous exposure to lead or other heavy metals
    c. Avoid situations where she would be exposed to "secondhand" smoke
    d. Not to be concerned because there are no genetic factors associated with lung cancer

90. The nurse has determined that a patient with COPD has the priority problem of impaired oxygenation related to reduced airway size, ventilatory muscle fatigue, and excessive mucus production. Which action is best to delegate to the nursing assistant?
    a. Observe the patient for fatigue, shortness of breath, or change of breathing pattern during ADLs.
    b. Report a respiratory rate of greater than 24/min at rest or 30/min after ambulating to the nurses' station.
    c. Encourage the patient to cough up sputum, and examine the color, consistency, and amount.
    d. Record and monitor the patient's intake and output, and give fluids to keep the secretions thin.

91. A patient is receiving a chemotherapy agent for lung cancer. The nurse anticipates that the patient is likely to have which common side effect?
    a. Diarrhea
    b. Nausea
    c. Flatulence
    d. Constipation

92. A patient is having pain resulting from bone metastases caused by lung cancer. What is the most effective intervention for relieving the patient's pain?
    a. Support the patient through chemotherapy.
    b. Handle and move the patient very gently.
    c. Administer analgesics around the clock.
    d. Reposition the patient, and use distraction.

93. A patient has a chest tube in place. What does the water in the water seal chamber do when the system is functioning correctly?
    a. Bubbles vigorously and continuously
    b. Bubbles gently and continuously
    c. Fluctuates with the patient's respirations
    d. Stops fluctuation, and bubbling is not observed

94. Which intervention promotes comfort in dyspnea management for a patient with lung cancer?
    a. Administer morphine only when the patient requests it.
    b. Place the patient in a supine position with a pillow under the knees and legs.
    c. Encourage coughing and deep-breathing and independent ambulation.
    d. Provide supplemental oxygen via cannula or mask.

95. A patient with repeated pleural effusions as a result of lung cancer is injected with a sclerosing agent. What is the nurse's role?
    a. Position the patient so that the affected lung is dependent while the drug is being injected.
    b. Ensure that the chest tube is securely clamped after the instillation of the drug.
    c. Instruct the patient to remain very still for at least 2 hours after the drug has been injected.
    d. Notify the respiratory therapist to administer respiratory therapy treatments.

96. A patient is diagnosed with cor pulmonale secondary to pulmonary hypertension and is receiving an infusion of epoprostenol (Flolan) through a small portable IV pump. What is the critical priority for this patient?
    a. Strict aseptic technique must be used to prevent sepsis.
    b. Infusion must not be interrupted, even for a few minutes.
    c. The patient must have a daily dose of warfarin (Coumadin).
    d. The patient must be assessed for angina-like chest pain and fatigue.

97. A patient has developed pulmonary hypertension. What is the goal of drug therapy for this patient?
    a. Dilate pulmonary vessels and prevent clot formation.
    b. Decrease pain and make the patient comfortable.
    c. Improve or maintain gas exchange.
    d. Maintain and manage pulmonary exacerbation.

True or False? *Read each statement about pulmonary hypertension and write T for true or F for false in the blanks provided. If the statement is false, correct the statement to make it true.*

_____ 98. Conditions such as COPD, pulmonary fibrosis, and pulmonary emboli can result in pulmonary hypertension.

_____ 99. When treating cor pulmonale, collaborative management is designed around the underlying cause of pulmonary hypertension.

100. A patient is newly diagnosed with sarcoidosis. Which statement by the patient indicates an understanding of the disease?
    a. "Corticosteroids are the main type of therapy for sarcoidosis."
    b. "Sarcoidosis is a type of lung cancer that is treatable if diagnosed early."
    c. "My condition can be treated with antibiotics."
    d. "Sarcoidosis is a type of pneumonia that is highly contagious."

101. The nurse is providing discharge instructions to a patient with pulmonary fibrosis and the family. What instructions are appropriate for this patient's diagnosis? *(Select all that apply.)*
    a. Using home oxygen
    b. Maintaining activity level as before
    c. Preventing respiratory infections
    d. Limiting fluid intake
    e. Energy conservation measures

102. A patient with a history of asthma enters the emergency department with severe dyspnea, accessory muscle involvement, neck vein distention, and severe inspiratory/expiratory wheezing. The nurse is prepared to assist the physician with which procedure if the patient does not respond to initial interventions?
    a. Emergency intubation
    b. Emergency needle thoracentesis
    c. Emergency chest tube insertion
    d. Emergency pleurodesis

103. A patient presents to the walk-in clinic with extremely labored breathing and a history of asthma that is unresponsive to prescribed inhalers or medications. What is the priority nursing action?
    a. Establish IV access to give emergency medications.
    b. Obtain the equipment and prepare the patient for intubation.
    c. Place the patient in a high Fowler's position, and start oxygen.
    d. Call 911 and report that the patient has probable status asthmaticus.

104. The nurse is instructing a patient to use a flutter-valve mucus clearance device. What should the patient be taught to do?
    a. Inhale deeply and exhale forcefully through the device.
    b. Use an inhalation technique that is similar to the handheld inhaler.
    c. Use pursed-lip breathing before and after usage.
    d. Exhale slowly through the nose, and then inhale by sniffing.

CASE STUDY: THE PATIENT WITH COPD (1)

Use a separate sheet of paper to answer the questions in this Case Study, or go to the "Prepare for Class" folder on your Evolve website at http://evolve.elsevier.com/Iggy/ to download and complete as a word processing file. Answer guidelines for this Case Study are also available on your Evolve website.

A 54-year-old man is admitted to the hospital for exacerbation of COPD. The nurse observes that the patient is sitting at the side of the bed leaning forward with both arms on a bedside tray. When asking the patient simple questions, he answers using one or two words with signs of dyspnea. He stops talking to rest for 20 to 40 seconds to relieve his dyspnea. He uses pursed-lip breathing when not talking and nods his head yes when he acknowledges to the nurse that he is short of breath. He has on oxygen at 2 L via nasal cannula. He has frequent episodes of a moderate amount (1 tbsp) of thick, pale-green sputum that he expectorates in tissues during the assessment. He reports that the coughing spells mostly occur in the morning. The patient's weight is 68 kg (149 lbs) and his height is 6'0". A previously recorded weight of the patient 6 months ago indicates an unplanned weight loss of 24 lbs. Further assessment reveals body odor and his underwear is soiled. Vital signs are: temp 37.1° C (98.9° F); heart rate 92/min in sinus rhythm; respirations 32/min; pulse oximetry 93% on 2 L O_2 nasal cannula at rest; blood pressure 130/65 mm Hg in a sitting position. The patient states, "I think a lot about how I have trouble breathing."

1. Document a nursing note based on the top two priority patient problems from the list below. Be sure to include Additional Notes pertinent to documentation.
    - Anxiety
    - Hypoxemia
    - Weight loss
    - Activity Intolerance

2. What in the assessment indicates that the patient is a smoker?

3. Why does the patient have weight loss?

4. Why does the patient prefer the position of sitting up rather than lying down? What is it called when the patient sleeps in a semi-sitting position?

CASE STUDY: THE PATIENT WITH COPD (2)

Use a separate sheet of paper to answer the questions in this Case Study, or go to the "Prepare for Class" folder on your Evolve website at http://evolve.elsevier.com/Iggy/ to download and complete as a word processing file. Answer guidelines for this Case Study are also available on your Evolve website.

The 72-year-old patient is being evaluated in his home by the home health nurse. He was admitted to the hospital for an exacerbation of his COPD and discharged 2 days ago. He states, "I feel a little more out of breath today than I usually do, but I am breathing better than I was when I went to the hospital." He is thin with a barrel-shaped chest. He is slow-moving and slightly stooped. He demonstrates rapid, shallow respirations at 30/min. He currently denies chest pain, but he reports feeling exhausted.

1. List at least eight questions the nurse could ask to evaluate this patient's current condition.

2. Describe how the nurse uses the following assessment tools to determine the severity of the dyspnea:
   a. Visual Analog Dyspnea Scale (VADS)
   b. Peak expiratory flowmeter
   c. Pulse oximetry (assume availability of portable unit)

3. Identify at least eight teaching points to help this patient conserve energy.

4. The patient tells the nurse that he has heard about pulmonary rehabilitation. He is not sure why his doctor did not suggest this for him, but he wonders if it is a possibility.
   a. What is pulmonary rehabilitation?
   b. Describe a typical simple rehabilitation plan.

5. Prepare and practice a dialogue for calling the physician to make an inquiry if pulmonary rehabilitation is appropriate for this patient.

33 CHAPTER

Care of Patients with Infectious Respiratory Problems

STUDY/REVIEW QUESTIONS

1. An adult patient diagnosed with rhinitis medicamentosa reports chronic nasal congestion. What does the nurse instruct the patient to do?
   a. Avoid exposure to older adults or immunosuppressed persons when symptoms flare.
   b. Damp-dust the house and clean the carpets to remove animal dander or mold.
   c. Discontinue the use of the current nose drops or sprays.
   d. Identify what triggers the hypersensitivity reaction by keeping a symptom diary.

2. The nurse notes that a patient has a disorder that contraindicates drug therapy that the physician has just prescribed for symptomatic relief of allergic rhinitis. Which disorder does the nurse report to the physician as a possible contraindication?
   a. Sleep apnea
   b. Valvular heart disease
   c. Ménière's disease
   d. Urinary retention

3. Drug therapy with antihistamines and decongestants to treat sinusitis are used with caution in the older adult because of which possible side effects? (Select all that apply.)
   a. Vertigo
   b. Hypotension
   c. Hypertension
   d. Insomnia
   e. Blurred vision

4. A patient comes to the walk-in clinic reporting seasonal nasal congestion, sneezing, rhinorrhea, and itchy watery eyes. The nurse identifies that the patient most likely has rhinitis and should also be assessed for sinusitis. How does the nurse assess for sinusitis?
   a. Observe the color and consistency of nasal secretions, and do a nasal swab.
   b. Ask the patient to speak, and listen for nasal sounds in the voice quality.
   c. Visually inspect the throat for redness or white patches, and take a throat culture.
   d. Use reflection of light through the tissues, and observe for a red glow on the cheek.

5. An 80-year-old man has a diagnosis of chronic rhinitis. Which statement is relevant to the care of this patient?
   a. Viral rhinitis is self-limiting and rarely leads to complications in the older adult.
   b. Antihistamines and decongestants should be used with caution.
   c. Antipyretics are rarely used because older adults are unlikely to have fever.
   d. Complementary and alternative therapies are not recommended for older adults.

6. A patient reports difficulty breathing, facial pain (especially when head is dependent), sneezing or coughing, green or bloody nasal drainage, productive cough, and low-grade fever. Which disorder does the nurse suspect?
   a. Rhinitis
   b. Tonsillitis
   c. Sinusitis
   d. Pneumonia

7. An older adult patient residing in a long-term care facility demonstrates new onset of coughing and sneezing and rhinorrhea after his grandchildren came to visit him. He denies pain or fever. Which infection control procedures does the nurse instruct the LPN to initiate in order to protect the other residents?
   a. Initiate the use of standard precautions when caring for the patient.
   b. Place the patient on droplet precautions for the first 2 to 3 days.
   c. Use gown and gloves when entering the room and perform hand hygiene.
   d. Instruct the patient to wash his hands after coughing or sneezing.

8. The nurse is assessing an older adult who has been diagnosed with bacterial pharyngitis. Which assessment finding is typically associated with this medical diagnosis, but may not be present in the older adult patient?
   a. Cough and rash
   b. High fever and elevated white blood cell (WBC) count
   c. Pain with speaking or swallowing
   d. Erythema of tonsils with yellow exudate

9. Which factors can contribute to acute pharyngitis? *(Select all that apply.)*
   a. Viruses
   b. Coughing
   c. Irritants
   d. Bacteria
   e. Alcohol

10. A patient reporting a "sore throat" also has a temperature of 101.4° F, scarlatiniform rash, and a positive rapid test throat culture. This patient will most likely be treated for which type of bacterial infection?
    a. Staphylococcus
    b. Pneumococcus
    c. Streptococcus
    d. Epstein-Barr virus

11. A patient reporting a soreness in the throat is diagnosed with "strep throat." To prevent complications such as rheumatic heart disease, this patient should receive antibiotic treatment within what time frame?
    a. 24 hours
    b. 48 hours
    c. 1 week
    d. 1 month

12. A child is diagnosed with a group B Streptococcus throat infection. In teaching the parents about treatment of the infection, what does the nurse instruct the parents?
    a. Need to complete penicillin or penicillin-like antibiotics
    b. Gradual return to activities until there are no physical complaints
    c. Purpose of a clear liquid diet until infection subsides
    d. Signs and symptoms of meningitis which is a common complication

13. Which patients are at risk for developing hospital-acquired pneumonia? *(Select all that apply.)*
    a. Confused patient
    b. Patient with atrial fibrillation who is alert and oriented
    c. Patient with gram-negative colonization of the mouth
    d. Patient with hyperthyroid disease
    e. Malnourished patient

14. The nurse is teaching the patient and family about care of a peritonsillar abscess at home. For what symptoms does the nurse indicate the need for the patient to go to the emergency department immediately? *(Select all that apply.)*
    a. Persistent cough
    b. Hoarseness
    c. Stridor
    d. Drooling
    e. Nausea and vomiting

15. A 35-year-old male patient with no health problems states that he had a flu shot last year and asks if it is necessary to have it again this year. What is the best response by the nurse?
    a. "No, because once you get a flu shot, it lasts for several years and is effective against many different viruses."
    b. "Yes, because the immunity against the virus wears off, increasing your chances of getting the flu."
    c. "Yes, because the vaccine guards against a specific virus and reduces your chances of acquiring flu."
    d. "No, flu shots are only for high-risk patients and you are not considered to be at high risk."

16. An active 45-year-old schoolteacher with chronic obstructive pulmonary disease (COPD) taking prednisone asks if it is necessary to get a flu shot. What is the best response by the nurse?
    a. "Yes, flu shots are highly recommended for patients with chronic illness and/or patients who are receiving immunotherapy."
    b. "No, flu shots are only recommended for patients 50 years old and older."
    c. "Yes, it will help minimize the risk of triggering an exacerbation of COPD."
    d. "No, patients who are active, not living in a nursing home, and not health care providers do not need a flu shot."

17. A patient who had sinus surgery has a surgical incision under the upper lip. The nurse intervenes when a well-intentioned family member performs which action in attempting to make the patient feel better?
    a. Uses the bed controls to move the patient to a semi-Fowler's position
    b. Hands the patient a tissue to blow the nose
    c. Brings the patient a special custard dessert from a nearby restaurant
    d. Gently helps the patient with oral hygiene during morning care

18. The nurse is giving discharge instructions to a patient diagnosed with a viral pharyngitis. Which statement by the patient indicates the need for further teaching?
    a. "I should try to rest, increase my fluid intake, and get a humidifier for the house."
    b. "I will wait for my test results, then I can get a prescription for antibiotics."
    c. "Over-the-counter analgesics, like Tylenol or ibuprofen, can be used for pain."
    d. "I should gargle several times a day with warm salt water and use throat lozenges."

19. A patient with COPD needs instruction in the measures to prevent pneumonia. What information does the nurse include? *(Select all that apply.)*
    a. Avoid going outside.
    b. Clean all respiratory equipment you have at home.
    c. Avoid indoor pollutants such as dust and aerosols.
    d. Get plenty of rest and sleep daily.
    e. Limit alcoholic beverages to 4-5 per week.

20. The nurse is taking a history on a patient who presents with symptoms of pharyngitis: sore throat with dry sensation, pain on swallowing, and low-grade fever. The patient mentions plans to take an overseas trip. Which immunization does the nurse suggest the patient should have, if not already received, before leaving?
    a. Tetanus toxoid
    b. Hepatitis B
    c. Diphtheria
    d. Yellow fever

21. A patient with a history of frequent and recurrent episodes of tonsillitis now reports a severe sore throat with pain that radiates behind the ear and difficulty swallowing. The nurse suspects the patient may have a peritonsillar abscess. On physical assessment, which deviated structure supports the nurse's supposition?
    a. Uvula
    b. Trachea
    c. Tongue
    d. Mucous membranes

22. A parent calls the emergency department (ED) about her child who reports a severe sore throat and refuses to drink fluids or to take liquid pain medication. What is the most important question for the nurse to ask in order to determine the need to seek immediate medical attention?
   a. "Does the child seem to be refusing fluids and medications because of the sore throat?"
   b. "Is the child drooling or do you hear stridor, a raspy rough sound when the child breathes?"
   c. "When did the symptoms start and how long have you been encouraging fluids?"
   d. "Is the throat red or do you see any white patches in the back of the throat?"

23. In a long-term care facility for older adults and immunocompromised patients, one employee and several patients have been diagnosed with influenza (flu). What does the supervising nurse do to decrease risk of infection to other patients?
   a. Ask employees who have flu to stay at home for at least 24 hours.
   b. Place any patient with a sore throat, cough, or rhinorrhea into isolation for 1 to 2 weeks.
   c. Ask employees with flu symptoms to stay at home for up to 5 days after onset of symptoms.
   d. Recommend that all patients and employees be immediately vaccinated for flu.

24. The nurse is giving discharge instructions to an adult patient diagnosed with the flu. The patient says, "I am generally pretty healthy, but I am concerned because my wife has several serious chronic health problems. What can I do to protect her from getting my flu?" What does the nurse instruct the patient to do? *(Select all that apply.)*
   a. Wash hands thoroughly after sneezing, coughing, or blowing nose.
   b. Avoid kissing, hugging, close face-to-face proximity, or hand-holding.
   c. If there is no tissue immediately available, cough or sneeze into your upper sleeve.
   d. Have the wife wear a respiratory filter mask until you stop coughing.
   e. Use disposable tissues rather than cloth handkerchiefs, and immediately dispose of tissues.

25. Number the events in sequential order as they pertain to the pathophysiologic process of pneumonia using the numbers 1 through 12.
   _____ a. Atelectasis
   _____ b. Possible septicemia
   _____ c. Decreased surfactant production and compliance
   _____ d. Arterial hypoxemia
   _____ e. Edema formation and inflammation
   _____ f. Tachypnea and tachycardia
   _____ g. Migration of WBCs to alveoli
   _____ h. Spread of organisms to other alveoli
   _____ i. Shunting of unoxygenated blood
   _____ j. Thickening of alveolar wall and stiffening of lungs
   _____ k. Diminished capillary blood flow in alveoli
   _____ l. Invasion of pulmonary tissue by pathogens

26. Which patient is at highest risk of developing pneumonia?
    a. Any hospitalized patient between the ages of 18 and 65 years
    b. 32-year-old trauma patient on a mechanical ventilator
    c. Disabled 54-year-old with osteoporosis; discharged to home
    d. Any patient who has not received the vaccine for pneumonia

27. Which statement best describes pneumonia?
    a. An infection of just the "windpipe" because the lungs are "clear" of any problems
    b. A serious inflammation of the bronchioles from various causes
    c. Only an infection of the lungs with mild to severe effects on breathing
    d. An inflammation resulting from lung damage caused by long-term smoking

28. A patient is seen in the health care provider's office and is diagnosed with community-acquired pneumonia. What are the most common symptoms the patient will have? *(Select all that apply.)*
    a. Dyspnea
    b. Abdominal pain
    c. Back pain
    d. Hypoxemia
    e. Chest discomfort

29. Which diagnostic tests are most likely to be done for a patient suspected of having community-acquired pneumonia? *(Select all that apply.)*
    a. Sputum gram stain
    b. Pulmonary function test
    c. Fluorescein bronchoscopy
    d. Peak flowmeter measurement
    e. Chest x-ray

30. The nurse is reviewing laboratory results for a patient who has pneumonia. Which laboratory value does the nurse expect to see for this patient?
    a. Decreased hemoglobin
    b. Increased red blood cells (RBCs)
    c. Decreased neutrophils
    d. Increased WBCs

31. A patient is diagnosed with pneumonia. During auscultation of the lower lung fields, the nurse hears coarse crackles and identifies the patient problem of impaired oxygenation. What is the underlying physiologic condition associated with the patient's condition?
    a. Hypoxemia
    b. Hyperemia
    c. Hypocapnia
    d. Hypercapnia

32. Which patient is the least likely to be at risk for developing pneumonia?
    a. Patient with a 5-year history of smoking
    b. Renal transplant patient
    c. Postoperative patient with a bedside commode
    d. Postoperative patient with a hip replacement

Matching. A patient is hospitalized and on a mechanical ventilator. Match the appropriate role to each person on the health professional team.

Health Professional
a. Nurse
b. Physician
c. Nonlicensed technician
d. Respiratory therapist

Role

_____ 33. Keep the head of bed elevated at 30 degrees per order

_____ 34. Order antimicrobial solution to swab the patient's mouth every 12 hours

_____ 35. Assess vital signs and pulse oximeter reading, and auscultate lung sounds

_____ 36. Keep tubing of mechanical ventilator changed as needed and per protocol

37. A patient is admitted to the hospital with pneumonia. What does the nurse expect the chest x-ray results to reveal?
    a. Patchy areas of consolidation
    b. Tension pneumothorax
    c. Thick secretions causing airway obstruction
    d. Large hyperinflated airways

38. What nursing intervention may help to prevent the complication of pneumonia for a surgical patient?
    a. Monitoring chest x-rays and white cell counts for early signs of infection
    b. Monitoring lung sounds every shift and encouraging fluids
    c. Teaching coughing, deep-breathing exercises, and use of incentive spirometry
    d. Encouraging hand hygiene among all caregivers, patients, and visitors

39. The nurse is conducting an in-service for the hospital staff about practices that help prevent pneumonia among at-risk patients. Which nursing intervention is encouraged as standard practice?
    a. Administering vaccines to patients at risk
    b. Implementing isolation for debilitated patients
    c. Restricting foods from home in immunosuppressed patients
    d. Decontaminating respiratory therapy equipment weekly

40. A patient hospitalized for pneumonia has the priority patient problem of Ineffective Airway Clearance related to fatigue, chest pain, excessive secretions, and muscle weakness. What nursing intervention helps to correct these problems?
    a. Administer oxygen to prevent hypoxemia and atelectasis.
    b. Push fluids to greater than 3000 mL/day to ensure adequate hydration.
    c. Administer respiratory therapy in a timely manner to decrease bronchospasms.
    d. Maintain semi-Fowler's position to facilitate breathing and prevent further fatigue.

41. A patient is admitted to the hospital for treatment of pneumonia. Which nursing assessment finding best indicates that the patient is responding to antibiotics?
    a. Wheezing, oxygen at 2 L/min, respiratory rate 26, no shortness of breath or chills
    b. Temperature 99° F, lung sounds clear, pulse oximetry on 2 L/min at 98%, cough with yellow sputum
    c. Cough, clear sputum, temperature 99° F, pulse oximetry at 96% on room air
    d. Feeling tired, respiratory rate 28 on 2 L/min of oxygen, audible breath sounds

42. The nurse is reviewing the laboratory results for an older adult patient with pneumonia. Which laboratory value frequently seen in patients with pneumonia may not be seen in this patient?
    a. RBC 4.0 to 5.0
    b. Hgb 12 to 16
    c. Hct 36 to 48
    d. WBC 12 to 18

43. A patient is admitted to the hospital to rule out pneumonia. Which infection control technique does the nurse maintain?
    a. Strict respiratory isolation and use of a specially designed facemask
    b. Respiratory isolation and contact isolation for sputum
    c. Respiratory isolation with a stock surgical mask
    d. Standard precautions and no respiratory isolation

44. A critical concern for a patient returning to the unit after a surgical procedure is related to impaired oxygenation caused by inadequate ventilation. Which arterial blood gas value and assessment finding indicates to the nurse that oxygen and incentive spirometry must be administered?
    a. Pao_2 is 90 mm Hg with crackles.
    b. Pao_2 is 90 mm Hg with wheezing.
    c. Pco_2 is 38 mm Hg with clear lung sounds.
    d. Pco_2 is 45 mm Hg with atelectasis.

45. The nurse has identified the priority patient problem of Ineffective Airway Clearance with bronchospasms for a patient with pneumonia. The patient has no previous history of chronic respiratory disorders. The nurse obtains an order for which nursing intervention?
    a. Increased liters of humidified oxygen via facemask
    b. Scheduled and PRN aerosol nebulizer bronchodilator treatments
    c. Handheld bronchodilator inhaler as needed
    d. Prednisone via inhaler or IV to reduce the inflammation

46. A patient is admitted to the hospital with pneumonia. Which approach to the administration of antibiotics does the nurse expect the physician to order?
    a. Start any antibiotic that is immediately available and follow up on culture results.
    b. Start broad-spectrum IV antibiotic therapy without delay.
    c. Wait for sputum culture results with specificity before starting antibiotic therapy.
    d. Obtain three sputum specimens before starting IV antibiotics to reduce risk of toxicity.

47. An older adult patient asks the nurse how often one should receive the pneumococcal vaccine for pneumonia prevention. What is the nurse's best response?
    a. "Every year, when the patient is receiving the 'flu shot.'"
    b. "The standard is vaccination every 3 years."
    c. "It is usually given once, but some older adults may need a second vaccination after 5 years."
    d. "There is no set schedule; it depends on the patient's history and risk factors."

48. The nurse is providing discharge instructions about pneumonia to a patient and family. Which discharge information is the nurse sure to include?
    a. Complete antibiotics as prescribed, rest, drink fluids, and minimize contact with crowds.
    b. Take all antibiotics as ordered, resume diet and all activities as before hospitalization.
    c. No restrictions regarding activities, diet, and rest because the patient is fully recovered when discharged.
    d. Continue antibiotics only until no further signs of pneumonia are present; avoid exposing immunosuppressed individuals.

49. A patient is admitted to the hospital with cough, purulent sputum production, temperature of 37.9° C (100.3° F), and reports of shortness of breath. In what sequence does the nurse provide these interventions to this patient? *(Select in order of priority.)*

    _____ a. Set up oxygen equipment and administer oxygen.

    _____ b. Instruct the patient about the importance of keeping the oxygen delivery device on.

    _____ c. Assess the need to suction for oral secretions.

    _____ d. Monitor the effectiveness of oxygen therapy (pulse oximetry, ABGs) as appropriate.

    _____ e. Monitor the patient's anxiety related to the need for oxygen delivery.

50. A patient has been treated for pneumonia and the nurse is preparing discharge instructions. The patient is capable of performing self-care and is anxious to return to his job at the construction site. Which instructions does the nurse give to this patient?
    a. "You are not contagious to others, so you can return to work as soon as you like."
    b. "You will continue to feel tired and will fatigue easily for the next several weeks."
    c. "Try to drink 4 quarts of water per day, especially if you are very physically active."
    d. "You should be able to return to work full-time in 2 weeks when your energy returns."

51. Which complication of pneumonia creates pain that increases on inspiration because of inflammation of the parietal pleura?
    a. Pleuritic chest pain
    b. Pulmonary emboli
    c. Pleural effusion
    d. Meningitis

52. Which conditions may cause patients to be at risk for aspiration pneumonia? *(Select all that apply.)*
    a. Continuous tube feedings
    b. Bronchoscopy procedure
    c. MRI procedure
    d. Decreased level of consciousness
    e. Stroke
    f. Chest tube

53. An older adult patient often coughs and chokes while eating or trying to take medication. The patient insists that he is okay, but the nurse identifies the priority patient problem of Risk for Aspiration. Which nursing interventions are used to prevent aspiration pneumonia? *(Select all that apply.)*
    a. Head of bed should always be elevated during feeding.
    b. Monitor the patient's ability to swallow small bites.
    c. Give thin liquids to drink in small frequent amounts.
    d. Consult a nutritionist and obtain swallowing studies.
    e. Monitor the patient's ability to swallow saliva.
    f. Place the patient on NPO status until swallowing is normal.

54. Which condition causes a patient to have the greatest risk for community-acquired pneumonia?
    a. Tube feedings
    b. History of tobacco use
    c. Poor nutritional status
    d. Altered mental status

55. In the event of a new SARS outbreak, what is the nurse's primary role?
    a. Immediately report new cases of SARS to the Centers for Disease Control and Prevention.
    b. Administer oxygen, standard antibiotics, and supportive therapies to patients.
    c. Prevent the spread of infection to other employees and patients.
    d. Initiate and strictly enforce contact isolation procedures.

56. The nurse is preparing a community information packet about "bird flu." What information does the nurse include for public dissemination? *(Select all that apply.)*
    a. In the event of an outbreak, do not eat any cooked or uncooked poultry products.
    b. Prepare a minimum of 2 weeks supply of food, water, and routine prescription drugs.
    c. Listen to public health announcements and early warning signs for disease outbreaks.
    d. Avoid traveling to areas where there has been a suspected outbreak of disease.
    e. Obtain a supply of antiviral drugs such as oseltamivir (Tamiflu).
    f. In the event of an outbreak, avoid going to public areas such as churches or schools.

57. A patient reports experiencing mild fatigue and a dry, harsh cough. There is a possibility of exposure to inhalation anthrax, but the patient currently reports feeling much better. What does the nurse advise the patient to do?
    a. Have a complete blood count to rule out the disease.
    b. Monitor for and immediately seek attention for respiratory symptoms.
    c. Consult a physician for diagnostic testing and antibiotic therapy.
    d. Stay at home, rest, increase fluid intake, and avoid public places.

58. A patient with HIV is admitted to the hospital with a temperature of 99.6° F, and reports of bloody sputum, night sweats, feeling of tiredness, and shortness of breath. What are these assessment findings consistent with?
    a. *Pneumocystis jiroveci* pneumonia (PCP)
    b. Tuberculosis
    c. Superinfection as a result of a low CD4 count
    d. Severe bronchitis

59. Which statement about the precautions of caring for a hospitalized patient with tuberculosis (TB) are true? *(Select all that apply.)*
    a. Health care workers must wear a mask that covers the face and mouth.
    b. Negative airflow rooms are required for these patients.
    c. Health care workers must wear a N95 or high-efficiency particulate air (HEPA) mask.
    d. Gown and gloves are included in appropriate barrier protection.
    e. Strict contact precautions must be maintained.

60. Tuberculosis is transmitted via the _____ route.

61. Which people are at greatest risk for developing TB in the United States? *(Select all that apply.)*
    a. An alcoholic homeless man who occasionally stays in a shelter
    b. A college student sharing a room in a dormitory
    c. A person with immune dysfunction or HIV
    d. A homemaker who does volunteer work at a homeless shelter
    e. Foreign immigrants (especially those from the Philippines and Mexico)

62. After several weeks of "not feeling well," a patient is seen in the physician's office for possible TB. If TB is present, which assessment findings does the nurse expect to observe? *(Select all that apply.)*
    a. Fatigue
    b. Weight gain
    c. Night sweats
    d. Chest soreness
    e. Low-grade fever

63. Which test result indicates a patient has clinically active TB?
    a. Induration of 12 mm and positive sputum
    b. Positive chest x-ray for TB
    c. Positive chest x-ray and clinical symptoms
    d. Sputum tests positive for blood

64. After receiving the subcutaneous Mantoux skin test, a patient with no risk factors returns to the clinic in the required 48 to 72 hours for the test results. Which assessment finding indicates a positive result?
   a. Test area is red, warm, and tender to touch
   b. Induration or a hard nodule of any size at the site
   c. Induration/hardened area measures 5 mm or greater
   d. Induration/hardened area measures 10 mm or greater

65. A patient has a positive skin test result for TB. What explanation does the nurse give to the patient?
   a. "There is active disease, but you are not yet infectious to others."
   b. "There is active disease and you need immediate treatment."
   c. "You have been infected but this does not mean active disease is present."
   d. "A repeat skin test is necessary because the test could give a false-positive result."

66. What is the *minimum* time period for treatment of TB? _____

67. A patient has been compliant with drug therapy for TB and has returned as instructed for follow-up. Which result indicates that the patient is no longer infectious/communicable?
   a. Negative chest x-ray
   b. No clinical symptoms
   c. Negative skin test
   d. Three negative sputum cultures

68. A patient diagnosed with TB agrees to take the medication as instructed and to complete the therapy. When does the nurse tell the patient is the best time to take the medication?
   a. Before breakfast
   b. After breakfast
   c. Midday
   d. Bedtime

69. A patient has an HIV infection, but the TB skin test shows an induration of less than 10 mm and no clinical symptoms of TB are present. Which medication does the patient receive for a period of 12 months to prevent TB?
   a. Bacille Calmette-Guérin (BCG) vaccine
   b. Isoniazid (INH)
   c. Ethambutol
   d. Streptomycin

70. The nurse is teaching a patient about the combination drug therapy that is used in the treatment of TB. Which patient statement indicates the nurse's instruction was effective?
   a. "I will take three drugs: isoniazid, rifampin, and pyrazinamide, then ethambutol may be added later."
   b. "Combining the drugs in one pill is a convenient way for me to take all the medications."
   c. "The isoniazid combines with the TB bacteria. I can take the rifampin and pyrazinamide if I continue to have symptoms."
   d. "Combining the medications means to take the isoniazid, rifampin, and pyrazinamide all at the same time."

71. A patient diagnosed with TB has been receiving treatment for 3 weeks and has clinically shown improvement. The family asks the nurse if the patient is still infectious. What is the nurse's reply?
   a. "The patient is still infectious until the entire treatment is completed."
   b. "The patient is not infectious but needs to continue treatment for at least 6 months."
   c. "The patient is infectious until there is a negative chest x-ray."
   d. "The patient may or may not be infectious; a PPD must be done."

Matching. *Match the nursing interventions with the medications to treat TB. Answers may be used more than once.*

TB Medications

a.   Isoniazid (INH)
b.   Rifampin
c.   Pyrazinamide
d.   Ethambutol

Nursing Interventions

_____ 72.   Teach women that this drug reduces the effectiveness of oral contraceptives and that another form of birth control should be used while on this therapy.

_____ 73.   Teach the patient that urine will be orange in color.

_____ 74.   Consult the physician when the patient complains of blurry vision after starting treatment.

_____ 75.   Teach the patient not to take medications such as Maalox with this medication.

_____ 76.   Avoid drinking alcoholic beverages.

_____ 77.   Take a multivitamin with B-complex.

_____ 78.   Teach the patient to take on an empty stomach 1 hour before or 2 hours after meals.

_____ 79.   Teach the patient to report an increased tendency to bruise or bleed.

_____ 80.   If going out into the sun, wear protective clothing and sunscreen.

_____ 81.   Teach patients to identify changes in the ability to differentiate colors.

82.   A patient with suspected TB is admitted to the hospital. Along with a private room, which nursing intervention is appropriate related to isolation procedures?
  a.   Respiratory isolation and contact isolation for sputum only
  b.   Strict respiratory isolation and use of specially designed facemasks
  c.   Respiratory isolation with surgical masks until diagnosis is confirmed
  d.   No respiratory isolation necessary until diagnosis is confirmed

83.   A patient is admitted to the hospital to rule out TB. What type of mask does the nurse wear when caring for this patient?
  a.   Surgical facemask
  b.   Surgical facemask with eye shield
  c.   HEPA respirator mask
  d.   Any type of mask that covers the nose and mouth

84. After being discharged from the hospital, a patient is diagnosed with TB at the outpatient clinic. What is the correct procedure regarding public health policy in this case?
    a. Contact the infection control nurse at the hospital because the hospital is responsible for follow-up of this case.
    b. There are no regulations because the patient was diagnosed at the clinic and not during hospitalization.
    c. Contact the public health nurse so that all individuals who have come in contact with the patient can be screened.
    d. Have the patient sign a waiver regarding the hospital and clinic's liability for treatment.

85. Which diagnostic test is *not* used to diagnose TB?
    a. Chest radiography
    b. Complete blood count
    c. Mantoux skin test
    d. Sputum culture

86. Patients who are at high risk for TB would be asked which questions upon assessment? *(Select all that apply.)*
    a. "What does your diet normally consist of?"
    b. "Do you have an immune dysfunction or HIV?"
    c. "Do you abuse alcohol or inject recreational drugs?"
    d. "Where do you live in the United States?"
    e. "Do you work in a crowded area such as a prison or mental health facility?"

87. After a motor vehicle accident, the patient is dependent on mechanical ventilation. The nurse initiates "ventilator bundle" precautions to prevent ventilator-associated pneumonia. Which actions does the nurse perform to initiate these precautions? *(Select all that apply.)*
    a. Elevate head of the bed to between 30 and 45 degrees whenever possible.
    b. Continuously remove subglottic secretions.
    c. Change the ventilator circuit every 24 hours.
    d. Perform handwashing before and after contact with each patient.
    e. No rings are worn when caring for ventilator patients.
    f. Perform meticulous oral care no less frequently than every 12 hours.

88. The nurse is making home visits to an older adult recovering from a hip fracture and identifies the priority patient problem of risk for respiratory infection. Which condition represents a factor of normal aging that would contribute to this increased risk?
    a. Inability to force a cough
    b. Decreased strength of respiratory muscles
    c. Increased elastic recoil of alveoli
    d. Increased macrophages in alveoli

CASE STUDY: THE OLDER ADULT PATIENT WITH TUBERCULOSIS

Use a separate sheet of paper to answer the questions in this Case Study, or go to the "Prepare for Class" folder on your Evolve website at http://evolve.elsevier.com/Iggy/ to download and complete as a word processing file. Answer guidelines for this Case Study are also available on your Evolve website.

The patient is a 65-year-old woman who shares a three-room inner-city apartment with two of her daughters and their seven children. She comes into the neighborhood walk-in clinic reporting extreme fatigue, a 30-pound weight loss, and a cough of 4 months' duration. A Mantoux test, sputum culture, and chest x-ray confirm a diagnosis of tuberculosis (TB). She is to begin a 12-month course of medication therapy with isoniazid (INH) 300 mg orally once a day, and rifampin (Rifadin) 600 mg orally once a day.

1. Discuss why one or more pharmacologic agents are used to treat TB.
2. When is the best time for this patient to take the chemotherapeutic agents to minimize the side effects?
3. Why should rifampin (Rifadin) be taken on an empty stomach?
4. What type of follow-up care should be planned for this patient?
5. How long will this patient be considered contagious?
6. What measures should be taken with the other family members? Explain your answer.
7. Develop a teaching-learning plan for this patient.

Three weeks after diagnosis, the patient returns to the clinic stating that she has stopped taking her medications because they made her sick to her stomach. She is unable to eat and has continued to lose weight.

8. Identify the relevant patient problems for this patient based on the above information.
9. Discuss what the nurse should do to assist this patient in taking her medications and eating a balanced diet.

CASE STUDY: THE YOUNG ADULT WITH TUBERCULOSIS

Use a separate sheet of paper to answer the questions in this Case Study, or go to the "Prepare for Class" folder on your Evolve website at http://evolve.elsevier.com/Iggy/ to download and complete as a word processing file. Answer guidelines for this Case Study are also available on your Evolve website.

A young adult male who is from Mexico was screened for TB as part of a health checkup for a job in Florida. He lives with his wife and one child. The patient's PPD test was positive for TB two weeks ago. The patient is hospitalized and has positive sputum cultures and chest x-ray to confirm the diagnosis of TB.

The patient has a cough with purulent sputum and states that he has experienced progressive fatigue, weight loss of 20 lbs in the last 3 months, and night sweats. On assessment, lungs are auscultated and reveal bronchial breath sounds and crackles, mostly on the left lung fields. On the right lung fields, lung sounds are clear to diminished. The patient is on 2 L O_2 per nasal cannula. Isolation precautions are in place which includes Airborne Precautions.

Vital signs are: temp 37.3° C (99.2° F); heart rate/rhythm 89/min sinus rhythm; respirations 24/min; pulse oximeter reading 93% on 2 L O_2 nasal cannula at rest.

1. Identify the top two patient problems from the list below, and document each using the information in the case study. Include Additional Notes in your documentation.
   - Hypoxemia
   - Impaired oxygenation
   - Inadequate nutrition
2. What first-line drugs will likely be used to treat this patient's tuberculosis?
3. What kind of isolation must this patient be placed in and why? What measures are taken in these isolation procedures?
4. Sputum cultures for acid-fast bacilli (AFB) are ordered. When is the best time to collect sputum?
5. Can sputum that contains saliva be sent to the laboratory?
6. Before the patient is discharged, what interventions must be done at his home in preparation for his return?

CASE STUDY: THE PATIENT WITH PNEUMONIA

Use a separate sheet of paper to answer the questions in this Case Study, or go to the "Prepare for Class" folder on your Evolve website at http://evolve.elsevier.com/Iggy/ to download and complete as a word processing file. Answer guidelines for this Case Study are also available on your Evolve website.

A 75-year-old married woman comes to the outpatient clinic with her husband reporting a severe cough, left-sided chest pain, and she holds her left side while coughing. She appears anxious and her face is flushed. Vital signs are temperature 102.6° F, pulse 118, apical; respirations 32, shallow; and blood pressure 120/80. A diagnosis of pneumonia is suspected. A sputum specimen, chest x-ray, arterial blood gases, and complete blood count are ordered.

1. What should this patient and her husband be taught about the sputum collection and x-ray?
2. What will likely be heard when the patient's lungs are auscultated? Explain your answer.

A diagnosis of pneumonia is confirmed by the chest x-ray and sputum cultures. Because the patient's blood gases are within normal limits, she will be managed on an outpatient basis.

3. Identify the relevant patient problems for this patient based on the above information.

The physician orders cefaclor (Ceclor) 500 mg orally every 8 hours and wants the patient to return to the clinic in 1 week. If her condition does not improve within 48 hours or she becomes short of breath, she should call or return to the clinic.

4. Develop teaching-learning and discharge care plans for the patient and her husband.

34 CHAPTER

Care of Critically Ill Patients with Respiratory Problems

STUDY/REVIEW QUESTIONS

1. What are the risk factors for pulmonary embolism (PE) and deep vein thrombosis (DVT)? *(Select all that apply.)*
   a. Trauma
   b. Swimming activity
   c. Heart failure
   d. Chronic obstructive pulmonary disease (COPD)
   e. Cancer (particularly lung or prostate)

2. What is the most common site of origin for a clot to occur, causing a PE?
   a. Right side of the heart
   b. Deep veins of the legs and pelvis
   c. Antecubital vein in upper extremities
   d. Subclavian veins

3. A(n) _____ _____ embolus carries a high mortality rate and occurs as a rare complication of childbirth, abortion, or amniocentesis.

4. Any substance can cause an embolism, but _____ _____ are the most common cause.

5. Which conditions define respiratory failure? *(Select all that apply.)*
   a. Ventilatory failure
   b. Circulatory failure
   c. Oxygenation failure
   d. Severe anemia
   e. Combination of ventilatory and oxygenation failure

6. A patient in the hospital being treated for a PE is receiving a continuous infusion of heparin. When the nurse comes to take vital signs, the patient has blood on the front of his chest and nose, and the patient is holding a tissue saturated with blood to his nose. What is the priority order of actions the nurse takes? *(Select in priority order.)*

   _____ a. Have the patient sit up and lean forward, pinching the nostrils.

   _____ b. Have a patient care technician set up oral suctioning to suction excess blood from patient's mouth.

   _____ c. Stop the heparin IV infusion.

   _____ d. Notify the physician.

   _____ e. Obtain laboratory results for prothrombin time and complete blood count.

7. The nurse's young neighbor who smokes is going on an overseas flight. The neighbor knows he is at risk for DVT and PE, and asks the nurse for advice. What does the nurse suggest?
   a. Exercise regularly and walk around before boarding the flight.
   b. Get a prescription for heparin therapy and take it before the flight.
   c. Drink water; get up every hour for at least 5 minutes during the flight.
   d. Elevate the legs as much as possible during and after the flight.

8. The nurse is caring for several postoperative patients at risk for developing PE. Which interventions does the nurse use to help prevent the development of PE in these patients? *(Select all that apply.)*
   a. Start passive and active range-of-motion exercises for the extremities.
   b. Ambulate postoperative patients soon after surgery.
   c. Use antiembolism devices postoperatively.
   d. Elevate legs in an extended position.
   e. Change patient position every 4 to 6 hours.
   f. Massage leg muscles.
   g. Administer drugs to prevent episodes of Valsalva maneuver.

9. The nurse suspects a patient has a PE and notifies the physician who orders an arterial blood gas. The physician is en route to the facility. The nurse anticipates and prepares the patient for which additional diagnostic test?
   a. CT scan
   b. Pulmonary angiography
   c. 12-lead ECG
   d. Ventilation and perfusion scan

10. The physician orders heparin therapy for a patient with a relatively small PE. The patient states, "I didn't tell the doctor my complete medical history." Which condition may affect the physician's decision to immediately start heparin therapy?
    a. Type 2 diabetes mellitus
    b. Recent cerebral hemorrhage
    c. Newly diagnosed osteoarthritis
    d. Asthma since childhood

11. A patient with a PE asks for an explanation of heparin therapy. What is the nurse's best response?
    a. "It keeps the clot from getting larger by preventing platelets from sticking together to improve blood flow."
    b. "It will improve your breathing and decrease chest pain by dissolving the clot in your lung."
    c. "It promotes the absorption of the clot in your leg that originally caused the PE."
    d. "It increases the time it takes for blood to clot, therefore preventing further clotting and improving blood flow."

12. A patient is being treated with heparin therapy for a PE. The patient has the potential for bleeding with the administration of heparin. What does the nurse monitor in relation to the heparin therapy?
    a. Lab values for any elevation of PT or PTT value
    b. PTT values for greater than 2.5 times the control and/or the patient for bleeding
    c. Occurrence of a pulmonary infarction by blood in sputum
    d. PT values for International Normalized Ratio (INR) for a therapeutic range of 2 to 3 and/or the patient for bleeding

13. Acute respiratory failure is classified by which critical values of $Paco_2$? *(Select all that apply.)*
    a. 39 mm Hg
    b. 52 mm Hg
    c. < 60 mm Hg
    d. 77 mm Hg
    e. >50 mm Hg with a pH value of < 7.3

14. Upon diagnosis of a PE, the nurse expects to perform which therapeutic intervention for the patient?
    a. Oral anticoagulant therapy
    b. Bedrest in the supine position
    c. Oxygen therapy via mechanical ventilator
    d. Parenteral anticoagulant therapy

15. The nurse is caring for a patient with a postoperative complication of PE. The patient has been receiving treatment for several days. Which factors are indicators of adequate perfusion in the patient? *(Select all that apply.)*
    a. Pulse oximetry of 95%
    b. Arterial blood gas, pH of 7.28
    c. Patient's subjective desire to go home
    d. Absence of pallor or cyanosis
    e. Mental status at patient's baseline

16. Which are extrapulmonary causes of ventilatory failure? *(Select all that apply.)*
    a. Stroke
    b. Use of opioid analgesics
    c. Pulmonary edema
    d. Chronic obstructive pulmonary disease
    e. Morbid obesity

17. The nurse is caring for several postoperative patients with high risk for a PE. All of these patients have pre-existing chronic respiratory problems. What is a unique assessment finding for a clot in the lung?
    a. Dyspnea
    b. Sudden dry cough
    c. Pursed-lip breathing
    d. Audible wheezing

18. The nurse is caring for several patients at risk for DVT and PE. Which condition causes the patient to be the most likely candidate for placement of a vena cava filter?
    a. Massive PE causing the patient to experience shock symptoms
    b. Multiple emboli with deteriorating cardiopulmonary status
    c. Recurrent bleeding while receiving anticoagulants
    d. No response to oxygen therapy and conservative management

19. A patient with a massive PE has hypotension and shock, and is receiving IV crystalloids. However, the patient's cardiac output is not improving. The nurse anticipates an order for which drug?
    a. Hydromorphone (Dilaudid)
    b. Alteplase (Activase, tPA)
    c. Diltiazem (Cardizem)
    d. Dobutamine (Dobutrex)

20. An older adult patient on anticoagulation therapy for a PE is somewhat confused and requires assistance with ADLs. Which instruction specific to this therapy does the nurse give to the unlicensed assistive personnel?
    a. Count and report episodes of urinary incontinence.
    b. Use a lift sheet when moving or turning the patient in bed.
    c. Assist with ambulation because the patient is likely to have dizziness.
    d. Give the patient an extra blanket, because the patient is likely to feel cold.

21. A patient with a PE is receiving anticoagulant therapy. Which assessment related to the therapy does the nurse perform?
    a. Measure abdominal girth because the medication causes fluid retention.
    b. Check skin turgor because dehydration contributes to anticoagulation.
    c. Monitor for nausea, vomiting, and diarrhea.
    d. Examine skin every 2 hours for evidence of bleeding.

22. What does the nurse monitor for in a patient with a PE? *(Select all that apply.)*
    a. Nausea and vomiting
    b. Cyanosis
    c. Rapid heart rate
    d. Dyspnea
    e. Paradoxical chest movement
    f. Crackles in the lung fields

23. After receiving IV heparin anticoagulant therapy, patients are generally not discharged from the hospital without a prescription and instructions for which drug?
    a. Protamine sulfate
    b. Prednisone (Deltasone)
    c. Warfarin (Coumadin)
    d. Oral heparin

24. A patient is following up on a postoperative complication of PE. The patient must have blood drawn to determine the therapeutic range for Coumadin. Which lab test determines this therapeutic range?
    a. PTT level
    b. Platelets
    c. PT and INR
    d. Coumadin peak and trough

25. The nurse is reviewing lab results for a patient with a new-onset PE. What is the INR therapeutic range?
    a. 1.0 to 1.5
    b. 2.0 to 3.0
    c. 3.0 to 4.5
    d. 5

26. A patient demonstrates chest pain, dyspnea, dry cough, and change in level of consciousness. The nurse suspects PE and notifies the health care provider who orders an arterial blood gas (ABG). In the early stage of a PE, what would ABG results probably indicate?
    a. Respiratory alkalosis
    b. Respiratory acidosis
    c. Metabolic acidosis
    d. Metabolic alkalosis

27. A patient recently received anticoagulant therapy for complications of PE after knee surgery. The patient is now in a rehabilitation facility and is receiving warfarin (Coumadin). What is the nursing responsibility related to Coumadin?
    a. Having protamine sulfate available as an antidote
    b. Administering NSAIDs or aspirin for pain related to the knee
    c. Teaching the patient about foods high in vitamin K
    d. Monitoring platelets for thrombocytopenia

28. In _____ _____, ventilation-perfusion ($\dot{V}/\dot{Q}$) mismatch is found in conditions where perfusion is normal and ventilation is inadequate.

29. Ventilatory failure is the result of what processes? *(Select all that apply.)*
    a. Hematologic disease
    b. Defect in the respiratory control center of the brain
    c. Physical problem of the lungs
    d. Poor function of the diaphragm
    e. Physical problem of the chest wall

30. In _____ _____, there is $\dot{V}/\dot{Q}$ mismatch in which air movement and oxygen intake are normal and lung perfusion is decreased.

31. The patient who is having an _____ attack is at risk for combined ventilatory and oxygenation failure.

32. Which conditions are related to acute respiratory distress syndrome (ARDS)? *(Select all that apply.)*
    a. Lung fluid increases
    b. A systemic inflammatory response occurs
    c. The lungs dry out and become stiff
    d. Lung volume is decreased
    e. Hypoxemia results

33. _____-_____ _____ _____ _____ is a noncardiogenic pulmonary edema associated with the activation of the inflammatory response due to a recent transfusion of plasma-containing products?

34. The nurse is reviewing the ABG results for a patient. The latest ABGs show pH 7.48, HCO_3^- 23 mEq/L, $Paco_2$ 25 mm Hg, Pao_2 98 mm Hg. What is the correct interpretation of these lab findings?
    a. Normal ABGs indicating adequate ventilation
    b. Acute respiratory alkalosis and hyperventilation
    c. Acute respiratory acidosis and hypoventilation
    d. Chronic respiratory acidosis and hypoventilation

35. The nurse is caring for a patient with acute hypoxemia. Which nursing interventions are best for the care of this patient? *(Select all that apply.)*
    a. Minimal self-care
    b. PRN sedatives
    c. Upright position
    d. Oxygen therapy
    e. Keep NPO while dyspneic
    f. Prescribed metered dose inhalers

36. A patient reports pain with inspiration after falling off a skateboard. The physician makes the diagnosis of rib fracture. The nurse prepares to do patient teaching for which treatment?
    a. Mechanical ventilation
    b. Tight bandage around chest
    c. Coughing and deep-breathing
    d. Potent analgesics for pain

37. The nurse is assessing a patient who sustained significant chest trauma during a motor vehicle accident. What significant assessment finding suggests tension pneumothorax?
    a. Tracheal deviation to the unaffected side
    b. Inspiratory stridor and respiratory distress
    c. Diminished breath sounds over the affected hemothorax
    d. Hyperresonant percussion note over the affected side

38. The nurse is assessing a patient with a hemothorax. When the nurse performs percussion of the chest on the affected side, what type of sound is expected?
    a. Hypertympanic
    b. Dull
    c. Hyperresonant
    d. Crackles

39. On arrival to the ED, the patient develops extreme respiratory distress and the physician identifies a tension pneumothorax. The nurse prepares to assist with which urgent procedure?
    a. Endotracheal intubation with mechanical ventilation
    b. Placement of a chest tube to reduce pneumothorax on the affected side
    c. Insertion of a 8-inch (20.3-cm), 16- or 18-gauge pericardial needle
    d. Insertion of a large-bore needle into the intercostal space on the affected side

40. The nurse is performing patient teaching for a patient who will be taking anticoagulants at home. What does the nurse include in the instructions? *(Select all that apply.)*
    a. Use a soft-bristled toothbrush and floss frequently.
    b. Do not take aspirin or any aspirin-containing products.
    c. Do not participate in activities that will cause bumps, scratches, or scrapes.
    d. If you are bumped, apply ice to the site for at least 24 hours.
    e. Eat warm, cool, or cold foods to avoid burning your mouth.
    f. Check your skin and mouth monthly for bruising or bleeding.
    g. If you must blow your nose, do so gently without blocking either nasal passage.

41. Which patient has the greatest risk for developing ARDS?
    a. 74-year-old who aspirates a tube feeding
    b. 34-year-old with chronic renal failure
    c. 56-year-old with uncontrolled diabetes mellitus
    d. 18-year-old with a fractured femur

42. Which assessment finding is considered an early sign of ARDS?
    a. Adventitious lung sounds
    b. Hyperthermia and hot, dry skin
    c. Intercostal and suprasternal retractions
    d. Heightened mental acuity and surveillance

43. A patient with which condition is a potential candidate for autotransfusion, should the need arise?
    a. Tension pneumothorax
    b. Hemothorax
    c. Abdominal bleeding
    d. Esophageal bleeding

44. A patient sustained a chest injury resulting from a motor vehicle accident. The patient is asymptomatic at first, but slowly develops decreased breath sounds, crackles, wheezing, and blood in the sputum. The mechanism of injury and physical findings are consistent with which condition?
    a. Flail chest
    b. Rib fractures
    c. Pneumothorax
    d. Pulmonary contusion

45. A patient is admitted after a near-drowning and develops ARDS which is confirmed by the physician. The nurse prepares equipment for which treatment?
    a. Oxygen therapy via CPAP
    b. Mechanical ventilation and endotracheal tube
    c. High-flow oxygen via facemask
    d. Tracheostomy tube

46. A 19-year-old patient was seen in the ED after a motorcycle accident for multiple rib fractures that resulted in free-floating ribs, paradoxical breathing, and inadequate oxygenation. What is this condition called?
    a. Tension pneumothorax
    b. Flail chest
    c. Pulmonary contusion
    d. Subcutaneous emphysema

47. The high-pressure alarm of a patient's mechanical ventilator goes off. What are the potential causes for this occurrence? *(Select all that apply.)*
    a. Mucus plug
    b. Patient is asleep
    c. Patient is fighting the ventilator
    d. Bronchospasm
    e. Patient is coughing

48. The low-pressure alarm of a patient's mechanical ventilator goes off. What are potential causes for this occurrence? *(Select all that apply.)*
    a. Blockage in the circuit
    b. Cuff leak in the endotracheal or tracheostomy tube
    c. Patient has stopped breathing
    d. Cuff of the endotracheal or tracheostomy tube is overinflated
    e. Leak in the circuit

49. A patient with ARDS is currently in the phase 1 management stage. What is the focus of the nursing assessment?
    a. Monitor closely for progressive hypoxemia.
    b. Note early changes in dyspnea and tachypnea.
    c. Review the x-ray reports for evidence of patchy infiltrates.
    d. Monitor for multiple organ dysfunction syndrome.

50. The nurse is caring for a patient at risk for pulmonary contusion. Why is this a potentially lethal chest injury?
    a. The patient could have broken ribs.
    b. The patient could develop laryngospasm.
    c. Respiratory failure develops over time.
    d. There is a risk of infection from chest tubes.

Matching. *Match each disorder or event that can cause patients to be at risk for acute respiratory failure with its corresponding type of respiratory failure. Answers may be used more than once.*

Types of Respiratory Failure
a. Ventilatory failure
b. Oxygenation failure
c. Combination of ventilatory and oxygenation failure

Disorders and Events
_____ 51. Cerebral edema
_____ 52. Bronchial asthma
_____ 53. Sleep apnea
_____ 54. Pulmonary embolism
_____ 55. Pneumonia
_____ 56. Chronic bronchitis
_____ 57. Gross obesity
_____ 58. Poliomyelitis
_____ 59. Smoke inhalation
_____ 60. Myasthenia gravis
_____ 61. Meningitis
_____ 62. Pulmonary emphysema
_____ 63. Carbon monoxide poisoning
_____ 64. Opioid overdose
_____ 65. Guillain-Barré syndrome

66. A patient has been successfully intubated by the physician, and the nurse and respiratory therapist are securing the tube in place. What does the nurse include in the documentation regarding the intubation procedure? *(Select all that apply.)*
    a. Presence of bilateral and equal breath sounds
    b. Level of the tube
    c. Changes in vital signs during the procedure
    d. Rate of the IV fluids
    e. Presence (or absence) of dysrhythmias
    f. Patient's speech quality during and after procedure
    g. Placement verification by end-tidal carbon dioxide levels

67. The nurse is assisting with an emergency intubation for a patient in severe respiratory distress. Although the physician is experienced, the procedure is difficult because the patient has severe kyphosis. At what point does the nurse intervene?
    a. First intubation attempt lasts longer than 15 seconds.
    b. First intubation attempt lasts longer than 30 seconds.
    c. Second intubation attempt is unsuccessful.
    d. Second intubation attempt causes the patient to struggle.

68. A patient in the ED required emergency intubation for status asthmaticus. Immediately after the insertion of an endotracheal tube (ET) tube, how does the nurse and/or physician verify correct placement?
    a. Observe for chest excursion.
    b. Listen for expired air from the ET tube.
    c. Check end-tidal CO_2 level.
    d. Wait for the results of the chest x-ray.

69. The nurse is caring for several patients on the medical-surgical unit who are experiencing acute respiratory problems. Which conditions may eventually require a patient to be intubated? *(Select all that apply.)*
    a. Trouble maintaining a patent airway because of mucosal swelling
    b. History of congestive heart failure and demonstrating orthopnea
    c. Copious secretions and lacking muscular strength to cough
    d. Pulse oximetry of 93% with a high-flow oxygen facemask
    e. Increasing fatigue because of the work of breathing

70. The nurse hears in report that a patient with ARDS has been intubated for 6 days and has progressive hypoxemia that responds poorly to high levels of oxygen. This patient is in which phase of ARDS case management?
    a. Phase 1
    b. Phase 2
    c. Phase 3
    d. Phase 4

71. A postoperative patient reports sudden onset of shortness of breath and pleuritic chest pain. Assessment findings include diaphoresis, hypotension, crackles in the left lower lobe, and pulse oximetry of 85%. What does the nurse suspect this patient has?
    a. Atelectasis
    b. Pneumothorax
    c. Pulmonary embolism
    d. Flail chest

72. The nurse hears in shift report that a patient has been agitated and pulling at the ET. Restraints have recently been ordered and placed, but the patient continues to move his head and chew at the tube. What does the nurse do to ensure proper placement of the ET tube?
    a. Suction the patient frequently through the oral airway.
    b. Talk to the patient and tell him to calm down.
    c. Mark the tube where it touches the patient's teeth.
    d. Auscultate for breath sounds every 4 hours.

73. The nurse is caring for a patient on a mechanical ventilator. What does the nurse monitor to assess for the most likely cardiac problem associated with this therapy?
    a. Check blood pressure.
    b. Check for ventricular dysrhythmias.
    c. Take an apical pulse before giving medications.
    d. Ask the patient about chest pain.

Matching. *Match the parts of an endotracheal tube (ET) with their descriptions.*

Parts of ET
a. Shaft
b. Cuff
c. Pilot balloon
d. Adapter

Descriptions

_____ 74. Device to provide a seal between the trachea and tube

_____ 75. Device to allow attachment of ET tube to ventilation source

_____ 76. Hollow tube extending from naso-oral cavity to just above the carina

_____ 77. Access site for inserting air into the cuff

78. A patient in the critical care unit requires an emergency ET intubation. The nurse immediately obtains and prepares which supplies to perform this procedure? *(Select all that apply.)*
    a. Tracheostomy tube or kit
    b. Resuscitation Ambu bag
    c. Source for 100% oxygen
    d. Suction equipment
    e. Insertion equipment (i.e., laryngoscope)
    f. Oral airway
    g. Bronchodilator inhaler

79. A patient on a ventilator is biting and chewing at the ET tube. Which nursing intervention is used for ET management?
    a. Reassure the patient that everything is okay.
    b. Administer a paralyzing agent.
    c. Insert an oral airway.
    d. Frequently suction the mouth.

80. The nurse is performing a check of the ventilator equipment. What is included during the equipment check?
    a. Drain the condensed moisture back into the humidifier.
    b. Empty the humidifier and the drainage tubing.
    c. Note the prescribed and actual settings.
    d. Turn off the alarms during the system check.

81. The nursing student is assisting in the care of a critically ill patient on a ventilator. Which action by the student nurse requires intervention by the supervising nurse?
    a. Deflates the cuff on the ET tube to check placement.
    b. Applies soft wrist restraints as ordered.
    c. Suctions the patient for 10 seconds at a time.
    d. Maintains the correct placement of the ET tube.

82. A patient has a history of chronic obstructive pulmonary disease (COPD) and had to be intubated for respiratory failure. The patient is currently on a mechanical ventilator. The nurse obtains an order for which type of dietary therapy for this patient?
    a. High-fat nutritional supplement
    b. High-protein nutritional supplement
    c. High-carbohydrate nutritional supplement
    d. High-calorie nutritional supplement

83. The nursing student is assisting in the care of a patient on a mechanical ventilator. Which action by the student contributes to the prevention of ventilator-assisted pneumonia?
    a. Suctions the patient frequently
    b. Performs oral care every 2 hours
    c. Encourages visitors to wear a mask
    d. Obtains a sputum specimen for culture

84. The nurse is caring for a patient on a mechanical ventilator. During the shift, the nurse hears the patient talking to himself. What does the nurse do next?
    a. See if the patient has a change of mental status.
    b. Check the inflation of the pilot balloon.
    c. Assess the pulse oximetry for saturation level.
    d. Evaluate the patient's readiness to be weaned.

85. The nurse notices that a patient has a gradual increase in peak inspiratory pressure over the last several days. What is the best nursing intervention for this patient?
    a. Assess for a reason such as ARDS or pneumonia.
    b. Continue to increase peak airway pressure as needed.
    c. Change to another mode such as IMV.
    d. Make arrangements for permanent ventilatory support.

86. A patient is intubated and has mechanical ventilation with positive end-expiratory pressure (PEEP). Because this patient is at risk for a tension pneumothorax, what is the nurse's priority action?
    a. Assess lung sounds every 30 to 60 minutes.
    b. Obtain an order for an arterial blood gas.
    c. Have chest tube equipment on standby.
    d. Direct the unlicensed assistive personnel to turn the patient every 2 hours.

87. The nurse is caring for a patient on a mechanical ventilator. Which assessments does the nurse perform for this patient? *(Select all that apply.)*
    a. Observe the patient's mouth around the tube for pressure ulcers.
    b. Auscultate the lungs for crackles, wheezes, equal breath sounds, and decreased or absent breath sounds.
    c. Assess the placement of the endotracheal tube.
    d. Check at least every 24 hours to be sure the ventilator settings are as prescribed.
    e. Check to be sure alarms are set.
    f. Ensure the endotracheal cuff is deflated.
    g. Observe the patient's need for tracheal, oral, or nasal suctioning every 2 hours.

88. What are the characteristics of a mechanical ventilator that is pressure-cycled? *(Select all that apply.)*
    a. Preset inspiration and expiratory rate is programmed with possible variation of tidal volume and pressure.
    b. It is a positive-pressure ventilator.
    c. It pushes air into the lungs until a preset airway pressure is reached.
    d. There is no need for an artificial airway such as a tracheostomy or endotracheal tube.
    e. Tidal volumes and inspiratory times are varied.

89. What are the characteristics of a mechanical ventilator that is time-cycled? *(Select all that apply.)*
    a. It needs an artificial airway such as a tracheostomy or endotracheal tube.
    b. It is a positive-pressure ventilator.
    c. Its tidal volumes are variable.
    d. Preset inspiration and expiration rate can be set with possible variation of tidal volume.
    e. Inspiratory time is variable.

90. What are the characteristics of a noninvasive pressure support (Bi-PAP) mechanical ventilator? *(Select all that apply.)*
    a. It uses positive airway pressure (Bi-PAP) for the inhalation mode of breathing assistance.
    b. Air is delivered at one pressure for inhaling and another pressure for exhaling.
    c. It administers consistent volume of positive pressure until a preset tidal volume is reached.
    d. It administers consistent oxygen concentration regardless of the patient's lung status.
    e. It is a negative-pressure ventilator.

Matching. *Match the ventilator terms and settings with their descriptions.*

Terms and Settings
a. Assist-control mode (AC)
b. Rate or breaths/minute (BPM)
c. Continuous positive airway pressure (CPAP)
d. Bi-level positive airway pressure (BiPAP)
e. Fraction of inspired oxygen (Fio_2)
f. Peak airway inspiratory pressure (PIP)
g. Positive end-expiratory pressure (PEEP)
h. Tidal volume (V_T)
i. Synchronized intermittent mandatory ventilation (SIMV)
j. Microprocessor ventilator

Descriptions
_____ 91. Pressure needed to deliver a set tidal volume

_____ 92. Positive pressure throughout the entire respiratory cycle to prevent alveolar collapse

_____ 93. Number of ventilations delivered per minute

_____ 94. Volume of air the patient receives with each breath

_____ 95. Set tidal volume and set rate delivered to the patient

_____ 96. Positive pressure exerted during expiration to keep lungs partially inflated

_____ 97. Oxygen concentration delivered to the patient

_____ 98. Noninvasive pressure support ventilation by nasal mask or facemask

_____ 99. Ventilator delivers mandatory breaths at a preset rate and allows the patient to breathe spontaneously between set rate

_____ 100. A computer monitors ventilatory functions, alarms, and patient condition

101. The nurse hears an alarm go off on a mechanical ventilator that signals the ventilator is not able to give the patient a breath. What are the possible reasons that would make this alarm go off? *(Select all that apply.)*
    a. The tubing has become disconnected.
    b. The patient is not breathing on his or her own.
    c. The pulse oximetry reading is below 90%.
    d. The patient has become disconnected from the ventilator.
    e. The patient needs to be suctioned.

102. A patient with a tracheostomy who is on a mechanical ventilator is beginning to take spontaneous breaths at his own rate and tidal volume between set ventilator breaths. Which mode is the ventilator on?
    a. Assist-control (AC) ventilation
    b. Bi-level positive airway pressure (Bi-PAP)
    c. SIMV (synchronized intermittent ventilation)
    d. Continuous flow (flow-by)

103. A patient who is on a mechanical ventilator needs a set volume and set rate delivered because the patient is not able to do the work of breathing. What mode must the ventilator be set at?
    a. Positive-end expiratory pressure (PEEP)
    b. Continuous positive airway pressure (CPAP)
    c. Bi-level positive airway pressure (Bi-PAP)
    d. Assist-control mode (AC)

104. The physician instructs the nurse to watch for and report signs and symptoms of improvement so the patient can be weaned from the ventilator. Which assessment finding indicates the patient is ready to be weaned?
    a. Indications that respiratory infection is resolving
    b. Showing signs of becoming ventilator-dependent
    c. Maintaining blood gases within normal limits
    d. Patient insisting that the ventilator is not necessary anymore

105. An older adult patient arrives in the ED after falling off a roof. The nurse observes "sucking inward" of the loose chest area during inspiration and a "puffing out" of the same area during expiration. ABG results show severe hypoxemia and hypercarbia. Which procedure does the nurse prepare for?
    a. Chest tube insertion
    b. Endotracheal intubation
    c. Needle thoracotomy
    d. Tracheostomy

106. The charge nurse in the intensive care unit is reviewing the patient census and caseload to identify staffing needs and potential transfers. Which patient might take the longest time to wean from a ventilator?
    a. 54-year-old man with metastatic colon cancer who has been intubated for 6 days
    b. 32-year-old woman recovering from a general anesthetic following a tubal ligation
    c. 25-year-old man intubated for 28 hours after an anaphylactic reaction
    d. 49-year-old man with a gunshot wound to the chest who was intubated for 8 hours

107. A patient is being extubated and the nurse has emergency equipment at the bedside. Which intervention is implemented during extubation?
    a. Ensure that the cuff is inflated at all times.
    b. Remove the tube during expiration.
    c. Instruct the patient to pant while the tube is removed.
    d. Instruct the patient to cough after tube is removed.

108. The nurse is caring for a patient who was recently extubated. What is an expected assessment finding for this patient?
    a. Stridor
    b. Dyspnea
    c. Restlessness
    d. Hoarseness

109. Place the steps for extubating a patient in the correct order using the numbers 1 through 8.
    _____ a. Hyperoxygenate the patient.
    _____ b. Rapidly deflate the cuff of the ET tube.
    _____ c. Immediately instruct the patient to cough.
    _____ d. Thoroughly suction both the ET tube and the oral cavity.
    _____ e. Give oxygen by facemask or nasal cannula.
    _____ f. Explain the procedure.
    _____ g. Set up oxygen; bring emergency reintubation equipment.
    _____ h. Remove the tube at peak inspiration.

110. Which patients on mechanical ventilators are at high risk for barotraumas? *(Select all that apply.)*
    a. Patient with ARDS
    b. Patient with underlying chronic airflow limitation
    c. Patient on BiPAP
    d. Patient on PEEP
    e. Patient on SIMV

111. The nurse is caring for a patient who has just been extubated. What interventions does the nurse use in caring for this patient? *(Select all that apply.)*
    a. Monitor vital signs every 30 minutes at first.
    b. Assess the ventilatory pattern for manifestations of respiratory distress.
    c. Place the patient in a recumbent position.
    d. Instruct the patient to take deep breaths every half hour.
    e. Encourage use of an incentive spirometer every 2 hours.
    f. Advise the patient to limit speaking right after extubation.

112. The nurse is assessing a patient who was extubated several hours ago. Which patient finding warrants notification of the Rapid Response Team?
    a. Hoarseness
    b. Report of sore throat
    c. Inability to expectorate secretions
    d. 90% saturation on room air

113. A patient is admitted to the trauma unit following a front-end motor vehicle collision. The patient is currently asymptomatic, but the physician advises the nurse that the patient has a high risk for pulmonary contusion. What does the nurse carefully monitor for?
    a. Tracheal deviation
    b. Paradoxical chest movements
    c. Progressive chest pain
    d. Decreased breath sounds

114. Which finding might delay weaning a patient from mechanical ventilation support?
    a. Hematocrit = 42%
    b. Arterial Po_2 = 70 mm Hg on a 40% Fio_2
    c. Apical heart rate = 72 beats per minute
    d. Oral temperature = 101° F

115. A patient in respiratory failure is diagnosed with a flail chest. After the patient is intubated, which treatment does the nurse expect to be implemented?
    a. PEEP
    b. SIMV
    c. BiPap
    d. PIP

116. A patient in a motor vehicle accident was unrestrained and appears to have hit the front dashboard. The patient has severe respiratory distress, inspiratory stridor, and extensive subcutaneous emphysema. The ED physician identifies tracheobronchial trauma. Which procedure does the nurse immediately prepare for?
    a. Cricothyroidotomy
    b. Chest tube insertion
    c. Cardiopulmonary resuscitation
    d. Pericardiocentesis

117. What causes the potential cardiac problems that can result from mechanical ventilation?
    a. Negative pressure increases in the chest
    b. Positive pressure increases in the chest
    c. Positive pressure decreases in the heart
    d. Negative pressure increases in the heart

118. What is the cardiac problem that can occur from mechanical ventilation?
    a. Hypotension
    b. Dehydration
    c. Bradycardia
    d. Hypertension

119. Which clinical manifestations can occur from cardiac problems due to mechanical ventilation? *(Select all that apply.)*
    a. Decreased cardiac output
    b. Diuresis
    c. Bradycardia
    d. Fluid retention
    e. Tachycardia

CASE STUDY: PNEUMONIA WITH RESPIRATORY FAILURE

Use a separate sheet of paper to answer the questions in this Case Study, or go to the "Prepare for Class" folder on your Evolve website at http://evolve.elsevier.com/Iggy/ to download and complete as a word processing file. Answer guidelines for this Case Study are also available on your Evolve website.

A 61-year-old man was hospitalized with a productive cough of thick, rust-colored sputum. The history of the patient includes COPD and NIDDM.

Previously in the ED, the patient went into respiratory failure. He was intubated with an endotracheal tube that has an inline suction catheter, and placed on a mechanical ventilator. The ventilator was set at AC = 14, TV = 350, and Fio_2 30%. An ABG that was done just before the patient was intubated revealed the following results: pH 7.30; $Paco_2$ = 68 mm Hg; Pao_2 = 65 mm Hg; HCO_3 = 29 mEq/L. On auscultation of the lungs, the upper anterior and posterior lobes were coarse, and the anterior and posterior lobes had diminished breath sounds. The patient is able to follow simple commands: he can squeeze hands with equal and strong hand grasps, open eyes, and can move all extremities.

The patient nods his head "no" when asked if he has pain. It appears that he is in no pain: there is no facial grimacing or restlessness. The pupils are equal and reactive to light at 2 mm. The patient is on a Flexicare mattress and assessment reveals that the skin is intact. The head of bed is elevated at 30 degrees. He is receiving nutrition from Glucerna infusing via pump through a PEG tube in the abdomen at 50 mL/hour. The PEG tube is checked every 4 hours for residuals, which have been less than 10 mL. Oral care has been done every 12 hours by toothbrushing with toothpaste, suctioning, and swabbing the mouth until clear with a tooth sponge moistened with water. Then 60 minutes later chlorhexidine 0.12% is used to swab the mouth and suction any excess to prevent aspiration.

Vital signs are: Temp 37.5° C (99.5° F); heart rate and rhythm 62/min, sinus rhythm with occasional PVCs; respirations 26/min; blood pressure 103/68 mm Hg.

1. Document a nursing note on this patient's top priority problem.
2. What measures to prevent ventilator-associated pneumonia have been taken for this patient?
3. What does the arterial blood gas reading of this patient indicate?

CASE STUDY: CHEST TRAUMA AND ADULT RESPIRATORY DISTRESS SYNDROME (ARDS)

Use a separate sheet of paper to answer the questions in this Case Study, or go to the "Prepare for Class" folder on your Evolve website at http://evolve.elsevier.com/Iggy/ to download and complete as a word processing file. Answer guidelines for this Case Study are also available on your Evolve website.

A 36-year-old woman is brought to the hospital following a head-on car accident. She was unrestrained and sustained a blunt injury to the chest from hitting the steering wheel. Initially, she is asymptomatic. Initial orders include a stat chest x-ray, arterial blood gases, and oxygen at 4 L/minute via Venturi mask.

1. What other assessments should be made when she arrives in the ED?

2. Gradually over the next 24 hours, she develops difficulty breathing, hypoxemia, and secretions increase. The nurse notifies the physician who orders an arterial blood gas and a chest x-ray. The chest x-ray obtained in the ED showed no abnormalities; however, the repeat x-ray now shows a hazy opacity in the lobes and the physician makes a diagnosis of pulmonary contusion. What physical assessments will accompany this diagnosis?

3. Arterial blood gas results show: Pao_2 68 mm Hg, $Paco_2$ 32 mm Hg, HCO_3 21 mEq/L, and pH 7.53. What do these values suggest?

4. What interventions should be implemented based on the laboratory results?

5. The patient temporarily responds to the high-flow oxygen therapy, but later the nurse notes that the patient demonstrates hyperpnea, grunting respiration, cyanosis, pallor, and intercostal and substernal retractions, with a change in mental status. The nurse suspects ARDS and calls the physician to obtain an order for which primary laboratory study used to establish this diagnosis?

6. Discuss the pathophysiology of ARDS.

7. The patient is intubated for respiratory failure. Describe how the nurse would secure the ET in place.

8. The patient is placed on a respirator with PEEP. Why is PEEP necessary?

9. Explain the rationale for the use of corticosteroids and antibiotics in the management of the patient with ARDS.

35 CHAPTER

Assessment of the Cardiovascular System

STUDY/REVIEW QUESTIONS

Matching. *Match each structure of the heart with its description.*

Structures of the Heart

a. Aortic valve
b. Atria
c. Chordae tendineae
d. Coronary arteries
e. Mitral valve
f. Pulmonic valve
g. Septum
h. Tricuspid valve
i. Ventricle

Descriptions

_____ 1. Muscular wall dividing the heart into halves

_____ 2. Upper heart chamber

_____ 3. Lower heart chamber

_____ 4. Valve between right atrium and ventricle

_____ 5. Valve between right ventricle and pulmonary artery

_____ 6. Valve between left atrium and ventricle, bicuspid valve

_____ 7. Filaments that secure the AV valve leaflets

_____ 8. Vessels that supply the heart with oxygenated blood

_____ 9. Valve from the left ventricle to the aorta

10. What are the three pacemaker sites in the heart? Name the pacer rate for each site.

    a. _____

    _____

    b. _____

    _____

    c. _____

    _____

Matching. *Match each variable that affects cardiac output with its description.*

Cardiac Output Variables
a. Afterload
b. Contractility
c. Heart rate
d. Impedance
e. Preload

Descriptions

_____ 11. Number of times ventricles contract per minute

_____ 12. Degree of myocardial fiber stretch at end of diastole and just before heart contracts

_____ 13. Amount of pressure or resistance that the ventricles must overcome to eject blood through the semilunar valves and into the peripheral blood vessels

_____ 14. Pressure that ventricle must overcome to open aortic valve

_____ 15. Force of contraction independent of preload

16. Which are risk factors for cardiovascular disease (CVD) in women? *(Select all that apply.)*
    a. Waist and abdominal obesity
    b. Excess fat in the buttocks, hips, and thighs
    c. Postmenopausal
    d. Diabetes mellitus
    e. Asian ethnicity

17. The nurse is assessing a patient's nicotine dependency. Which questions does the nurse ask for an accurate assessment? *(Select all that apply.)*
    a. "How soon after you wake up in the morning do you smoke?"
    b. "What kind of cigarettes do you smoke?"
    c. "Do you inhale deeply when you smoke?"
    d. "Do you find it difficult not to smoke in places where smoking is prohibited?"
    e. "Do you smoke when you are ill?"
    f. "What happened the last time you tried to quit smoking?"

18. The nurse is talking to a patient who has been trying to quit smoking. Which statement by the patient indicates an understanding of cigarette usage as it relates to reducing cardiovascular risks?
    a. "I need to be completely cigarette-free for at least 3 years."
    b. "I don't smoke as much as I used to; I'm down to one pack a day."
    c. "I started smoking a while ago, but I'll quit in a couple of years."
    d. "I only smoke to relax, when I drink, or when I go out with friends."

19. When disease or other disorders of the cardiovascular system occur, and _____ decrease.

20. The nurse is providing health teaching for a patient at risk for heart disease. Which factor is the most modifiable, controllable risk factor?
    a. Obesity
    b. Diabetes mellitus
    c. Ethnic background
    d. Family history of cardiovascular disease

21. The nurse is giving a community presentation about heart disease in women. What information does the nurse include in the presentation? *(Select all that apply.)*
    a. Dyspnea on exertion may be the first and only symptom of heart failure.
    b. Symptoms are subtle or atypical.
    c. Pain is often relieved by rest.
    d. Having waist and abdominal obesity is a higher risk factor than having fat in buttocks and thighs.
    e. Pain always responds to nitroglycerin.
    f. Common symptoms include back pain, indigestion, nausea, vomiting, and anorexia.

22. Which blood pressure readings require further prehypertensive assessment? *(Select all that apply.)*
    a. 125 mm Hg systolic
    b. 139 mm Hg systolic
    c. 115 mm Hg systolic
    d. 60 mm Hg diastolic
    e. 100 mm Hg diastolic

23. The nurse working in the public health department is reviewing data for populations at risk for CVD. Which group has the greatest need for intervention to reduce CVD risk?
    a. Government employees who make approximately $40,000 a year
    b. Part-time fast-food workers who make approximately $9,000 a year
    c. Hospital-employed nurses who make approximately $52,000 a year
    d. Chain retail employees who make approximately $18,000 a year

24. The _____ system slows the heart rate, whereas _____ stimulation increases the heart rate.

25. Which category of cardiovascular drugs increases heart rate and contractility?
    a. Diuretics
    b. Beta blockers
    c. Catecholamines
    d. Benzodiazepines

26. Which category of cardiovascular drugs blocks the sympathetic stimulation to the heart and decreases the heart rate?
    a. Beta blockers
    b. Catecholamines
    c. Steroids
    d. Benzodiazepines

27. What different pathophysiologic conditions can the healthy heart adapt to? *(Select all that apply.)*
    a. Menses
    b. Stress
    c. Gastroesophageal reflux disease
    d. Infection
    e. Hemorrhage

28. Which statements about blood pressure are accurate? *(Select all that apply.)*
    a. Pulse pressure is the difference between the systolic and diastolic pressures.
    b. The right ventricle of the heart generates the greatest amount of blood pressure.
    c. Diastolic blood pressure is primarily determined by the amount of peripheral vasoconstriction.
    d. To maintain adequate blood flow through the coronary arteries, diastolic blood pressure must be at least 60 mm Hg.
    e. Diastolic blood pressure is the highest pressure during contraction of the ventricles.

29. The nurse is assessing a 62-year-old native Hawaiian woman. She is postmenopausal, diabetic for 10 years, smokes 1 pack a day of cigarettes for 20 years, walks twice a week for 30 minutes, is an administrator, and describes her lifestyle as sedentary. For her weight and height she has a body mass index of 32. Which risk factors for this patient are uncontrollable, and which are controllable for cardiovascular disease?

    Uncontrollable risk factors:

    Controllable risk factors:

True or False? *Read each statement about the various components of blood pressure and write T for true or F for false in the blanks provided. If the statement is false, correct the statement to make it true.*

_____ 30. The right ventricle of the heart generates the greatest amount of blood pressure.

_____ 31. To maintain adequate blood flow through the coronary arteries, diastolic blood pressure must be at least 60 mm Hg.

32. Place the steps for checking a patient for postural hypotension in the correct order, using the numbers 1 through 5.

_____ a. Patient changes position to sitting or standing.

_____ b. Measure the blood pressure when the patient is supine.

_____ c. Have the patient remain supine for at least 3 minutes.

_____ d. Observe and record any signs or symptoms of dizziness.

_____ e. Wait for at least 1 minute before auscultating blood pressure and counting the radial pulse.

33. While taking a patient's blood pressure, the nurse observes a weak pulse that alternates with a strong pulse despite a regular heart rhythm. What does the nurse do to exclude a false reading?
   a. Repeat the blood pressure on the other arm with a different cuff.
   b. Palpate the radial or brachial artery.
   c. Repeat the blood pressure and ask the patient to hold his or her breath.
   d. Place the patient on a cardiac monitor.

34. In a hypovolemic patient, stretch receptors in the blood vessels sense a reduced volume or pressure and send fewer impulses to the central nervous system. As a result, which sign/symptoms does the nurse expect to observe in the patient?
   a. Reddish mottling to skin and a blood pressure elevation
   b. Cool, pale skin and tachycardia
   c. Warm, flushed skin with low blood pressure
   d. Pale pink skin with bradycardia

35. What term describes the difference between systolic and diastolic values, which is an indirect measure of cardiac output?
   a. Paradoxical blood pressure
   b. Pulse pressure
   c. Ankle-brachial index
   d. Normal blood pressure

36. The nurse is performing a dietary assessment on a 45-year-old business executive at risk for CVD. Which assessment method used by the nurse is the most reliable and accurate?
   a. Ask the patient to identify foods he or she eats that contain sodium, sugar, cholesterol, fiber, and fat.
   b. Ask the patient's spouse, who does the cooking and shopping, to identify the types of foods that are consumed.
   c. Ask the patient how cultural beliefs and economic status influences the choice of food items.
   d. Ask the patient to recall the intake of food, fluids, and alcohol during a typical 24-hour period.

37. Based on the physiologic force that propels blood forward in the veins, which patient has the greatest risk for venous stasis?
   a. Older adult patient with hypertension who rides a bicycle daily
   b. Middle-aged construction worker taking Coumadin
   c. Bedridden patient in the end stage of Alzheimer's disease
   d. Teenage patient with a broken leg who sits and plays videogames

38. Which statement about the peripheral vascular system is true?
    a. Veins are equipped with valves that permit one-way flow of blood toward the heart.
    b. The velocity of blood flow depends on the diameter of the vessel lumen.
    c. Blood flow decreases and blood tends to clot as the viscosity decreases.
    d. The parasympathetic nervous system has the largest effect on blood flow to organs.

39. A patient comes to the clinic stating "my right foot turns a darkish red color when I sit too long, and when I put my foot up, it turns pale." Which conditions does the nurse suspect?
    a. Central cyanosis
    b. Peripheral cyanosis
    c. Arterial insufficiency
    d. Venous insufficiency

40. Which exercise regimen for an older adult meets the recommended guidelines for physical fitness to promote heart health?
    a. 6-hour bike ride every Saturday
    b. Golfing for 4 hours two times a week
    c. Running for 15 minutes three times a week
    d. Brisk walk 30 minutes every day

41. Calculate the number of pack-years for a patient who has smoked half a pack of cigarettes per day for 2 years. _____

42. In assessing a patient who has come to the clinic for a physical exam, the nurse sees that the patient has pallor. What is this finding most indicative of?
    a. Anemia
    b. Thrombophlebitis
    c. Heart disease
    d. Stroke

43. Emergency personnel discovered a patient lying outside in the cool evening air for an unknown length of time. The patient is in a hypothermic state and the metabolic needs of the tissues are decreased. What other assessment finding does the nurse expect to see?
    a. Blood pressure and heart rate lower than normal
    b. Heart rate and respiratory rate higher than normal
    c. Normal vital signs due to compensatory mechanisms
    d. Gradually improved vital signs with enteral nutrition

44. The advanced-practice nurse is assessing the vascular status of a patient's lower extremities using the ankle-brachial index. What is the correct technique for this assessment method?
    a. A blood pressure cuff is applied to the lower extremities and the systolic pressure is measured by Doppler ultrasound at both the dorsalis pedis and posterior tibial pulses.
    b. The dorsalis pedis and posterior tibial pulses are manually palpated and compared bilaterally for strength and equality and compared to the standard index.
    c. A blood pressure cuff is applied to the lower extremities to observe for an exaggerated decrease in systolic pressure by more than 10 mm Hg during inspiration.
    d. Measure blood pressure on the legs when the patient is supine; then have the patient stand for several minutes and repeat blood pressure measurement in the arms.

45. What is the correct technique for assessing a patient with arterial insufficiency in the right lower leg?
    a. Use the Doppler to find the dorsalis pedis and posterior tibial pulses on the right leg.
    b. Palpate the peripheral arteries in a head-to-toe approach with a side-to-side comparison.
    c. Check all the pulse points in the right leg in dependent and supine positions.
    d. Palpate the major arteries, such as the radial and femoral, and observe for pallor.

46. The nurse is performing a cardiac assessment on an older adult. What is a common assessment finding for this patient?
    a. S_4 heart sound
    b. Leg edema
    c. Pericardial friction rubs
    d. Change in point of maximum impulse location

47. A patient's chart notes that the examiner has heard S_1 and S_2 on auscultation of the heart. What does this documentation refer to?
    a. First and second heart sounds
    b. Pericardial friction rub
    c. Murmur
    d. Gallop

48. The nurse is taking report on a patient who will be transferred from the cardiac intensive care unit to the general medical-surgical unit. The reporting nurse states that S_4 is heard on auscultation of the heart. This indicates that the patient has which condition?
    a. Heart murmur
    b. Pericardial friction rub
    c. Ventricular hypertrophy
    d. Normal heart sounds

49. Which patient has an abnormal heart sound?
    a. S_1 in a 45-year-old patient
    b. S_2 in a 30-year-old patient
    c. S_3 in a 15-year-old patient
    d. S_3 in a 54-year-old patient

50. The nurse is caring for a patient at risk for heart problems. What are normal findings for the cardiovascular assessment of this patient? *(Select all that apply.)*
    a. Presence of a thrill
    b. Splitting of S_2; decreases with expiration
    c. Jugular venous distention to level of the mandible
    d. Point of maximal impulse (PMI) in fifth intercostal space at midclavicular line
    e. Paradoxical chest movement with inspiration and expiration

51. The nurse practitioner reads in a patient's chart that a carotid bruit was heard during the last two annual checkups. Today on auscultation, the bruit is not present. How does the nurse practitioner evaluate this data?
    a. The problem has resolved spontaneously.
    b. There may have been an anomaly in previous findings.
    c. The occlusion of the vessel may have progressed past 90%.
    d. The antiplatelet therapy is working.

52. In assessing a patient, the nurse finds that the PMI appears in more than one intercostal space, and has shifted lateral to the midclavicular line. How does the nurse interpret this data?
    a. Left ventricular hypertrophy
    b. Superior vena cava obstruction
    c. Pulmonary hypertension
    d. Constrictive pericarditis

53. In the illustration below, locate and describe the sites for auscultation of the heart sounds and pulse points listed.
    a. Aortic area
    b. Pulmonic area
    c. Right ventricular area
    d. Epigastric area
    e. Mitral area
    f. Tricuspid area

True or False? Read each statement about performing a pericardium assessment and write T for true or F for false in the blanks provided. If the statement is false, correct the statement to make it true.

_____ 54. The assessment begins with auscultation.

_____ 55. The patient is in a supine position with the head of bed elevated for comfort and ease of breathing.

_____ 56. Inspect for PMI or pulsations at the apex of the heart.

_____ 57. Murmurs and rubs are detected by palpation.

_____ 58. Inspect the chest from the side, at a right angle, and downward over areas of the precordium where vibrations are visible.

_____ 59. The first heart sound is heard best at the base of the heart.

_____ 60. When auscultating, use the diaphragm of the stethoscope to listen for low-frequency sounds.

_____ 61. The skill of accurately auscultating sounds requires a good stethoscope and lots of practice.

Matching. Match each source of chest pain with its assessment findings. Each source of chest pain may be used more than once.

Sources of Chest Pain
a. Angina
b. Myocardial infarction
c. Pericarditis
d. Esophageal-gastric
e. Anxiety
f. Pleuropulmonary

Assessment Findings
_____ 62. Sudden onset
_____ 63. Moderate ache, worse on inspiration
_____ 64. Substernal, may spread to shoulders or abdomen
_____ 65. Intermittent, relieved with sitting upright
_____ 66. Substernal, may spread across chest, back, arms
_____ 67. Usually lasts less than 15 minutes
_____ 68. Continuous until underlying condition is treated
_____ 69. Intense, stabbing, vice-like pain
_____ 70. Dull ache to sharp stabbing, may have numbness of fingers
_____ 71. Sudden onset, often in early morning
_____ 72. May be in response to stress
_____ 73. Sharp stabbing, moderate to severe
_____ 74. Squeezing, heartburn, variable in severity

75. The nurse working in a women's health clinic is reviewing the risk factors for several patients for stroke and myocardial infarction (MI). Which patient has the highest risk for MI?
    a. 49-year-old on estrogen replacement therapy
    b. 40-year-old taking oral contraceptives who smokes
    c. 23-year-old with diabetes that is currently not well-controlled
    d. 60-year-old with well-controlled hypertension

76. A patient comes to the emergency department (ED) reporting chest pain. In evaluating the patient's pain, which questions does the nurse ask the patient? *(Select all that apply.)*
    a. "How long does the pain last and how often does it occur?"
    b. "How do you feel about the pain?"
    c. "Is the pain different from any other episodes of pain you've had?"
    d. "What activities were you doing when the pain first occurred?"
    e. "Where is the chest pain? What does it feel like?"
    f. "Have you had other signs and symptoms that occur at the same time?"
    g. "How can we help you to alleviate the pain?"

77. The nurse is instructing a patient with congestive heart failure (CHF) on what signs to look for when experiencing an exacerbation of CHF. Which are appropriate teaching points for this patient? *(Select all that apply.)*
    a. It is possible to gain up to 10 to 15 lbs before edema develops.
    b. Notify the physician of a weight loss of 3 to 5 lbs within 2 weeks.
    c. Notify the physician of a weight gain of 2 lbs within 1-2 days.
    d. Notify the physician if you notice that your shoes or rings feel tight.
    e. Notify the physician if your skin becomes dry and scaly.

78. A 65-year-old patient comes to the clinic reporting fatigue and tiredness. The patient would like to start an exercise program, but thinks "anemia might be causing the fatigue." What is the nurse's first action?
    a. Advise the patient to start out slowly and gradually build strength and endurance.
    b. Obtain an order for a complete blood count and nutritional profile.
    c. Assess the onset, duration, and circumstances associated with the fatigue and tiredness.
    d. Perform a physical assessment to include testing of muscle strength and tone.

79. A young patient reports having frequent episodes of palpitations but denies having chest pain. Which follow-up question does the nurse ask to assess the patient's symptom of palpitations?
    a. "Have you noticed a worsening of shortness of breath when you are lying flat?"
    b. "Do your shoes feel unusually tight, or are your rings tighter than usual?"
    c. "Do you feel dizzy or have you lost consciousness with the palpitations?"
    d. "Does anyone in your family have a history of palpitations?"

80. Syncope in the aging person can likely occur with which actions by the patient? *(Select all that apply.)*
    a. Laughing
    b. Turning the head
    c. Performing a Valsalva maneuver
    d. Walking briskly for 20 to 30 minutes
    e. Shrugging the shoulders

81. Syncope in the older adult may result from _____ of the carotid sinus bodies in the carotid arteries.

True or False? *Read each statement and write T for true or F for false in the blanks provided.*

_____ 82. Dyspnea that is associated with activity, such as climbing stairs, is referred to as *dyspnea on exertion.*

_____ 83. Paroxysmal nocturnal dyspnea occurs when the patient has been sitting for a prolonged period of time.

_____ 84. Severity of orthopnea is measured by the length of time it takes to recover after exertion.

_____ 85. Dyspnea on exertion may be the only sign of early heart failure in women.

86. The nurse performing a physical assessment on a patient with a history of CVD observes that the patient has ascites, jaundice, and anasarca. How does the nurse interpret these findings?
    a. Late signs of severe right-sided heart failure
    b. Early signs of mild right-sided heart failure
    c. Late signs of mild left-sided heart failure
    d. Early signs of left- and right-sided heart failure

87. The nurse is performing an assessment on a patient brought in by emergency personnel. The nurse immediately observes that the patient has spontaneous respirations and the skin is cool, pale, and moist. What is the priority patient problem?
    a. Abnormal body temperature
    b. Impaired oxygenation
    c. Altered skin integrity
    d. Potential for peripheral neurovascular dysfunction

88. The nurse is caring for a patient at risk for MI. For what primary reason does the nurse plan interventions to prevent anxiety or overexertion?
    a. An increase in heart rate increases myocardial oxygen demand.
    b. A release of epinephrine and norepinephrine causes MI.
    c. An increase in activity or emotion effects preload and afterload.
    d. Cardiac output is decreased by anxiety or physical stress.

89. The nurse is caring for a patient with the priority problem of Decreased Cardiac Output. Which situation may result in decreased myocardial contractility that will further lower cardiac output?
    a. Administration of a positive inotropic medication
    b. Hyperventilation to correct respiratory acidosis
    c. Frequent endotracheal suctioning that results in hypoxemia
    d. Administration of IV fluids to correct underlying hypovolemia

90. A patient reports severe cramping in the legs while attempting to walk for exercise. The physician diagnoses the patient with intermittent claudication. What does the nurse advise the patient to do?
    a. Elevate the legs on a pillow.
    b. Buy and wear supportive shoes.
    c. Massage the legs before walking.
    d. Rest the legs in a dependent position.

91. A patient entering the cardiac rehabilitation unit seems optimistic and at times unexpectedly cheerful and upbeat. Which statement by the patient causes the nurse to suspect a maladaptive use of denial in the patient?
    a. "I am sick and tired of talking about these dietary restrictions. Could we talk about it tomorrow?"
    b. "Oh, I don't really need that medication information. I'm sure that I'll soon be able to get by without it."
    c. "This whole episode of heart problems has been an eye-opener for me, but I really can't wait to get out of here."
    d. "That doctor is really driving me crazy with all his instructions. Could you put all that information away in my suitcase?"

92. The nurse taking a medical history of a patient makes a special notation to follow up on valvular abnormalities of the heart. Which recurrent condition in the patient's history causes the nurse to make this notation?
    a. Streptococcal infections of the throat
    b. Staphylococcal infections of the skin
    c. Vaginal yeast infections
    d. Fungal infections of the feet or inner thighs

Matching. Match each serum lipid value with the serum lipid laboratory test used to determine the value in an adult.

Name of Lipid Test
a. Total cholesterol
b. Triglycerides
c. Plasma high-density lipoproteins (HDLs)
d. Plasma low-density lipoproteins (LDLs)
e. HDL:LDL ratio

Normal Laboratory Value
_____ 93. Less than 70 mg/dL in high-risk cardiovascular patients, less than 100 mg/dL in patients with moderate risk factors, and less than 130 mg/dL in patients with no risk factors

_____ 94. Less than 150 mg/dL

_____ 95. 122 to 200 mg/dL; older adults is 144 to 280 mg/dL

_____ 96. 3:1

_____ 97. Greater than 45 mg/dL

98. What is the most significant laboratory cardiac marker in a patient who has had an MI?
a. Presence of troponin T and I
b. Elevation of myoglobin levels
c. Creatine kinase levels
d. Elevation of the white count

99. A patient in the ED with chest pain has a possible MI. Which laboratory test is done to determine this diagnosis?
a. Troponin T and I
b. Serum potassium
c. Homocysteine
d. Highly sensitive C-reactive protein

100. Which laboratory tests are used to predict a patient's risk for coronary artery disease (CAD)? *(Select all that apply.)*
a. Cholesterol level
b. Triglyceride level
c. Prothrombin time
d. Low-density lipoprotein level
e. Albumin level

101. A patient is undergoing diagnostic testing for reports of chest pain. Which test is done to determine the location and extent of CAD?
a. Electrocardiogram (ECG)
b. Echocardiogram
c. Cardiac catheterization
d. Chest x-ray

102. Microalbuminuria has been shown to be a clear marker of widespread endothelial dysfunction in cardiovascular disease. Which conditions should prompt patients to be tested annually for microalbuminuria? *(Select all that apply.)*
a. Hypertension
b. Metabolic syndrome
c. Smoker
d. Diabetes mellitus
e. Use of anticoagulant therapy

103. A patient is being discharged with a prescription for warfarin (Coumadin). Which test does the nurse instruct the patient to routinely have done for follow-up monitoring?
a. Prothrombin time (PT) and International Normalized Ratio (INR)
b. Partial thromboplastin time (PTT)
c. Complete blood count and platelet count
d. Sodium and potassium levels

104. What is the significance of a sodium level of 130 mEq/L for a patient with heart failure?
a. Increased risk for ventricular dysrhythmias
b. Dilutional hyponatremia and fluid retention
c. Potential for electrical instability of the heart
d. Slowed conduction of impulse through the heart

105. Which test is performed to determine valve disease of the mitral valve, left atrium, or aortic arch?
    a. Transesophageal echocardiogram
    b. ECG
    c. Myocardial nuclear perfusion imaging (MNPI)
    d. Phonocardiography

106. A patient is scheduled to have an exercise electrocardiography test. What instruction does the nurse provide to the patient before the procedure takes place?
    a. Have nothing to eat or drink after midnight.
    b. Avoid smoking or drinking alcohol for at least 2 weeks before the test.
    c. Wear comfortable, loose clothing and rubber-soled, supportive shoes.
    d. Someone must drive you home because of possible sedative effects of the medications.

107. A nurse is monitoring the patient's blood pressure and ECG during a stress test. Which parameter indicates the patient should stop exercising?
    a. Increase in heart rate
    b. Increase in blood pressure
    c. ECG showing the PQRS complex
    d. ECG showing ST-segment depression

108. What measures are taken to prepare a patient for a pharmacologic stress echocardiogram? *(Select all that apply.)*
    a. Patient can eat his/her diet as ordered
    b. IV access needs to be present
    c. Oxygen at 2 L per nasal cannula is placed on patient 3 hours prior to test
    d. An oral laxative is given the day before the test
    e. Patient is to be NPO for 3 to 6 hours before the test

True or False? *Read each statement and write T for true or F for false in the blanks provided. If the statement is false, correct the statement to make it true.*

_____ 109. Echocardiograms require an informed consent.

_____ 110. MNPI is a radioactive technique used to view cardiovascular abnormalities.

_____ 111. Technetium scanning is effective for diagnosing old infarctions.

_____ 112. After an MNPI, the patient is placed in isolation because of radioactive isotopes.

_____ 113. Thallium imaging can be done with the patient at rest or during exercise.

_____ 114. For patients who cannot perform a treadmill stress test, vasodilating drugs can simulate the effects of exercise.

_____ 115. During a thallium imaging scan, patients should be aware that vasodilators can cause flushing, headache, dyspnea, and chest tightness a few moments after the injection.

_____ 116. An echocardiogram is a risk-free, pain-free test that uses sound waves to assess cardiac structure and mobility, particularly that of the valves.

_____ 117. A PET scan takes 2 to 3 hours and a patient may be asked to use a treadmill.

_____ 118. During multigated blood pool scanning, several blood samples are taken for measurement of oxygen saturation.

_____ 119. Electronic beam computed tomography (EBCT) can look for calcifications within the arteries.

_____ 120. During an electrophysiologic study (EPS), programmed electrical stimulation of the heart is used to induce and evaluate lethal dysrhythmias and conduction abnormalities.

_____ 121. MRI is not useful in evaluating disorders of the cardiac system.

122. The nurse is obtaining a pulmonary artery wedge pressure (PAWP) from a patient. During recording, at what position must the transducer be?
   a. External jugular axis
   b. Aortic axis
   c. Superior vena cava axis
   d. Phlebostatic axis

123. A patient is being hemodynamically monitored via a pulmonary artery catheter. There is a right atrial pressure (RAP) reading of less than 9 mm Hg. How does the nurse interpret this finding?
   a. Right-sided heart failure
   b. Left-sided heart failure
   c. Cardiac tamponade
   d. Hypovolemia

124. A patient's Svo_2 (mixed venous oxygen saturation) is 70%. What is the nurse's interpretation of this finding?
   a. Oxygen demand is balanced by the oxygen supply.
   b. Oxygen demand exceeds the available oxygen supply.
   c. Available oxygen supply exceeds the current oxygen demand.
   d. Venous oxygen saturation is equal to the arterial oxygen saturation.

125. What are the purposes of an angiogram? (Select all that apply.)
   a. Determine an abnormal structure of the heart
   b. Identify an arterial obstruction
   c. Assess the cardiovascular response to increased workload
   d. Identify an arterial narrowing
   e. Identify an aneurysm

126. What is included in postprocedural care of a patient after a cardiac catheterization? (Select all that apply.)
   a. Patient remains on bedrest for 12 to 24 hours.
   b. Patient is placed in a high-Fowler's position.
   c. Dressing is assessed for bloody drainage or hematoma.
   d. Peripheral pulses in the affected extremity, as well as skin temperature and color, are monitored with every vital sign check.
   e. Patient is assessed for pain at the insertion site.
   f. Adequate oral and IV fluids are provided for hydration.
   g. Intake and output are monitored because the dye is an osmotic diuretic.
   h. Vital signs are monitored every hour for 24 hours.

127. Which assessment finding in a patient who has had a cardiac catheterization does the nurse report immediately to the physician?
   a. Pain at the catheter insertion site
   b. Catheterized extremity dusky with decreased peripheral pulses
   c. Small hematoma at the catheter insertion site
   d. Pulse pressure of 40 mm Hg with a slow, bounding pulse

128. The critical care nurse has just taken a reading of the patient's PAWP. The balloon remains in the wedge position after the reading. What does the nurse do next? *(Select all that apply.)*
   a. Elevate the head of the bed to 45 degrees.
   b. Ask the patient to cough.
   c. Notify the physician immediately.
   d. Assist the patient to change positions.
   e. Place the transducer at the level of the phlebostatic axis.

129. What are possible complications associated with a pulmonary artery catheter? *(Select all that apply.)*
   a. Ventricular dysrhythmias
   b. Pneumonia
   c. MI
   d. Pulmonary infarction
   e. Infection

CASE STUDY: ASSESSMENT OF THE CARDIOVASCULAR SYSTEM (1)

Use a separate sheet of paper to answer the questions in this Case Study, or go to the "Prepare for Class" folder on your Evolve website at http://evolve.elsevier.com/Iggy/ to download and complete as a word processing file. Answer guidelines for this Case Study are also available on your Evolve website.

A 67-year-old Mexican-American woman is admitted to the hospital for dyspnea and progressive fatigue. The patient's history reveals that she is 45 lbs overweight from her previously recorded weight one year ago. She has had insulin-dependent diabetes for 23 years that is controlled with daily insulin. A 24-hour account by the patient of her diet reveals an intake of high-sodium and high-cholesterol foods. Her exercise routine includes walking a half-mile for 20 minutes 1 to 2 times a week. She states she smokes one pack per day and has done so for 40 years. She reports no alcohol consumption. At night she sleeps with three pillows and gets up urgently to void at least once each night.

The patient is slightly dyspneic while speaking one to two sentences and then must stop to rest for 2 minutes before she can resume answering questions. On assessment she has anasarca and ascites. Jugular vein distension is 4 mm above the sternal angle with the head of bed elevated at 45 degrees. A right ventricular heave is observed at the sternal border with the patient in a semi-Fowler's position. Her skin is pale and cool to the touch. Her apical pulse is not palpable. Radial pulses are 1+ bilaterally and pedal pulses are 1+ bilaterally on palpation. Auscultation of the heart reveals S_1, S_2, and S_3. She denies any chest pain.

Vital signs are: pulse oximeter reading 90%, but after administering 2 L of oxygen per nasal cannula the pulse oximeter reading elevates to 93%; temp 36.3° C (97.3° F); heart rate and rhythm 88/min, sinus arrhythmia with occasional PVCs; respirations 28/min.

1. Document the case study above using the format of 1) History, 2) Inspection, 3) Palpation, 4) Auscultation, and 5) Additional Notes.

2. What kind of heart failure (which side) does this patient's assessment reveal?

3. What does the auscultation of S_3 indicate?

4. The patient reports that she sleeps on three pillows at night. What does this indicate?

CASE STUDY: ASSESSMENT OF THE CARDIOVASCULAR SYSTEM (2)

Use a separate sheet of paper to answer the questions in this Case Study, or go to the "Prepare for Class" folder on your Evolve website at http://evolve.elsevier.com/Iggy/ to download and complete as a word processing file. Answer guidelines for this Case Study are also available on your Evolve website.

The patient is a 72-year-old man who had an extensive left ventricular myocardial infarction (MI) at 36 years of age. At the time of his MI, he was overweight by 50 pounds and smoked two packs of unfiltered cigarettes per day. He had smoked for 20 years. Alcohol consumption was part of his ethnic background; it was customary for him to drink one or two beers per day and several mixed drinks per week. His father had also suffered an MI at the age of 48, and was a chain smoker. The patient slowly recovered from his MI, gave up smoking, and lost weight. His weight stabilized within 15 pounds of the upper limit of his ideal weight. His wife became an active participant in his recovery by changing her style of cooking and virtually eliminating saturated fats from their diets. He no longer drank beer, but he continued to consume an average of two mixed drinks per day. He began a moderate exercise program that included walking several miles at least three times a week. He has had stable angina for many years and has annual physical checkups and ECGs at the cardiologist's office. He took up the hobby of downhill skiing at the age of 66, with his cardiologist's approval. He is a retired accountant with a type A personality. Over the past 6 months, he has experienced infrequent periods of lightheadedness. He has "blacked out" on at least one occasion and was unable to remember any details of what happened. A second episode of loss of consciousness occurred on a clear, cold winter day while he was skiing. He revived spontaneously. The next day, he scheduled an appointment with his physician.

1. Which lifestyle changes decreased the patient's risk status after his MI? Which habits increased his risk status?

2. Compare and contrast the risk factors of CV disease for a 36-year-old man and a 72-year-old man.

3. The cardiologist performs an ECG and orders bloodwork drawn for serum lipids, troponins, AST, CK and CK-MB, LDH and isoenzymes, serum potassium, and C-reactive protein. What is the purpose of these tests?

4. The ECG and bloodwork are inconclusive, but the physician is concerned about the patient's symptoms. Discuss why there is reason for concern.

5. The patient is scheduled for an inpatient cardiac catheterization. The physician tells him that, based on the findings at the time of the catheterization, he may go ahead and perform an angioplasty. Develop a teaching-learning plan for this patient.

6. What are postprocedural nursing responsibilities?

7. What are home instructions and risk factor modifications the nurse should relay to the patient before discharge?

(Continued on next page.)

8. The cardiac catheterization is completed, and a 95% blockage of the left anterior descending (LAD) artery is seen along with an 80% blockage of the circumflex artery. A balloon angioplasty is performed in the catheterization laboratory. After the procedure, the LAD has a 40% blockage, and the circumflex has a 25% blockage. The physician counsels the patient to resume activity gradually. A stress test will be scheduled in several weeks for further evaluation of his exercise tolerance and cardiac status. Develop a teaching-learning plan for this patient to prepare him for the upcoming tests.

36 CHAPTER

Care of Patients with Dysrhythmias

STUDY/REVIEW QUESTIONS

Fill in the blank.

1. The primary pacemaker of the heart is the
   _____.

2. The electrical impulse of the heart moves through the ventricles from the _____ to right and left bundle branches to the _____.

3. The function of the atrioventricular (AV) node is to _____ impulses between the atria and ventricles.

4. The ability of all cardiac cells to initiate an impulse spontaneously and repetitively is called _____.

5. _____ is the ability of atrial and ventricular muscle cells to shorten their fiber length in response to electrical stimulation.

6. The transmitting of electrical impulses from cardiac cell to cardiac cell is called _____.

7. The ability of a cell to respond to a stimulus by initiating an impulse is called _____.

8. _____ contributes additional blood volume for a greater cardiac output.

9. What does stimulation of the sympathetic nervous system produce?
   a. Delayed electrical impulse that causes hypotension and bradypnea
   b. Contractility and dilation of coronary vessels and increased heart rate
   c. Virtually no effect on the ventricles of the heart or vital signs
   d. A slowed AV conduction time that results in a slow heart rate

10. The primary pacemaker of the heart, the sinoatrial (SA) node, is functional if a patient's pulse is at what regular rate?
    a. Fewer than 60 beats/min
    b. 60 to 100 beats/min
    c. 80 to 100 beats/min
    d. Greater than 100 beats/min

11. The nurse is taking vital signs and reviewing the electrocardiogram (ECG) of a patient who is training for a marathon. The heart rate is 45 beats/min and the ECG shows sinus bradycardia. How does the nurse interpret this data?
    a. A rapid filling rate that lengthens diastolic filling time and leads to decreased cardiac output
    b. The body's attempt to compensate for a decreased stroke volume by decreasing the heart rate
    c. An adequate stroke volume that is associated with cardiac conditioning
    d. A common finding in the healthy adult that would be considered normal

12. The nurse is performing the shift assessment on a cardiac patient. In order to determine if the patient has a pulse deficit, what does the nurse do?
    a. Take the patient's blood pressure and subtract the diastolic from the systolic pressure.
    b. Take the patient's pulse in a supine position and then in a standing position.
    c. Assess the apical and radial pulses for a full minute and observe for differences.
    d. Take the radial pulse, have the patient rest for 15 minutes, and then retake the pulse.

Matching. *Match the placements with the correct limb leads for ECG monitoring.*

Limb Lead
a. Lead I
b. Lead II
c. Lead III
d. aVr
e. aVL
f. aVF

Placement
_____ 13. Right arm (+)

_____ 14. Right arm (−), left arm (+)

_____ 15. Left arm (−), left leg (+)

_____ 16. Left leg (+)

_____ 17. Left arm (+)

_____ 18. Right arm (−), left leg (+)

19. Identify the components of a normal ECG.

20. What does the P wave in an ECG represent?
    a. Atrial depolarization
    b. Atrial repolarization
    c. Ventricular depolarization
    d. Ventricular repolarization

21. What is the normal measurement of the PR interval in an ECG?
    a. Less than 0.11 second
    b. 0.06 to 0.10 second
    c. 0.12 to 0.20 second
    d. 0.16 to 0.26 second

22. What is the QRS complex in an ECG normally?
    a. Less than 0.12 second
    b. 0.10 to 0.16 second
    c. 0.12 to 0.20 second
    d. 0.16 to 0.24 second

23. What is the ST segment in an ECG normally?
    a. Isoelectric
    b. Elevated
    c. Depressed
    d. Biphasic

24. What is the total time required for ventricular depolarization and repolarization as represented on the ECG?
    a. PR interval
    b. QRS complex
    c. ST segment
    d. QT interval

25. The nurse is performing a 12-lead ECG on a patient with chest pain. Because the positioning of the electrodes is crucial, how does the nurse place the ECG components?
    a. Four leads are placed on the limbs and six are placed on the chest.
    b. The negative electrode is placed on the left arm and the positive electrode is placed on the right leg.
    c. Four leads are placed on the limbs and four are placed on the chest.
    d. The negative electrode is placed on the right arm and the positive electrode is placed on the left leg.

26. Where does the nurse place the electrodes on a patient who requires continuous ECG monitoring?
    a. On the right arm, left arm, and left foot
    b. On the left arm, left leg, and right arm
    c. Below the clavicles and on the lowest ribs
    d. With regular spacing across the anterior chest

27. Cardiac dysrhythmias are abnormal rhythms of the heart's electrical system. How does this affect the heart's function?
    a. It cannot oxygenate the blood throughout the body.
    b. It cannot remove carbon dioxide from the body.
    c. It cannot effectively pump oxygenated blood throughout the body.
    d. It cannot effectively conduct impulses with increased activity.

28. The nurse is caring for several patients in the telemetry unit who are being remotely watched by a monitor technician. What is the nurse's primary responsibility in the monitoring process of these patients?
    a. Watching the bank of monitors on the unit
    b. Printing ECG rhythm strips routinely and as needed
    c. Interpreting rhythms
    d. Assessment and management

29. A patient in the telemetry unit is having continuous ECG monitoring. The patient is scheduled for a test in the radiology department. Who is responsible for determining when monitoring can be suspended?
    a. Telemetry technician
    b. Charge nurse
    c. Physician
    d. Primary nurse

30. The nurse is reviewing preliminary ECG results of a patient admitted for mental status changes. The nurse alerts the provider about ST elevation or depression in the patient because it is an indication of which condition?
    a. Myocardial injury or ischemia
    b. Ventricular irritability
    c. Subarachnoid hemorrhage
    d. Prinzmetal's angina

31. The nurse is reviewing ECG results of a patient admitted for fluid and electrolyte imbalances. The T waves are tall and peaked. The nurse reports this finding to the provider and obtains an order for which serum level test?
    a. Sodium
    b. Glucose
    c. Potassium
    d. Phosphorus

32. The nurse is notified by the telemetry monitor technician about a patient's heart rate. Which method does the nurse use to confirm the technician's report?
    a. Count QRS complexes in a 6-second strip and multiply by 10.
    b. Analyze an ECG rhythm strip by using an ECG caliper.
    c. Run an ECG rhythm strip and use the memory method.
    d. Assess the patient's heart rate directly by taking an apical pulse.

33. Place the six steps of analyzing an ECG rhythm strip in the correct order using the numbers 1 through 6.

    _____ a. Interpret the rhythm

    _____ b. Analyze the P waves

    _____ c. Determine the heart rate

    _____ d. Measure the QRS duration

    _____ e. Measure the PR interval

    _____ f. Determine the heart rhythm

34. A patient's ECG rhythm strip is irregular. Which method does the nurse use for an accurate assessment?
    a. 6-second strip method
    b. Memory method
    c. Big block method
    d. Commercial ECG rate ruler

35. The nurse is assessing a patient's ECG rhythm strip and checking the regularity of the atrial rhythm. What is the correct technique?
    a. Place one caliper point on a QRS complex; place the other point on the precise spot on the next QRS complex.
    b. Place one caliper point on a P wave; place the other point on the precise spot on the next P wave.
    c. · Place one caliper point at the beginning of the P wave; place the other point at the end of the P-R segment.
    d. Place one caliper point at the beginning of the QRS complex; place and the other point where the S-T segment begins.

36. The nurse is assessing a patient's ECG rhythm strip and analyzing the P waves. Which questions does the nurse use to evaluate the P waves? *(Select all that apply.)*
    a. Are P waves present?
    b. Are the P waves occurring regularly?
    c. Does one P wave follow each QRS complex?
    d. Are the P waves greater than 0.20 second?
    e. Do all the P waves look similar?
    f. Are the P waves smooth, rounded, and upright in appearance?

37. The nurse is assessing a patient's ECG rhythm strip and notes that occasionally the QRS complex is missing. How does the nurse interpret this finding?
    a. A junctional impulse
    b. A supraventricular impulse
    c. Ventricular tachycardia
    d. A dysrhythmia

38. The student nurse is looking at a patient's ECG rhythm strip and suspects a normal sinus rhythm (NSR). Which ECG criteria are included for NSR? *(Select all that apply.)*
    a. Rate: Atrial and ventricular rates of 40 to 120 beats/min
    b. Rhythm: Atrial and ventricular rhythms regular
    c. P waves: Present, consistent configuration, one P wave before each QRS complex
    d. P-R interval is nondetermined
    e. QRS duration: 0.04 to 0.10 second and constant

39. What does the P wave on an ECG represent?
    a. Atrial depolarization
    b. The period of time from the firing of the SA node to just before ventricular depolarization
    c. The period between ventricular depolarization and beginning of ventricular repolarization
    d. When depolarization occurs in the ventricles

40. The heart monitor of a patient shows a rhythm that appears as a wandering or fuzzy baseline. What is the priority action for the nurse?
    a. Immediately obtain a 12-lead ECG to assess the actual rhythm.
    b. Assess the patient to differentiate artifact from actual lethal rhythms.
    c. Check to see if the patient has a do-not-resuscitate order.
    d. Ask the patient care technician to take vital signs on the patient.

41. When depolarization occurs in the ventricles, the _____ _____ is formed on the ECG.

42. The period between ventricular depolarization and the beginning of ventricular repolarization is known as the _____ _____.

43. What does the T wave on an ECG represent?
    a. Ventricular depolarization
    b. Atrial repolarization
    c. Atrial depolarization
    d. Ventricular repolarization

44. The amplitude of the wave on a ECG reflects the _____ _____ of the contraction.

True or False? *Read each statement about characteristics of an ECG complex and write T for true or F for false in the blanks provided. If the statement is false, correct the statement to make it true.*

_____ 45. The P-R interval is the period of time from the firing of the SA node to just before ventricular depolarization.

_____ 46. The period between ventricular depolarization and the beginning of ventricular repolarization is the S-T segment.

_____ 47. The T wave represents ventricular repolarization.

_____ 48. Q-T interval is the total time it takes the depolarization and repolarization of atria and ventricles to occur.

49. The remote telemetry technician calls the nurse to report that a patient's ECG signal transmission is not very clear. What does the nurse do to enhance the transmission?
    a. Clean the skin with povidone-iodine solution before applying the electrodes.
    b. Ensure that the area for electrode placement is dry and non-hairy.
    c. Apply tincture of benzoin to the electrode sites and allow it to dry.
    d. Abrade the skin by rubbing briskly with a rough washcloth.

50. With the speed set for 25 mm/second, the segment between the dark lines on a monitor ECG strip represents how many seconds?
    a. 3
    b. 6
    c. 10
    d. 20

51. Which components measure ECG waveforms?
    a. Blood pressure (BP) and cardiac output (CO)
    b. Seconds (sec) and minutes (min)
    c. Heart rate per minute (HR/min)
    d. Amplitude (voltage) and duration (time)

52. Calculate the heart rate from an ECG strip when there are 25 small blocks from one R wave to the next R wave.

53. Calculate the heart rate shown on a 6-second ECG strip when the number of R-R intervals is 5. What is this rhythm?

54. How does the nurse interpret the measurement of the P-R interval when the interval to be measured is six small boxes on the ECG strip?
    a. Atrium is taking longer to repolarize.
    b. Longer than normal impulse time from the SA node to the ventricles is shown.
    c. There is a problem with the length of time the ventricles are depolarizing.
    d. This is the normal length of time for the P-R interval.

55. The nurse is reviewing a patient's ECG and interprets a wide distorted QRS complex of 0.14 second followed by a P wave. What does this finding indicate?
    a. Wide but normal complex, and no cause for concern
    b. Premature ventricular contraction
    c. Problem with the speed set on the ECG machine
    d. Delayed time of the electrical impulse through the ventricles

56. Which clinical manifestations are reflections of sustained tachydysrhythmias and bradydysrhythmias? *(Select all that apply.)*
    a. Weakness and fatigue
    b. Warm, dry skin
    c. Dyspnea
    d. Hypertension
    e. Decreased urine output

Matching. *Match each type of dysrhythmia with its description. Answers may be used more than once.*

Types of Dysrhythmias
a. Sinus tachycardia
b. Atrial flutter
c. Atrial fibrillation
d. First-degree atrioventricular block
e. Ventricular tachycardia
f. Ventricular fibrillation
g. Asystole
h. Third-degree heart block

Descriptions

_____ 57. A straight line or wavy line on the cardiac monitor

_____ 58. Sinus impulses are delayed, but all eventually reach the ventricles

_____ 59. A ventricular rhythm that in most cases results in loss of consciousness

_____ 60. Rapidly fatal if not corrected in 3 to 5 minutes

_____ 61. Complete heart block

_____ 62. Results in asynchrony of atrial contraction and decreased cardiac output

_____ 63. May result from sympathetic nervous system stimulation of the heart or vagal inhibition

_____ 64. Characterized by rapid atrial depolarization occurring at a rate of 250 to 350 times per minute

_____ 65. Causes the ventricles to quiver, resulting in absence of cardiac output

66. The nurse hears in report that a patient has sinus arrhythmia. In order to validate that this is associated with the changes in intrathoracic pressure, what does the nurse do next?
    a. Count the respiratory and pulse rate at rest and then count both rates after moderate exertion.
    b. Observe that the heart rate increases slightly during inspiration and decreases slightly during exhalation.
    c. Ask the patient to hold the breath and take an apical pulse; then have the patient resume normal breathing.
    d. Have the patient take a deep breath and count the patient's apical pulse rate while the patient slowly exhales.

67. The nurse is caring for a patient with coronary artery disease (CAD). The patient reports palpitations and chest discomfort and the nurse notes a tachydysrhythmia on the ECG monitor. What does the nurse do next?
    a. Analyze the ECG strip.
    b. Notify the health care provider.
    c. Give supplemental oxygen.
    d. Administer a narcotic analgesic.

68. The nurse is taking the initial history and vital signs on a patient with fatigue. The nurse notes a regular apical pulse of 130 beats/min. Which contributing factors does the nurse assess for? *(Select all that apply.)*
    a. Anxiety or stress
    b. Fever
    c. Hypovolemia
    d. Anemia or hypoxemia
    e. Hypothyroidism
    f. Constipation

69. The nurse is taking a history and vital signs on a patient who has come to the clinic for a routine checkup. The patient has a pulse rate of 50 beats/min, but denies any distress. What does the nurse do next?
    a. Give supplemental oxygen.
    b. Establish IV access.
    c. Complete the health history.
    d. Check the blood pressure.

70. The nurse is reviewing the monitored rhythms of several patients in the cardiac stepdown unit. The patient with which cardiac anomaly has the greatest need of immediate attention?
    a. Chronic atrial fibrillation
    b. Paroxysmal supraventricular tachycardia that is suddenly terminated
    c. Sustained rapid ventricular response
    d. Sinus tachycardia with premature atrial complexes

71. A patient is diagnosed with recurrent supraventricular tachycardia (SVT). What does the nurse do in order to accomplish the preferred treatment?
    a. Place the patient on the cardiac monitor and perform carotid massage.
    b. Give oxygen and establish IV access for antidysrhythmic drugs.
    c. Assist the physician in attempting atrial overdrive pacing.
    d. Provide information about radiofrequency catheter ablation therapy.

72. Based on the prevalence and risk factors for atrial fibrillation (AF), which patient group is at highest risk for AF?
    a. Older adults
    b. Diabetics
    c. Substance abusers
    d. Pediatric cardiology patients

73. What are the risk factors for atrial fibrillation (AF) in the patient group identified in the previous question? *(Select all that apply.)*
    a. Chronic obstructive pulmonary disease (COPD)
    b. Hypertension
    c. Peripheral vascular disease
    d. Diabetes mellitus
    e. Valvular disease

74. A patient with AF suddenly develops shortness of breath, chest pain, hemoptysis, and a feeling of impending doom. The nurse recognizes these symptoms as which complication?
    a. Pulmonary embolism
    b. Embolic stroke
    c. Absence of atrial kick
    d. Increased cardiac output

75. A patient scheduled to have elective cardioversion for AF will receive drug therapy for about 6 weeks before the procedure. What information about the drug therapy does the nurse teach the patient?
    a. Managing orthostatic hypotension
    b. Watching for bleeding signs
    c. Eating potassium-rich food sources
    d. Reporting muscle weakness or tremors

76. The bedside cardiac monitor of a postoperative patient who becomes confused shows sinus rhythm, but there is no palpable pulse. How does the nurse interpret these findings?
    a. ECG monitor artifact or dysfunction
    b. Pulseless electrical activity with inadequate perfusion
    c. A paced rhythm with hypotension
    d. Idioventricular rhythm as seen in the dying heart

77. The remote telemetry technician alerts the nurse to the presence of premature ventricular contractions (PVCs) in a newly admitted patient. How does the nurse assess whether the premature complexes perfuse to the extremities?
    a. Palpate peripheral arteries while observing the monitor for widened complexes.
    b. Auscultate for the apical heart sounds and listen for irregularities or pauses.
    c. Check the color and temperature of extremities, and capillary refill of fingers and toes.
    d. Assess the ECG strip for regularity and width of QRS complexes.

78. What is the primary significance of ventricular tachycardia (VT) in a cardiac patient?
    a. It increases the ventricular filling time, therefore increasing cardiac output.
    b. It signals that the patient needs potassium supplement for replacement.
    c. It warrants immediate initiation of cardiopulmonary resuscitation.
    d. It is commonly the initial rhythm before deterioration into ventricular fibrillation.

79. The nurse is interviewing a patient who suddenly becomes faint, immediately loses consciousness, and becomes pulseless and apneic. There is no blood pressure, and heart sounds are absent. What does the nurse do next?
    a. Request the defibrillator.
    b. Start cardiopulmonary resuscitation (CPR).
    c. Establish or ensure IV access.
    d. Give supplemental oxygen.

80. A patient is in full cardiac arrest and CPR is in progress. The ECG monitor shows ventricular asystole. What does the nurse do next?
    a. Assist with or administer defibrillation.
    b. Assess another ECG lead to ensure the rhythm is asystole and not fine VF.
    c. Assist the physician with noninvasive pacing or invasive transvenous pacing.
    d. Encourage the family's presence during the resuscitation.

81. Traditionally, what medications will most likely be ordered for a patient with atrial fibrillation? *(Select all that apply.)*
    a. Diltiazem hydrochloride (Cardizem)
    b. Furosemide (Lasix)
    c. Heparin
    d. Enoxaparin (Lovenox)
    e. Sodium warfarin (Coumadin)

82. A patient is diagnosed with torsades de pointes. The nurse prepares to administer which emergency medication?
    a. Magnesium sulfate
    b. Epinephrine (Adrenalin)
    c. Adenosine (Adenocard)
    d. Calcium chloride

83. In a patient's record, the nurse notes frequent episodes of bradycardia and hypotension related to unintended vagal stimulation. Which instruction for this patient's care does the nurse relay to the unlicensed assistive personnel (UAP)?
    a. Avoid raising the patient's arms above the head during hygiene.
    b. Ambulate the patient slowly and stop frequently for brief rests.
    c. Generously lubricate rectal thermometer probes and insert very cautiously.
    d. Monitor the heart rate and rhythm if the patient is vomiting.

84. Depending on the degree, which interventions may be used for a patient with AV block? *(Select all that apply.)*
    a. Oxygen
    b. Defibrillation
    c. Pacing
    d. Drug therapy
    e. Permanent pacemaker

85. Excessive vagal stimulation to the heart causes the rate to (increase or decrease) from the sinus node discharge.

86. Excessive vagal stimulation can result from which activities? *(Select all that apply.)*
    a. Jogging
    b. Carotid sinus massage
    c. Suctioning
    d. Voiding
    e. Valsalva maneuver

87. What are two clinical findings that result from excessive vagal stimulation?

True or False? Read each statement about heart block and write T for true or F for false in the blanks provided. If the statement is false, correct the statement to make it true.

_____ 88. In *second-degree* heart block, some sinus impulses reach the ventricles, but others do not because they are blocked.

_____ 89. First-degree heart block is the complete blockage of impulses from the SA node.

_____ 90. Third-degree AV block results in ventricular rhythm.

_____ 91. A characteristic feature of third-degree block is that none of the sinus impulses reaches the ventricles.

92. The nurse is caring for several patients who have a dysrhythmia. What does the nurse instruct these patients to do?
    a. Stay at least 4 feet away from a microwave oven that is operating.
    b. Avoid electronic metal detectors, such as those at airports.
    c. Learn the procedure for assessing the pulse.
    d. Purchase an automatic external defibrillator for home use.

93. A patient reports chest pain and dizziness after exertion, and the family reports a concurrent new onset of mild confusion in the patient as well as difficulty concentrating. What is the priority problem for this patient?
    a. Activity Intolerance
    b. Decreased Cardiac Output
    c. Acute Confusion
    d. Inadequate Oxygenation

Matching. *Using the Vaughn-Williams classification of antidysrhythmics, match the class of drug with its action.*

Class
a.   Class I
b.   Class II
c.   Class III
d.   Class IV

Action

_____ 94.   Lengthens the absolute refractory period and prolongs repolarization and the action potential duration of ischemic cells

_____ 95.   Impedes the flow of calcium into the cell during depolarization, thereby depressing the automaticity of SA and AV nodes and decreasing heart rate

_____ 96.   Membrane-stabilizing agents used to decrease automaticity

_____ 97.   Controls dysrhythmias associated with excessive beta-adrenergic stimulation by competing for receptor sites, and thereby decreasing heart rate and conduction velocity

98.   According to the Vaughn-Williams classification of antidysrhythmics, which class II drug controls dysrhythmias associated with excessive beta-adrenergic stimulation?
a.   Amiodarone hydrochloride (Cordarone)
b.   Propranolol hydrochloride (Inderal)
c.   Diltiazem (Cardizem)
d.   Verapamil hydrochloride (Calan)

99.   Which drug for symptomatic bradycardia does the nurse prepare to administer to a patient with a bradydysrhythmia?
a.   Epinephrine
b.   Atropine
c.   Calcium
d.   Lidocaine

100.   Which medication does an adult patient with ventricular fibrillation or pulseless ventricular tachycardia receive?
a.   Propranolol (Inderal)
b.   Adenosine (Adenocard)
c.   Diltiazem hydrochloride (Cardizem)
d.   Epinephrine (Adrenalin Chloride)

101.   The respiratory therapist (RT) and the medical student are ventilating a patient in cardiac arrest, while the nurse and physician are preparing the patient and equipment for intubation. At which point does the nurse intervene?
a.   The RT inserts an oropharyngeal airway.
b.   The medical student sets the oxygen flow meter at 2 L/min.
c.   The RT ventilates with a manual resuscitation bag and mask.
d.   The medical student uses the chin-lift position on the patient.

102.   After advanced cardiac life support (ACLS) is performed, a patient who experienced ventricular fibrillation has a return of spontaneous circulation. To protect the patient's nervous system, which intervention does the nurse anticipate will be performed?
a.   Neurologic checks every 4 hours
b.   Administration of IV mannitol
c.   Application of a cooling blanket
d.   Continuous ECG monitoring

103. The nurse discovers a patient is unconscious and without palpable pulses and immediately initiates CPR. For what reason is CPR started on this patient?
    a. To identify the underlying heart rhythm
    b. For the rapid return of a pulse, blood pressure, and consciousness
    c. To prevent rib fractures or lacerations of the liver and spleen
    d. To mimic cardiac function until the defibrillator arrives

104. Automatic external defibrillator (AED) electrodes are placed on a patient who is unconscious and pulseless. The nurse prepares to immediately defibrillate if the monitor shows which cardiac anomaly?
    a. Third-degree heart block
    b. Pulseless electrical activity
    c. Ventricular fibrillation
    d. Idioventricular rhythm

105. A patient is found pulseless and the cardiac monitor shows a rhythm that has no recognizable deflections, but instead has coarse "waves" of varying amplitudes. What is the priority ACLS intervention for this rhythm?
    a. Immediate defibrillation
    b. Administration of epinephrine IVP
    c. Administration of lidocaine IVP
    d. Noninvasive temporary pacing

106. What other actions are essential interventions for the patient in the question number 105? *(Select all that apply.)*
    a. Providing effective CPR
    b. Supplying a temporary pacemaker
    c. Administrating epinephrine, vasopressin, and atropine, as appropriate
    d. Identifying and correcting the cause of the pulseless rhythm
    e. Providing continuous ECG monitoring

107. A patient has no pulse and the cardiac monitor shows ventricular fibrillation. Which drugs does the nurse prepare to administer during the resuscitation? *(Select all that apply.)*
    a. Lidocaine
    b. Epinephrine
    c. Calcium chloride
    d. Amiodarone hydrochloride (Cordarone)
    e. Dopamine hydrochloride (Intropin)
    f. Magnesium sulfate
    g. Dobutamine hydrochloride (Dobutrex)
    h. Vasopressin (Pitressin)

108. The nurse is placing the electrodes on a patient for cardioversion. What is the correct placement for the electrodes?
    a. One electrode is placed on the upper left chest and the other is placed on the lower left chest in a midaxillary line.
    b. One electrode is placed the upper right chest below the clavicle and the other is placed on the back.
    c. One electrode is placed to the left of the precordium, and the other is placed on the right next to the sternum and below the clavicle.
    d. One electrode is placed on the sternum and the other is placed on the lower left chest in a midaxillary line.

109. A patient is in ventricular fibrillation. The nurse sets the biphasic defibrillator to deliver how many joules?
    a. 100
    b. 200
    c. 300
    d. 360

110. A patient is about to undergo elective cardioversion. The nurse sets the defibrillator for synchronized mode so that the electrical shock is not delivered on the T wave. This is done to avoid which complication?
    a. Electrical burns to the skin
    b. Ventricular standstill
    c. Arcing from the electrodes
    d. Ventricular fibrillation

111. The nurse is performing external defibrillation. Which step is most vital this procedure?
    a. Place the gel pads anterior over the apex and posterior for better conduction.
    b. Do not administer a second shock for 1 minute to allow for recharging.
    c. No-one must touch the patient at the time a shock is delivered.
    d. Continuously ventilate the patient via endotracheal tube during the defibrillation.

Matching. *Match the terms with their correct definitions.*

Terms
a. Capture
b. Atrial overdrive pacing
c. Synchronous (demand) pacing mode
d. Asynchronous (fixed-rate) pacing mode
e. Noninvasive temporary pacing (NTP)
f. Invasive temporary pacemaker

Definitions
_____ 112. The pacemaker continues to fire at a fixed rate as set on the generator.

_____ 113. Electrical pulses are transmitted through two large external electrodes, then transcutaneously to stimulate ventricular depolarization.

_____ 114. Indicating that the pacemaker has successfully depolarized, or captured, the chamber.

_____ 115. Rapidly pacing the atrium to control depolarization, followed by no pacing, to allow the sinus node to regain control of the heart.

_____ 116. External battery-operated pulse generator on one end and wires in contact with the heart on the other end.

_____ 117. The pacemaker's sensitivity is set to sense the patient's own beats.

118. The nurse is assisting the physician to perform temporary pacing for a patient who has third-degree heart block. What are the desired outcomes for this patient as evidenced by the cardiac monitor? *(Select all that apply.)*
    a. A spike followed by a P wave, indicating atrial depolarization
    b. No spike, but a complete QRS complex indicating atrial depolarization
    c. A spike followed by a QRS complex indicating ventricular depolarization
    d. Two spikes, followed by a QRS complex indicating ventricular depolarization
    e. A spike before and after a QRS complex indicating atrial depolarization

119. The physician has completed the placement of lead wires for the invasive temporary pacemaker in a patient who is asystolic. In turning on the pacing unit, which setting does the nurse use?
    a. Synchronous pacing mode
    b. Demand pacing mode
    c. Asynchronous pacing mode
    d. Temporary pacing mode

120. The nurse in the telemetry unit may have to perform NTP in nonemergent situations. Place the steps of this procedure in sequential order using the numbers 1 through 7.

_____ a. Explain NTP to the patient and family and prepare the equipment.

_____ b. Apply the electrodes on the chest according to package instructions.

_____ c. Set milliamperes (mA) output 2 mA above where consistent capture is observed.

_____ d. Turn the pacer on; set the pacing rate as ordered.

_____ e. Establish the stimulation threshold.

_____ f. Palpate the right radial or carotid pulse and assess the blood pressure.

_____ g. Wash the skin with soap and water.

121. The nurse in the telemetry unit must perform NTP. How does the nurse position the electrodes?
    a. One over breast tissue on the right side and one over breast tissue on left side
    b. One on the upper chest to the left of the sternum and one beneath the left scapula
    c. One on the upper chest to the right of the sternum and one over the heart apex
    d. One over the sternum and one on the left anterior lateral chest

122. The nurse has been taking postprocedure vital signs of a patient with NTP. The patient is now stable and vital sign monitoring can be delegated to UAP. Which instruction does the nurse give the UAP regarding this patient's vital signs?
    a. Assess blood pressure using the patient's right arm and check the right radial pulse.
    b. Assess blood pressure using the patient's left arm and check the left carotid pulse.
    c. Set the automatic blood pressure cuff to cycle every 15 minutes on either arm.
    d. Do not use the pulse oximeter because of the danger of electromagnetic interference.

123. A patient has an invasive temporary pacemaker. In what ways does the nurse ensure the patient's safety related to electrical issues with the pacemaker? *(Select all that apply.)*
    a. Ensure that external ends of the lead wires are insulated with rubber gloves.
    b. Loop the wire ends and cover with nonconductive tape.
    c. Ensure that no electrical equipment is used in the patient's room.
    d. Report frayed wire to the biomedical engineering department.
    e. Wash hands before touching any of the wires.

124. What effects does dobutamine (Dobutrex) have on the heart? *(Select all that apply.)*
    a. Decreases myocardial contractility
    b. Stimulates beta-adrenergic receptors
    c. Improves myocardial contractility
    d. Depresses stimulation of beta-adrenergic receptors
    e. May cause dysrhythmias

125. The nurse administers a class III antidysrhythmic to a patient with _____ dysrhythmias.

126. Which descriptions are characteristic of a class III antidysrhythmic? *(Select all that apply.)*
    a. Lengthens the absolute refractory period
    b. Is a beta blocker
    c. Includes hypertension as a side effect
    d. Prolongs repolarization
    e. Includes bradycardia as a side effect

True or False? *Read each statement and write T for true or F for false in the blanks provided. If the statement is false, correct the statement to make it true.*

_____ 127. The implantable cardioverter defibrillator (ICD) treats bradydysrhythmias.

_____ 128. Ventricular aneurysms are a complication of MI.

129. A patient has an implantable cardioverter de-fibrillator (ICD). In cardioversion shock, the defibrillator is set in the synchronized mode to do what?
    a. Avoid discharging the shock during the T wave
    b. Discharge the shock during the R wave
    c. Discharge the shock during the T wave
    d. Avoid dischargsing the shock during the Q wave

130. The nurse caring for a patient with an NTP will assess for which common complications? *(Select all that apply.)*
    a. Chills
    b. Diaphoresis
    c. Chest pain
    d. Skin irritation
    e. Discomfort from muscle stimulation

131. A patient with atrial fibrillation is scheduled to have an elective cardioversion. The nurse ensures that the patient has a prescription for a 4-6 week supply of which type of medication?
    a. Anticoagulants
    b. Digitalis
    c. Diuretics
    d. Potassium supplements

132. The nurse is teaching a patient with an ICD. What instruction does the nurse emphasize to the patient?
    a. Rest for several hours after an internal de-fibrillator shock before resuming activities.
    b. Have family members step away during the internal defibrillator shock for safety.
    c. Expect that the shock may feel like a thud or a painful kick in the chest.
    d. Report any pulse rate higher than what is set on the pacemaker.

133. A patient has had synchronized cardioversion for unstable ventricular tachycardia. Which interventions does the nurse include in this patient's care after the procedure? *(Select all that apply.)*
    a. Administer therapeutic hypothermia.
    b. Assess vital signs and the level of con-sciousness.
    c. Administer antidysrhythmic drug therapy.
    d. Monitor for dysrhythmias.
    e. Monitor for loss of capture.
    f. Assess for chest burns from electrodes.

134. The nurse is teaching a community group how to use an automatic external defibrillator (AED). Place the steps of using an AED in sequential order using the numbers 1 through 5.
    _____ a. Rescuer presses the "analyze" button on the machine.
    _____ b. Place the patient on a firm, dry surface.
    _____ c. Rescuer stops CPR and directs anyone present to move away.
    _____ d. The machine advises if a shock is necessary.
    _____ e. Place two large adhesive-patch electrodes on the patient's chest.

135. A patient has had a permanent pacemaker surgically implanted. What are the nursing re-sponsibilities for the care of this patient related to the surgery? *(Select all that apply.)*
    a. Administer short-acting sedatives.
    b. Assess the implantation site for bleeding, swelling, redness, tenderness, or infection.
    c. Teach about and monitor for the initial ac-tivity restrictions.
    d. Observe for overstimulation of the chest wall which could lead to pneumothorax.
    e. Monitor the ECG rhythm to check that the pacemaker is working correctly.

136. The nurse is interviewing a patient with spontaneous ventricular tachycardia who may be a possible candidate for an ICD. The nurse senses that the patient is anxious. What is the nurse's most therapeutic response?
    a. "Your feelings are natural; patients report psychological distress related to ICD."
    b. "ICD is similar to defibrillation which saved your life during the last episode."
    c. "You seem anxious. What are your concerns about having this therapy?"
    d. "Would you like to talk to the doctor about the details of the procedure?"

137. The nurse is teaching a patient with a permanent pacemaker. What information about the pacemaker does the nurse tell the patient? *(Select all that apply.)*
    a. Report any pulse rate lower than what is set on the pacemaker.
    b. If the surgical incision is near the shoulder, avoid overextending the joint.
    c. Keep handheld cellular phones at least 6 inches away from the generator.
    d. Avoid sources of strong electromagnetic fields, such as magnets.
    e. Avoid strenuous activities that may cause the device to discharge inappropriately.
    f. Carry a pacemaker identification card and wear a medical alert bracelet.

Interpret each ECG strip below. Write your answers in the blanks provided.

138. _____

RATE _____ RHYTHM _____ P WAVES _____

PR INTERVAL _____ QRS DURATION _____

INTERPRETATION _____

139. _____

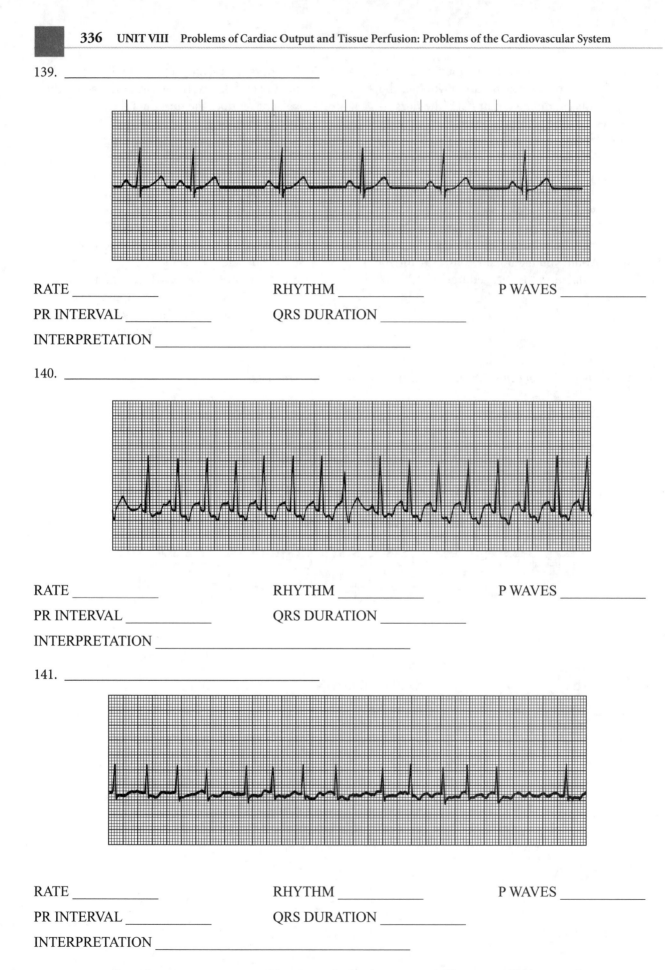

RATE _____   RHYTHM _____   P WAVES _____

PR INTERVAL _____   QRS DURATION _____

INTERPRETATION _____

140. _____

RATE _____   RHYTHM _____   P WAVES _____

PR INTERVAL _____   QRS DURATION _____

INTERPRETATION _____

141. _____

RATE _____   RHYTHM _____   P WAVES _____

PR INTERVAL _____   QRS DURATION _____

INTERPRETATION _____

142. _____

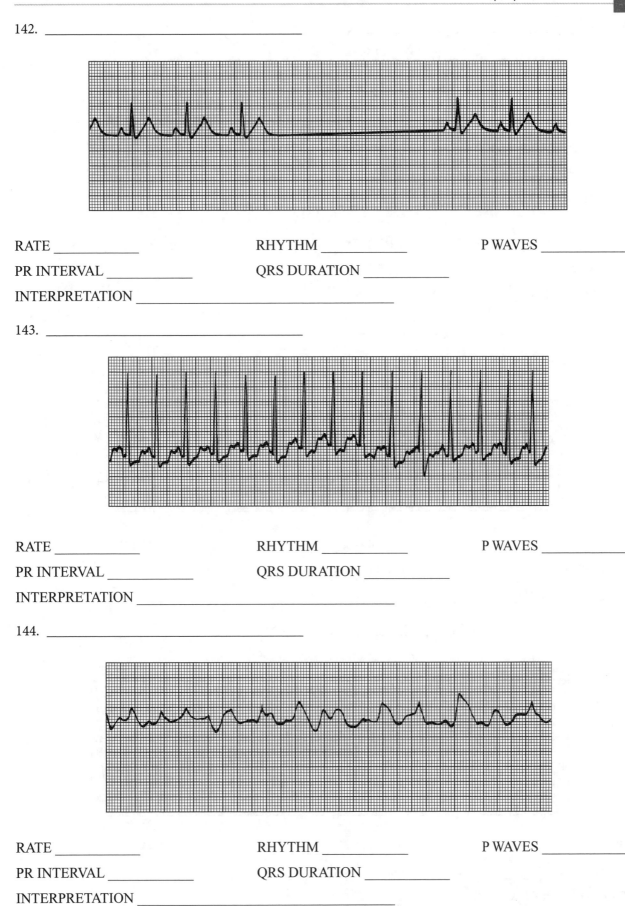

RATE _____ RHYTHM _____ P WAVES _____

PR INTERVAL _____ QRS DURATION _____

INTERPRETATION _____

143. _____

RATE _____ RHYTHM _____ P WAVES _____

PR INTERVAL _____ QRS DURATION _____

INTERPRETATION _____

144. _____

RATE _____ RHYTHM _____ P WAVES _____

PR INTERVAL _____ QRS DURATION _____

INTERPRETATION _____

145. _____

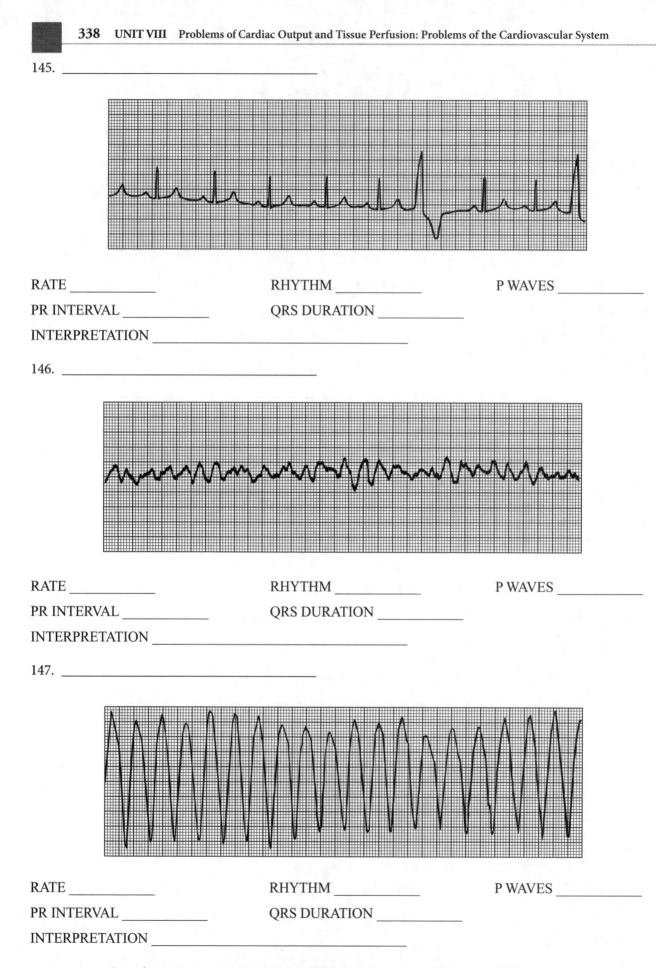

RATE _____   RHYTHM _____   P WAVES _____

PR INTERVAL _____   QRS DURATION _____

INTERPRETATION _____

146. _____

RATE _____   RHYTHM _____   P WAVES _____

PR INTERVAL _____   QRS DURATION _____

INTERPRETATION _____

147. _____

RATE _____   RHYTHM _____   P WAVES _____

PR INTERVAL _____   QRS DURATION _____

INTERPRETATION _____

148. _____

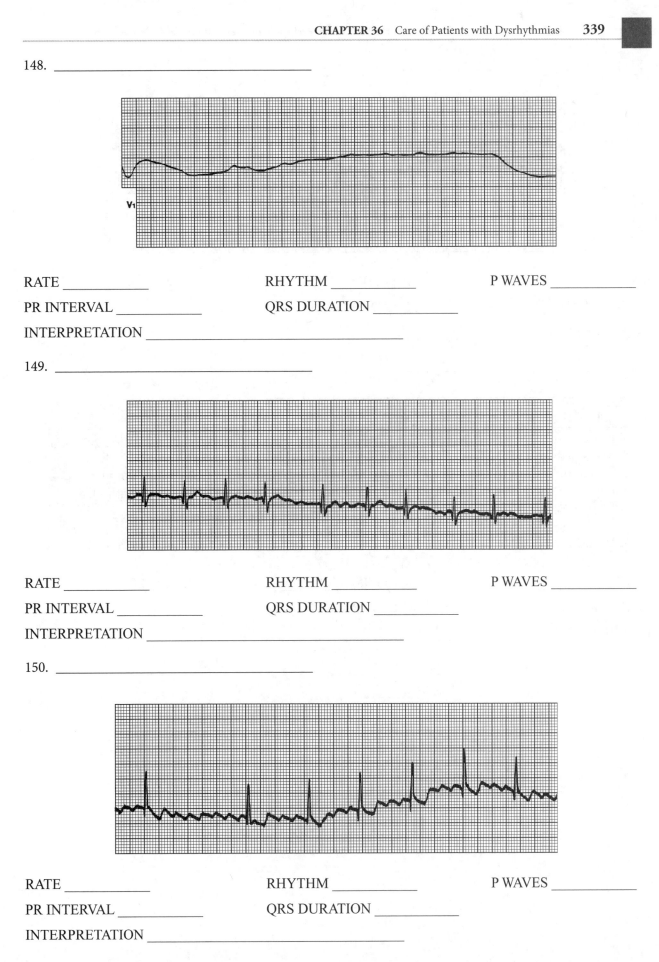

RATE _____ RHYTHM _____ P WAVES _____

PR INTERVAL _____ QRS DURATION _____

INTERPRETATION _____

149. _____

RATE _____ RHYTHM _____ P WAVES _____

PR INTERVAL _____ QRS DURATION _____

INTERPRETATION _____

150. _____

RATE _____ RHYTHM _____ P WAVES _____

PR INTERVAL _____ QRS DURATION _____

INTERPRETATION _____

151. _____

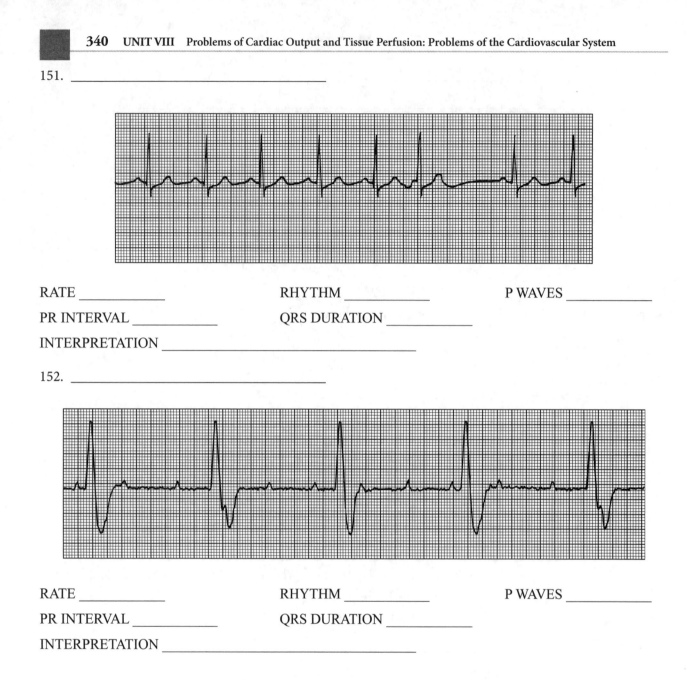

RATE _____   RHYTHM _____   P WAVES _____

PR INTERVAL _____   QRS DURATION _____

INTERPRETATION _____

152. _____

RATE _____   RHYTHM _____   P WAVES _____

PR INTERVAL _____   QRS DURATION _____

INTERPRETATION _____

CASE STUDY: THE PATIENT WITH BRADYCARDIA

Use a separate sheet of paper to answer the questions in this Case Study, or go to the "Prepare for Class" folder on your Evolve website at http://evolve.elsevier.com/Iggy/ to download and complete as a word processing file. Answer guidelines for this Case Study are also available on your Evolve website.

A patient in a critical care unit on telemetry develops the following rhythm: normal P waves at a regular rate of 88 beats per minute. There is a separate ventricular regular rate of 55 with a normal QRS complex.

1. What can be determined about the relationship of the P wave and the QRS complexes?
2. Based on this ECG, what assessment findings might be identified with this dysrhythmia?
3. What would make a difference in the physical findings?
4. What type of heart block has been identified?
5. What interventions are necessary for this patient?
6. Differentiate between invasive and noninvasive temporary pacing. Describe the two types of invasive temporary pacing.
7. Identify the three complications that can occur with noninvasive pacemaker therapy.
8. Briefly describe what the synchronous, or demand, mode means regarding pacemaker therapy.
9. Would the patient have a temporary or permanent pacemaker?
10. What would be included in a teaching plan for a patient with a pacemaker?

CASE STUDY: THE PATIENT WITH A DYSRHYTHMIA (1)

Use a separate sheet of paper to answer the questions in this Case Study, or go to the "Prepare for Class" folder on your Evolve website at http://evolve.elsevier.com/Iggy/ to download and complete as a word processing file. Answer guidelines for this Case Study are also available on your Evolve website.

A 71-year-old man is admitted to the telemetry unit from the ED for treatment and monitoring of atrial fibrillation. The patient was at work when he suddenly experienced palpitations and light-headedness. An ECG revealed he was in rapid atrial fibrillation. The patient's history reveals alcohol intake of 2 to 3 beers per day, coronary artery bypass graft (CABG) 6 months ago, and hypertension.

Further assessment indicates that the patient is alert and oriented to person, place, and time. His Glasgow coma scale rating is 15. He appears anxious and asks how long he will be in the hospital and whether he can call his wife. He has trace edema of the bilateral lower extremities. Pulses are palpated at 2+ radial bilaterally and 1+ pedal bilaterally. Auscultation of heart tones reveals that S_1 and S_2 are irregular. Auscultation of the lungs reveals the upper lobes, anterior and posterior, are clear, and bases of the posterior lobes have fine crackles bilaterally. The patient has a nonproductive cough. The abdomen is soft and nontender to light palpation with bowel sounds auscultated in all four quadrants.

Vital signs are: Temp 36.7° C (98.0° F); heart rate/rhythm 139 to 147/min, rapid atrial fibrillation; respirations 29/min; blood pressure 111/67 mm Hg. Pulse oximetry is 94% on 2 L of oxygen per nasal cannula at rest.

1. Document a nursing note for the patient using the following format:
   - History
   - Cardiac
   - Neurologic
   - Respiratory
   - Abdomen
   - Additional notes
2. What is the initial treatment for this patient?
3. What is a potential risk for this cardiac dysrhythmia? What are the preventive measures?
4. What are additional treatments for this patient if medication does adequately treat this dysrhythmia?

CASE STUDY: THE PATIENT WITH A DYSRHYTHMIA (2)

Use a separate sheet of paper to answer the questions in this Case Study, or go to the "Prepare for Class" folder on your Evolve website at http://evolve.elsevier.com/Iggy/ to download and complete as a word processing file. Answer guidelines for this Case Study are also available on your Evolve website.

A 78-year-old woman is admitted to a telemetry unit directly from her physician's office for evaluation and management of congestive heart failure. She has a history of systemic hypertension and chronic moderate mitral regurgitation. Her medication orders include furosemide (Lasix) 80 mg orally four times a day, digoxin 0.125 mg orally daily, and diltiazem (Cardizem) 60 mg orally three times a day. The initial assessment of the patient reveals a pulse rate that is rapid and very irregular. The patient is restless, her skin is pale and cool, she states she is dizzy when she stands up, and she is slightly short of breath and anxious. Her blood pressure is 106/88 mm Hg. Her ECG monitor pattern shows uncontrolled atrial fibrillation, with a rate ranging from 150 to 170 beats/min. Her oxygen saturation level is 90%.

1. Given the assessment findings, what should the nurse do first?

2. What additional physical assessment techniques would the nurse perform?

3. Because the length of time the patient has been in atrial fibrillation is unknown, what potential complication may occur if cardioversion is attempted?

4. What should be done before elective cardioversion is attempted?

5. Later that evening, the patient calls the nurse because she feels "like something terrible is going to happen." She reports chest pain, has increased shortness of breath, and has coughed up blood-tinged sputum. What should the nurse suspect? What is the first thing the nurse should do, and what further assessments should be performed at this time?

37 CHAPTER

Care of Patients with Cardiac Problems

STUDY/REVIEW QUESTIONS

Matching. Match the terms with their correct definitions.

Terms
a. Right-sided heart (ventricular) failure
b. Left-sided heart (ventricular) failure
c. High-output failure
d. Ejection fraction
e. Pulsus alternans
f. Renin-angiotensin system (RAS)

Definitions

_____ 1. Decreased tissue perfusion from poor cardiac output and pulmonary congestion from increased pressure in the pulmonary vessels

_____ 2. Alternate in strength

_____ 3. Can occur when cardiac output remains normal or above normal

_____ 4. Percentage of blood ejected from the heart during systole

_____ 5. Activated by reduced blood flow to the kidneys

_____ 6. Increased volume and pressure develop and result in peripheral edema

Fill in the blanks.

7. Most heart failure begins with failure of the _____ and progresses to failure of both ventricles.

8. As the ejection fraction decreases, tissue perfusion _____ and blood accumulates in the _____ vessels.

9. B-type natriuretic peptide (BNP) is produced and released by the ventricles when the patient has _____ as a result of heart failure.

10. Cardiac output (CO) is the product of heart rate (HR) and stroke volume (SV), and an increase in HR results in an immediate _____ in cardiac output.

11. The initial compensatory mechanism of the heart that maintains cardiac output is increased _____ _____.

12. The nurse is taking a history on a patient recently diagnosed with heart failure. The patient admits to "sometimes having trouble catching my breath," but is unable to provide more specific details. What question does the nurse ask to gather more data about the patient's symptoms?
    a. "Do you have any medical problems, such as high blood pressure?"
    b. "What did your doctor tell you about your diagnosis?"
    c. "What was your most strenuous activity in the past week?"
    d. "How do you feel about being told that you have heart failure?"

13. The night shift nurse is listening to report and hears that a patient has paroxysmal nocturnal dyspnea. What does the nurse plan to do next?
    a. Instruct the patient to sleep in a side-lying position and then check on the patient every 2 hours to help with switching sides.
    b. Make the patient comfortable in a bedside recliner with several pillows to keep the patient more upright throughout the night.
    c. Check on the patient several hours after bedtime and assist the patient to sit upright and dangle the feet when dyspnea occurs.
    d. Check the patient frequently because the patient has insomnia due to a fear of suffocation.

14. The nurse is assessing a patient with right-sided heart failure. Which assessment findings does the nurse expect to see in this patient? *(Select all that apply.)*
    a. Dependent edema
    b. Weight loss
    c. Polyuria at night
    d. Hypotension
    e. Hepatomegaly
    f. Angina

15. The nurse is assessing a patient with left-sided heart failure. Which assessment findings does the nurse expect to see in this patient? *(Select all that apply.)*
    a. Displacement of the apical impulse to the left
    b. S_3 heart sound
    c. Paroxysmal nocturnal dyspnea
    d. Jugular venous distention
    e. Oliguria during the day
    f. Wheezes or crackles

16. Based on the etiology and the main cause of heart failure, which patient has the greatest need for health promotion measures to prevent heart failure?
    a. Alzheimer's patient
    b. Patient with cystitis
    c. Patient with asthma
    d. Patient with hypertension

17. What is an early sign of left ventricular failure that a patient is most likely to report?
    a. Nocturia
    b. Weight gain
    c. Swollen legs
    d. Nocturnal coughing

18. The nurse is reviewing diagnostic test results for a patient who is hypertensive. Which laboratory result is an early warning sign of decreased heart compliance, and prompts the nurse to immediately notify the health care provider?
    a. Normal B-type natriuretic peptide
    b. Decreased hemoglobin and hematocrit
    c. Elevated thyroxine (T_4)
    d. Presence of microalbuminuria

19. The nurse is interviewing a patient with a history of high blood pressure and heart problems. Which statement by the patient causes the nurse to suspect the patient may have heart failure?
    a. "I noticed a very fine red rash on my chest."
    b. "I had to take off my wedding ring last week."
    c. "I've had fever quite frequently."
    d. "I have pain in my shoulder when I cough."

20. A patient who was admitted for newly diagnosed heart failure is now being discharged. The nurse instructs the patient and family on how to manage heart failure at home. What five major self-management categories should the nurse include?

    a. _____

    b. _____

    c. _____

    d. _____

    e. _____

21. List one teaching component for each of the self-management categories you identified in the previous question.

    a. _____
       _____
       _____

    b. _____
       _____
       _____

    c. _____
       _____
       _____
       _____

    d. _____
       _____
       _____

    e. _____
       _____
       _____

22. A patient's bilateral radial pulses are occasionally weak and irregular. Which assessment technique does the nurse use first to investigate this finding?
    a. Check the color and the capillary refill in the upper extremities.
    b. Check the peripheral pulses in the lower extremities.
    c. Take the apical pulse for 1 minute, noting any irregularity in heart rhythm.
    d. Check the cardiac monitor for irregularities in rhythm.

23. A patient is at risk for heart failure, but currently has no official medical diagnosis. While assessing the patient's lungs, the nurse hears fine profuse crackles. What does the nurse do next?
    a. Report the finding to the health care provider.
    b. Document the finding as a baseline for later comparison.
    c. Give the patient low-flow supplemental oxygen.
    d. Ask the patient to cough and reauscultate the lungs.

24. A patient is admitted for heart failure and has edema, neck vein distention, and ascites. What is the most reliable way to monitor fluid gain or loss in this patient?
    a. Check for pitting edema in the dependent body parts.
    b. Auscultate the lungs for crackles or wheezing.
    c. Assess skin turgor and the condition of mucous membranes.
    d. Weigh the patient daily at the same time with the same scale.

25. The home health nurse is evaluating a patient being treated for heart failure. Which statement by the patient is the best indicator of hope and well-being as a desired psychological outcome?
    a. "I'm taking the medication and following the doctor's orders."
    b. "I'm looking forward to dancing with my wife on our wedding anniversary."
    c. "I'm planning to go on a long trip; I'll never go back to the hospital again."
    d. "I want to thank you for all that you have done. I know you did your best."

26. The nurse is reviewing the laboratory results for a patient whose chief complaint is dyspnea. Which diagnostic test best differentiates between heart failure and lung dysfunction?
    a. Arterial blood gas
    b. B-type natriuretic peptide
    c. Hemoglobin and hematocrit
    d. Serum electrolytes

27. The nursing student is assisting in the care of a patient with advanced right-sided heart failure. In addition to bringing a stethoscope, what additional piece of equipment does the student bring in order to assess this patient?
    a. Tape measure
    b. Glasgow Coma Scale
    c. Portable Doppler
    d. Bladder ultrasound scanner

28. Which test is the best tool for diagnosing heart failure?
    a. Echocardiography
    b. Pulmonary artery catheter
    c. Radionuclide studies
    d. Multigated angiographic (MUGA) scan

29. A patient with heart failure has inadequate tissue perfusion. Which nursing interventions are included in the plan of care for this patient? *(Select all that apply.)*
    a. Monitor respiratory rate, rhythm, and quality every 1 to 4 hours.
    b. Auscultate breath sounds every 4 to 8 hours.
    c. Provide supplemental oxygen to maintain oxygen saturation at 90% or greater.
    d. Place the patient in a supine position with pillows under each leg.
    e. Assist the patient in performing coughing and deep-breathing exercises every 2 hours.

30. Which interventions are effective for a patient with a potential for pulmonary edema caused by heart failure? *(Select all that apply.)*
    a. Sodium and fluid restriction
    b. Slow infusion of hypotonic saline
    c. Administration of potassium
    d. Administration of loop diuretics
    e. Position in semi-Fowler's to high-Fowler's position
    f. Weekly weight monitoring

31. An older adult patient with heart failure is volume depleted and has a low sodium level. The health care provider has ordered valsartan (Diovan), an angiotensin-receptor blocker (ARB). After the initial dose, what does the nurse carefully monitor this patient for?
    a. Hypotension
    b. Cough
    c. Fluid retention
    d. Chest pain

32. The health care provider has ordered an ARB for a patient with heart failure. The parameters are to maintain a systolic blood pressure ranging from 90 to 110 mm Hg. Today the patient has a blood pressure of 110/80 mm Hg, but shows acute confusion. What is the nurse's priority action?
    a. Give the medication because blood pressure is within the parameters.
    b. Call the health care provider about the new onset of confusion.
    c. Hold the medication and document the new findings.
    d. Assess the patient for other symptoms of decreased tissue perfusion.

33. A patient with heart failure has excessive aldosterone secretion and is therefore experiencing thirst and continuously asking for water. What does the nurse instruct the unlicensed assistive personnel (UAP) to do?
    a. Severely restrict fluid to 500 mL plus output from the previous 24 hours.
    b. Give the patient as much water as desired to prevent dehydration.
    c. Restrict fluid to a normal 2 L daily, with accurate intake and output.
    d. Frequently offer the patient ice chips and moistened toothettes.

34. A patient is prescribed diuretics for treatment of heart failure. Because of this therapy, the nurse pays particular attention to which laboratory test level?
    a. Peak and trough of medication
    b. Serum potassium
    c. Serum sodium
    d. PT and PTT

35. An older adult patient is taking digoxin for treatment of heart failure. What is the priority nursing action for this patient related to the medication therapy?
    a. Give the medication in conjunction with an antacid.
    b. Keep the patient on the cardiac monitor and observe for ventricular dysrhythmias.
    c. Check that the dose is in the lowest possible range for therapeutic effect.
    d. Advise the patient that there is increased mortality related to toxicity.

36. A patient is receiving digoxin therapy for heart failure. What assessment does the nurse perform before administering the medication?
    a. Auscultate the apical pulse rate and heart rhythm.
    b. Assess for nausea and abdominal distention.
    c. Auscultate the lungs for crackles.
    d. Check for increased urine output.

37. The nurse is reviewing the ECG of a patient on digoxin therapy. What early sign of digitalis toxicity does the nurse look for?
    a. Tachycardia
    b. Peaked T wave
    c. Atrial fibrillation
    d. Loss of P wave

38. Which laboratory test monitors for potential cardiac problems and digoxin toxicity?
    a. Complete blood count
    b. BUN and creatinine level
    c. Serum potassium level
    d. Prothrombin time and INR

39. A patient is receiving an infusion of nesiritide (Natrecor) for treatment of heart failure. What is the priority nursing assessment while administering this medication?
    a. Monitor for hypotension.
    b. Assess for cardiac dysrhythmias.
    c. Observe for respiratory depression.
    d. Monitor for peripheral vasoconstriction.

40. A patient has recently been diagnosed with acute heart failure. Which medication order does the nurse question?
    a. Dobutamine (Dobutrex), a beta-adrenergic agonist
    b. Milrinone (Primacor), a phosphodiesterase inhibitor
    c. Levosimendan (Simdax), a positive inotropic
    d. Carvedilol (Coreg), a beta blocker

41. A patient has an ejection fraction of less than 30%. The nurse prepares to provide patient education about which potential treatment?
    a. Automatic implantable cardio-defibrillator
    b. Heart transplant
    c. Mechanical implanted pump
    d. Ventricular reconstructive procedures

42. The nurse identifies a priority problem of fatigue and weakness for the patient with heart failure. After ambulating 200 feet down the hall, the patient's blood pressure change is more than 20 mm Hg. How does the nurse interpret this data?
    a. The patient is building endurance.
    b. The activity is too stressful.
    c. The patient could walk farther.
    d. The activity is appropriate.

43. A patient with heart failure is anxious to recover quickly. After ambulating with the UAP, the nurse observes that the patient has dyspnea. The nurse asks the patient to rate her exertion on a scale of 1 to 20 and the patient says, "I can keep going. It's only about a 15." What is the nurse's best response?
    a. "Slow down a bit; ideally you should be less than 12."
    b. "As long as you are less than 18, you can keep going."
    c. "Stop right now; you should not tax your heart beyond 5."
    d. "You should go slower; you cannot reach level 0 in one day."

44. Why does the nurse document the precise location of crackles auscultated in the lungs of a patient with heart failure?
    a. Crackles will eventually change to wheezes as the pulmonary edema worsens.
    b. The level of the fluid spreads laterally as the pulmonary edema worsens.
    c. The level of the fluid ascends as the pulmonary edema worsens.
    d. Crackles will eventually diminish as the pulmonary edema worsens.

45. A patient comes to the ED extremely anxious, tachycardic, and struggling for air with a moist cough productive of frothy, blood-tinged sputum. What is the priority nursing intervention?
    a. Apply a pulse oximeter and cardiac monitor.
    b. Administer high-flow oxygen therapy via facemask.
    c. Prepare for continuous positive airway pressure ventilation.
    d. Prepare for intubation and mechanical ventilation.

46. A patient is treated for acute pulmonary edema. Which medications does the nurse prepare to administer to this patient? *(Select all that apply.)*
    a. Sublingual nitroglycerin
    b. IV Lasix
    c. IV morphine sulfate
    d. IV beta blocker
    e. IV nitroglycerin

47. What is the expected outcome for the collaborative problem *potential for pulmonary edema*?
    a. No dysrhythmias
    b. Clear lung sounds
    c. Less fatigue
    d. No disorientation

48. The nurse is teaching a patient with heart failure about signs and symptoms that suggest a return or worsening of heart failure. What does the nurse include in the teaching? *(Select all that apply.)*
    a. Rapid weight loss of 3 lbs in a week
    b. Increase in exercise tolerance lasting 2 to 3 days
    c. Cold symptoms (cough) lasting more than 3 to 5 days
    d. Excessive awakening at night to urinate
    e. Development of dyspnea or angina at rest or worsening angina
    f. Increased swelling in the feet, ankles, or hands

49. A patient is prescribed bumetanide (Bumex). What is an important teaching point for the nurse to include about this medication?
    a. Caution to move slowly when changing positions, especially from lying to sitting
    b. Information about potassium-rich foods to include in the diet
    c. Written instructions on how to count the radial pulse rate
    d. Information about low-sodium diets and reading food labels for sodium content

50. The nurse is teaching a patient about the treatment regimen for heart failure. Which statement by the patient indicates a need for further instruction?
    a. "I must weigh myself once a month and watch for fluid retention."
    b. "If my heart feels like it is racing, I should call the doctor."
    c. "I'll need to consider my activities for the day and rest as needed."
    d. "I'll need periods of rest and activity, and I should avoid activity after meals."

Matching. Match the types of valvular disease with their characteristics. Answers may be used more than once.

Types of Valvular Disease
a.   Mitral valve stenosis
b.   Mitral valve insufficiency
c.   Mitral valve prolapse
d.   Aortic stenosis
e.   Aortic insufficiency

Characteristics
_____ 51.   Usually coexists with some degree of mitral stenosis
_____ 52.   Classic signs of dyspnea, angina, and syncope
_____ 53.   Hepatomegaly is a late sign
_____ 54.   A high-pitched, blowing decrescendo diastolic murmur
_____ 55.   Irregular rhythm; atrial fibrillation can cause emboli
_____ 56.   Most patients are asymptomatic
_____ 57.   Right-side heart failure; later cardiac output fails
_____ 58.   The patient may experience palpitations while lying on left side
_____ 59.   Symptom-free for decades, later related to left ventricle failure
_____ 60.   Rumbling apical diastolic murmur
_____ 61.   Right-sided failure results in neck vein distention
_____ 62.   Leaflets enlarge and fall back into left atrium during systole
_____ 63.   Normal heart rate and blood pressure
_____ 64.   Becoming a disorder of aging populations
_____ 65.   Murmur, systolic crescendo-decrescendo
_____ 66. S_3 often present due to severe regurgitation

67.   A patient is diagnosed with moderate mitral valve stenosis. Which findings is the nurse most likely to encounter during the physical assessment of this patient? *(Select all that apply.)*
a.   Dyspnea on exertion
b.   Orthopnea
c.   Palpitations
d.   Asymptomatic
e.   Neck vein distention

68.   The nurse hears in report that a patient has been diagnosed with mitral insufficiency. Which early symptom is most likely to be first reported by the patient?
a.   Atypical chest pain
b.   Chronic weakness
c.   Anxiety
d.   Dyspnea

69.   A patient is diagnosed with mitral valve stenosis. Which finding warrants immediate notification of the health care provider because of potential for decompensation?
a.   Irregularly irregular heart rhythm signifying atrial fibrillation
b.   Slow, bounding peripheral pulses associated with bradycardia
c.   An increase and decrease in pulse rate that follows inspiration and expiration
d.   An increase in pulse rate and blood pressure after exertion

70.   The nurse is assessing the pulses of a patient with valvular disease and finds "bounding" arterial pulses. What is this finding most characteristic of?
a.   Aortic regurgitation
b.   Aortic stenosis
c.   Mitral valve prolapse
d.   Mitral insufficiency

71. A patient with a history of valvular heart disease requires a routine colonoscopy. The nurse notifies the health care provider to obtain a patient prescription for which type of medication?
    a. Anticoagulants
    b. Antihypertensives
    c. Antibiotics
    d. Antianginals

72. What is the most common preventable cause of valvular heart disease?
    a. Congenital disease or malformation
    b. Calcium deposits and thrombus formation
    c. Beta-hemolytic streptococcal infection
    d. Hypertension or Marfan syndrome

73. The nurse is assessing a patient at risk for valvular disease and finds pitting edema. This finding is a sign for which type of valvular disease?
    a. Mitral valve stenosis and insufficiency
    b. Aortic valve stenosis and insufficiency
    c. Tricuspid valve prolapse
    d. Mitral valve prolapse

74. The health care provider recommends to a patient that diagnostic testing be performed to assess for valvular heart disease. The nurse teaches the patient about which test that is commonly used for this purpose?
    a. Echocardiography
    b. Electrocardiography
    c. Exercise testing
    d. Thallium scanning

75. Long-term anticoagulant therapy for a patient with valvular heart disease and chronic atrial fibrillation includes which drug?
    a. Heparin sodium
    b. Warfarin sodium (Coumadin)
    c. Diltiazem (Cardizem)
    d. Enoxaparin (Lovenox)

76. The surgical noninvasive intervention of a balloon valvuloplasty is often used for which type of patient?
    a. Young adults with a genetic valve defect
    b. Older adults who are nonsurgical candidates
    c. Adults whose open-heart surgery failed
    d. Older adults who need replacement valves

77. The nurse is caring for a patient who had a valvuloplasty. The nurse monitors for which common complication in the postprocedural period?
    a. Myocardial infarction
    b. Angina
    c. Bleeding and emboli
    d. Infection

78. A patient with a prosthetic valve replacement must understand that postoperative care will include lifelong therapy with which type of medication?
    a. Antibiotics
    b. Anticoagulants
    c. Immunosuppressants
    d. Pain medication

79. A patient is a candidate for a xenograft valve. The nurse emphasizes that this type of valve does not require anticoagulant therapy, but will require which intervention?
    a. Replacement in about 7 to 10 years
    b. An exercise program to develop collateral circulation
    c. Daily temperature checks to watch for signs of rejection
    d. Frequent monitoring for pulmonary edema

80. A patient is scheduled for valve surgery. Which medication does the nurse advise the patient to discontinue for several days before the procedure?
    a. Antihypertensives
    b. Diuretics
    c. Anticoagulants
    d. Antibiotics

81. What is the most common problem for the patient with valvular heart disease?
    a. Reduced cardiac output
    b. Difficulty coping
    c. Shortness of breath
    d. Altered body image

82. The nurse is giving discharge instructions to a patient who had valve surgery. Which home care instructions does the nurse include in the teaching plan? *(Select all that apply.)*
    a. Increase consumption of foods high in vitamin K.
    b. Use an electric razor to avoid skin cuts.
    c. Report any bleeding or excessive bruising.
    d. Avoid invasive dental procedures unless absolutely necessary.
    e. Watch for and report any fever, drainage, or redness at the site.
    f. Avoid heavy lifting for 3 to 6 months.
    g. Report dyspnea, syncope, dizziness, edema, and palpitations.
    h. Avoid any procedure using magnetic resonance if a prosthetic valve was used.

Matching. Match each description to its corresponding key feature/finding of cardiac disease.

Key Features/Findings
a. Percardial friction rub
b. Splinter hemorrhages
c. Petechiae
d. Systemic emboli
e. Pulsus paradoxus
f. Aschoff bodies
g. Cardiac tamponade

Descriptions
_____ 83. Vegetation fragments in circulation resulting in a cerebrovascular accident (CVA) or transient ischemic attack (TIA)
_____ 84. Red, flat pinpoint spots/lesions in mucous membrane and conjunctivae
_____ 85. Small red streaks or black longitudinal lines of nail beds
_____ 86. Having a systolic blood pressure higher on expiration than on inspiration
_____ 87. Scratchy, high-pitched sound heard at left lower sternal border
_____ 88. Small nodules on myocardium replaced by scar tissue
_____ 89. Excess fluid in the pericardial cavity

Matching. Match each assessment finding with its corresponding inflammatory cardiac disease. Answers will be used more than once.

Inflammatory Cardiac Disease
a. Endocarditis
b. Pericarditis
c. Rheumatic carditis

Assessment Finding
_____ 90. Grating pain that is aggravated by breathing
_____ 91. A new, regurgitant murmur
_____ 92. Janeway's lesions
_____ 93. Streptococcal infection
_____ 94. Osler's nodes
_____ 95. Scratchy, high-pitched sound heard on auscultation over left lower sternal border
_____ 96. Petechiae
_____ 97. Aschoff's bodies

98. Which patients are at greatest risk of developing infective endocarditis? *(Select all that apply.)*
    a. IV drug user
    b. Patient with pancreatitis
    c. Patient with a myocardial infarction
    d. Patient with a prosthetic mitral valve replacement, postoperative
    e. Patient with mitral stenosis who recently had an abscessed tooth removed
    f. Older adult patient with urinary tract infection and valve damage
    g. Patient with cardiac dysrhythmias

99. A patient with aortic valve endocarditis reports fatigue and shortness of breath. Crackles are heard on lung auscultation. What do these assessment findings likely indicate?
    a. Emboli to the lung
    b. Valve incompetence resulting in heart failure
    c. Valve stenosis resulting in increased chamber size
    d. Coronary artery disease

100. A patient is admitted for possible infective endocarditis. Which test does the nurse anticipate will be performed to confirm a positive diagnosis?
    a. CT scan
    b. MRI
    c. Blood cultures
    d. Echocardiogram

101. A patient is diagnosed with new-onset infective endocarditis. Which recent procedure is the patient most likely to report?
    a. Teeth cleaning
    b. Urinary bladder catheterization
    c. Chest radiography
    d. ECG

102. In what way does arterial embolization to the brain manifest itself in a patient with infective endocarditis?
    a. Dysarthria
    b. Dysphagia
    c. Atelectasis
    d. Electrolyte imbalances

103. Which treatment intervention applies to a patient with infective endocarditis?
    a. Administration of oral penicillin for 6 weeks or more
    b. Hospitalization for initial IV antibiotics, possibly with a central line
    c. Complete bedrest for the duration of treatment
    d. Long-term anticoagulation therapy with heparin

104. What is the definitive treatment for a patient with chronic constrictive pericarditis?
    a. Antibiotic therapy
    b. Surgical excision of the pericardium
    c. Administration of beta blockers and corticosteroids
    d. Pericardiocentesis

105. Dressler's syndrome can occur after a myocardial infarction. The syndrome is characterized by which symptoms? *(Select all that apply.)*
    a. Fever
    b. Productive cough
    c. Pericarditis
    d. Epigastric pain
    e. Pleural effusions

106. A patient is admitted to the unit with assessment findings that include substernal pain that radiates to the left shoulder. The pain is described by the patient to be grating, and is worse with inspiration and coughing. What likely is the cause of this patient's symptoms?
    a. Chronic constrictive pericarditis
    b. Cardiac tamponade
    c. Hypertrophic cardiomyopathy
    d. Acute pericarditis

107. Which signs/symptoms occur with chronic constrictive pericarditis? *(Select all that apply.)*
    a. Pericardium becomes rigid
    b. Heart valves stiffen
    c. Ventricles inadequately fill
    d. Signs of left-sided heart failure appear
    e. Heart failure eventually occurs

108. A patient with pericarditis develops a pericardial effusion. This can result in another complication called _____ _____.

109. The nurse is assessing a patient with pericarditis. In order to hear a pericardial friction rub, which technique does the nurse use?
    a. Place the diaphragm at the apex of the heart.
    b. Place the diaphragm at the left lower sternal border.
    c. Place the bell just below the left clavicle.
    d. Place the bell at several points while the patient holds his or her breath.

110. A patient is admitted for pericarditis. In order to assist the patient to feel more comfortable, what does the nurse instruct the patient to do?
    a. Sit in a semi-Fowler's position with pillows under the arms.
    b. Lie on the side in a fetal position.
    c. Sit up and lean forward.
    d. Lie down and bend the legs at the knees.

111. The nurse is reviewing the ECG of a patient admitted for acute pericarditis. Which ECG change does the nurse anticipate?
    a. Normal ECG
    b. ST-T spiking
    c. Peaked T waves
    d. Wide QRS complexes

112. A patient is admitted for pericarditis. How will the patient likely describe his pain?
    a. Grating substernal pain that is aggravated by inspiration.
    b. Sharp pain that radiates down the left arm.
    c. Dull ache that feels vaguely like indigestion.
    d. Continuous boring pain that is relieved with rest.

113. Which patient is at greatest risk for developing viral pericarditis?
    a. 35-year-old woman with tuberculosis
    b. 45-year-old man who has had radiation therapy for lung cancer
    c. 30-year-old man with a respiratory infection
    d. 50-year-old woman with chest trauma

114. What is the common treatment for rheumatic carditis?
    a. Pericardiocentesis
    b. Antibiotics for 10 days
    c. Pain medication for substernal pain control
    d. Rest with observation for further necessary treatment

115. Which medication is used to treat rheumatic carditis?
    a. Antibiotic (penicillin)
    b. NSAIDs
    c. Pain medications (opioids)
    d. Steroids

116. Assessment findings for a patient with acute pericarditis indicate neck vein distention, clear lungs, muffled heart sounds, tachycardia, tachypnea, and a greater than 10 mm Hg difference in systolic pressure on inspiration than on expiration. What is the nurse's first response to these assessment findings?
    a. Continue to monitor the patient; these are normal signs of pericarditis.
    b. Administer oxygen and immediately report the findings to the health care provider.
    c. Monitor oxygen saturation and seek order for pain medication to control symptoms.
    d. Check ECG, administer morphine for pain, and administer diuretics.

117. A patient had an emergency pericardiocentesis for cardiac tamponade. Which nursing interventions are included in the postprocedural care for this patient? *(Select all that apply.)*
    a. Closely monitor for the recurrence of tamponade.
    b. Be prepared to provide adequate fluid volumes to increase cardiac output.
    c. Be prepared to assist in emergency sternotomy if tamponade recurs.
    d. Administer diuretics to decrease fluid volumes around the heart.
    e. Send the pericardial effusion specimen to the laboratory for culture.

118. Which is a characteristic of dilated cardiomyopathy (DCM)?
    a. Results from replacement of myocardial tissue with fibrous tissue
    b. Causes stiff ventricles that restrict filling during diastole
    c. Causes symptoms of left ventricular failure
    d. Causes a stiff left ventricle

119. Which type of cardiomyopathy results from replacement of myocardial tissue with fibrous and fatty tissue?
    a. Hypertrophic cardiomyopathy
    b. Arrhythmogenic right ventricular cardiomyopathy
    c. Dilated cardiomyopathy
    d. Restrictive cardiomyopathy

120. A patient may die without any symptoms of which type of cardiomyopathy?
    a. Dilated cardiomyopathy
    b. Arrhythmogenic right ventricular cardiomyopathy
    c. Restrictive cardiomyopathy
    d. Hypertrophic cardiomyopathy

121. The cause of dilated cardiomyopathy may include which factors? *(Select all that apply.)*
    a. Alcohol abuse
    b. Sedentary lifestyle
    c. Infection
    d. Chemotherapy
    e. Poor nutrition

122. Which descriptions accurately characterize restrictive cardiomyopathy? *(Select all that apply.)*
    a. Prognosis is poor.
    b. Symptoms are similar to left or right heart failure.
    c. Some patients die without any symptoms.
    d. It is the most common type of cardiomyopathy.
    e. It is the rarest of cardiomyopathies.

123. A patient who reports having a sore throat 2 weeks ago now reports chest pain. On physical assessment, the nurse hears a new murmur, pericardial friction rub, and tachycardia. ECG shows a prolonged P-R interval. What condition does the nurse suspect in this patient?
    a. Rheumatic carditis
    b. Heart failure
    c. Cardiomyopathy
    d. Aortic stenosis

124. A patient has received a heart transplant for dilated cardiomyopathy. Because the patient has a high risk for cardiac tamponade, of which sign/symptoms does the nurse immediately notify the provider?
    a. Crackles and wheezes of the lungs
    b. Pulsus paradoxus and muffled heart sounds
    c. Hepatomegaly and ascites
    d. Dependent edema and fluid retention

125. The nurse is assessing a patient who has received a heart transplant. Which clinical manifestations suggest transplant rejection? *(Select all that apply.)*
    a. Shortness of breath
    b. Depression
    c. Fluid loss or dehydration
    d. Severe abdominal pain
    e. New bradycardia
    f. Hypotension
    g. Decreased ejection fraction

CASE STUDY: THE PATIENT WITH AORTIC STENOSIS

Use a separate sheet of paper to answer the questions in this Case Study, or go to the "Prepare for Class" folder on your Evolve website at http://evolve.elsevier.com/Iggy/ to download and complete as a word processing file. Answer guidelines for this Case Study are also available on your Evolve website.

A 49-year-old woman is admitted to the hospital for a report of syncope and dyspnea on exertion. The patient states that after she ambulates 20 to 30 feet she has difficulty breathing and stops to rest for 1 to 2 minutes. In the past month the patient reports experiencing marked fatigue with her daily routine.

Assessment reveals 2+ edema of the bilateral lower extremities. Radial pulses are 2+ bilaterally and pedal pulses are 1+ bilaterally. Capillary refill of the fingernail beds is less than 3 seconds. Auscultation of heart sounds reveals a systolic murmur. Her abdomen is soft and nontender with bowel sounds auscultated in all four abdominal quadrants. The skin is warm, dry, and intact. The patient is alert and oriented to person, place, and time.

Auscultation of the lungs is clear in the upper lobes anteriorly and the posteriorly with fine crackles in the anterior and the posterior bases. It is noted that the patient has a dry, nonproductive cough. At night the patient says she sleeps in a recliner and has been doing this for several months.

A history of the patient includes endocarditis 10 years ago that was treated with antibiotics. Vital signs are: temp 37.1° C (98.7° F); heart rate/rhythm 72/min and sinus rhythm with first degree A-V block; respirations 22/min; pulse oximeter reading 92% on room air at rest.

The physician has confirmed the diagnosis of aortic stenosis from the following procedures:
- Echocardiography
- Transesophageal echocardiography (TEE)
- ECG
- Stress echocardiography

    1. Of the following, what are the top three patient problems in this case study?
        - Inadequate oxygenation related to cardiac problem
        - Decreased Cardiac Output
        - Fatigue and weakness related to cardiac problem
        - Insufficient knowledge related to the new diagnosis
        - Possible risk of neurologic problems
    2. Document a chart note based on the priority patient problems from the previous question. Include any Additional Notes pertinent to documentation.

CASE STUDY: THE PATIENT WITH HEART FAILURE

Use a separate sheet of paper to answer the questions in this Case Study, or go to the "Prepare for Class" folder on your Evolve website at http://evolve.elsevier.com/Iggy/ to download and complete as a word processing file. Answer guidelines for this Case Study are also available on your Evolve website.

A 74-year-old woman is admitted to the hospital with heart failure. She had been growing progressively weaker and had ankle edema, dyspnea on exertion, and three-pillow orthopnea. On admission, she is severely dyspneic and can answer questions only with one-word phrases. She is diaphoretic, with a heart rate of 132 beats/min, and blood pressure 98/70 mm Hg. She is extremely anxious.

1. Because this patient cannot breathe or talk easily, prioritize the immediate nursing assessments upon admission.

2. Considering the process of congestive heart failure, explain the symptoms she is having.

3. Based on assessment, identify the priority problems for this patient.

The physician orders a treatment plan for this patient: Start an IV, then give dobutamine 3 mg/kg/hr IV; furosemide (Lasix) 40 mg IV stat; digoxin 0.5 mg orally stat, then 0.125 every 6 hours for three doses, with ECG before doses 3 and 4; morphine 2 mg IV stat and then 2 mg IV every 1 to 2 hours PRN; oxygen 4 L/min per nasal cannula; schedule for an echocardiogram; no added salt diet; weigh daily and monitor input and output.

4. Explain the rationale for these medications and treatments.

5. What should the nurse include in the discharge instructions for self-care for patients with heart failure? What will the nurse teach about the digoxin therapy?

6. The home health nurse is making an initial visit to the patient. What would the nurse include in the home care assessment?

Care of Patients with Vascular Problems

STUDY/REVIEW QUESTIONS

True or False? *Read each statement and write T for true or F for false in the blanks provided. If the statement is false, correct the statement to make it true.*

_____ 1. Atherosclerosis progresses for years before clinical manifestations are evident.

_____ 2. An example of a step one diet is 630 calories a day of fat in a 2100 calorie/ day diet.

_____ 3. Patients with low-density lipoprotein (LDL) values of 130 to 159 are advised to follow a fat-modified diet.

_____ 4. Generally, medications for hyperlipidemia should be taken with meals.

5. Atherosclerosis affects which larger arteries? *(Select all that apply.)*
    a. Renal
    b. Femoral
    c. Coronary
    d. Brachial cephalic
    e. Aorta

6. An African-American man is being seen for a right toe blister. He has a 20-year history of insulin-dependent diabetes mellitus, and states that both his biological parents have diabetes mellitus. He is 35 lbs overweight and reports he is sedentary in his work and home life. What factors increase this patient's risk for developing atherosclerosis?

7. Which factors can increase systemic arterial pressure? *(Select all that apply.)*
    a. Decreased cardiac output
    b. Increased heart rate
    c. Increased peripheral vascular resistance
    d. Increased stroke volume
    e. Decreased blood pressure

8. The effects of hyperglycemia in diabetes can result in which conditions? *(Select all that apply.)*
    a. Intimal arterial damage
    b. Severe atherosclerosis
    c. Decreased cardiac output
    d. Premature atherosclerosis
    e. Decreased total peripheral vascular resistance

9. A patient is admitted with a vascular problem. Based on the pathophysiology of systemic arterial pressure, what is the systemic arterial pressure a product of? *(Select all that apply.)*
    a. Cardiac output
    b. Peripheral vascular volume
    c. Preload
    d. Peripheral vascular resistance

10. A patient's cholesterol screening shows a high-density lipoprotein (HDL) value greater than 40, and a total serum cholesterol level of 188. The patient has no other cardiac or vascular risk factors. What does the nurse advise the patient to do?
    a. Modify the diet to exclude fats and increase fiber, then repeat tests.
    b. Contact the physician for a prescription of antilipemic medication.
    c. Repeat total and HDL cholesterol testing in 6 to 12 weeks.
    d. Repeat total and HDL cholesterol testing during the next routine exam.

11. The nurse is counseling a group of women about triglyceride levels. For women, what is a normal triglyceride level?
    a. Over 150 mg/dL
    b. Under 135 mg/dL
    c. Over 100 mg/dL
    d. Under 70 mg/dL

12. A patient has an elevated homocysteine level. Potentially, this may be lowered by what type of nutritional modification?
    a. Including enriched cereals that contain folic acid, vitamin B_6, and vitamin B_{12}
    b. A total fat intake of less than 30% of total calories
    c. Up to 10% of total calories from polyunsaturated fat
    d. Increasing fiber up to 25 to 35 g in the daily diet

13. The nurse is conducting dietary teaching with a patient. Which statement by the patient indicates an understanding of fat sources and the need to limit saturated fats?
    a. "Coconut oil has a rich flavor and is a good cooking oil."
    b. "Sunflower oil is high in saturated fats, so I should avoid it."
    c. "Meat and eggs mostly contain unsaturated fats."
    d. "Canola oil has monounsaturated fat and is recommended."

14. The nurse educates and advises a patient to follow the National Cholesterol Education Program (NCEP) Therapeutic Lifestyle Changes (TLC) diet. Which instruction does the nurse give to the patient?
    a. Review the literature and see what aspects of the program fit into the patient's current lifestyle.
    b. Return for serum cholesterol levels at 6 and 12 weeks after starting the diet.
    c. Record dietary intake and weight for 12 weeks and then call the physician.
    d. Weigh self once a week for 6 weeks and consult the physician if not losing weight.

15. A patient is prescribed atorvastatin (Lipitor). The nurse instructs the patient to watch for and report which side effect?
    a. Nausea and vomiting
    b. Cough
    c. Headaches
    d. Muscle cramps

16. A patient gets a new prescription for Pravigard for treatment of high cholesterol. Because this is a combination drug, the nurse alerts the physician when the patient discloses an allergy to which drug?
    a. Sulfa
    b. Aspirin
    c. Some calcium channel blockers
    d. Some diuretics

17. A patient is prescribed niacin (Niaspan) to lower low-density lipoprotein cholesterol (LDL-C) and very-low-density lipoprotein (VLDL). Why are lower doses prescribed to the patient?
    a. To prevent an elevation of hepatic enzymes
    b. To prevent muscle myopathies
    c. To prevent elevation of blood pressure
    d. To prevent undesirable hypokalemia

18. The nurse is conducting an initial cardiac-vascular assessment on a middle-aged patient. What techniques does the nurse include in the assessment? *(Select all that apply.)*
    a. Take blood pressure on the dominant arm.
    b. Palpate pulses at all of the major sites.
    c. Palpate for temperature differences in the lower extremities.
    d. Perform bilateral but separate palpation on the carotid arteries.
    e. Auscultate for bruits in the radial and brachial arteries.

19. The nurse is performing blood pressure screening at a community center. Which patients are referred for evaluation of their blood pressure? *(Select all that apply.)*
    a. Diabetic patient with a blood pressure of 118/78 mm Hg
    b. Patient with heart disease with a blood pressure of 134/90 mm Hg
    c. Patient with no known health problems who has a blood pressure of 125/86 mm Hg
    d. Diabetic patient with a blood pressure of 180/80 mm Hg
    e. Patient with no known health problems who has a blood pressure of 106/70 mm Hg

20. The home health nurse is making the initial visit to an older adult patient with hypertension. The nurse recommends that the patient obtain which item for home use?
    a. Ambulatory blood pressure monitoring device
    b. Exercise bicycle
    c. Blood glucose monitor scale
    d. Food scale

21. The nurse is evaluating the blood pressure of a 75-year-old woman. Based on current research, which finding is the better indicator of heart disease risk for this patient?
    a. Diastolic of 86 mm Hg
    b. Systolic of 160 mm Hg
    c. Blood pressure of 138/68 mm Hg
    d. Blood pressure of 110/90 mm Hg

22. A 32-year-old patient with diabetes reports sudden onset of headaches, blurred vision, and dyspnea. The patient's blood pressure is normally 120/80 mm Hg, but today is 200/130 mm Hg. What condition does the nurse suspect?
    a. Sustained hypertension
    b. Malignant hypertension
    c. Primary hypertension
    d. Secondary hypertension

23. Which are risk factors for hypertension? *(Select all that apply.)*
    a. Age greater than 40 years
    b. Family history of hypertension
    c. Excessive calorie consumption
    d. Physical inactivity
    e. Excessive alcohol intake
    f. Hypolipidemia
    g. High intake of salt or caffeine
    h. Increased intake of potassium, calcium, or magnesium

24. A patient's blood pressure reading is 128/80 mm Hg. Two weeks later, the patient's blood pressure is 130/84 mm Hg. One month later, the reading is unchanged. How is this patient's blood pressure classified?
    a. Normal
    b. Prehypertension
    c. Stage 1 hypertension
    d. Stage 2 hypertension

25. The nurse is taking a blood pressure on a new patient who reports headaches and dizziness. What technique does the nurse use to perform the blood pressure procedure?
    a. Take blood pressure readings in both arms; two or more readings are averaged as the value for the visit.
    b. Take the blood pressure in sitting and standing positions, with 15 minutes between position changes.
    c. Take the blood pressure with an automatic cuff, then retake it with a manual cuff to validate readings.
    d. Delegate the procedure to the unlicensed assistive personnel (UAP) and direct him or her to record the findings on the graphic sheet.

26. The nurse is reviewing the laboratory results of urine tests for a patient with a medical diagnosis of essential hypertension. The presence of catecholamines in the urine is evidence of which disorder?
    a. Renal failure
    b. Primary aldosteronism
    c. Cushing's syndrome
    d. Pheochromocytoma

27. The nurse is reviewing the electrocardiogram (ECG) for a patient with a medical diagnosis of essential hypertension. What is the first ECG sign of heart disease resulting from hypertension?
    a. Left atrial and ventricular hypertrophy
    b. Right atrial and ventricular atrophy
    c. Malfunction of the sinoatrial (SA) node
    d. Malfunction of the atrioventricular (AV) node

28. Which blood pressure findings for an adult patient with no other medical problems are evaluated further for hypertension? *(Select all that apply.)*
    a. 118/78 mm Hg
    b. 124/86 mm Hg
    c. 138/78 mm Hg
    d. 140/96 mm Hg
    e. 110/90 mm Hg

29. A middle-aged patient with no health insurance has tried lifestyle modifications to control uncomplicated hypertension, but continues to struggle. What is considered a first drug of choice for this patient?
    a. Calcium channel blocker
    b. Alpha blocker
    c. Thiazide-type diuretic
    d. Angiotensin-converting enzyme (ACE) inhibitor

30. The nurse is reviewing the medication schedule for an older adult patient who needs medication for hypertension. The patient lives alone, but is able to manage self-care. What frequency of drug therapy does the nurse advocate for this patient?
    a. Once a day
    b. Two times a day
    c. Three times a day
    d. Four times a day

31. The nurse is reviewing prescriptions for a patient recently diagnosed with hypertension. The nurse questions a prescription for which type of drug?
    a. Aldosterone receptor antagonist
    b. Alpha blocker
    c. Thiazide-type diuretic
    d. ACE inhibitor

32. For which patient does the nurse question the use of hydrochlorothiazide (HydroDIURIL)?
    a. Asthmatic patient
    b. Patient with chronic airway limitation
    c. Patient with hyperkalemia
    d. Patient with hyponatremia

33. The nurse is teaching a patient about taking hydrochlorothiazide (HydroDIURIL). Which food does the nurse instruct the patient to eat in conjunction with the use of this drug?
    a. Bananas and oranges
    b. Milk and cheese
    c. Cranberries and prunes
    d. Cabbage and cauliflower

34. A patient reports dizziness when she changes positions from sitting to standing and a sudden cough after starting a prescription for captopril (Capoten). Which nursing intervention is most useful for this patient?
    a. Instruct the patient to change positions slowly and take an over-the-counter cough syrup.
    b. Tell the patient to take the medication at bedtime and use over-the-counter throat lozenges.
    c. Notify the prescribing physician because the medication should be discontinued.
    d. Teach the patient to increase her fluid intake.

35. Which intervention renders angiotensin II receptor blockers (ARBs) and angiotensin-converting enzyme (ACE) inhibitors effective in African Americans?
    a. Take with diuretics, a beta blocker, or calcium channel blocker.
    b. Give at a much higher dosage than for other ethnic groups.
    c. Combine with a rigorous lifestyle modification compliance.
    d. Take around the clock on a very individualized schedule.

36. The nurse is reviewing antihypertensive medication orders for a patient with asthma. The nurse questions the use of which type of medication?
    a. Cardioselective beta blockers because they reduce cardiac output
    b. Non-cardioselective beta blockers because they may cause bronchoconstriction
    c. ACE inhibitors because they cause a nagging cough
    d. Thiazide diuretics because they promote potassium excretion

37. The nurse prepares to teach a patient recovering from a myocardial infarction (MI) about combination drug therapy based on "best practice" for controlling hypertension. Which drugs does the nurse include in the teaching plan? *(Select all that apply.)*
    a. Beta blockers
    b. ACE inhibitors or ARBs
    c. Aldosterone antagonists
    d. Central alpha agonists
    e. NSAIDs
    f. Aspirin

38. The student nurse is giving a patient with benign prostatic hyperplasia a morning dose of terazosin (Hytrin). The student says, "This is your blood pressure medicine," but the patient responds, "I don't have high blood pressure." What does the student nurse do next?
    a. Explain to the patient that his blood pressure is not high because the drug is controlling it.
    b. Stop and recheck the medication administration record and then do additional drug research.
    c. Recheck the blood pressure, then hold the drug if blood pressure is not elevated.
    d. Contact the charge nurse for advice about how to handle the patient's refusal.

39. A patient admits to difficulty with long-term compliance to antihypertensive therapy. Which nursing interventions promote compliance for this patient? *(Select all that apply.)*
    a. Carefully review all the medication instructions with the patient.
    b. Give the patient a list of resources for which to find information on the medications.
    c. Reinforce the fact that damage to organs occurs even if there are no symptoms.
    d. Teach the patient about the continuous ambulatory blood pressure monitoring device.
    e. Assess the patient's resources to obtain medications.

40. The nurse is reviewing medical records for several patients with kidney problems and actual or potential for hypertension. Which patient does the nurse expect to be screened for renal artery stenosis?
    a. Patient with a history of kidney stones
    b. Patient taking three categories of antihypertensive drugs at high doses
    c. Patient with newly diagnosed hypertension
    d. Patient with a history of frequent urinary tract infections

41. A patient with hypertension also has heart disease and type 2 diabetes mellitus. What is the blood pressure goal for this patient?
    a. 120/80 mm Hg
    b. 125/80 mm Hg
    c. 135/90 mm Hg
    d. 140/90 mm Hg

42. The nurse assesses a patient and documents the following findings: "edema 2+ bilateral ankles, brown pigmentation of lower extremities skin, aching pain of lower extremities when standing that is relieved with elevation." What condition does the patient likely have?
    a. Deep vein thrombosis
    b. Venous insufficiency
    c. Peripheral arterial disease (PAD)
    d. Raynaud's syndrome

43. The nurse assesses a patient and documents the following findings: "decreased pedal and posterior tibial pulses bilateral (1+), skin is cool-to-cold to touch, loss of hair on lower extremities, patient reports that lower extremity pain is reproducible when walking and relieved by rest, and also noted are thickened toenails." What condition does the patient likely have?
    a. Peripheral vascular disease
    b. Deep vein thrombosis
    c. Raynaud's syndrome
    d. PAD

44. The nurse documents the following findings of a patient on assessment: "paresthesia in lower extremities, dependent rubor color of the skin, and pain in the distal portion of the extremity." These findings are likely indicative of which disorder?
    a. Arterial aneurysm
    b. Peripheral arterial disease
    c. Deep vein thrombosis
    d. Peripheral vascular disease

45. Which patients are at risk for PAD? *(Select all that apply.)*
    a. Hypertensive patient
    b. Patient with diabetes mellitus
    c. Patient who is a cigarette smoker
    d. Anemic patient
    e. Patient who is very thin
    f. African-American patient

46. Which symptom is the most common initial manifestation of PAD?
    a. Intermittent claudication
    b. Pain at rest
    c. Redness in the extremity
    d. Muscle atrophy

47. The nurse is caring for a patient with a medical diagnosis of inflow PAD. Which symptom does the nurse expect the patient to report?
    a. Very frequent episodes of rest pain
    b. Discomfort in the lower back, buttocks, or thighs after walking
    c. Burning or cramping in the calves, ankles, feet, or toes after walking
    d. Waking frequently at night to hang the feet off the bed

48. The nurse is assessing the lower extremity of a patient with PAD. What does the nurse palpate?
    a. Posterior tibial pulse of the affected leg
    b. Pedal pulses in both feet
    c. All pulses in both legs
    d. Strength of the pulses in the affected leg

49. While assessing a patient, the nurse sees a small, round ulcer with a "punched out" appearance and well-defined borders on the great toe. The patient reports the ulcer is painful. How does the nurse interpret this finding?
    a. Venous stasis ulcer
    b. Diabetic ulcer
    c. Gangrenous ulcer
    d. Arterial ulcer

50. A patient is undergoing diagnostic testing for pain and burning sensation in the legs. What does an ankle-brachial index (ABI) of less than 0.9 in either leg indicate?
    a. Normal arterial circulation to the lower extremities
    b. Presence of PAD
    c. Severe venous disease of the lower extremities
    d. Need for immediate surgical intervention

51. The nurse is consulting with the physical therapist to design an exercise program for patients with peripheral vascular disease. Which patient is a candidate for an exercise program?
    a. Patient with severe rest pain
    b. Patient with intermittent claudication
    c. Patient with gangrene
    d. Patient with venous ulcers

52. A patient with PAD asks, "Why should I exercise when walking several blocks seems to make my leg cramp up?" What is the nurse's best response?
    a. "Exercise may improve blood flow to your leg because small vessels will compensate for blood vessels that are blocked off."
    b. "This type of therapy is free and you can do it by yourself to improve the muscles in your legs."
    c. "The cramping will eventually stop if you continue the exercise routine. If you have too much pain, just rest for a while."
    d. "Exercise is a noninvasive nonsurgical technique that is used to increase arterial flow to the affected limb."

53. The nurse is teaching a patient with PAD about positioning and position changes. What suggestion does the nurse give to the patient?
    a. Sit upright in a chair if legs are not swollen.
    b. Sleep with legs above the heart level if legs are swollen.
    c. Avoid crossing the legs at all times.
    d. Change positions slowly when getting out of bed.

54. The nurse is instructing a patient with PAD about ways to promote vasodilation. What information does the nurse include? *(Select all that apply.)*
    a. Maintain a warm environment at home.
    b. Wear socks or insulated shoes at all times.
    c. Apply direct heat to the limb by using a heating pad.
    d. Prevent cold exposure of the affected limb.
    e. Limit fluids to prevent increased blood viscosity.
    f. Completely abstain from smoking or chewing tobacco.

55. A patient reports numbness or burning pain that is severe enough to disturb sleep at night. The patient also has dependent rubor. Which stage of PAD does the nurse suspect in this patient?
    a. I
    b. II
    c. III
    d. IV

56. The nurse is assessing a patient at risk for peripheral vascular disease. Which assessment finding indicates arterial ulcers rather than diabetic or venous ulcers?
    a. Ulcer located over the pressure points of the feet
    b. Ulcer of deep, pale color with even edges and little granulation tissue
    c. Severe pain or discomfort occurring at the ulcer site
    d. Associated ankle discoloration and edema

57. Which are complications that can result from severe PAD? *(Select all that apply.)*
    a. Gangrene
    b. Varicose veins
    c. Septicemia
    d. Amputation
    e. Ulcer formation

58. Which drugs are used to promote circulation in a patient with chronic PAD? *(Select all that apply.)*
    a. Pentoxifylline (Trental)
    b. Propranolol hydrochloride (Inderal)
    c. Aspirin
    d. Clopidogrel (Plavix)
    e. Ezetimibe (Zetia)

59. Which statements pertaining to a percutaneous transluminal balloon angioplasty are correct? *(Select all that apply.)*
    a. One or more arteries are dilated with a balloon catheter to open the vessel.
    b. It is a minor surgical procedure.
    c. Stents may be placed to ensure adequate blood flow.
    d. Placement of stents results in a longer hospital stay.
    e. Some patients are occlusion-free for 3 to 5 years.

60. Which statements about care of a patient who has undergone a percutaneous transluminal balloon angioplasty procedure are correct? *(Select all that apply.)*
    a. Distal pulses of the procedure limb are checked frequently.
    b. The patient is on bedrest with the limb straight for 6 to 8 hours.
    c. Vital signs are taken frequently until the patient is stable.
    d. The nurse monitors for the primary complication of bleeding at the puncture site.
    e. Only a liquid diet is allowed for 12 hours after the procedure.

61. A patient with PAD is scheduled to have percutaneous transluminal angioplasty (PTA). What information does the nurse give the patient about this procedure?
    a. It is usually used when amputation is inevitable.
    b. Reocclusion may occur afterwards and the procedure may be repeated.
    c. Most patients are occlusion-free afterwards, particularly if stents are placed.
    d. It is painless and there are very few risks or dangers.

62. A patient has returned to the unit after having PTA. What does the nurse include in the postprocedural care of this patient? *(Select all that apply.)*
    a. Observe for bleeding at the puncture site.
    b. Observe vital signs frequently.
    c. Perform frequent checks of the distal pulses in both limbs.
    d. Encourage bedrest with the limb straight for about 1 to 2 hours.
    e. Administer anticoagulant therapy such as heparin.
    f. Provide supplemental oxygen via nasal cannula.

63. A patient has returned to the unit after surgery for arterial revascularization with graft placement. The nurse monitors for graft occlusion which is most likely to occur within what time frame?
    a. First 2 hours
    b. First 24 hours
    c. Next 2 days
    d. First week

64. A patient is in the postanesthesia care unit (PACU) after surgery for arterial revascularization with graft placement. Which procedure does the nurse use to check the patency of the graft?
    a. Check the extremity every 15 minutes for the first hour, then hourly, for changes in color, temperature, and pulse intensity.
    b. Check the dorsalis pedis pulse every 15 minutes for the first hour, then hourly.
    c. Ask the patient if there is any pain or loss of sensation anywhere in the extremity, and withhold patient-controlled analgesia.
    d. Gently palpate the site every 15 minutes for the first hour and assess for warmth, redness, and edema.

65. A patient has returned to the unit after a PTA. What is the postprocedural nursing priority?
    a. Pain management
    b. Check the distal pulses
    c. Early ambulation to prevent complications
    d. Monitoring for bleeding at the puncture site

66. The student nurse is assisting in the care of a patient returning from the PACU after aorto-femoral bypass. The nurse intervenes when the student performs which action?
    a. Offers to obtain a meal tray for the patient
    b. Demonstrates to the patient how to use the incentive spirometer
    c. Encourages the patient to deep-breathe every 1 to 2 hours
    d. Explains to the patient the purpose of 24-hour bedrest

67. A patient has had surgery for arterial revascularization with graft placement. The nurse notes swelling, tenseness of the skin tissue, and the patient reports an increasing pain with numbness and tingling as well as a decrease in the ability to wiggle toes and ankles. What does the nurse suspect is occurring with this patient?
    a. Graft infection
    b. Compartment syndrome
    c. Graft occlusion
    d. Reaction to thrombolytic therapy

68. A patient has had aortoiliac bypass surgery with graft placement. The nurse notes induration, erythema, tenderness, warmth, edema, and drainage at the site. Before calling the physician, what additional assessment does the nurse perform?
    a. Palpates the patient's abdomen and checks for the last bowel movement
    b. Auscultates the patient's lung sounds and checks the pulse oximeter reading
    c. Assesses the patient for signs of occult bleeding and looks at the PT results
    d. Checks the patient's temperature and looks at the white blood cell results

69. A patient is admitted with a medical diagnosis of acute arterial occlusion. What documentation does the nurse expect to see in this patient's medical record?
    a. Acute MI and/or atrial fibrillation within the previous weeks
    b. History of chronic venous stasis disease treated with débridement and wound care
    c. History of Marfan syndrome or Ehlers-Danlos syndrome
    d. Episode of blunt trauma that occurred several months ago

70. A patient with an acute arterial occlusion requires abciximab (ReoPro). What nursing responsibilities are associated with the administration of this platelet inhibitor?
    a. Platelet counts must be monitored at 3, 6, and 12 hours after the start of the infusion.
    b. For platelet counts over 100,000/mm³, infusion must be readjusted or discontinued.
    c. Monitor for manifestations of rash, itching, or swelling.
    d. Monitor for edema, pain on passive movement, or poor capillary refill.

71. Which is a postoperative nursing intervention for a patient with arterial revascularization?
    a. Promote graft patency by limiting IV fluid infusion.
    b. Instruct the patient to avoid bending at the hips or knees.
    c. Resume regular diet immediately after surgery.
    d. Avoid coughing and deep-breathing exercises.

Matching. Match the types of aneurysms with their descriptions.

Types of Aneurysms
a. Dissecting aneurysm
b. Saccular
c. Fusiform

Descriptions
_____ 72. Involves the entire circumference of the artery

_____ 73. Involves a distinct portion of the artery

_____ 74. Is caused by blood in the wall of the artery

75. What is the most common location for an aneurysm?
    a. Abdominal aorta
    b. Thoracic aorta
    c. Femoral arteries
    d. Popliteal arteries

76. What is the most common cause of an aneurysm?
    a. Emboli
    b. Trauma
    c. Atherosclerosis
    d. Thrombus formation

77. A patient is suspected to have an abdominal aortic aneurysm (AAA). What does the nurse assess for?
   a. Abdominal, flank, or back pain
   b. Chest pain and shortness of breath
   c. Hoarseness and difficulty swallowing
   d. Disruption of bowel and bladder patterns

78. A 75-year-old man with a history of atherosclerosis comes to the emergency department (ED) with abdominal pain. What findings indicate a possible AAA? *(Select all that apply.)*
   a. Left-sided chest pain
   b. Abdominal, flank, or back pain
   c. Visible pulsation on the upper abdominal wall
   d. Hoarseness
   e. Difficulty swallowing

79. A patient with an AAA is admitted to the hospital. Which tests does the physician order to confirm an accurate diagnosis as well as to determine the size and location of the AAA? *(Select all that apply.)*
   a. Abdominal x-rays
   b. Ultrasound
   c. Electrocardiogram
   d. Magnetic resonance imaging
   e. Computed tomography

80. A patient is diagnosed with a small 3 cm AAA. What is the best nonsurgical intervention to decrease the risk of rupture of an aneurysm and to slow the rate of enlargement?
   a. Maintenance of normal blood pressure and avoidance of hypertension
   b. Bedrest until there is shrinkage of the aneurysm
   c. Heparin and Coumadin therapy to decrease clotting
   d. Intra-arterial thrombolytic therapy

81. A patient with a ruptured aneurysm may exhibit which symptoms? *(Select all that apply.)*
   a. Bradypnea
   b. Tachycardia
   c. Increased systolic pressure
   d. Decreased blood pressure
   e. Severe pain
   f. Diaphoresis
   g. Loss of pulses distal to rupture
   h. Decreased level of consciousness

82. Which action does the nurse take first if a patient has a suspected aneurysm rupture?
   a. Start an IV infusion with a large-bore needle.
   b. Assess baseline measurements of blood pressure and pulse rate.
   c. Palpate the pulsating abdominal mass to determine its size.
   d. Assess all peripheral pulses to use as a baseline for comparison.

83. A patient has had a repair of an AAA. For what reason is this patient being monitored postoperatively for urinary output and renal function studies (creatinine and BUN)?
   a. The patient was probably in shock preoperatively, and there may be glomerular damage.
   b. The patient is usually in a critical care nursing unit where this is done routinely.
   c. The aorta was clamped during the surgery and the kidneys may have been inadvertently damaged.
   d. Repair of the aneurysm improves renal perfusion and the urinary output should increase.

84. A patient has had an aneurysm repair. Which activity does the nurse suggest as an example of appropriate exercise during the recovery period?
   a. Playing golf
   b. Washing dishes
   c. Raking leaves
   d. Driving a car

85. A patient is admitted for a medical diagnosis of detectable AAA. What does the nurse expect to find documented in the patient's description of symptoms?
   a. Hematuria and painful urination that started very suddenly
   b. Steady and gnawing abdominal pain unaffected by movement and lasting for days
   c. No subjective complaints of pain, but episodes of dizziness
   d. Pain in the lower extremities exacerbated by walking and relieved by rest

86. While assessing a patient with AAA, the nurse notes a pulsation in the upper abdomen slightly to the left of the midline between the xyphoid process and the umbilicus. What does the nurse do next?
    a. Measure the mass with a ruler.
    b. Palpate the mass for tenderness.
    c. Percuss the mass to determine the borders.
    d. Auscultate for a bruit over the mass.

87. A patient was admitted for AAA with a pulsating abdominal mass. The nurse notes a sudden onset of diaphoresis, decreased level of consciousness, a blood pressure of 88/60 mm Hg, and an irregular apical pulse. Oxygen is in place via mask. What is the priority nursing action?
    a. Establish IV access.
    b. Alert the Rapid Response Team.
    c. Auscultate for a bruit and assess the mass.
    d. Place the patient on the cardiac monitor.

88. The nurse is reviewing the radiologist's report of the abdominal x-ray of a patient suspected of having AAA. The report notes an "eggshell" appearance. How does the nurse interpret this data?
    a. Validates the presence of an aneurysm
    b. Suggests an artifact; therefore, the x-ray must be repeated
    c. Indicates a congenital anomaly that will obscure the aneurysm
    d. Indicates the aneurysm is the size of an egg

89. The nurse is designing a teaching plan for a patient with a small (4 cm) AAA. The patient is currently asymptomatic. What is the nurse's goal for nonsurgical management of this patient?
    a. Teach lifestyle modifications that will minimize the growth of the aneurysm.
    b. Monitor the growth of the aneurysm and follow the antihypertensive medication regimen.
    c. Encourage compliance with anticoagulant drugs and laboratory follow-up appointments.
    d. Stabilize the patient's condition and improve overall health so surgery can be safely performed.

90. The nurse is performing preoperative care for a patient who is having an elective surgery for AAA resection. What is included in this patient's care? *(Select all that apply.)*
    a. Bowel preparation
    b. Instruction on coughing and deep-breathing
    c. Blood type and cross-match
    d. Administration of a large volume IV fluid bolus
    e. Assessment of all peripheral pulses
    f. Use of a marker to note where the pulse is palpated or heard by Doppler

91. A patient who has had AAA surgical repair develops chest pain, shortness of breath, diaphoresis, anxiety, and restlessness. These symptoms are consistent with which postoperative complication?
    a. Myocardial infarction
    b. Graft occlusion
    c. Renal failure
    d. Paralytic ileus

92. The nurse notes a change in pulses, a cool extremity below the graft, bluish discoloration to the flanks, and abdominal distention in a patient who has had AAA surgical repair. These symptoms are consistent with which postoperative complication?
    a. Ischemic colitis
    b. Cerebral and spinal cord ischemia
    c. Graft occlusion or rupture
    d. Thoracic outlet syndrome

93. A patient is admitted through the ED for emergency surgery of a ruptured aneurysm. Why does the nurse monitor the patient for renal failure?
    a. A Foley catheter was inserted under potentially nonsterile conditions.
    b. Aggressive fluid management in the ED could overload the kidneys.
    c. Hypovolemia associated with rupture can result in acute tubular necrosis.
    d. Medications used in the emergency procedure are nephrotoxic.

94. A patient who had surgery for an AAA was just extubated. What does the nurse do in caring for this patient for the next 24 hours?
    a. Assess respiratory rate and depth every hour.
    b. Turn and suction the patient every 2 hours.
    c. Discourage coughing and deep-breathing.
    d. Assist the patient to a bedside chair.

95. The nurse is performing an assessment on a patient who had AAA repair the day before. The nurse does not hear any bowel sounds when auscultating the abdomen. What does the nurse do next?
    a. Continue to monitor the patient; paralytic ileus is expected for 2 to 3 days.
    b. Obtain an order for a nasogastric tube set to low suction.
    c. Report assessment findings immediately to the surgeon.
    d. Palpate for distention and ask the patient to ambulate.

96. The nurse is assessing a patient with a ruptured AAA. Which assessment finding is most likely to be present?
    a. Retroperitoneal hemorrhage
    b. Mass may be visible above the suprasternal notch
    c. Hoarseness and difficulty swallowing
    d. Disruption of bowel and bladder patterns

97. A patient who had a thoracic aortic aneurysm repair has been progressing well for several days after the surgery, but today tells the nurse, "My toes and lower legs feel a little numb and tingly." What does the nurse do next?
    a. Encourage the patient to do active range-of-motion exercises in bed.
    b. Help the patient get up, dangle the legs, and then ambulate.
    c. Assess extremities for sensation, movement, or pulse changes.
    d. Instruct UAP to assist the patient in elevating the legs.

98. The nurse is caring for a patient who had a repair of a thoracic aneurysm. What does the nurse monitor for in this patient? *(Select all that apply.)*
    a. Cardiac dysrhythmias
    b. Paraplegia
    c. Respiratory distress
    d. Hemorrhage
    e. Pericarditis

99. A patient has had a repair of a thoracic aneurysm. What does the nurse monitor for in this patient and immediately report to the surgeon?
    a. Productive cough when using the incentive spirometer
    b. Increased drainage from chest tubes
    c. Sternal pain with coughing and deep-breathing
    d. Increased urinary output from the indwelling catheter

100. A patient is considering endovascular stent grafts. What is one of the advantages of this procedure?
    a. Decreased length of hospital stay
    b. Less risk for hemorrhage
    c. Decreased incidence of postprocedural rupture
    d. Use of local, rather than general, anesthesia

101. The home health nurse is making the first visit to a patient who had a surgical aneurysm repair. In evaluating the home situation, what does the nurse observe that is cause for concern?
    a. The patient has been having groceries delivered for several weeks.
    b. There is a calendar hanging on the refrigerator with medication times.
    c. The patient's bedroom and bathroom access are on the ground floor.
    d. The patient decides to vacuum the house and clean out the garage.

102. A patient comes to the ED with anterior chest pain described as a "tearing" sensation. The patient is diaphoretic, nauseated, faint, apprehensive, and blood pressure is 200/130 mm Hg. Which medication is most likely to be ordered for this patient?
    a. Antianginal such as nitroglycerin (Nitrobid)
    b. Antihypertensive such as sodium nitroprusside (Nipride)
    c. Calcium channel antagonist such as amlodipine (Norvasc)
    d. Beta blocker such as propranolol (Inderal)

103. Indicate whether the signs and symptoms below are related to Buerger's disease (BD) or Raynaud's disease (RD).
    _____ a. Occurs in smokers and often in young males
    _____ b. Occurs in both sexes, predominately female
    _____ c. Episodic, causing white then blue fingers
    _____ d. Triggered by exposure to tobacco
    _____ e. Occurs in medium and small arteries and veins
    _____ f. Severe episodes may lead to gangrene

Matching. Match the physical findings with their related arterial disorders.

Arterial Disorders
a. Popliteal entrapment
b. Subclavian steal
c. Thoracic outlet syndrome

Physical Findings
_____ 104. Blood pressure different in each arm
_____ 105. Intermittent claudication in one or both legs
_____ 106. Intermittent neck and shoulder pain

107. A young male patient is diagnosed with early stage Buerger's disease. What assessment finding does the nurse expect to find in the patient's record?
    a. Claudication of the arch of the foot
    b. Intolerance of warm environments
    c. Dizziness and lightheadedness
    d. Pain in the lower back with ambulation

108. The nurse is teaching a patient with Buerger's disease about self-care. What is the most important point that the nurse emphasizes?
    a. Lower intake of fat and reducing cholesterol to reverse the disease process.
    b. Perform daily exercise of fingers or toes to slow the progress of the disease.
    c. Limit exposure to extreme or prolonged cold temperatures because of vasoconstriction.
    d. Cease cigarette smoking and tobacco use to arrest the disease process.

109. A patient reports tiredness in the arm with exertion, paresthesia, dizziness, and exercise-induced pain in the forearm when the arms are elevated. The nurse suspects subclavian steal. What physical assessment does the nurse perform?
    a. Check blood pressure in both arms.
    b. Auscultate for a carotid bruit.
    c. Check for orthostatic hypotension.
    d. Observe the arm for redness or edema.

110. A patient who is an avid golfer is diagnosed with thoracic outlet syndrome. What does the nurse advise the patient that is specific to this syndrome?
    a. Rest if shortness of breath occurs.
    b. Avoid walking long distances.
    c. Avoid elevating the arms.
    d. Perform deep-breathing exercises.

111. A 25-year-old woman reports bilateral blanching of both upper extremities that occurs in cold temperatures. She reports numbness and cold sensation, and afterwards the arms become very red. What are these symptoms consistent with?
    a. Raynaud's disease
    b. Buerger's disease
    c. Subclavian steal
    d. Raynaud's phenomenon

112. Which medication is a patient with Raynaud's disease most likely to be prescribed?
    a. Lovastatin (Mevacor)
    b. Coumadin (Warfarin)
    c. Nifedipine (Procardia)
    d. Captopril (Capoten)

113. A patient has been on bedrest following a motor vehicle accident. The nurse notes on assessment that the patient's left lower extremity has edema and is warm to the touch. The patient reports the calf of the left leg is slightly painful. The nurse suspects that this assessment may indicate which disorder?
    a. Raynaud's syndrome
    b. Cellulitis
    c. Aneurysm
    d. Deep vein thrombosis

114. Which diagnostic tests will likely be ordered to confirm diagnosis for the patient in question 113?
    a. Venous duplex ultrasonography
    b. Venogram
    c. X-ray films
    d. CT scan

True or False? *Read each statement about venous disorders and write T for true or F for false in the blanks provided. If the statement is false, correct the statement to make it true.*

_____ 115. The focus of treatment for a DVT is to prevent complications and increase in size of the thrombus.

_____ 116. DVTs are often treated medically with rest, anticoagulants, elevation of legs, and compression stockings.

_____ 117. Thrombolytic therapy must be initiated within 24 hours of symptom onset.

_____ 118. To prevent leg edema, elevate legs when in bed or in a chair.

_____ 119. Thrombus formation has been associated with hyperlipidemia, hyperglycemia, and/or hypertension, known as *Virchow's triad.*

_____ 120. The highest incidence of clot formation occurs in patients who have undergone hip surgery, total knee replacement, or open prostate surgery.

_____ 121. Severe infections, systemic lupus erythematosus, polycythemia vera, oral contraceptives, and trauma have also been linked to thrombosis.

_____ 122. Cancer, especially adenocarcinoma of the visceral organs, is the most common malignancy associated with DVT.

_____ 123. Unfractionated heparin (UFH) is an anticoagulant agent that will break up the clot.

124. A patient is admitted to the hospital with a DVT. Which drug therapy does the nurse expect the health care provider to order?
    a. Heparin 5000 units subcutaneously twice a day
    b. Loading high dose of Coumadin, then smaller doses on following days
    c. Alternate heparin and Coumadin depending on the laboratory values
    d. Heparin via IV infusion, with Coumadin therapy started at the same time

125. What test is the most definitively preferred noninvasive test to diagnose a DVT?
    a. Venogram
    b. Duplex ultrasonography
    c. X-ray films
    d. CT scan

126. The patients with which conditions are candidates for an inferior vena cava filter placement? *(Select all that apply.)*
    a. Abdominal aorta aneurysm
    b. Chronic obstructive pulmonary disease
    c. Recurrent deep vein thrombosis
    d. No response to medical treatment
    e. Intolerance to anticoagulation drug therapy

127. What is the recommended therapeutic range for the International Normalized Ratio (INR) that is done along with prothrombin time in a patient receiving warfarin sodium (Coumadin)?
    a. 0.5 to 1.0
    b. 1.0 to 1.5
    c. 1.5 to 2.0
    d. 2.0 to 2.5

128. A patient prescribed warfarin sodium (Coumadin) is instructed that certain foods decrease the effect of the drug. Which foods, if eaten, must be consumed in consistent and small amounts each day?
    a. Fresh fruits
    b. Chicken and beef
    c. Spinach and asparagus
    d. Milk and cheese

129. The nurse is teaching a patient who is at risk for venous thromboembolism (VTE). The patient is currently asymptomatic and is living in the community. What interventions does the nurse instruct the patient to do to minimize the risk of VTE? *(Select all that apply.)*
    a. Avoid oral contraceptives.
    b. Drink adequate fluids to avoid dehydration.
    c. Exercise the legs during long periods of bedrest or sitting.
    d. Arise early in the morning for ambulation.
    e. Use a venous plexus foot pump.

130. The nurse is reviewing the diagnostic test results for a patient suspected of having a DVT. The results show a negative D-dimer test. How does the nurse interpret this data?
    a. The test excludes DVT.
    b. Venous duplex ultrasonography is needed.
    c. The patient has arterial disease.
    d. Impedance plethysmography is needed.

131. The health care provider has ordered unfractionated heparin (UFH) for a patient with DVT. Before administering the drug, the nurse ensures that which laboratory tests were obtained for baseline measurement? *(Select all that apply.)*
    a. Prothrombin time (PT)
    b. Activated partial thromboplastin time (APTT or aPTT)
    c. International Normalized Ratio (INR)
    d. Complete blood count (CBC) with platelet count
    e. Arterial blood gas
    f. Creatinine level
    g. Urinalysis

132. The nurse notes that the platelet count for a patient who is to receive unfractionated heparin (UFH) is 100,000/mm^3. How does the nurse interpret this result?
    a. It is slightly lowered and worth monitoring for trends.
    b. It is significantly low, so the health care provider should be notified.
    c. It is insignificant unless other values such as PT or APTT are abnormal.
    d. It is higher than expected, but within normal limits for therapy.

133. The medication order for unfractionated heparin (UFH) is for 80 units/kg of body weight. How does the nurse interpret this order?
    a. Appropriate dose for the continuous IV infusion
    b. Higher than expected dose for the initial IV bolus
    c. Appropriate dose for the initial IV bolus
    d. Appropriate dose for maintenance therapy

134. A patient is receiving unfractionated heparin (UFH) therapy. The nurse instructs the UAP in which task related to the unfractionated heparin (UFH) therapy?
    a. Observe the skin for ecchymosis, bruising, and petechiae during AM hygiene.
    b. Replace the antiembolism devices after bathing or ambulating.
    c. Check on the patient every 2 hours and report changes in mental status.
    d. Watch for and report blood in the stool when assisting the patient with toileting.

135. A patient receiving unfractionated heparin (UFH) therapy is ordered to discontinue the therapy and begin low–molecular-weight heparin (LMWH) and enoxaparin (Lovenox). What is the priority nursing intervention?
    a. Discontinue the unfractionated heparin (UFH) at least 30 minutes before the first LMWH injection.
    b. Check the APTT results after giving the first LMWH injection.
    c. Assess the patient's IV site before starting the LMWH.
    d. Check the PT and INR results before giving the first LMWH injection.

136. What are the contraindications for thrombolytic therapy for DVT? *(Select all that apply.)*
    a. Recent surgery
    b. Trauma
    c. Stroke
    d. Diabetes mellitus
    e. Spinal injury

137. A patient is receiving thrombolytic therapy. How does the nurse monitor for the most serious complication from thrombolytic therapy?
    a. Performing neurologic checks and monitoring for level of consciousness
    b. Auscultating for breath sounds and counting respiratory rates
    c. Assessing the IV site and watching for infiltration and swelling
    d. Checking patency of the Foley catheter and monitoring urinary output

138. The nurse is teaching a patient about the side effects and potential problems associated with taking warfarin sodium (Coumadin). Which statement by the patient indicates a correct understanding of the nurse's instruction?
    a. "If I notice bleeding of the gums, I should skip one or two doses of the medication."
    b. "I should eat a lot of cabbage, cauliflower, and broccoli to prevent bleeding."
    c. "For injury and bleeding, I should apply direct pressure and seek medical assistance."
    d. "I should avoid going to the dentist while I am taking this medication."

139. A patient with a history of vascular disease as a result of diabetes has developed a peripheral neuropathy. This patient is at risk for which problem?
    a. Fatigue
    b. Severe pain
    c. Injury
    d. Poor circulation

140. The nurse is instructing a patient and caregiver on warfarin (Coumadin) therapy at home. Which items does the nurse include in the teaching plan? *(Select all that apply.)*
    a. Eat small amounts of broccoli and spinach.
    b. Avoid beta-blockers and ACE inhibitors.
    c. Inform your dentist of taking warfarin prior to treatment.
    d. Eat small amounts of oranges and bananas.
    e. Avoid NSAIDs and birth control pills.

141. Which statements pertaining to the use of the Unna boot are correct? *(Select all that apply.)*
    a. It is used to heal peripheral arterial disease ulcers.
    b. It is applied from the toes to the knee.
    c. The patient is instructed on the signs and symptoms of arterial occlusion.
    d. It is changed by a health care provider every 3 to 4 days.
    e. It is used to heal venous stasis ulcers.

142. List three goals for managing venous stasis ulcers.

143. The nurse is assessing an obese patient's lower leg and notes a small irregular-shaped ulcer over the medial malleolus with brownish discoloration. The patient reports that the "leg has been that way for a long time." What do these findings suggest to the nurse?
    a. Varicose vein
    b. Venous stasis ulcer
    c. Phlebitis
    d. Raynaud's phenomenon

144. The nurse is consulting with the registered dietitian about diet therapy for a patient with chronic venous stasis ulcers. What are the dietary recommendations to help this patient promote wound healing?
    a. High-protein foods
    b. Vitamin D and B supplements
    c. Low-fat foods
    d. High-calcium foods

145. A patient has a venous stasis ulcer that requires a dressing. Which dressing materials are selected for this type of wound? *(Select all that apply.)*
    a. Oxygen-permeable polyethylene film
    b. Oxygen-impermeable hydrocolloid dressing
    c. Dry gauze dressings
    d. Artificial skin products
    e. Unna boot
    f. Vacuum-assisted wound closure

146. The nurse is assessing a patient with distended, protruding veins. In order to assess for varicose veins, what technique does the nurse use?
    a. Place the patient in a supine position with elevated legs; as the patient sits up, observe the veins filling from the proximal end.
    b. Place the patient in the Trendelenburg position and observe the distention and protruding of the veins.
    c. Ask the patient to stand and observe the leg veins; then ask the patient to sit or lie down and observe the veins.
    d. Ask the patient to walk around the room and observe the veins; then have the patient rest for several minutes and reassess the veins.

147. A patient with varicose veins asks the nurse to provide a list of all available treatment options. What does the nurse include on the list? *(Select all that apply.)*
    a. Elastic stockings and elevation of the extremities
    b. Sclerotherapy
    c. Stab avulsion technique
    d. Vein stripping
    e. Application of radiofrequency (RF) energy
    f. Endovenous laser treatment
    g. Anticoagulant therapy

148. The nurse is assessing the IV site of a patient who has been receiving a normal saline infusion. There is redness, warmth radiating up the arm with pain, soreness, and swelling. What does the nurse do next?
    a. Discontinue the IV and apply warm, moist soaks.
    b. Slow the infusion rate and reassess within 1 hour.
    c. Discontinue the IV and apply a cold pack.
    d. Contact the health care provider for an order for an antidote.

149. Which patient has the greatest risk for a pulmonary embolus related to a venous disorder?
    a. Patient with bilateral varicose veins
    b. Patient with phlebitis of superficial veins
    c. Patient with thrombophlebitis in a deep vein of the lower extremity
    d. Patient with venous insufficiency throughout the leg

150. What information does the nurse include when teaching a patient with chronic venous stasis? *(Select all that apply.)*
    a. Elevate the legs when sitting.
    b. Avoid crossing the legs.
    c. Wear antiembolic stockings at night during sleep.
    d. Avoid standing still for any length of time.
    e. Avoid wearing tight girdles, tight pants, and narrow-banded knee-high socks.

151. Which patient is at greatest risk for developing varicose veins?
    a. 37-year-old mail carrier
    b. 19-year-old retail store clerk
    c. 40-year-old operating room scrub technician
    d. 25-year-old pregnant woman in the first trimester

152. What is the preferred treatment for phlebitis?
    a. Dry heat
    b. Ice packs
    c. Warm, moist packs
    d. Massage and elevation

153. Which type of vascular injury is most likely to result from blunt trauma?
    a. Arteriovenous fistula
    b. Hematoma
    c. Dissection
    d. Incompetent valves

154. Which patient with vascular trauma is a candidate for immediate emergency surgery?
    a. 54-year-old with fractured humerus
    b. 36-year-old with a ruptured renal artery
    c. 18-year-old with a contusion of the pelvis
    d. 67-year-old with a chronic subdural hematoma

155. A patient arrives in the ED with severe trauma from a gunshot wound. Identify in order of priority the management of vascular trauma using the numbers 1 through 6.

    _____ a. Prepare the patient for arteriography.

    _____ b. Restore blood flow.

    _____ c. Control bleeding.

    _____ d. Ask about mechanism of injury, blood loss, and symptoms after the injury.

    _____ e. Assess for circulatory, sensory, or motor impairment.

    _____ f. Establish patent airway.

156. The nurse observes diminished pulses, cold skin, and a pulsatile mass over the femoral artery in a patient reporting pain in the right leg. What condition does the nurse suspect in this patient?
    a. Venous thromboembolism
    b. Buerger's disease
    c. Femoral aneurysm
    d. Popliteal entrapment

CASE STUDY: THE PATIENT WITH DEEP VEIN THROMBOSIS (1)

Use a separate sheet of paper to answer the questions in this Case Study, or go to the "Prepare for Class" folder on your Evolve website at http://evolve.elsevier.com/Iggy/ to download and complete as a word processing file. Answer guidelines for this Case Study are also available on your Evolve website.

A 62-year-old woman is hospitalized for surgical repair of an abdominal aneurysm. The patient is 3 days postoperative. The patient is alert and oriented to person, place, and time, and is cooperative and pleasant. The abdomen midline incision has a nonadherent dressing covering that is clean, dry, and intact.

The dressing is untaped at the top to assess the incision, which is dry, approximated, and with staples. The dressing is then resecured. Auscultation of the abdomen reveals bowel sounds in all four quadrants. The patient reports that she has "passed gas" but has not had a bowel movement yet. She states that she is still slightly tender at the incision site, rating her pain a 2 when turning or coughing (on a pain scale of 0 to 10, 0 being no pain and 10 being the worst pain imaginable). The patient has refused the need for any pain medication at this time. The patient is instructed to call the nurse if pain medication is needed before the nurse goes on rounds again in one hour or less. The patient states understanding.

Lung sounds per auscultation are clear in anterior and posterior upper lobes, and diminished in bases anterior and posterior. Radial pulses are bilateral 2+ and pedal pulses left 2+ and right 1+. Right lower extremity from the foot to the distal aspect of the knee has 2+ edema. Left lower extremity has no edema. Vital signs are: temp 37.2° C (98.9° F); heart rate/rhythm 79/min and sinus rhythm with occasional PACs; respirations 20/min; and pulse oximeter 96% on room air.

The patient asks the nurse after the assessment is complete if she can get up and ambulate in the hallway.

1. What should the nurse's response be to the patient's request to ambulate in the hallway?
2. What specific diagnostic test would be ordered to verify the presence or absence of a DVT?
3. If a DVT is present in the right lower extremity, what specific treatment may be ordered?
4. Document this patient's case using the below categories in order of priority.
   - Gastrointestinal
   - Cardiovascular
   - Pulmonary
   - Neurologic
   - Surgical incision
   - Alteration in comfort

CASE STUDY: THE PATIENT WITH HYPERTENSION

Use a separate sheet of paper to answer the questions in this Case Study, or go to the "Prepare for Class" folder on your Evolve website at http://evolve.elsevier.com/Iggy/ to download and complete as a word processing file. Answer guidelines for this Case Study are also available on your Evolve website.

The patient is a 64-year-old African-American man who is diagnosed with hypertension. He is 6 feet tall and weighs 300 lbs. He smokes two packs of cigarettes per day. He works as a salesman and has two to three alcoholic drinks a week. He admits that he does not get as much exercise as he used to when he was 40 years old. His mother and brother have high blood pressure, and his father died of a heart attack at age 68.

1. Does he have essential or secondary hypertension? Can this be determined at this point? Give a rationale for the answer.

2. What diseases would have made this patient at risk for developing secondary hypertension?

3. What cultural aspects need to be considered in controlling his hypertension?

4. How does this patient's age impact the diagnosis and treatment of hypertension?

5. During the initial workup for hypertension, what laboratory testing would be ordered? Explain.

6. An interdisciplinary team consult was completed. What assessment findings would indicate successful outcomes have been met?

7. This patient was later seen in the ED with severe headache, extremely high blood pressure, dizziness, blurred vision, and disorientation. His diagnosis is malignant hypertension. Describe the medical interventions for this problem.

CASE STUDY: THE PATIENT WITH DEEP VEIN THROMBOSIS (2)

Use a separate sheet of paper to answer the questions in this Case Study, or go to the "Prepare for Class" folder on your Evolve website at http://evolve.elsevier.com/Iggy/ to download and complete as a word processing file. Answer guidelines for this Case Study are also available on your Evolve website.

A 58-year-old woman was discharged from the hospital 4 days ago after lower abdominal surgery. She has been readmitted for pain and edema in her right calf. She has a tentative diagnosis of thrombophlebitis.

1. Discuss the probable etiology of this patient's thrombophlebitis.

2. The physician prescribes heparin sodium 1000 units per hour intravenously for this patient, and also begins therapy with warfarin (Coumadin). Discuss the purpose of these medications, the nursing precautions, and laboratory tests to monitor their effectiveness.

3. The patient asks, "Which medication dissolves the clot? The IV or the pill?" What does the nurse say to her? How does heparin differ from warfarin in the treatment of thrombophlebitis?

4. This patient is placed on strict bedrest with her legs elevated, and a warm, moist pack is to be applied. What are the purposes of these interventions?

5. The following morning, the patient reports leg cramps and asks the nurse to massage her calf because it is "cramping." Should the nurse comply with this request? Why or why not?

6. The patient's activated partial thromboplastin time is 70 seconds (normal range is 22.1 to 34.1 seconds) and the INR is 1. Discuss the significance of these test results.

7. The patient's laboratory values are now within therapeutic ranges, and the patient is being discharged from the hospital on Coumadin. Develop a teaching-learning plan for this patient.

CASE STUDY: THE PATIENT WITH BYPASS SURGERY FOR PAD

Use a separate sheet of paper to answer the questions in this Case Study, or go to the "Prepare for Class" folder on your Evolve website at http://evolve.elsevier.com/Iggy/ to download and complete as a word processing file. Answer guidelines for this Case Study are also available on your Evolve website.

A 77-year-old woman has just had femoral-popliteal bypass surgery to treat severe arterial disease.

1. What are the six Ps that are assessed for after femoral-popliteal bypass surgery in relation to arterial flow and lack of oxygenation to the tissues? Indicate techniques, equipment, and principles that are used by the nurse to assess these findings.

2. Which of the six Ps written above is often the first indicator of a graft site occlusion and requires immediate attention from the physician? Give an explanation for the answer.

3. What is the procedure to be followed if a graft occlusion occurs?

4. What is compartment syndrome? What assessments should be performed to detect compartment syndrome?

5. The patient is discharged home and a home health nurse is coming to make the initial visit. What type of assessments should the nurse make?

39 CHAPTER

Care of Patients with Shock

STUDY/REVIEW QUESTIONS

Matching. Match the terms with their correct definitions.

Terms

a. Dilation
b. Sympathetic tone
c. Exogenous
d. Endogenous
e. Anaphylaxis
f. Sepsis
g. Capillary leak syndrome
h. Anoxic
i. Ischemic
j. Vasoconstriction

Definitions

_____ 1. Allergic reactions that result in widespread loss of blood vessel tone and decreased cardiac output

_____ 2. Increase in diameter of vessel walls by relaxing the smooth muscle

_____ 3. Widespread infection that triggers a whole-body inflammatory response

_____ 4. State of partial blood vessel constriction

_____ 5. No oxygen

_____ 6. Originate outside the body

_____ 7. Substances normally found in the body

_____ 8. Cell dysfunction or death from lack of oxygen

_____ 9. Mediators change blood vessel integrity and allow fluid to shift from the vascular space to the interstitial tissues

_____ 10. Decrease in diameter by contracting the muscle

11. Which statements about shock are true? *(Select all that apply.)*
    a. Shock is a whole-body response to body tissues not receiving enough oxygen.
    b. Shock is widespread abnormal cellular metabolism.
    c. Shock only occurs in the acute care setting.
    d. Shock may occur in older adults in response to urinary tract infections.
    e. Shock is mostly classified as a disease.

12. Which hormones are released in response to decreased mean arterial pressure (MAP)? *(Select all that apply.)*
    a. Insulin
    b. Renin
    c. Antidiuretic hormone (ADH)
    d. Epinephrine
    e. Aldosterone
    f. Serotonin

13. The patient has decreased oxygenation and impaired tissue perfusion. Which clinical manifestations are evidence of one of the nonprogressive or compensatory stages of shock? *(Select all that apply.)*
    a. Decreased urine output
    b. Low-grade fever
    c. Change of mental status
    d. Decreased heart rate
    e. Increased heart rate

14. Which statement about the systemic effects of shock is correct?
    a. The liver is essentially unaffected, but liver enzymes may be lower than normal.
    b. The current heart rate and blood pressure indicate cardiac system is at baseline.
    c. The brain and neurologic system can withstand 10 to 15 minutes of severe hypoperfusion.
    d. The kidneys can tolerate hypoxia and anoxia up to 1 hour without permanent damage.

15. Which patients are at risk for shock related to fluid shifts? *(Select all that apply.)*
    a. Hypoglycemic patient
    b. Severely malnourished patient
    c. Patient with paralytic ileus
    d. Patient with kidney disease
    e. Patient with minor burns
    f. Patient with large wounds

16. A young woman comes to the emergency department (ED) with lightheadedness and "a feeling of impending doom." Pulse is 110 beats/min; respirations 30/min; blood pressure 140/90 mm Hg. Which factors does the nurse ask about that could contribute to shock? *(Select all that apply.)*
    a. Recent accident or trauma
    b. Prolonged diarrhea or vomiting
    c. History of depression or anxiety
    d. Possibility of pregnancy
    e. Use of over-the-counter medications

17. The nurse is caring for a patient with cardiogenic shock. What is the priority for managing this patient?
    a. Prepare for open heart surgery.
    b. Insert an intra-aortic balloon pump.
    c. Administer a thromboembolic agent.
    d. Determine and treat the cause of the shock.

18. Which patients are at risk for cardiogenic shock? *(Select all that apply.)*
    a. Patient with a history of angina
    b. Patient with a recent myocardial infarction
    c. Patient with chronic atrial fibrillation
    d. Patient with a functional pacemaker
    e. Patient with a history of congestive heart failure

19. A patient has cardiac dysrhythmias and pulmonary problems as a result of receiving an IV antibiotic. What type of shock does this represent?
    a. Hypovolemic
    b. Cardiogenic
    c. Anaphylactic
    d. Septic

20. A patient with a head injury was treated for a cerebral hematoma. After surgery, this patient is at risk for what type of shock?
    a. Obstructive
    b. Cardiogenic
    c. Distributive-chemical
    d. Distributive-neural

21. The nurse is performing the AM shift assessment on several patients. The nurse is immediately concerned about decreased tissue perfusion if the capillary refill time was delayed for which patient?
    a. Patient with diabetes mellitus
    b. Anemic patient
    c. Patient with peripheral vascular disease
    d. Asthmatic patient

22. The nursing student takes the morning blood pressure of a postoperative patient and the reading is 90/50 mm Hg. What does the student do next? *(Select all that apply.)*
    a. Report the reading to the primary nurse as a possible sign of hypovolemia.
    b. Assess the patient for subjective feelings of dizziness or shortness of breath.
    c. Check the patient's chart for trends of morning vital sign readings.
    d. Notify the instructor to verify the significance of the finding.
    e. Call a "code blue."

23. A patient at risk for shock has had some small and subtle changes in behavior within the past hour. How does the nurse evaluate the patient's mental status throughout the night?
    a. Assess the patient while he or she is awake, and then allow him or her to sleep until morning.
    b. Ask the patient and family to describe the patient's normal sleep and behavioral patterns.
    c. Periodically attempt to awaken the patient and document how easily he or she is aroused.
    d. Allow the patient to sleep, but assess respiratory effort and skin temperature.

Matching. *Match the overall pathophysiology response that occurs with various types of shock.*

Types of Shock
a. Hypovolemic
b. Cardiogenic
c. Distributive
d. Obstructive

General Pathophysiology Responses
_____ 24. Total body fluid volume not affected

_____ 25. Fluid shifted from central vascular space

_____ 26. Total body fluid decreased (in all fluid compartments)

_____ 27. Direct pump failure

Matching. *Match either the colloid or crystalloid solution with each of the indications. Answers will be used more than once.*

Solutions
a. Colloid
b. Crystalloid

Indications
_____ 28. Hemorrhagic shock

_____ 29. Fluid replacement

_____ 30. Restore osmotic pressure

_____ 31. Carries oxygen to peripheral tissues

_____ 32. Does not cause allergic reactions

_____ 33. Substitute for blood

34. Identify solutions as colloids (Col) or crystalloids (Cry).

    _____ a. Normal saline

    _____ b. Hetastarch

    _____ c. Packed red cells

    _____ d. Ringer's lactate

    _____ e. Fresh frozen plasma (FFP)

35. The nurse is caring for a patient at risk for hypovolemic shock. Which indicators of shock does the nurse monitor for? *(Select all that apply.)*
    a. Elevated body temperature
    b. Increased peristalsis
    c. Decreasing urine output
    d. Vasodilation
    e. Increasing heart rate

36. Assessment findings of a patient with trauma injuries reveals cool, pale skin; reported thirst, urine output 100 mL/8 hr, blood pressure 122/78 mm Hg, pulse 102 beats/min, respirations 24/min with decreased breath sounds. This patient is in what phase of shock?
    a. Compensatory/nonprogressive
    b. Progressive
    c. Refractory
    d. Multiple organ dysfunction

37. A patient with blunt trauma to the abdomen has been NPO for several hours in preparation for a procedure and now reports subjective thirst. What is the nurse's priority action?
    a. Get the patient a few ice chips or a moistened toothette.
    b. Obtain an order for a stat hematocrit and hemoglobin.
    c. Take the patient's vital signs and compare to baseline.
    d. Obtain an order to increase the IV rate.

38. A patient is brought to the ED with a gunshot wound. The nurse closely monitors the patient for early signs of hypovolemic shock. What early signs does the nurse look for? *(Select all that apply.)*
    a. Elevated serum potassium level
    b. Marked decrease in blood pressure
    c. Decrease in oxygen saturation
    d. Increase in heart rate
    e. Increase in respiratory rate

39. The unlicensed assistive personnel (UAP) reports repeatedly and unsuccessfully trying to take a patient's blood pressure with the electronic and manual devices. The nurse notes that the patient's apical pulse is elevated and the patient is at risk for hypovolemic shock. The patient begins to deteriorate. What is the quickest way for the nurse to determine the systolic blood pressure?
    a. Apply the electronic device to a lower extremity.
    b. Instruct the UAP to immediately get the Doppler.
    c. Apply the manual cuff and palpate for the systolic.
    d. Tell the UAP to try the electronic device on the other arm.

40. The nurse identifies signs and symptoms of internal hemorrhage in a postoperative patient. What is included in the care of this patient in hypovolemic shock? *(Select all that apply.)*
    a. Elevate the feet with the head flat or elevated 30 degrees.
    b. Monitor vital signs every 5 minutes until they are stable.
    c. Administer clotting factors or plasma.
    d. Administer heparin.
    e. Provide oxygen therapy.
    f. Ensure IV access.
    g. Notify the Rapid Response Team.

41. A young trauma patient is at risk for hypovolemic shock related to occult hemorrhage. What baseline indicator allows the nurse to recognize the early signs of shock?
    a. Urine output
    b. Pulse rate
    c. Fluid intake
    d. Skin color

42. Which patient is most likely to show elevated hemoglobin and hematocrit during shock?
    a. Patient with severe vomiting and large watery diarrheal stools
    b. Patient with a large wound with copious drainage
    c. Patient who was stable after surgery, but is now decompensating
    d. Patient with a hemothorax and chest tube

43. A patient in hypovolemic shock is receiving sodium nitroprusside (Nitropress) to enhance myocardial perfusion. What is an important nursing implication for administering this drug?
    a. Assess the patient for headache because it is an early symptom of drug excess.
    b. Assess blood pressure at least every 15 minutes because hypertension is a symptom of overdose.
    c. Assess blood pressure at least every 15 minutes because systemic vasodilation can cause hypotension.
    d. Assess the patient every 30 minutes for extravasation because nitroprusside can cause severe vasoconstriction and tissue ischemia.

44. A patient is at risk for hypovolemia secondary to large amounts of watery diarrhea and vomiting. The patient reports feeling a little thirsty and a slightly lightheaded. What does the nurse do next?
    a. Take the blood pressure and pulse and compare results to the patient's baseline.
    b. Obtain an order to start a sodium nitroprusside (Nipride) IV infusion.
    c. Have the patient rest in bed and take small frequent sips of water.
    d. Compare the patient's intake to the urinary output.

45. A patient with hypovolemia is restless and anxious. The skin is cool and pale, pulse is thready at a rate of 135 beats/min; blood pressure is 92/50 mm Hg; respirations are 32/min. What actions does the nurse take? *(Select all that apply.)*
    a. Obtain a stat order for an IV normal saline bolus.
    b. Administer supplemental oxygen.
    c. Notify the Rapid Response Team.
    d. Place the patient in a semi-Fowler's position.
    e. Call a "code blue."

46. A patient is showing early clinical manifestations of hypovolemic shock. The physician orders an arterial blood gas (ABG). Which ABG values in does the nurse expect to see in hypovolemic shock?
    a. Increased pH with decreased Pao_2 and increased $Paco_2$
    b. Decreased pH with decreased Pao_2 and increased $Paco_2$
    c. Normal pH with decreased Pao_2 and normal $Paco_2$
    d. Normal pH with decreased Pao_2 and decreased $Paco_2$

47. The nurse finds a patient on the bathroom floor. There is a large amount of blood on the floor and on the patient's hospital gown. Which actions does the nurse take? *(Select all that apply.)*
    a. Elevate the patient's legs.
    b. Establish large-bore IV access.
    c. Look for the source of the bleeding.
    d. Ensure a patent airway.
    e. Begin a nitroprusside (Nitropress) infusion.

48. The nurse is caring for a postoperative patient who had major abdominal surgery. Which assessment finding is consistent with hypovolemic shock?
    a. Pulse pressure of 40 mm Hg
    b. A rapid, weak, and thready pulse
    c. Warm, flushed skin
    d. Increased urinary output

49. Which IV therapy results in the greatest increase in oxygen-carrying capacity for a patient with hypovolemic shock?
    a. Lactated Ringer's solution
    b. Hetastarch
    c. FFP
    d. Packed red cells

50. A patient comes to the ED with severe injury and significant blood loss. The nurse anticipates that resuscitation will begin with which fluid?
    a. Whole blood
    b. 0.5% dextrose in water
    c. 0.9% sodium chloride
    d. Plasma protein fractions

51. Which change in the skin is an early indication of hypovolemic shock?
    a. Pallor or cyanosis in the mucous membranes
    b. Color changes in the trunk area
    c. Axilla and groin feel moist or clammy
    d. Generalized mottling of skin

52. A patient is in hypovolemic shock related to hemorrhage from a large gunshot wound. Which order does the nurse question?
    a. Establish a large-bore peripheral IV and give crystalloid bolus.
    b. Give furosemide (Lasix) 20 mg slow IVP.
    c. Insert a Foley catheter and monitor intake and output.
    d. Give high-flow oxygen via mask at 10 L/min.

53. The nurse is performing a psychosocial assessment on a patient who is at risk for shock. Which statement made by the patient is of greatest concern to the nurse?
    a. "Do you have any idea when I might go home? No one is feeding my cat."
    b. "Something feels wrong, but I'm not sure what is causing me to feel this way."
    c. "I live alone in my house and my family lives in a different state."
    d. "I would usually go golfing with my friends today. I hope they're not worried about me."

54. A patient has a systemic infection with a fever, increased respiratory rate, and change in mental status. Which laboratory values does the nurse seek out that are considered "hallmark" of sepsis?
    a. Increased white blood count and increased glucose level
    b. Increased serum lactate level and rising band neutrophils
    c. Increased oxygen saturation and decreased clotting times
    d. Decreased white blood count with increased hematocrit

55. The nurse is caring for an older adult patient at risk for shock. What is an early sign of shock in this patient?
    a. Cool, clammy skin
    b. Decreased urinary output
    c. Restlessness
    d. Hypotension

56. The nurse is caring for a patient with sepsis. At the beginning of the shift, the patient is in a hypodynamic state. Several hours later, the patient's blood pressure is elevated and pulse is bounding. How does the nurse interpret this change?
    a. A positive response and a signal of recovery
    b. Temporary situation that is likely to normalize
    c. Worsening of the condition rather than improvement
    d. Expected response to standard therapies

57. The nurse is caring for a patient with sepsis. What is a late clinical manifestation of shock?
    a. Drop in blood pressure
    b. MAP is decreased by less than 10 mm Hg
    c. Tachycardia with a bounding pulse
    d. Increased urine output

58. The nurse is caring for a patient at risk for sepsis. Why does the nurse closely monitor the patient for early signs of shock?
    a. The patient is unable to self-identify or report these early signs.
    b. Distributive shock usually begins as a bacterial or fungal infection.
    c. Prevention of septic shock is easier to achieve in the early phase.
    d. There is widespread vasodilation and pooling of blood in some tissues.

59. A patient has a localized infection. What assessment findings are considered evidence of a beneficial inflammatory response?
    a. Decreased urine output which normalizes after fluid bolus
    b. Pulse rate of 120 beats/min related to increased metabolic activity
    c. Decreased oxygen saturation which responds to supplemental O_2
    d. Redness and edema that appear but subside in several days

60. The student nurse is assessing a patient's mental status because of the patient's risk for decreased tissue perfusion. The supervising nurse intervenes when the student nurse asks the patient which question?
    a. "What is today's date?"
    b. "Who is the president of this country?"
    c. "Where are we right now?"
    d. "Is your name Mr. John Smith?"

61. The nurse is caring for a patient at risk for septic shock from a wound infection. In order to prevent systemic inflammatory response syndrome, the nurse's priority is to monitor which factor?
    a. Patient's pulse rate and quality
    b. Patient's electrolyte imbalance
    c. Localized infected area
    d. Patient's intake and output

62. The nurse is evaluating the care and treatment for a patient in shock. Which finding indicates that the patient is having an appropriate response to the treatment?
    a. Blood pH of 7.28
    b. Arterial Po_2 of 65 mm Hg
    c. Distended neck veins
    d. Increased urinary output

63. The nurse is caring for a patient with septic shock. Which therapy specific to the management of shock for this patient does the nurse anticipate will be used?
    a. Inotropics
    b. Antibiotics
    c. Colloids
    d. Antidysrhythmics

64. A patient receives dopamine 20 mcg/kg/min IV for the treatment of shock. What does the nurse assess for while administering this drug?
    a. Decreased urine output and decreased blood pressure
    b. Increased respiratory rate and increased urine output
    c. Chest pain and hypertension
    d. Bradycardia and headache

65. When administering norepinephrine (Levophed), what does the nurse monitor for in the patient?
    a. Extravasation
    b. Profuse sweating
    c. High output renal failure
    d. Cough

66. The nurse is caring for a patient in septic shock. The nurse notes that the rate and depth of respirations is markedly increased. The nurse interprets this as a possible manifestation of the respiratory system compensating for which condition?
    a. Metabolic acidosis
    b. Metabolic alkalosis
    c. Respiratory acidosis
    d. Respiratory alkalosis

67. The ICU nurse observes petechiae, ecchymoses, and blood oozing from gums and other mucous membranes of a patient with septic shock. How does the nurse interpret this finding?
    a. Pulmonary emboli (PE)
    b. Acute respiratory distress syndrome (ARDS)
    c. Systemic inflammatory response syndrome (SIRS)
    d. Disseminated intravascular coagulation (DIC)

68. The nurse is reviewing the laboratory results of a patient with a systemic infection. What is the significance of a "left shift" in the differential leukocyte count?
    a. Expected finding because the patient has a serious infection.
    b. Indication that the infection is progressing toward resolution.
    c. Indication that the infection is outpacing the white cell production.
    d. Important to watch for trends, but otherwise not urgently significant.

69. The ICU nurse is caring for a patient with septic shock. Which IV infusion order for this patient does the nurse question?
    a. Antibiotics
    b. Insulin
    c. 10% dextrose in water
    d. Synthetic activated C protein

70. The nurse is preparing a teaching session for a patient at risk for septic shock. Which topics does the nurse include in this teaching? *(Select all that apply.)*
    a. Wash hands frequently using antimicrobial soap.
    b. Avoid aspirin and aspirin-containing products.
    c. Avoid large crowds or gatherings where people might be ill.
    d. Do not share utensils; wash toothbrushes in a dishwasher.
    e. Take temperature once a week.
    f. Do not change pet litter boxes.

71. A patient is at risk for sepsis. Which assessment finding is most indicative of the hyperdynamic activity that occurs in septic shock?
    a. Crackles in lung bases
    b. Weak, rapid peripheral pulses
    c. Cool, clammy, and cyanotic skin
    d. Increased pulse rate with warm, pink skin

72. The home health nurse is visiting a frail older adult patient at risk for sepsis because of failure to thrive and immunosuppression. What does the nurse assess this patient for? *(Select all that apply.)*
    a. Signs of skin breakdown and presence of redness or swelling
    b. Cough or any other symptoms of a cold or the flu
    c. Appearance and odor of urine, and pain or burning during urination
    d. Patient's and family's understanding of isolation precautions
    e. Presence of pets, especially cats, rodents, or reptiles
    f. Availability and type of facilities for hand-washing

73. A postoperative hospitalized patient has a decrease in MAP of greater than 20 mm Hg from baseline value; elevated, thready pulse; decreased blood pressure; shallow respirations of 26/min; pale skin; moderate acidosis; and moderate hyperkalemia. This patient is in what phase of shock?
    a. Compensatory/nonprogressive
    b. Progressive
    c. Refractory
    d. Multiple organ dysfunction

74. A 70-year-old man is admitted to the hospital with an infected finger of several days' duration. He is lethargic, confused, and has a temperature of 101.3° F. Other assessment findings include blood pressure of 94/50 mm Hg, pulse 105 beats/min, respirations 40, and shallow breathing. Pulmonary arterial wedge pressure (PAWP) is 4 mm Hg. These assessment findings indicate what type of shock?
    a. Hypovolemic
    b. Cardiogenic
    c. Anaphylactic
    d. Septic shock

75. The clinical manifestations in the first phase of sepsis-induced distributive shock results from the body's reaction to which factor?
    a. Leukocytes
    b. Endotoxins
    c. Hemorrhage
    d. Hypovolemia

76. What factor increases an older adult's risk for distributive (septic) shock?
    a. Reduced skin integrity
    b. Diuretic therapy
    c. Cardiomyopathy
    d. Musculoskeletal weakness

True or False? *Read each statement about shock and write T for true or F for false in the blanks provided. If the statement is false, correct the statement to make it true.*

_____ 77. Regardless of the cause, the pathophysiologic cellular response is the same for all types of shock.

_____ 78. When shock occurs, the body fails and death is the inevitable result.

_____ 79. The most reliable indicator that causes the nurse to suspect shock in the patient is changes in the systolic blood pressure.

_____ 80. Anaphylaxis results in widespread loss of blood vessel tone and decreased cardiac output.

_____ 81. Oxygen administration is appropriate therapy for any type of shock.

_____ 82. Examples of external causes of hypovolemic shock are trauma, wounds, and surgery.

_____ 83. Dehydration as a result of decreased fluid intake or increased fluid loss can cause hypovolemic shock.

_____ 84. Distributive shock is a result of a decrease in the MAP caused by a loss of sympathetic tone, blood vessel dilation, pooling of blood in venous and capillary beds, and increased blood vessel permeability (leak).

_____ 85. During the hyperdynamic phase of septic shock, the endotoxins cause a decrease in cardiac output.

_____ 86. The clinical manifestations of the first phase of septic shock are unique, often opposite to other types of shock.

Matching. *Match each type of patient who may be at risk with the corresponding type of shock. Answers may be used more than once.*

Types of Shock
a. Hypovolemic
b. Cardiogenic
c. Distributive-neurogenic
d. Obstructive
e. Distributive-chemical
f. Distributive-septic

Types of Patients

_____ 87. Patient with cardiac tamponade

_____ 88. Older adult with urinary tract infection

_____ 89. Patient who had an allergic reaction to a medication

_____ 90. Patient who had a myocardial infarction

_____ 91. Patient who had a ruptured aortic aneurysm

_____ 92. Patient with tension pneumothorax

_____ 93. Patient with insect bites

_____ 94. Patient with ruptured spleen resulting from trauma

_____ 95. Patient with pneumonia

_____ 96. Patient with pulmonary hypertension

_____ 97. Patient receiving heparin therapy

_____ 98. Older adult who has a spinal cord reunion

_____ 99. Patient with dehydration

_____ 100. Patient with diabetes insipidus

_____ 101. Older adult with sacral pressure ulcers

_____ 102. Patient who has upper GI bleeding, with a nasogastric tube

_____ 103. Patient with methicillin-resistant *Staphylococcus aureus* (MRSA) infection

_____ 104. Patient receiving excessive diuretic therapy

CASE STUDY: THE PATIENT WITH HYPOVOLEMIC SHOCK

Use a separate sheet of paper to answer the questions in this Case Study, or go to the "Prepare for Class" folder on your Evolve website at http://evolve.elsevier.com/Iggy/ to download and complete as a word processing file. Answer guidelines for this Case Study are also available on your Evolve website.

A 38-year-old female patient returned to the postanesthesia recovery area 2 hours ago after undergoing a tubal ligation by colposcopy (through the back wall of the vagina behind the cervix). Her last documented vital signs taken 30 minutes ago were blood pressure = 102/80 mm Hg, pulse = 88 beats/min, and respirations = 22/min. The nurse now notes that her face is pale and the skin around her lips has a bluish cast. She reports some back pain. Her vital signs are now blood pressure = 90/76 mm Hg, pulse = 98 beats/min, and respirations = 28/min.

1. What additional assessment data would the nurse want to obtain?
2. Where would the nurse look for the hemorrhage?

The nurse reassesses the patient 15 minutes later. Vital signs are blood pressure = 88/70 mm Hg, pulse = 102 beats/min, and respirations = 30/min. She awakens when the nurse shakes her arm and reports increased back pain and thirst.

3. Given these findings, which actions would be priority actions for the nurse?
4. What expected outcomes would be specific to this situation?
5. The primary health care provider has arrived in the PACU. Document the SBAR report that the nurse would give in the handoff.

CASE STUDY: THE PATIENT WITH SEPTIC SHOCK

Use a separate sheet of paper to answer the questions in this Case Study, or go to the "Prepare for Class" folder on your Evolve website at http://evolve.elsevier.com/Iggy/ to download and complete as a word processing file. Answer guidelines for this Case Study are also available on your Evolve website.

A 72-year-old male patient has been living in an assisted-living center. He is generally alert, cheerful, and ambulatory with a walker. He has had frequent bouts of urinary tract infections secondary to prostate problems and is being treated for high blood pressure. He was discovered today by one of the UAPs in his room in a lethargic and confused state. He was easily aroused, but irritable and uncooperative with simple commands. He is transported to the ED for an acute change in mental status. On arrival to the ED, vital signs are 110/70 mm Hg, pulse = 120 beats/min, respirations = 30/min, and temperature is 101° F.

1. What does the term *SIRS* stand for? Discuss how this patient meets or does not meet the criteria for SIRS. If the patient meets the criteria, what are the initial indicators of SIRS for this patient? Based on the criteria, what additional assessments and diagnostic tests should be performed?

2. Explain why a patient in severe septic shock could "look" better and have a warm flushed appearance?

3. Explain why the patient can have a massive infection with a low white count.

4. What is the purpose of the sepsis resuscitation and management bundles? Discuss the care and interventions of the patient using the bundle approach.

5. The patient recovers and is discharged back to the assisted-living facility. What types of information would the hospital nurse give to the nurse at the assisted-living facility regarding the patient? Use the SBAR format to document this handoff report.

40 CHAPTER

Care of Patients with Acute Coronary Syndromes

STUDY/REVIEW QUESTIONS

Matching. *Match the terms with their correct descriptions.*

Terms

a. Ischemia
b. Infarction
c. Angina pectoris
d. New-onset angina
e. Variant (Prinzmetal's) angina
f. Pre-infarction angina
g. Transmural myocardial infarction (MI)
h. Ventricular remodeling
i. Zone of necrosis
j. Zone of injury
k. Zone of ischemia

Descriptions

_____ 1. Chest pain that occurs in the days or weeks before an MI

_____ 2. Necrosis or cell death

_____ 3. All three layers of heart are involved

_____ 4. First angina symptoms, usually after exertion or other increased demands on the heart

_____ 5. "Strangling of the chest"

_____ 6. Scar tissue permanently changes the size and shape of the entire left ventricle

_____ 7. Tissue that is oxygen-deprived

_____ 8. Around the initial area of infarction

_____ 9. Chest pain or discomfort from coronary artery spasm; typically occurs after rest

_____ 10. Tissue that is injured but not necrotic

_____ 11. Occurs when insufficient oxygen is supplied to meet the requirements of the myocardium

12. The nurse is interviewing a patient reporting chest discomfort that occurs with moderate to prolonged exertion. The patient describes the pain as being "about the same over the past several months and going away with nitroglycerin or rest." Based on the patient's description of symptoms, what does the nurse suspect in this patient? *(Select all that apply.)*
    a. Chronic stable angina (CSA)
    b. Unstable angina
    c. Acute coronary syndrome (ACS)
    d. Acute myocardial infarction (MI)
    e. Coronary artery disease (CAD)

13. A patient with a history of angina is admitted for surgery. The patient reports nausea, pressure in the chest radiating to the left arm, appears anxious, skin is cool and clammy, blood pressure is 150/90 mm Hg, pulse is 100, and respiratory rate is 32. What are the priorities of nursing care for this patient? *(Select all that apply.)*
    a. Relieve anxiety
    b. Maintain NPO status
    c. Improve coronary perfusion
    d. Improve coronary oxygenation
    e. Relieve chest pain

14. A patient has been admitted for acute angina. Which diagnostic test identifies if the patient will benefit from further invasive management after acute angina or an MI?
    a. Exercise tolerance test
    b. Cardiac catheterization
    c. Thallium scan
    d. Multigated angiogram (MUGA) scan

15. The nurse is talking to a patient with angina about resuming sexual activity. Which statement by the patient indicates a correct understanding about the effects of angina on sexual activity?
    a. "I won't be able to resume the same level of physical exertion as I did before I had chest pain."
    b. "I will discuss alternative methods with my partner since I will no longer be able to have sexual intercourse."
    c. "If I cannot walk a mile, I am not strong enough to resume intercourse."
    d. "I can resume sexual activity after a rest period."

16. A patient with angina is prescribed nitroglycerin tablets. What information does the nurse include when teaching the patient about this drug? *(Select all that apply.)*
    a. "If one tablet does not relieve the angina after 5 minutes, take two pills."
    b. "You can tell the pills are active when your tongue feels a tingling sensation."
    c. "Keep your nitroglycerin with you at all times."
    d. "The prescription should last about 6 months before a refill is necessary."
    e. "If pain doesn't go away, just wait; the medication will eventually take effect."
    f. "The medication can cause a temporary headache or a flushed face."

17. A patient reports chest pain that is unrelieved with sublingual nitroglycerin. What drug does the nurse administer to this patient next?
    a. Valium intramuscularly
    b. Morphine sulfate IV
    c. Supplemental oxygen
    d. Chewable aspirin

18. A patient is hypertensive and continues to have angina despite therapy with beta blockers. The nurse anticipates which type of drug will be prescribed for this patient?
    a. Calcium channel blocker
    b. Digoxin
    c. Angiotensin-converting enzyme (ACE) inhibitor
    d. Dopamine

19. The nurse has just given a patient two doses of sublingual nitroglycerin for anginal pain. The patient's blood pressure is typically 130/80 mm Hg. Which finding warrants immediate notification of the health care provider?
    a. Patient reports a headache.
    b. Systolic pressure is 140 mm Hg.
    c. Systolic pressure is 90 mm Hg.
    d. Anginal pain continues but is somewhat relieved.

20. A patient is admitted for unstable angina. The patient is currently asymptomatic and all vital signs are stable. Which position does the nurse place the patient in?
    a. Any position of comfort
    b. Supine
    c. Sitting in a chair
    d. Fowler's

21. Place the steps for administering sublingual nitroglycerin to a patient with episodes of angina in the correct order using the numbers 1 through 5.

    _____ a. In 5-minute increments, a total of three doses may be administered in an attempt to relieve angina pain.

    _____ b. For no relief after dosing, immediately inform the health care provider and prepare the patient for transfer to a specialized unit.

    _____ c. Hold the tablet under the tongue so the tablet can dissolve.

    _____ d. After 5 minutes, recheck pain intensity and vital signs.

    _____ e. If the patient is experiencing some, but not complete, relief and vital signs remain stable, another tablet may be used.

22. Indicate whether the characteristics listed below are angina (A) or myocardial infarction (MI).

    _____ a. Pain is precipitated by exertion or stress.

    _____ b. Pain occurs without cause, usually in the morning.

    _____ c. Pain is relieved only by opioids.

    _____ d. Pain is relieved by nitroglycerin or rest.

    _____ e. Nausea, diaphoresis, feelings of fear, and dyspnea may occur.

    _____ f. There are few associated symptoms.

    _____ g. Pain lasts less than 15 minutes.

    _____ h. Pain lasts 30 minutes or more.

    _____ i. Pain radiates to left arm, back, or jaw.

True or False? Read each statement and write T for true or F for false in the blanks provided. If the statement is false, correct the statement to make it true.

_____ 23. Ischemia that occurs with angina is limited in duration and does not cause permanent damage of myocardial tissue.

_____ 24. Studies have shown that endothelial dysfunction may be the cause of CAD in women.

_____ 25. Postmenopausal women in their 70s have a higher incidence of MI than men.

_____ 26. Many patients suffering sudden cardiac arrest die before reaching the hospital due to ventricular fibrillation.

27. A patient is admitted for acute MI, but the nurse notes that the traditional manifestation of ST elevation MI (STEMI) is not occurring. What other evidence for acute MI does the nurse expect to find in the patient? *(Select all that apply.)*
    a. Positive troponin markers
    b. Chronic stable angina
    c. Non-ST elevation MI (non-STEMI)
    d. Cardiac dysrhythmia
    e. Heart failure

28. People should seek treatment for symptoms of MI rather than delay because physical changes will occur approximately how many hours after an infarction?
    a. 3
    b. 6
    c. 12
    d. 24

29. The nurse is caring for a patient admitted with unstable angina and elevated lipid levels. What does the nurse include in teaching this patient about his or her elevated lipid levels? *(Select all that apply.)*
    a. Begin a vigorous exercise program.
    b. Avoid trans-fatty acids.
    c. Reduce intake of saturated fats.
    d. Monitor the amount of cholesterol ingested, staying below 200 mg/day.
    e. Decrease weight.

30. The nurse is auscultating the heart of a patient who had an MI. Which finding most strongly indicates heart failure?
    a. Murmur
    b. S_3 gallop
    c. Split S_1 and S_2
    d. Pericardial friction rub

31. Which diagnostic tests are used to assess myocardial damage caused by an MI? *(Select all that apply.)*
    a. Positive chest x-ray
    b. Creatine kinase (CK) elevation
    c. ECG: ST depression
    d. CK-MB isoenzymes elevation
    e. Troponin I isoenzyme elevation

32. A patient has heart failure related to MI. What intervention does the nurse plan for this patient's care?
    a. Administering digoxin (Lanoxin) 1.0 mg as a loading dose and then daily
    b. Infusing IV fluids to maintain a urinary output of 60 mL/hr
    c. Titrating vasoactive drugs to maintain a sufficient cardiac output
    d. Observing for such complications as hypertension and flushed, hot skin

33. Which patient has the highest risk for death because of ventricular failure and dysrhythmias related to damage to the left ventricle?
    a. Patient with an anterior wall MI (AWMI)
    b. Patient with a posterior wall MI (PWMI)
    c. Patient with a lateral wall MI (LWMI)
    d. Patient with an inferior wall MI (IWMI)

34. A patient had an IWMI. The nurse closely monitors the patient for which dysrhythmia associated with IWMI?
    a. Bradycardia and second-degree heart block
    b. Premature ventricular contractions
    c. Supraventricular tachycardia
    d. Atrial fibrillation

35. The nurse is giving a community presentation about heart disease. Because 95% of sudden cardiac arrest victims die of ventricular fibrillation before reaching the hospital, which teaching point does the nurse emphasize?
    a. Controlling alcohol consumption and quitting cigarette smoking
    b. Modifying risk factors such as diet and weight, and blood pressure medication compliance
    c. Recognizing the difference between chronic stable angina and unstable angina
    d. Learning to operate the automatic external defibrillators (AEDs) in the workplace

36. What are indicators of metabolic syndrome, which increases the risk for coronary heart disease? *(Select all that apply.)*
    a. Triglyceride level of 170 mg/dL
    b. HDL cholesterol level of 45 mg/dL in a male
    c. HDL cholesterol level of 45 mg/dL in a female
    d. Blood pressure of 130/86 mm Hg
    e. Fasting blood sugar level of 120 mg/dL

37. A patient has high risk for CAD. What is the goal for this patient's LDL level?
    a. Less than 70 mg/dL
    b. Less than 100 mg/dL
    c. Below 135 mg/dL
    d. Below 200 mg/dL

38. A patient is trying to make dietary modifications to reduce lipid levels. The patient would like information about omega-3 fatty acid food sources. What best source does the nurse recommend?
    a. Flaxseed
    b. Flaxseed oil
    c. Fish
    d. Walnuts

True or False? Read each statement about CAD and write T for true or F for false in the blanks provided. If the statement is false, correct the statement to make it true.

_____ 39. Tobacco use, especially cigarette smoking, accounts for over 90% of deaths from CAD.

_____ 40. A person who stops smoking may decrease the risk of CAD by as much as 80% in 1 year.

_____ 41. Reducing the tar and nicotine content of the cigarettes smoked reduces the risk of CAD.

_____ 42. Less active, less fit people have a 30% to 50% greater risk of developing high blood pressure which predisposes to CAD.

_____ 43. Physical activity increases collateral circulation and reduces the size of existing plaques.

44. A patient comes to the walk-in clinic reporting left anterior chest discomfort with mild shortness of breath. The patient is alert, oriented, diaphoretic, and anxious. What is the priority action for the nurse?
    a. Obtain a complete cardiac history to include a full description of the presenting symptoms.
    b. Place the patient in Fowler's position and start supplemental oxygen.
    c. Instruct the patient to go immediately to the closest full-service hospital.
    d. Immediately alert the physician and establish IV access.

45. A patient reports having chest discomfort that started during exercise. The patient is currently pain-free, but "is concerned." What questions does the nurse ask to assess the patient's pain episode? *(Select all that apply.)*
    a. "When did the pain start and how long did it last?"
    b. "What were you doing when the pain started?"
    c. "What did you do to alleviate the pain?"
    d. "How did you feel about the pain?"
    e. "Did the pain radiate to other locations?"
    f. "Was the pain sharp and stabbing?"
    g. "On a scale of 0 to 10 with 10 as the worst pain, what number would you use to categorize the pain?"

46. A patient is currently pain- and symptom-free, but reports having intermittent episodes of chest pain over the past week. The nurse asks about which associated symptoms? *(Select all that apply.)*
    a. Nausea
    b. Diarrhea
    c. Diaphoresis
    d. Dizziness
    e. Joint pain
    f. Palpitations
    g. Shortness of breath

47. The emergency department (ED) nurse is assessing an 86-year-old patient with acute confusion, increased respiratory rate, anxiety, and chest pain. The nurse finds a respiratory rate of 36/min with crackles and wheezes on auscultation. How does the nurse interpret these findings?
    a. Left sided-heart failure
    b. Atypical angina
    c. CAD
    d. Unstable angina

48. The nurse is assessing a middle-aged woman with diabetes who denies any history of known heart problems. However, on auscultation of the heart the nurse hears an S₄ heart sound. The nurse alerts the physician and obtains an order for which diagnostic test?
    a. Blood glucose level
    b. ECG
    c. Chest x-ray
    d. Echocardiogram

49. A middle-aged African-American patient with no known medical problems has acute onset chest pain and dyspnea. In order to rule out acute MI, the nurse obtains orders for which diagnostic tests? *(Select all that apply.)*
    a. Myoglobin
    b. Triglyceride levels and C-reactive protein
    c. Chest x-ray, arterial blood gas
    d. Pulmonary function testing
    e. Total serum cholesterol, low-density lipoprotein, high-density lipoprotein
    f. Troponin T and I
    g. Creatine kinase-MB, myoglobin

50. A patient had severe chest pain several hours ago but is currently pain-free and has a normal ECG. Which statement by the patient indicates a correct understanding of the significance of the ECG results?
    a. "I'll go home and make an appointment to see my family doctor next week."
    b. "The ECG could be normal since I am currently pain-free."
    c. "A normal ECG means I am okay."
    d. "I have always had a strong heart, low blood pressure, and a normal ECG."

51. Which statement about silent MI is correct?
    a. In a silent MI, the patient does not have any pain, so there is less myocardial damage.
    b. Diabetic patients are prone to silent MI that goes undiagnosed without complications.
    c. Silent MI increases the incidence of new coronary events.
    d. In silent MI, the myocardium is oxygenated by increased collateral circulation.

52. The ED nurse is caring for a patient with acute pain associated with MI. What are the purposes of collaborative management that address the patient's pain? *(Select all that apply.)*
    a. Return the vital signs and cardiac rhythm to baseline, so the patient can resume activities of daily living.
    b. Prevent further damage to the cardiac muscle by decreasing myocardial oxygen demand and increasing myocardial oxygen supply.
    c. Aggressively diagnose and treat life-threatening cardiac dysrhythmias and restore pulmonary wedge pressure.
    d. Closely monitor the patient for accompanying symptoms such as nausea and vomiting or indigestion.
    e. Eliminate discomfort by providing pain relief modalities, decrease myocardial oxygen demand, and increase myocardial oxygen supply.

53. The ED nurse caring for a patient with severe chest pain and ECG changes gives supplemental oxygen to the patient as ordered. Which other medications does the nurse anticipate giving to this patient? *(Select all that apply.)*
    a. IV nitroglycerin
    b. Beta blocker
    c. IV morphine
    d. Oral aspirin
    e. ACE inhibitor

54. The nurse is caring for a hospitalized patient being treated initially with IV nitroglycerin. What intervention does the nurse include in this patient's care?
    a. Increase the dose rapidly to achieve pain relief.
    b. Assist the patient to the bathroom as needed.
    c. Monitor blood pressure continuously.
    d. Elevate the head of the bed to 90 degrees

55. A patient is currently on oxygen therapy for chest pain. The pulse oximetry is on and signals an abrupt drop from 93% to 89%. What is the priority action for the nurse?
    a. Alert the Rapid Response Team.
    b. Troubleshoot the oxygen setup and the pulse oximeter sensor.
    c. Increase the oxygen flow rate and elevate the head of the bed.
    d. Advise the patient to watch the monitor and take several deep breaths.

56. The home health nurse receives a call from a patient with CAD who reports having new onset of chest pain and shortness of breath. What does the nurse direct the patient to do?
    a. Rest quietly until the nurse can arrive at the house to check the patient.
    b. Chew 325 mg of aspirin and immediately call 911.
    c. Use supplemental home oxygen until symptoms resolve.
    d. Take three nitroglycerin tablets and have family drive the patient to the hospital.

57. A patient is newly diagnosed with cardiovascular disease. What psychosocial reactions does the nurse assess for? *(Select all that apply.)*
    a. Fear
    b. Anxiety
    c. Anger
    d. Suspicion
    e. Denial
    f. Euphoria
    g. Depression

58. Which drug is given within 1 to 2 hours of an MI, if the patient is hemodynamically stable, to help the heart to perform more work without ischemia?
    a. Vasodilators, such as sublingual or spray nitroglycerin (NTG)
    b. Beta-adrenergic blocking agents, such as metoprolol (Lopressor)
    c. Antiplatelet agents, such as clopidogrel (Plavix)
    d. Calcium channel blockers, such as diltiazem (Cardizem)

59. Which statements are true about the use of thrombolytic agents for a patient with an acute MI? *(Select all that apply.)*
    a. A patient who has received a thrombolytic agent must be continuously monitored before and after the medication is given.
    b. Thrombolytic therapy is indicated for chest pain of longer than 30 minutes duration that is unrelieved by other medications.
    c. There are no contraindications to thrombolytic therapy if the patient is having an acute MI as evidenced by cardiac enzymes and ECG.
    d. Bleeding is a risk for patients receiving thrombolytic therapy.
    e. The nurse need only monitor clotting studies of the patient who has received thrombolytic therapy. No further assessment is needed.

60. The health care provider is considering use of thrombolytic therapy for a patient. What is the criterion for this therapy?
    a. Chest pain of greater than 15 minutes' duration that is unrelieved by nitroglycerin
    b. Indications of transmural ischemia and injury as shown by the ECG
    c. Ventricular dysrhythmias shown on the cardiac monitor
    d. History of chronic, severe, poorly controlled hypertension

61. A patient is being evaluated for thrombolytic therapy. What are contraindications for this procedure? *(Select all that apply.)*
    a. Ischemic stroke within 3 months
    b. Pregnancy
    c. Surgery within the last 10 days
    d. Major trauma in the last 12 months
    e. Intracranial hemorrhage
    f. Malignant intracranial neoplasm
    g. Deep vein thrombosis

62. A patient has received thrombolytic therapy for treatment of acute MI. What are post-administration nursing responsibilities for this treatment? *(Select all that apply.)*
    a. Document the patient's neurologic status.
    b. Observe all IV sites for bleeding and patency.
    c. Monitor WBC count and differential.
    d. Monitor clotting studies.
    e. Monitor hemoglobin and hematocrit.
    f. Test stools, urine, and emesis for occult blood.

63. A patient is receiving beta-blocker therapy for treatment of MI. What does the nurse monitor for in relation to this therapy? *(Select all that apply.)*
    a. Tachycardia
    b. Hypotension
    c. Decreased level of consciousness
    d. Chest discomfort
    e. Increased urinary output

64. A patient is being treated with medication therapy following an acute MI. The nurse questions the order for which type of drug?
    a. Calcium channel blocker
    b. Beta-blocker
    c. Angiotensin-converting enzyme (ACE) inhibitor
    d. Angiotensin receptor blocker (ARB)

65. A patient with angina is taking calcium channel blockers. What does the nurse monitor the patient for?
    a. Wheezes
    b. Hypotension
    c. Bradycardia
    d. Forgetfulness

66. Which diagnostic test is performed after angina or MI to determine cardiac changes that are consistent with ischemia, to evaluate medical interventions, and to determine whether invasive intervention is necessary?
    a. Stress test
    b. ECG
    c. Echocardiography
    d. Chest x-ray

67. The nurse is monitoring a patient who had fibrinolytics and percutaneous transluminal coronary angioplasty (PTCA). What is an indication that the clot has lysed and the artery reperfused?
    a. Abrupt increase of pain or discomfort
    b. Sudden onset of ventricular dysrhythmias
    c. Appearance of ST-segment depression
    d. Obvious T wave inversion

68. A patient has had an MI. The nurse anticipates which type of drug will be prescribed within 48 hours to prevent the development of heart failure?
    a. Calcium channel blockers
    b. ACE inhibitor
    c. Beta blockers
    d. Digoxin

69. The nurse has identified the priority problem of Activity Intolerance for a patient who had an acute MI. What is the best expected outcome for this patient?
    a. Patient will walk at least 200 feet four times a day without chest discomfort or shortness of breath.
    b. Patient will name three or four activities that will not cause shortness of breath or chest pain.
    c. Nurse will teach the patient to exercise and to take the pulse if symptoms of shortness of breath or pain occur.
    d. Nurse will assist the patient with ADLs until shortness of breath or pain resolves.

70. A patient is in the acute phase (phase 1) of cardiac rehabilitation. Which task is best to delegate to the unlicensed assistive personnel (UAP)?
    a. Assist the patient to ambulate approximately 200 feet three times a day.
    b. Assist the patient with ambulation to the bathroom.
    c. Assess heart rate, blood pressure, respiratory rate, and fatigue with each higher level of activity.
    d. Assist the patient into the bathtub.

71. A patient in the cardiac rehabilitation facility is having difficulty coping with the changes in her health status. Which statement by the patient is the strongest indicator of ineffective or harmful coping?
    a. "I don't mind going to therapy, but I'm not sure if I'm getting any benefit from it."
    b. "I'll take the pills and just do whatever you want me to do."
    c. "I don't want to go to therapy; I had a bad experience yesterday with the therapist."
    d. "I know I need to talk about going home soon, but could we discuss it later?"

72. A post-MI patient in phase 1 cardiac rehabilitation is encouraged to perform which activity?
    a. Range-of-motion exercises
    b. Modified weight training
    c. Stair climbing
    d. Jogging

73. The nurse is caring for a patient admitted for an inferior wall MI. The patient develops heart block with bradycardia. Because the patient's pulse rate is low and the blood pressure is unstable, which procedure is the nurse prepared to assist with?
    a. Temporary pacemaker
    b. Defibrillation
    c. 16-lead ECG
    d. Percutaneous intervention

74. The nurse is contacted by the cardiac monitoring technician who says a patient is having a dysrhythmia. What does the nurse do next?
    a. Identify the dysrhythmia.
    b. Administer antidysrhythmic medication.
    c. Evaluate for chest pain or discomfort.
    d. Double-check the lead placement.

75. The nurse is evaluating a patient with CAD. What is an expected patient outcome that demonstrates hemodynamic stability?
    a. Blood pressure and pulse within range and adequate for metabolic demands
    b. An increase in urine output
    c. Regular P waves and no abnormal heart sounds
    d. Verbal understanding of risk factors and need for compliance

76. The nurse is assessing a patient at risk for left ventricular failure and inadequate organ perfusion. Which signs and symptoms signal decreased cardiac output? *(Select all that apply.)*
    a. Change in orientation or mental status
    b. Urine output less than 1 mL/kg (2.2 lbs)/hr or less than 30 mL/hr
    c. Hot, dry skin with flushed appearance
    d. Cool, clammy extremities with decreased or absent pulses
    e. Unusual fatigue
    f. Recurrent chest pain

77. The nurse is reviewing medication orders for several cardiac patients. There is an order for beta-adrenergic blocking agent metoprolol XL (Toprol XR) once a day. This drug order is most appropriate for which class of patients according to the Killip classification system?
    a. All classes
    b. Class I only
    c. Class II and III
    d. Class IV only

78. The nurse is caring for a patient with an anterior wall MI (AWMI). The patient develops tachycardia, hypotension, urine output of 10 mL/hr, cold and clammy skin with poor peripheral pulses, and agitation. What does the nurse suspect in this patient?
    a. Ventricular dysrhythmia
    b. Cardiogenic shock
    c. Post-pericardiotomy syndrome
    d. Acute coronary syndrome

79. The nurse is assessing a cardiac patient and finds a paradoxical pulse, clear lungs, and jugular venous distention that occurs when the patient is in a semi-Fowler's position. What are these findings consistent with?
    a. Right ventricle failure
    b. Unstable angina
    c. CAD
    d. Valvular disease

80. The intensive care nurse is monitoring a patient with a right ventricular MI. The pulmonary artery wedge pressure (PAWP) reading is 30 mm Hg. What does the nurse do next?
    a. Increase the IV fluid rate to 200 mL/hour.
    b. Auscultate the lungs to assess for left-sided heart failure.
    c. Perform an ECG using right-sided precordial leads.
    d. Place the patient in semi-Fowler's position.

81. A patient continues to have chest pain despite compliance with medical therapy. The nurse teaches the patient about which diagnostic test?
    a. Left-sided cardiac catheterization with coronary angiogram
    b. PTCA
    c. Coronary artery bypass grafting (CABG)
    d. Stent placement in coronary artery

82. Immediate reperfusion is an invasive intervention that shows some promise for managing which disorder?
    a. Right ventricular failure
    b. Metabolic syndrome
    c. Cardiogenic shock
    d. Acute coronary syndrome

83. A patient is scheduled to have PTCA. The nurse anticipates that an initial dose of which medication will be given before the procedure?
    a. Clopidogrel (Plavix)
    b. Nitroglycerin (Nitrostat)
    c. Isosorbide mononitrate (Imdur)
    d. Carvedilol (Coreg)

84. A patient has angina and is scheduled for PTCA. Based on outcomes of the PTCA, the nurse prepares the patient for immediate transfer to undergo which procedure?
    a. Intra-aortic balloon pump
    b. CABG
    c. Cardiac catheterization
    d. Carotid endarterectomy

85. The nurse is caring for a patient who had PTCA. Which symptom indicates acute closure of the vessel and therefore warrants immediate notification of the health care provider?
    a. Chest pain
    b. Hyperkalemia
    c. Bleeding at the insertion site
    d. Cough and shortness of breath

86. Which patients may be potential candidates for CABG? *(Select all that apply.)*
    a. Patient with angina and greater than 50% occlusion of left main coronary artery that cannot be stented
    b. Patient with unstable angina with moderate vessel disease appropriate for stenting
    c. Patient with valvular disease
    d. Patient with coronary vessels unsuitable for PTCA
    e. Patient with acute MI responding to therapy
    f. Patient with signs of ischemia or impending MI after angiography or PTCA

87. A patient is trying to decide whether to consent to a CABG. What information does the nurse give the patient? *(Select all that apply.)*
    a. CABG improves the quality of life for most patients.
    b. Most patients are pain-free at 1 year after surgery.
    c. 70% of patients will remain permanently pain-free.
    d. Most patients have a decreased quality of life after 15 years.
    e. Most patients remain pain-free 5 years after surgery, but some patients experience some pain after 5 years.

88. A patient is having an elective CABG with a minimally invasive surgical technique. What does the nurse include in the preoperative teaching?
    a. Prevention of edema and scarring at the harvest site
    b. Protection and splinting of the chest incision while coughing
    c. Availability of analgesics if needed, but probably unnecessary
    d. Limitation of ambulation for several days after the procedure

89. A patient is having a CABG with the traditional surgical procedure. What does the nurse include in the preoperative teaching? *(Select all that apply.)*
    a. Expect a small 1- to 2-inch incision on the leg.
    b. There will be a sternal incision.
    c. Expect one, two, or three chest tubes.
    d. An indwelling urinary catheter will be placed.
    e. An endotracheal tube will prevent talking.

90. The intensive care nurse is caring for a patient who has just had a CABG. The nurse notes that the patient has edema. In order to adjust fluid administration, the nurse collects which additional information and then consults the health care provider? *(Select all that apply.)*
    a. Blood pressure
    b. PAWP
    c. Skin turgor
    d. Cardiac output
    e. Blood loss
    f. Urine output

91. A potassium bolus of 80 mEq mixed in 100 mL of IV solution at a rate of 40 mEq/hr is ordered for a patient in the critical care unit. What does the nurse do next?
    a. Contact the health care provider because the order exceeds the recommended amount.
    b. Give the infusion; the order exceeds the recommended amount, but is within acceptable standards of practice for critical care patients.
    c. Contact the health care provider because even though the dosage is acceptable, the rate is too fast.
    d. Consult with the pharmacist because even though the rate is acceptable, the mixture is too concentrated.

92. The intensive care nurse is caring for a patient who has just had a CABG. The patient has a systolic blood pressure of 80 mm Hg. What is the primary concern related to this patient's hypotension?
    a. It is associated with warm cardioplegia.
    b. It may result in the collapse of the graft.
    c. It will result in acute tubular necrosis.
    d. It is related to mechanical ventilation.

93. Following a CABG, a patient has a body temperature below 96.8° F (36° C). What measures (if any) should be used to rewarm the patient?
    a. Infuse warm IV fluids.
    b. Do not rewarm; cold cardioplegia is protective.
    c. Place the patient in a warm fluid bath.
    d. Use lights or thermal blankets.

94. The intensive care nurse is caring for a patient who has just had a CABG. What does the nurse do to assess for postoperative bleeding?
   a. Measure mediastinal and pleural chest tube drainage at least hourly and report drainage amounts over 150 mL/hr to the surgeon.
   b. Measure mediastinal and pleural chest tube drainage at least once a shift and report drainage amounts over 50 mL/hr to the surgeon.
   c. Assess the dressing over the sternal site every 4 hours and reinforce the dressing with sterile gauze as needed.
   d. Assess the donor site every 4 hours and report serous drainage and increasing pain to the surgeon.

95. Following a CABG, a patient in the ICU on a mechanical ventilator suddenly decompensates. The health care provider makes a diagnosis of cardiac tamponade. The nurse prepares the patient for which emergency procedure?
   a. Chest tube
   b. Sternotomy
   c. Pericardiocentesis
   d. Thoracentesis

96. The nurse is assessing a patient who had a CABG. Which finding is a permanent deficit that is associated with an intraoperative stroke?
   a. Decreased level of consciousness that resolves when body temperature is normal
   b. Arousal from anesthesia which takes several hours
   c. Inability to speak clearly and coherently immediately after surgery
   d. Generalized seizure activity

97. A patient reports pain after a CABG. Which statement by the patient suggests that the pain is related to the sternotomy and not anginal in origin?
   a. "The pain goes down my arm or sometimes into my jaw."
   b. "My pain increases when I cough or take a deep breath."
   c. "The nitroglycerin helped to relieve the pain."
   d. "I feel nausea and shortness of breath when the pain occurs."

98. A patient with a CABG is transferred from the ICU to the intermediate care unit. Which activity does the nurse assist the patient with?
   a. Ambulating 25 to 100 feet three times a day as tolerated
   b. Turning the patient every 2 hours for the first 48 hours
   c. Dangling and turning every 2 hours for at least 24 hours
   d. Coughing and deep-breathing three times a day

99. A patient had CABG with the radial artery used as a graft. The nurse performs which assessment specific to this patient?
   a. Check the blood pressure every hour on the unaffected arm or use the legs.
   b. Check the fingertips, hand, and arm for sensation and mobility every shift.
   c. Assess hand color, temperature, ulnar/radial pulses, and capillary refill every hour initially.
   d. Note edema, bleeding, and swelling at the donor site, which are expected.

100. A patient with a CABG has been diagnosed with mediastinitis. What information does the nurse expect to find in the patient's assessment documentation? *(Select all that apply.)*
   a. Fever continuing beyond the first 4 days after CABG
   b. Bogginess of the sternum
   c. Redness and drainage from suture sites
   d. Decreased white blood cell count
   e. Induration or swelling at the suture sites
   f. Anginal-type chest pain

101. A patient had a CABG with a vein graft. To help prevent collapse of the graft, what assessment does the nurse perform?
   a. Auscultate lung sounds
   b. Monitor for hypotension
   c. Assess for motion and sensation
   d. Observe for generalized hypothermia

102. The nurse is caring for a patient who had a CABG. The nurse pays close attention to which electrolyte levels for this postoperative patient? *(Select all that apply.)*
    a. Sodium
    b. Potassium
    c. Calcium
    d. Magnesium
    e. Phosphorus

103. After a CABG, a postoperative patient suddenly has a decrease in mediastinal drainage, jugular vein distention with clear lung sounds, pulsus paradoxus, and equalizing PAWP and right atrial pressure. Of what does the nurse suspect these are signs?
    a. Acute MI
    b. Occlusion at the donor site
    c. Cardiac tamponade
    d. Prinzmetal's angina

104. The nurse coming on duty receives the change of shift report. Which patient is assessed first by the nurse?
    a. Patient with anxiety, nausea, diaphoresis, and shortness of breath
    b. Patient with diabetes mellitus and elevated serum lipid levels
    c. Patient with a friction rub and elevated temperature
    d. Patient with fever, instability of sternum, and increased white blood cell count

105. The nurse is caring for a patient who had a minimally invasive direct coronary artery bypass (MIDCAB). Which sign/symptom prompts the nurse to immediately contact the health care provider?
    a. Acute incisional pain
    b. ST-segment changes in the V leads
    c. Drainage from the chest tubes
    d. Problems with coughing

106. A patient has discrete, proximal, noncalcified lesions of only one or two vessels. Which procedure is most likely to be recommended for this patient?
    a. PTCA
    b. Stress test
    c. Immediate reperfusion
    d. Thrombolytic therapy

107. The nurse is caring for a patient who had a PTCA. Which postoperative interventions are included in the care for this patient? *(Select all that apply.)*
    a. Monitor for acute closure of the vessel.
    b. Observe for bleeding from the insertion site.
    c. Assess for reaction to the dye.
    d. Observe for hypotension, hypokalemia, and dysrhythmias.
    e. Teach about medications such as aspirin and beta blockers or ACE inhibitors.
    f. Instruct about lifestyle changes relating to CAD.

108. Treatment of hypothermia, a common problem after CABG surgery, with warming blankets is necessary because this condition may cause a patient to be at risk for which condition?
    a. Hypotension
    b. Hypertension
    c. Heart failure
    d. Loss of consciousness

109. Which statement is true about post-pericardiotomy syndrome?
    a. It is a psychological disorder for which the patient needs emotional support.
    b. It is generally mild and self-limiting.
    c. It places the patient at high risk for cardiac tamponade.
    d. It can be prophylactically managed with antibiotics

Matching. Match the different types of therapy with the correct descriptions.

Terms

a. Minimally invasive direct coronary artery bypass (MIDCAB)
b. Endovascular (endoscopic) vessel harvesting (EVH)
c. Transmyocardial laser revascularization
d. Off-pump coronary artery bypass (OPCAB)
e. Robotic heart surgery

Descriptions

_____ 110. Eliminates tremors that can exist with human hands, increases the ability to reach inaccessible sites, and improves depth perception and visual acuity.

_____ 111. Patient has one or two very small incisions in the leg or arm.

_____ 112. Cardiopulmonary bypass (CPB) is not required.

_____ 113. Creates channels that will eventually allow oxygenated blood to flow during diastole from the left ventricle to nourish the muscle.

_____ 114. Procedure in which open heart surgery is performed without the use of a heart-lung bypass machine.

CASE STUDY: THE PATIENT WITH ANGINA

Use a separate sheet of paper to answer the questions in this Case Study, or go to the "Prepare for Class" folder on your Evolve website at http://evolve.elsevier.com/Iggy/ to download and complete as a word processing file. Answer guidelines for this Case Study are also available on your Evolve website.

A 68-year-old woman arrives in the emergency department stating to the nurse, "I think I had a heart attack." She states that earlier that day while on her daily 3-mile walk, she had an episode of chest pain that lasted a couple of minutes but was resolved with rest. The pain returned shortly after arriving home. Again the pain was relieved with rest. On admission to the ED her ECG rhythm is normal sinus rhythm. She has no abnormal heart sounds or laboratory values. VS are stable. Po_2 by pulse oximetry is 97% on room air. She is diagnosed with angina. The patient is seen by a cardiologist who prescribes nitroglycerin tablets and one aspirin per day.

1. What differences in assessment/clinical data would the nurse expect if the patient was experiencing a myocardial infarction?
2. What would the nurse explain to the patient about the diagnosis of angina?
3. What teaching would the nurse provide for this patient regarding her diagnosis of angina?
4. What instructions should this patient have received regarding managing her chest pain at home?

Six months later the patient returns to the ED via EMS, reporting sudden onset midsternal chest pain radiating to the jaw. The pain occurred without activity and is unrelieved with two sublingual nitroglycerin tablets. EMS initiated two IV sites in the right and left AC spaces with 20-gauge angiocatheters. Infusing to each is 1000 mL of 0.9% normal saline KVO. Oxygen is delivered via nasal cannula at 2 L/min. Initial vital signs are blood pressure 175/99 mm Hg, heart rate 102, respirations 24, temperature 99° F, pulse oximetry 98% on 2 L of oxygen. The patient is diaphoretic, short of breath, and states she has felt nauseated for several hours. An ECG is completed and reviewed by the physician who states there are elevated ST segments across the precordium. A STEMI alert is called, and blood is drawn for cardiac enzymes and routine admission lab work.

The patient receives two doses of 81 mg of aspirin PO. Sublingual nitroglycerin is administered without relief. Next, 4 mg of MSO_4 slow IV push is administered via the right IV site for which the patient states relief of pain. The patient's belongings are given to a family member. The physician and nurse discuss percutaneous transluminal coronary angioplasty with the patient and family, the patient agrees to the procedure, and a consent form is signed. The patient is transferred to the cath lab with both side rails elevated.

5. Document in free-text timeframes the above episode as the patient is admitted to the PCU.

CASE STUDY: THE PATIENT WITH CORONARY ARTERY DISEASE

Use a separate sheet of paper to answer the questions in this Case Study, or go to the "Prepare for Class" folder on your Evolve website at http://evolve.elsevier.com/Iggy/ to download and complete as a word processing file. Answer guidelines for this Case Study are also available on your Evolve website.

The patient is a 40-year-old African-American man with a history of hypertension. He is in for an annual physical and admits that he has experienced chest pain "a time or two" when he takes the stairs at work, so lately he has avoided the stairs. The chest pain subsided once he rested for a few minutes in his office. He smokes one pack of cigarettes per day. He is 5' 8" and weighs 250 lbs. He takes hydrochlorothiazide and metoprolol (Lopressor) for his hypertension. His last serum cholesterol level was 220 mg/dL, with the HDL 35 mg/dL and LDL 105 mg/dL. His father died of an MI at age 54 and his mother has hypertension. He works 50 hours a week as a lawyer and takes occasional walks on weekends.

1. What are this patient's modifiable risks for CAD? What are his nonmodifiable risks for CAD?

2. What patient education would you provide for this patient?

3. Explain to this patient his risk factors for developing CAD.

41 CHAPTER

Assessment of the Hematologic System

STUDY/REVIEW QUESTIONS

True or False? *Read each statement about blood components and write T for true or F for false in the blanks provided. If the statement is false, correct the statement to make it true.*

_____ 1.   Erythrocytes are the largest proportion of blood cells.

_____ 2.   Blood is composed of plasma and cells.

_____ 3.   The three major types of plasma proteins are albumin, globulins, and fibrinogen.

_____ 4.   Globulins increase the osmotic pressure of the blood, preventing plasma from leaking into the tissues.

_____ 5.   Healthy mature RBCs have a life span of about 30 days.

_____ 6.   Iron is an essential part of hemoglobin.

_____ 7.   The most important feature of hemoglobin is its ability to combine loosely with oxygen.

_____ 8.   Erythropoiesis is the selective growth of stem cells into mature erythrocytes.

_____ 9.   The liver produces RBC growth factor erythropoietin at the same rate as RBC destruction or loss occurs to maintain a constant normal level of circulating RBCs.

_____ 10.   Leukocytes perform actions important for protection through inflammation and immunity.

_____ 11.   Platelets are the largest of the blood cells.

_____ 12.   Platelets perform most of their functions by aggregation.

_____ 13.   The spleen is the site for production of prothrombin and most blood clotting factors.

_____ 14.   Vitamin D is the vitamin that plays the most important role in the production of blood clotting factors VII, IX, and X and prothrombin.

_____ 15.   After a splenectomy, patients are less able to rid themselves of disease-causing organisms and are at greater risk for infection and sepsis.

True or False? *Read the statements about hemostasis and blood clotting and write T for true or F for false in the blanks provided. If the statement is false, correct the statement to make it true.*

_____ 16. Platelets normally circulate as individual cell-like structures and do not aggregate until activated.

_____ 17. Platelet plugs are clots that provide complete hemostasis.

_____ 18. Substances that cause platelets to clump include adenosine diphosphate (ADP), calcium, thromboxane A_2, and collagen.

_____ 19. The blood clotting cascade is triggered by the formation of a platelet plug.

_____ 20. Extrinsic factors that induce platelet plugs to form are usually the result of changes in blood vessels rather than in the blood.

_____ 21. Fibrin clot formation is the last phase of blood clotting.

_____ 22. Fibrinolysis prevents overenlargement of the fibrin clot.

_____ 23. Plasmin is a protein that digests fibrin.

_____ 24. A person who has a deficiency of any anti-clotting factor has an increased risk for pulmonary embolism, myocardial infarction, and stroke.

25. The nurse is performing a hematologic assessment in the older adult patient. Which findings does the nurse identify as normal changes in the older adult? *(Select all that apply.)*
    a. Progressive loss of body hair
    b. Thickened or discolored nails
    c. Yellowing of the skin
    d. Dryness of the skin
    e. Ecchymosis

26. Which statement about hematologic changes associated with aging is true?
    a. The older adult has increased blood volume.
    b. The older adult has increased levels of plasma proteins.
    c. Platelet counts decrease with age.
    d. Antibody levels and responses are lower and slower in older adults.

27. The nurse is interviewing the patient who reports dizziness and lightheadedness, and bleeding gums every time she brushes her teeth. Based on Gordon's Functional Health Patterns, which questions does the nurse ask the patient in order to focus in on the problem? *(Select all that apply.)*
    a. "How often do you take aspirin or any other nonsteroidal anti-inflammatory drug?"
    b. "How often do you eat salads or other green leafy vegetables?"
    c. "How much meat do you eat in a week?"
    d. "How much exercise do you get?"
    e. "Does your heart ever seem to pound?"

28. Which drug disrupts platelet action?
    a. Vitamin K
    b. Ibuprofen
    c. Methyldopa
    d. Azathioprine

True or False? *Read each statement and write T for true or F for false in the blanks provided. If the statement is false, correct the statement to make it true.*

_____ 29. Anticoagulants break down existing clots.

_____ 30. Anticoagulant drugs are classified as thrombin inhibitors, vitamin K antagonists, and indirect factor X inhibitors.

_____ 31. Platelet inhibitors are drugs that either prevent platelets from becoming active or prevent activated platelets from clumping together.

_____ 32. Aspirin inhibits the production of substances that can trigger platelet activation such as thromboxane.

_____ 33. The use of fibrinolytic drugs is limited to 6 hours because the drugs are inactive after this time.

_____ 34. Fibrinolytic drugs are used for the treatment of embolic strokes.

35. Which symptom is the single most common symptom of anemia?
    a. Fatigue
    b. Dizziness
    c. Palpitations
    d. Tinnitus

36. When assessing the patient with darker skin for pallor and cyanosis, which parts of the body does the nurse examine? *(Select all that apply.)*
    a. Palms of the hands
    b. Soles of the feet
    c. Outer surface of the cheeks
    d. Oral mucous membranes
    e. Conjunctiva of the eye

37. Severe anemia could cause enlargement of which organs? *(Select all that apply.)*
    a. Heart
    b. Kidneys
    c. Spleen
    d. Liver
    e. Gallbladder
    f. Colon

38. Which statement is true about tests to measure bleeding and coagulation?
    a. Heparin therapy is monitored using PT levels.
    b. The International Normalized Ratio (INR) measures the same process as the PTT.
    c. The partial thromboplastin time (PTT) assesses the extrinsic clotting cascade.
    d. Platelet aggregation is tested by mixing the patient's plasma with a substance called *ristocetin*.

True or False? *Read the statements about bone marrow aspiration and biopsy and write T for true or F for false in the blanks provided. If the statement is false, correct the statement to make it true.*

_____ 39. An informed consent is needed for a bone marrow aspiration and biopsy.

_____ 40. The patient should be told that a heavy sensation of pressure and pushing will be felt while the needle is being inserted.

_____ 41. The most common site for bone marrow aspiration and biopsy is the sternum.

_____ 42. Aspirin is commonly used to treat the discomfort often experienced by patients after a bone marrow aspiration and biopsy.

_____ 43. If the iliac crest is used for the bone marrow biopsy or aspiration, the patient should be placed in the prone or side-lying position.

CASE STUDY: HEMATOLOGIC ASSESSMENT

Use a separate sheet of paper to answer the questions in this Case Study, or go to the "Prepare for Class" folder on your Evolve website at http://evolve.elsevier.com/Iggy/ to download and complete as a word processing file. Answer guidelines for this Case Study are also available on your Evolve website.

The patient is a 45-year-old woman who is married to a career military officer. Her father was a miner, leading an itinerant life as he worked in uranium mines. She grew up in a western state and remembers playing with other children on slag heaps from the mines. She recalls being ill often as a child and attributes this to being chronically undernourished. The family was often cold during the winter months when there was no money to buy warm clothing or fuel for heat.

Over the past 6 months, the patient has had episodes of epistaxis and prolonged bleeding after having her teeth cleaned by a dental hygienist. She has also noticed that she seems to bruise easily; there are multiple ecchymotic areas on her legs and arms. She reported to the military hospital for a checkup and was referred to a regional civilian hospital for further evaluation. During the admission history, she tells the nurse that she tires easily and often has little energy. Her husband and children are worried about her.

1. What additional assessment data should the nurse elicit from the patient at this time?

2. As part of the diagnostic workup, the patient is scheduled to have blood work drawn for CBC, PT, PTT, INR, and TIBC. Discuss these laboratory studies to include what they measure.

3. The results of the laboratory tests and bone scan indicate that the patient has depressed bone marrow function. The hematologist discusses plans to perform a bone marrow aspiration with her. Document the preprocedure care and patient teaching that would be provided for this patient.

4. What is the postprocedure nursing care that will follow the bone marrow aspiration?

42 CHAPTER

Care of Patients with Hematologic Problems

STUDY/REVIEW QUESTIONS

1. The nurse is interviewing a patient who is newly admitted to the unit with a diagnosis of anemia. Which assessment findings does the nurse expect? *(Select all that apply.)*
   a. Dyspnea on exertion
   b. Orthostatic hypotension
   c. Intolerance to cold temperatures
   d. Clublike appearance of the nails
   e. Pallor of the ears
   f. Headache

2. A patient with sickle cell crisis is admitted to the hospital. Which questions does the nurse ask the patient to elicit information about the cause of the current crisis? *(Select all that apply.)*
   a. Ask the patient about recent airplane travel.
   b. Determine the patient's perceived energy level using a scale ranging from 0 to 10.
   c. Review all activities and events during the past 24 hours.
   d. Ask the patient about ability to climb stairs.
   e. Ask the patient about symptoms of infection.

3. A patient is scheduled to undergo laboratory testing to diagnose sickle cell anemia. For which diagnostic tests does the nurse provide patient teaching? *(Select all that apply.)*
   a. Bone marrow biopsy
   b. White blood cell count
   c. MRI
   d. Hemoglobin S
   e. Red blood cell count

4. The student nurse is caring for a patient with sickle cell crisis. Which action by the student nurse warrants intervention by the supervising nurse?
   a. Keeping the patient's room cold
   b. Using distraction and relaxation techniques
   c. Positioning painful areas of the patient with support
   d. Use of therapeutic touch

5. A patient with vitamin B_{12} deficiency anemia is being discharged home with primary care responsibility being assumed by the family. The nurse has taught the patient and family about dietary modifications to manage this condition. Which statement by the family indicates additional teaching is needed about dietary modification? *(Select all that apply.)*
   a. "Dairy products will be omitted from the diet."
   b. "Dried beans will be a part of the diet."
   c. "Animal protein will be a part of the diet."
   d. "Citrus fruit will be omitted from the diet."
   e. "Nuts will be part of the diet."
   f. "Green leafy vegetables will be omitted from the diet."

6. Which statement is true about the pattern of inheritance for sickle cell disease?
   a. If a patient with sickle cell disease has children, each child will have sickle cell disease.
   b. If a patient with sickle cell trait has children, the children will have sickle cell disease.
   c. If a patient with sickle cell disease has children, each child will inherit one of the two abnormal gene alleles and at least have the sickle cell trait.
   d. If a patient has sickle cell disease, it was the result of an autosomal dominant pattern of inheritance.

7. The nurse is caring for a patient in sickle cell crisis. Which are priority interventions for this patient? *(Select all that apply.)*
   a. Pain management
   b. Teaching the patient long-term management of the disease
   c. Smoking cessation
   d. Administration of the pneumonia vaccine
   e. Assessing oxygen saturation

8. The nurse's aide is providing care to a patient in sickle cell crisis. Which action by the nurse's aide requires intervention by the supervising nurse?
   a. Elevating the head of the bed to 25 degrees
   b. Keeping the foot of the bed flat
   c. Obtaining the patient's blood pressure with an external cuff
   d. Offering the patient her beverage of choice

9. A patient admitted for sickle cell crisis is being discharged home. Which statement by the patient indicates the need for further post-discharge instruction?
   a. "I will no longer run 2 miles every morning."
   b. "I will visit my friends in Denver."
   c. "I will avoid the sauna at the gym."
   d. "I will not drink alcoholic beverages."

10. When reviewing the procedure for administering intramuscular medications by the Z-track method, which statement by the student nurse indicates that further instruction is needed?
    a. "I will discard the needle used to draw up the medication."
    b. "I will use the ventral gluteal site for the injection."
    c. "I will pull the skin and subcutaneous tissue sideways away from the muscle."
    d. "I will not massage the injection site."

11. A patient with polycythemia vera is being cared for by a nurse's aide. Which action by the nurse's aide requires intervention by the supervising nurse?
    a. Assisting the patient to floss his teeth
    b. Using an electric shaver on the patient
    c. Using a soft-bristled toothbrush on the patient
    d. Assisting the patient to wear support hose

12. A patient with a low white blood cell count is being discharged home. In which situations will the patient be instructed by the nurse to contact his or her health care provider? *(Select all that apply.)*
    a. For a temperature greater than 100° F (38° C)
    b. If a persistent cough develops with or without sputum
    c. If pus or foul-smelling drainage develops from any open skin area or normal body opening
    d. If a boil or abscess develops
    e. For urine that is cloudy or foul-smelling, or if burning on urination is experienced

13. Which food should a patient with a low white blood cell count be encouraged to eat?
    a. Fresh strawberries
    b. Raw carrots
    c. Pepper
    d. Well-done steak

14. The nurse is caring for a patient with acute leukemia. Which characteristics does the nurse assess the patient for? *(Select all that apply.)*
    a. Hematuria
    b. Orthostatic hypotension
    c. Bone pain
    d. Joint swelling
    e. Fatigue
    f. Weight gain

15. Which factors are associated with an increased risk for lymphoma? *(Select all that apply.)*
    a. Autoimmune disease and immunosuppressive disorders
    b. Chronic infection from *Helicobacter pylori*
    c. Epstein-Barr viral infection
    d. Inherited gene damage
    e. Pesticides and insecticides

16. Which disorder makes a patient at highest risk for the development of infection?
    a. Sickle cell crisis
    b. Vitamin B_{12} deficiency anemia
    c. Polycythemia vera
    d. Thrombocytopenia

17. Which medication places a patient at risk for infection?
    a. Steroids
    b. Diuretics
    c. ACE inhibitors
    d. Beta blockers

18. The nurse is caring for a patient with thrombocytopenia. Which order does the nurse question?
    a. Test all urine and stool for the presence of occult blood.
    b. Avoid IM injections.
    c. Administer enemas.
    d. Apply ice to areas of trauma.

19. A patient undergoing bone marrow/stem cell transplantation reports severe fatigue. To assist the patient with energy management, what does the nurse encourage the patient to do? *(Select all that apply.)*
    a. Verbalize feelings about limitations.
    b. Monitor nutritional intake to ensure adequate energy resources.
    c. Avoid napping throughout the day.
    d. Limit the number of visitors as appropriate.
    e. Plan activities for periods when the patient has the most energy.
    f. Monitor overall response to self-care activities.

20. The home care nurse is visiting a patient who had a stem cell transplant. Which observation by the nurse requires immediate action?
    a. The patient's grandson is visiting after receiving a MMR vaccine.
    b. The patient bumps his toe on a chair and applies pressure to the toe for 10 minutes.
    c. The patient with a platelet count of 48,000/mm^3 follows platelet precautions.
    d. The patient avoids going grocery shopping in the winter months.

21. A patient has been taught how to care for his central venous catheter at home. Which statements by the patient indicate that further instruction is necessary? *(Select all that apply.)*
    a. "I will flush the catheter with heparin three times a day."
    b. "I will change the Luer-Lok cap on each catheter daily."
    c. "I will tape the catheter to my skin."
    d. "If the catheter lumen breaks or punctures, I will immediately clamp the catheter between myself and the opening."
    e. "I will wash my hands before working with the catheter."

22. The nurse has instructed a patient at risk for bleeding about techniques to manage this condition. Which statements by the patient indicate that teaching has been successful? *(Select all that apply.)*
    a. "I will take a stool softener to prevent straining during a bowel movement."
    b. "I won't take aspirin or aspirin-containing products."
    c. "I won't participate in any contact sports."
    d. "I will report a headache that is not responsive to acetaminophen."
    e. "I will avoid bending over at the waist."
    f. "If I am bumped, I will apply ice to the site for at least 10 minutes."

23. The new registered nurse is giving a blood transfusion to a patient. Which statement by the new nurse indicates the need for action by the supervising nurse?
    a. "I will be sure to complete the red blood cell transfusions within 6 hours of removal from refrigeration."
    b. "I will check the patient verification with another registered nurse."
    c. "I will use normal saline solution to dilute the blood."
    d. "I will remain with the patient for the first 15 to 30 minutes of the infusion."

24. The new registered nurse is identifying a patient for blood transfusion. Which action by the new nurse warrants intervention by the supervising nurse?
    a. Checks the physician's prescription before the blood transfusion.
    b. Determines the patient's identity and whether the hospital identification band name and number are identical to those on the blood component tag.
    c. Uses the patient's room number as a form of identification.
    d. Examines the blood bag tag, the attached tag, and the requisition slip to ensure that the ABO and Rh types are compatible.

25. A patient receiving a stem cell transplant from an identical twin is receiving which type of transplant?
    a. Allogeneic
    b. Syngeneic
    c. Autologous
    d. Human leukocyte antigen (HLA)

26. A patient with hemophilia VIII will most likely receive which component of blood for management of the disease?
    a. Pooled platelets
    b. Fresh frozen plasma
    c. Cryoprecipitate
    d. Washed red blood cells

27. Patients with sickle cell disease are more susceptible to infections, specifically *Streptococcus pneumoniae* and *Haemophilus influenzae*. Which actions help prevent infection? *(Select all that apply.)*
    a. Consistent good handwashing technique
    b. Yearly flu vaccination
    c. Twice-daily oral penicillin
    d. NSAIDs three times a day
    e. Monitoring CBC
    f. Assessment of vital signs at least every 4 hours

Matching: Match the source with the type of transplant.

Types
a.   Allogeneic
b.   Autologous
c.   Syngeneic

Sources
_____ 28.   From a sibling or HLA match
_____ 29.   From an identical twin
_____ 30.   From own stem cells

31.   The nurse is caring for a patient who has donated bone marrow. In addition to having the aspiration sites monitored, the nurse will anticipate the need for which interventions? *(Select all that apply.)*
a.   Fluid for hydration
b.   Pain management
c.   Possible RBC infusion
d.   Antibiotic therapy
e.   Assessment for complications of anesthesia

32.   When caring for a patient after bone marrow stem cell transplantation, when does the nurse expect engraftment (the settling in of stem cells and the start of producing new cells) to occur?
a.   8 to 12 hours after infusion
b.   7 days after infusion
c.   12 to 28 days after infusion
d.   6 weeks after infusion

33.   A patient is at high risk for the development of veno-occlusive disease (VOD). What assessments does the nurse perform for early detection of this disorder? *(Select all that apply.)*
a.   Jaundice
b.   Weight loss
c.   Hepatomegaly
d.   Right upper quadrant abdominal pain
e.   Ascites

Matching: Match each characteristic with the corresponding disease. Diseases will be used more than once.

Disease
a.   Hodgkin's lymphoma
b.   Non-Hodgkin's lymphoma

Characteristics
_____ 34.   Pain in lymph nodes brought on or made worse with ingestion of alcohol
_____ 35.   One of the most treatable types of cancer
_____ 36.   Fevers, drenching night sweats, and unexplained weight loss
_____ 37.   Viral infections (Epstein-Barr, HTLV, and HIV) and exposure to chemical agents
_____ 38.   Over 60 subtypes
_____ 39.   Reed-Sternberg cell
_____ 40.   Enlarged painless lymph node or nodes
_____ 41.   Associated with autoimmune disorders
_____ 42.   More common in teens

For questions 43 through 51, indicate whether each characteristic corresponds to autoimmune thrombolytic purpura (ATP) or thrombotic thrombocytopenic purpura (TTP).

_____ 43. Also called idiopathic

_____ 44. Platelets clump

_____ 45. Antibodies directed against own platelets

_____ 46. Inappropriate aggregation of platelets

_____ 47. Women 20 to 40 years of age

_____ 48. Pre-existing autoimmune condition

_____ 49. Plasmapheresis

_____ 50. Immunosuppressive therapy to reduce intensity

_____ 51. Corticosteroids and azathioprine (Imuran)

52. While being interviewed for admission, a patient tells the nurse that he has Christmas disease. What does the nurse document this as?
    a. Hemophilia A
    b. Hemophilia B
    c. Thrombocytopenia
    d. Sickle cell disease

53. Which characteristics describe patients who have hemophilia? *(Select all that apply.)*
    a. Bleeding more often
    b. Bleeding more rapidly
    c. Bleeding for a longer period
    d. Are not able to form platelet plugs
    e. Exhibit abnormal bleeding in response to any trauma

54. What size of intravenous needle is best for administering a blood transfusion?
    a. 22-gauge needle
    b. 20-gauge needle
    c. 19-gauge needle
    d. Butterfly needle

55. A patient is receiving a blood transfusion. Which solution does the nurse administer with the blood?
    a. Ringer's lactate
    b. Normal saline
    c. Dextrose in water
    d. Dextrose in saline

56. A nursing student asks the registered nurse why D_5W is contraindicated when transfusing blood. How does the nurse respond?
    a. "It causes hemolysis of blood cells."
    b. "It dilutes the cells."
    c. "It shrinks the blood cells."
    d. "It causes blood cells to coagulate."

57. A patient is receiving a blood transfusion through a single lumen peripherally inserted central catheter. The patient has two other peripheral IVs: one is capped and the other has D_5/.45 NS running at a rate of 50 mL/hr. What infusion is acceptable to add to the blood products?
    a. Normal saline
    b. Piggyback of 10 mEq potassium chloride
    c. Total parenteral nutrition
    d. Furosemide (Lasix) 5 mg IV push

58. The nurse realizes that hemolytic reactions to blood transfusions occur most often within the first ____ mL of the infusion.
    a. 5
    b. 50
    c. 100
    d. 150

59. Which type of medication is used for patients receiving a platelet transfusion as a premedication to prevent a reaction?
    a. Demerol and Vistaril
    b. Valium and aspirin
    c. Benadryl and Tylenol
    d. Hydrocortisone and Demerol

60. A patient has been receiving frequent blood transfusions. Soon after this transfusion has begun, the patient develops a fever and reports a "racing heart," but does not report any pain. The nurse notes that the patient is also hypotensive. These clinical manifestations may be the cause of which types of transfusion reaction? *(Select all that apply.)*
    a. Hemolytic
    b. Allergic
    c. Bacterial
    d. Febrile
    e. Transfusion-associated graft versus host disease

CASE STUDY: HODGKIN'S AND NON-HODGKIN'S LYMPHOMAS

Use a separate sheet of paper to answer the questions in this Case Study, or go to the "Prepare for Class" folder on your Evolve website at http://evolve.elsevier.com/Iggy/ to download and complete as a word processing file. Answer guidelines for this Case Study are also available on your Evolve website.

The nurse is providing patient care on a unit which specializes in the care of patients with malignant lymphomas. One of the patients is DS, a 19-year-old college freshman who has been diagnosed with Hodgkin's lymphoma. The other patient is EM, a 60-year-old woman who has been diagnosed with an indolent non-Hodgkin's lymphoma. EM tells the nurse, "I know there is nothing that can really be done for me. My sister died of the same thing 16 years ago." DS appears frightened and confused when the nurse asks him if he has any questions about the treatment plan. DS tells the nurse, "I have a girlfriend, but we're not that serious, and I'm still young. Will I ever be able to have children?"

1. Compare malignant lymphoma and leukemia. How do they differ?

2. Compare and contrast the etiology, pathophysiology, and clinical manifestations of Hodgkin's lymphoma and non-Hodgkin's lymphoma.

3. When planning care for DS, what nursing interventions will the nurse focus on to deal with the side effects of therapy?

4. EM states that she does not understand the term "indolent." How should the nurse respond?

5. Document the patient teaching between the nurse and EM and family regarding the current treatment of non-Hodgkin's lymphoma.

6. How should the nurse address DS's concerns about having children?

43 CHAPTER

Assessment of the Nervous System

STUDY/REVIEW QUESTIONS

Matching: *Match the cerebral areas with their functions.*

Cerebral Areas

a. Motor cortex of the frontal lobe
b. Broca's area
c. Occipital lobe
d. Parietal lobe
e. Limbic lobe
f. Wernicke's area
g. Temporal lobe

Functions

_____ 1. Speech center

_____ 2. Visual center

_____ 3. Initiate voluntary movement

_____ 4. Process language

_____ 5. Spatial perception

_____ 6. Complicated memory patterns

_____ 7. Emotional and visceral patterns

8. The nurse is performing a mental status examination on a patient. Which question best assesses recall memory?
   a. "How did you get to the hospital?"
   b. "What city were you born in?"
   c. "What is your mother's maiden name?"
   d. "How many children do you have?"

9. A patient has sustained trauma affecting Broca's area of the brain. Which intervention does the nurse use to assist the patient to compensate for deficits related to damage in this area?
   a. Obtain an erasable white board and a pen for communication.
   b. Use a picture board to relate the spoken word to a visual picture.
   c. Move into the patient's visual field on the unaffected side.
   d. Put up the side rails and turn on the bed alarm.

10. Which type of stroke or stroke damage is most likely to cause problems with respiratory distress related to neurologic function?
    a. Frontal lobe damage
    b. Thalamic stroke
    c. Affected temporal lobe
    d. Involvement of medulla and pons

11. With what will a patient with a cerebellar dysfunction most likely need assistance?
    a. Orientation to place and time
    b. Buttoning the shirt
    c. Verbal communication
    d. Mood and pain control

12. Identify which substances pass through the blood-brain barrier with a "P" and which are blocked by the barrier with a "B."

_____ a. Oxygen

_____ b. Albumin

_____ c. Most bacteria

_____ d. Alcohol

_____ e. Water

_____ f. Anesthetics

_____ g. Many antibiotics

_____ h. Carbon dioxide

Matching: *Match the spinal tract with its function.*

Spinal Tracts

a. Spinothalamic
b. Spinocerebellar
c. Fasciculus gracilis or cuneatus
d. Corticospinal

Functions

_____ 13. Proprioception

_____ 14. Voluntary movement

_____ 15. Carry sensations of pain, temperature, pressure

_____ 16. Vibratory sense

Identify whether each description corresponds to the parasympathetic nervous system (PNS) or the sympathetic nervous system (SNS).

_____ 17. Has cell bodies in the gray matter of the spinal cord from S2 to S4

_____ 18. "Fight or flight" system

_____ 19. Has some sensory function

_____ 20. Is part of cranial nerves III, VII, IX, and X

_____ 21. Causes the heart to pump faster

_____ 22. Constricts pupils

23. The nurse is teaching an older adult patient about medication and healthy lifestyle. Which teaching strategy is the best to use with this patient?
    a. Give limited and simplified information.
    b. Do the teaching late in the afternoon.
    c. Relate the information to recent events.
    d. Allow extra time for teaching and questions.

24. The nurse is caring for an older adult patient who is at risk for falling related to altered balance and decreased coordination. Which initial interventions does the nurse employ for this patient? *(Select all that apply.)*
    a. Instruct the patient to move slowly when changing positions.
    b. Instruct the patient to call for assistance before getting out of bed.
    c. Put up all the side rails and place the bed in the lowest position.
    d. Place the call bell and personal items within the patient's reach.
    e. Store personal items out of sight and instruct the patient to call for help.
    f. Assign a sitter to stay with the patient and assist as needed.

25. The nurse is obtaining baseline information from an older adult patient at risk for a neurologic disorder about his ability to perform activities of daily living (ADLs). Why does the nurse ask whether the patient is right- or left-handed?
    a. The patient may be somewhat stronger on the dominant side, which is expected.
    b. Effects of a neurologic event will be worse if the nondominant side is involved.
    c. This information is part of any standardized database for patients with neurologic disorders.
    d. The patient should be encouraged to strengthen and rely on the dominant side.

26. The nurse is taking shift report on several patients with changes in functional health patterns. The levels are based on Gordon's Functional Assessment. Which level will require the most assistance during the shift?
    a. Level 0 for toileting
    b. Level I for general mobility
    c. Level II for grooming
    d. Level III for feeding

27. Which statement is included in an assessment of a patient's mental status?
    a. Reports of pain, discomfort, or weakness
    b. Ability to hear and see within normal limits
    c. Appropriateness of clothes to weather conditions
    d. Ability to push and pull against resistance

28. An older adult patient is brought to the clinic by the family who reports that "Dad doesn't seem to be quite like himself." Which behavior is an early sign of a neurologic problem?
    a. Inability to remember a trip that he took last week
    b. Failure to remember his mother's maiden name
    c. Failure to recall where he went to high school
    d. Inability to describe his favorite hobby

29. In performing a mental status examination on a patient, the nurse asks, "What would you do if you saw a fire in the wastebasket?" What is the nurse assessing with this question?
    a. Judgment
    b. Level of consciousness
    c. Memory
    d. Orientation

30. Which neurologic disorder is most likely to require hourly sensory assessments of a patient?
    a. Parkinson disease
    b. Alzheimer's disease
    c. Guillain-Barré syndrome
    d. Huntington disease

31. Which sensory assessment technique is correct?
    a. Separate assessments for pain and temperature
    b. Assessment of only the affected or injured side
    c. Assessment of the proximal and distal areas of extremities
    d. Assessment of sharp and dull senses by using a paper clip

32. The nurse is caring for several older adult patients in a long-term care facility. In planning care with consideration for the sensory changes related to aging, which intervention does the nurse implement?
    a. Controls environmental odors because older adults have a heightened sense of smell
    b. Plans simple teaching sessions because of the decline in intellectual ability
    c. Increases the ambient lighting because of the decrease in pupil size
    d. Limits physical contact because the touch sensation increases

33. The nurse is taking an initial history on a patient whose chief complaint is a headache that seems to be associated with blurred vision. The patient also reports several chronic health problems. Which chronic condition is most likely to impact neurologic function?
    a. Hypertension
    b. Obesity
    c. Crohn's disease
    d. Coronary artery disease

34. An older adult patient is admitted into a long-term care facility and the nurse is performing a baseline physical assessment that includes neurologic and sensory function. What is the purpose of the assessment?
    a. Determine a level of function for later comparison
    b. Show the family what problems the older adult has
    c. Gain information on past sensory changes
    d. Determine rehabilitation potential

Matching: *Match each mental and cognitive status assessment question/task to the type of information sought.*

Information Sought
a. Attention span
b. Recent memory
c. Remote memory
d. New memory
e. Language comprehension
f. Cognitive skills

Questions
_____ 35. Repeat three unrelated words.
_____ 36. "What is your birth date?"
_____ 37. Follow simple instructions.
_____ 38. "What health care providers have you seen during the last year?"
_____ 39. Repeat a series of numbers.
_____ 40. "Tell me about your hobbies."

41. The nurse is assessing the sensory functions of a patient with Guillain-Barré syndrome (GBS). The nurse makes a clinical judgment to forgo assessing for light touch discrimination. Why does the nurse make this decision?
    a. The patient's pain and temperature sensations are intact.
    b. Sensory testing is done routinely every 4 hours.
    c. Only patients with spinal trauma require this assessment.
    d. The patient with GBS will be too confused to respond appropriately.

42. The nurse is testing a patient for touch discrimination by touching the patient on both shoulders. What is a normal finding for this assessment?
    a. Pointing to where each shoulder was touched
    b. Moving the shoulders against resistance
    c. Describing the touch as sharp or dull
    d. Sensing touch on the unaffected side

Matching: *Match the component of motor testing with the corresponding test performed.*

Test Component
a. Brainstem integrity
b. Coordination
c. Muscle strength
d. Gait
e. Equilibrium

Test Performed
_____ 43. Patient walks across the room, and returns.
_____ 44. Patient stands, eyes open, feet close together.
_____ 45. Patient holds the arms perpendicular to the body, eyes closed.
_____ 46. Patient grasps and squeezes the nurse's fingers.
_____ 47. With arms out to the side, the patient touches the nose two to three times.

48. The nursing student is performing a neurologic assessment on a patient who sustained a stroke. The nurse observes the student evaluating grip and hand strength only on the affected side. What is the nurse's first action?
    a. Give the student positive feedback for performing the assessment correctly.
    b. Remind the student that strength testing needs to be done bilaterally.
    c. Redo the entire assessment and instruct the student to watch the process.
    d. Suggest to the instructor that the student needs remediation for assessment.

49. A patient is admitted to a rehabilitation center following a stroke that has left him with residual weakness on his left side. The nurse has completed the physical and neurologic assessment. Which documentation note best communicates the patient's progress?
    a. Shows progress and 3+ strength in left leg
    b. Demonstrates 5/5 in left leg and 5/5 in right leg against resistance
    c. Demonstrates 30-degree abduction of left leg
    d. Able to push against resistance with equal power in both legs

50. While assessing a patient's gait and equilibrium, the nurse observes that the patient has Romberg's sign. What is the priority patient problem associated with this objective data?
    a. Potential for falls related to dysfunctions in awareness of body position
    b. Inability to perform ADLs related to decreased muscle strength
    c. Incontinence related to inability to ambulate to bathroom
    d. Potential for falls related to unsteady gait

51. Which statement about the Glasgow Coma Scale (GCS) is correct?
    a. It is a thorough neurologic assessment tool.
    b. It establishes a baseline for eye opening and motor and verbal response.
    c. It establishes a baseline cognitive function.
    d. A score of 15 indicates serious neurologic impairment with poor prognosis.

52. The nurse is attempting to assess a coma patient's response to pain. Which technique does the nurse try first?
    a. Gently shake the patient, similar to attempting to wake a sleeping child.
    b. Speak to the patient and call his or her name using a normal tone of voice.
    c. Face the patient and speak loudly and clearly, similar to a hearing-impaired patient.
    d. Apply supraorbital pressure by placing the thumb under the orbital rim.

53. The nurse is assessing response to painful stimuli in a patient. What is the maximum length of time to apply the stimulus in the comatose patient?
    a. 1 to 2 seconds
    b. 5 to 10 seconds
    c. 20 to 30 seconds
    d. 40 to 60 seconds

54. The nurse is assessing several patients using the GCS. Which factors indicate the most serious neurologic presentation based on the GCS information?
    a. Eye opening to sound, localizes pain, confused conversation
    b. Eye opening to sound, obeys commands, inappropriate words
    c. Eye opening spontaneous, obeys commands, confused conversation
    d. Eye opening to pain, abnormal flexion, incomprehensible sounds

55. The nurse is performing neurologic checks every 4 hours for a patient who sustained a head injury. Which early sign indicates a decline in neurologic status?
    a. Nonreactive, dilated pupils
    b. Change in level of consciousness
    c. Decorticate posturing
    d. Loss of remote memory

56. The nursing student is talking to the patient and family about diagnostic testing. Which statement by the nursing student indicates the need for further study about the understanding of diagnostic procedures?
    a. "You are scheduled for a magnetic resonance imaging (MRI). Do you have a cardiac pacemaker?"
    b. "You are scheduled for a computed tomography (CT) of the head. Are you wearing hairpins?"
    c. "You are to have x-rays of the skull. Are you allergic to iodine?"
    d. "You are to have a cerebral angiography. Do you take medication for diabetes?"

57. Which statement about lumbar puncture is true?
    a. It is indicated for patients with infections at or near the puncture site.
    b. It is done at the T1 to T3 spinal level.
    c. It requires the patient to lie flat for 24 to 48 hours after the procedure.
    d. It is done with the patient in the "fetal" position.

58. The nurse is reviewing the results of a lumbar puncture test. Which cerebrospinal fluid result does the nurse point out to the physician as a significant abnormal finding?
    a. Protein 500-700 mg/100 mL
    b. Cells 0-5 small lymphocytes/mm³
    c. Color straw-yellow
    d. Glucose 50 to 75 mg/100 mL

59. A patient is scheduled for an EEG. How does the nurse prepare the patient for this diagnostic test?
    a. Giving a sedative before bedtime
    b. Having the patient drink extra fluids before the test
    c. Keeping the patient NPO after midnight
    d. Keeping the patient awake from 2 AM until the scheduled test time

60. A patient arrives on the unit alert and oriented after undergoing cerebral angiography. The report from the radiology nurse indicates the catheter was inserted into the left femoral artery. For which postprocedural order does the nurse call for clarification?
    a. Keep the left leg straight and immobilized.
    b. Maintain an ice pack and pressure dressing to the insertion site x 2 hours.
    c. IV and oral fluid restrictions for a total of 1000 mL/24 hours.
    d. Neurocirculation checks every 15 minutes x 2 hours; then every hour x 4 hours.

61. A patient is scheduled to have a CT with contrast media and the nurse is reviewing the patient's laboratory results. Which laboratory result could impact the procedure, prompting the nurse to notify the radiology department and the health care provider?
    a. Creatinine level
    b. White blood count
    c. Blood glucose
    d. Urobilinogen level

62. The nurse has instructed the patient and family on information about positron emission tomography (PET). However, the patient is suspected of having early signs of Alzheimer's disease. Which statement by the patient indicates he did not understand the information?
    a. "I may be asked to add or subtract numbers or to remember things during the test."
    b. "I am a little bit nervous about the idea of being blindfolded. Could you tell me about that?"
    c. "They will not give me my insulin shot on the morning of the test."
    d. "I will be asleep during most of the test; I will get a mild medication to help me relax."

63. Which factors are potential contraindications for having an MRI? *(Select all that apply.)*
    a. Cardiac pacemaker
    b. Implanted infusion pump
    c. Ferromagnetic aneurysm clip
    d. Confusion or agitation
    e. Pregnancy
    f. Continuous life support
    g. Recent tattoo

64. A patient is scheduled for a cerebral blood flow evaluation with use of radioactive substance. Which medications does the nurse anticipate the physician will likely withhold from the patient for 24 hours before the test?
    a. Central nervous system depressants and stimulants
    b. Insulin or oral hypoglycemics
    c. Antihypertensives and diuretics
    d. Anticoagulants and antiplatelets

CASE STUDY: NEUROLOGIC ASSESSMENT

Use a separate sheet of paper to answer the questions in this Case Study, or go to the "Prepare for Class" folder on your Evolve website at http://evolve.elsevier.com/Iggy/ to download and complete as a word processing file. Answer guidelines for this Case Study are also available on your Evolve website.

The patient is a 48-year-old man, married, and the father of three children. He works as a draftsman, designing decorative iron and other metal products. He is scheduled for a neurologic diagnostic workup. Over the past month, he has noticed that he has had difficulty drawing figures accurately. At times, he has been unable to hold a pencil with sufficient strength to mark the drawing paper. He denies visual changes; however, at times he has difficulty walking without tripping. Physical examination reveals that the patient is oriented to person, place, time, and situation, PERRLA, has a steady gait, upper extremity hand grip is equal and strong, strength against resistance reveals R hand 4/5 and L hand 5/5. A lumbar puncture is scheduled following x-rays of the skull and spine.

1. What additional data should the nurse collect initially?

2. Describe the preparation of the patient for the x-ray studies.

3. Identify at least four priority patient problems that are appropriate for the patient who is scheduled to have a lumbar puncture.

4. The hospital requires that a consent form be signed by the patient before the lumbar puncture. What is the purpose of this document?

5. The patient asks about complications from the procedure. He asks, "Will the test make my symptoms worse? I don't need any more problems right now." How do you reply to the patient?

6. The lumbar puncture is performed and five tubes of cerebrospinal fluid (CSF) are collected. The CSF pressure is 165 cm H_2O. What is the significance of this finding?

(Continued on next page.)

7. The physician orders that the specimens be analyzed for cells, protein, and glucose. The laboratory results are:
   - Color: straw
   - Cells: 7 lymphocytes/mm^3
   - RBCs: absent
   - Protein: 60 mg/100 mL
   - Glucose: 68 mg/100 mL

   Which of the laboratory findings are normal? Which are abnormal?

8. What assessments should the nurse make following the procedure?

9. The patient calls the nurse and says that he has a throbbing headache. What interventions are indicated to help make the patient more comfortable?

10. Document the patient's Glasgow Coma Score based on the assessment findings. (*Circle the correct number for each category.*)

Eye Opening	
Spontaneous	4
To sound	3
To pain	2
Never	1
Motor Response	
Obeys commands	6
Localizes pain	5
Normal flexion (withdrawal)	4
Abnormal flexion	3
Extension	2
None	1
Verbal Response	
Oriented	5
Confused	4
Inappropriate words	3
Incomprehensible sounds	2
None	1

What is the score for this patient?_____

44 CHAPTER

Care of Patients with Problems of the Central Nervous System: The Brain

STUDY/REVIEW QUESTIONS

Matching. Match the current pathophysiology theories with the corresponding type of headache.

Type of Headache
a.   Migraine
b.   Cluster headache

Pathophysiology

_____ 1.   Blood vessels in the brain overreact to a triggering event

_____ 2.   Increase in hypothalamic size

_____ 3.   Attributed to vasoreactivity and neurogenic inflammation

_____ 4.   Spasm in the arteries at the base of the brain

_____ 5.   May be caused by hyperexcitability of nerves

_____ 6.   Serotonin, a vasoconstrictor, is released

_____ 7.   Related to an overactive hypothalamus

_____ 8.   A decrease in cerebral blood flow; cerebral hypoxia may occur

_____ 9.   Prostaglandins, chemicals that cause inflammation and swelling

Matching. Match each characteristic with the corresponding type of headache.

Type of Headache
a. Migraine
b. Cluster headache

Characteristics
_____ 10. Familial disorder

_____ 11. Occurs more often in men

_____ 12. Associated with runny nose and ptosis

_____ 13. Has no known cause

_____ 14. May be caused by hyperexcitability of nerves

_____ 15. Patient may walk or rock

_____ 16. May last for several days

_____ 17. Duration limited to 30 minutes to 2 hours

_____ 18. Occurs at regular intervals with long remission periods

_____ 19. Occurs more often in women

20. A patient arrives at the clinic with a chief complaint of headache. He is irritable and impatient to receive treatment, but he is alert and oriented, his speech is clear, and he is able and willing to answer the nurse's questions. Which questions does the nurse ask to solicit additional relevant information about this patient's headache? *(Select all that apply.)*
    a. "When do the headaches occur?"
    b. "How often do the headaches occur?"
    c. "Why do you have headaches?"
    d. "Did you eat an unusually large meal just before your headache?"
    e. "Do you experience other symptoms with the headache?"
    f. "Have there been any recent changes in your headaches?"

21. A patient with a history of migraine headaches reports his current headache as "my usual throbbing pain, but today it is behind my left eye." Which question does the nurse ask to elicit information about trigger factors?
    a. "Do you have a history of illicit substance abuse?"
    b. "Do you smoke cigars or cigarettes?"
    c. "Are you having any trouble with your vision?"
    d. "Did you drink wine or coffee before the headache occurred?"

22. Which type of medication can be used to prevent migraines?
    a. Lamotrigine (Lamictal)
    b. Metoclopramide (Reglan)
    c. Sumatriptan (Imitrex)
    d. Propranolol (Inderal)

23. During a patient's last visit, the nurse instructed the patient about headaches and techniques to manage this condition. Which statement by the patient indicates teaching has been successful?
    a. "I have been keeping track of when my headaches occur."
    b. "My doctor told me that my headaches were not very serious."
    c. "My spouse knows the instructions that you gave me."
    d. "I have not had any headaches since we last talked."

24. A patient with a history of migraine headaches reports that noise makes her "head hurt worse." How does the nurse document this subjective finding?
    a. "Patient reports photophobia."
    b. "Patient reports phonophobia."
    c. "Patient reports vertigo."
    d. "Patient reports diplopia."

25. A patient is prescribed ergotamine with caffeine for migraine headaches. Which statement by the patient indicates the patient is experiencing a side effect of this drug?
    a. "My headache is initially relieved by the medication, but then it returns."
    b. "I seem to be gaining weight since I started taking this medication."
    c. "My headache seems worse in the morning when I take the medication."
    d. "I notice that I bruise more easily and my skin seems fragile and dry."

26. A patient has received a prescription for sumatriptan (Imitrex) for the treatment of migraine headaches. The patient tells the nurse that she elected not to tell the physician about all of her health conditions "because I just wanted treatment for my headaches and I didn't want to go into everything else." What is the nurse's response?
    a. The drug is contraindicated for patients who have glaucoma.
    b. It is necessary to monitor laboratory values such as PT, PTT, and electrolytes.
    c. The drug is contraindicated in actual or suspected ischemic heart disease.
    d. The dosage is calculated by using relevant factors from the health history.

Matching. *Match the type of generalized seizure with its correct definition.*

Types of Generalized Seizures
a. Tonic-clonic
b. Absence
c. Myoclonic
d. Atonic

Definitions
_____ 27. Brief jerking of extremities, singly or in groups
_____ 28. Brief period of staring or loss of consciousness
_____ 29. Rigidity followed by rhythmic jerking
_____ 30. Sudden loss of body tone

31. An elementary school teacher has just been informed that her student's brother has absence seizures. The teacher is fearful that her student may have the same type of seizures and is unsure what to expect. Which signs does the school nurse advise the teacher to look for?
    a. Brief jerking or stiffening of muscles that lasts only a few seconds
    b. Loss of consciousness and rhythmic jerking of extremities
    c. Brief loss of consciousness that may appear as daydreaming or blank staring
    d. "Blackout" that lasts 10 to 30 minutes with loss of memory and disorientation

32. What is the priority patient problem for atonic (akinetic) seizures?
    a. Potential for injury related to falls
    b. Organ ischemia related to neuromuscular dysfunction
    c. Confusion related to postictal state
    d. Limited mobility related to atonicity of muscles

33. Which tests does the nurse anticipate will be ordered for a patient to confirm a suspected diagnosis of epilepsy?
    a. Electrocardiogram (ECG) and positron emission tomography (PET)
    b. Electroencephalogram (EEG) and computed tomography (CT)
    c. Lumbar puncture (LP) and magnetic resonance imaging (MRI)
    d. Complete series of skull x-rays and neuroimaging

34. The nursing student is caring for a patient with absence seizures. Which statement by the student indicates an understanding of absence seizures?
    a. "The patient should be placed in a vest when sitting in a chair."
    b. "There is no medical treatment for absence seizures."
    c. "I should have a padded tongue blade at the bedside."
    d. "The patient may repeatedly pick at the linens."

35. An older adult patient is brought to the emergency department from the local mall after bystanders saw her "having a seizure." The patient is currently responsive to voice, but is lethargic, confused, and unable to give an accurate history. Which aspect of this patient's health history is the most important to verify with the family?
    a. History of acute or chronic respiratory problems
    b. General ability to answer questions accurately
    c. Likelihood of the patient shopping at the mall alone
    d. Patient's doctor's name

36. A patient is treated in the emergency department for status epilepticus and is admitted to the hospital. The physician has ordered seizure precautions. What equipment does the nurse place in the room before the patient's arrival?
    a. Cardiac monitor and a pulse oximeter
    b. Penlight and a neurologic assessment flow sheet
    c. Padded tongue blades and padding for side rails
    d. Oxygen and suction equipment

Matching. *Match each factor with its associated type of meningitis.*

Types of Meningitis
a. Bacterial
b. Viral
c. Fungal

Factors

_____ 37. Condition is usually self-limiting; full recovery is expected.

_____ 38. Manifestations vary according to the state of the immune system.

_____ 39. Cerebrospinal fluid (CSF) is hazy.

_____ 40. No organisms grow from the CSF.

_____ 41. Outbreaks occur in crowded conditions such as dormitories.

42. The nurse is caring for a patient who was admitted for a diagnosis of meningococcal meningitis. Which nursing action is specific to this type of meningitis?
    a. Administer an antifungal agent such as amphotericin B as ordered.
    b. Observe the patient for genital lesions.
    c. Place the patient in isolation per hospital procedure.
    d. Check to see if the patient is HIV positive.

43. The nurse is reviewing the electrolyte values for a patient with bacterial meningitis and notes that the serum sodium is 126 mEq/L. How does the nurse interpret this finding?
    a. Within normal limits considering the diagnosis of bacterial meningitis
    b. Evidence of syndrome of inappropriate antidiuretic hormone (SIADH) which is a complication of bacterial meningitis
    c. A protective measure that causes increased urination and therefore reduces the risk of increased intracranial pressure (ICP)
    d. An early warning sign that the electrolyte imbalances will potentiate an acute myocardial infarction (AMI) or shock

44. A patient with meningitis reports a headache, and the nurse gives the appropriate IV push PRN medication. Several hours later, the patient reports pain in the left hand; the radial pulse is very weak, the hand feels cool, and capillary refill is sluggish compared to the left. What does the nurse suspect is occurring in this patient?
   a. Stroke secondary to increased ICP resulting from meningitis
   b. Sickle cell crisis associated with an increased risk of meningitis
   c. Septic emboli causing vascular compromise
   d. Local phlebitis from the IV push pain medication that was given

45. A patient arrives in the emergency department reporting headache, fever, nausea, and photosensitivity. The patient has been living in close proximity with two people who were diagnosed with meningitis. Which diagnostic test does the nurse anticipate the physician will order to rule out meningitis?
   a. X-rays of the skull
   b. Lumbar puncture
   c. Myelography
   d. Cerebral angiogram

46. The nurse is caring for a patient who has symptoms and risk factors for bacterial meningitis. For which symptom must the nurse alert the physician?
   a. Capillary refill of 3 seconds
   b. Headache with nausea and vomiting
   c. Inability to move eyes laterally
   d. Oral temperature of 101.6° F

47. The nurse is carefully monitoring a patient with a severe case of encephalitis for signs of increased ICP. What vital sign changes are associated with increased ICP?
   a. Tachycardia and shallow, rapid respirations
   b. Increased core temperature and bradycardia
   c. Decreased pulse pressure and tachypnea
   d. Widened pulse pressure and bradycardia

48. The student nurse is caring for a patient with encephalitis. Which action by the student nurse warrants intervention by the supervising nurse?
   a. Performs deep suctioning for copious secretions
   b. Elevates the head of bed to 30 degrees after a lumbar puncture
   c. Turns the patient every 2 hours
   d. Performs a neurologic assessment every 2 hours

49. The nurse is assessing a patient with Parkinson disease. Which cardinal findings does the nurse expect to observe? *(Select all that apply.)*
   a. Tremors
   b. Rigidity
   c. Dementia
   d. Aphasia
   e. Postural instability
   f. Slow movements

50. A patient with Parkinson disease is being discharged on selegiline (Eldepryl), which is a selective monamine oxidase type B (MAO-B) inhibitor. What information does the nurse include for safe medication administration?
   a. Take the medication with meals.
   b. Avoid driving or operating heavy machinery for several hours after taking the medication.
   c. Avoid tyramine-rich foods such as aged or cured foods.
   d. Take the medication daily at bedtime.

51. During the nurse's assessment of a patient with Parkinson disease, the nurse notes that the patient has a masklike facies. What functional assessment is now a priority?
   a. Ability to hear normal voice tones
   b. Ability to chew and swallow
   c. Ability to sense pain in the facial area
   d. Visual acuity

52. The home health nurse is visiting an older adult patient with Stage 1 Parkinson disease. He demonstrates some trembling and weakness in his right hand and arm, and reports he occasionally gets dizzy when he first stands up. The patient is currently living by himself and has no family in the immediate area. What is the priority patient problem?
    a. Decreased ability to perform ADLs
    b. Feeling of isolation
    c. Potential for falls
    d. Decreased nutritional status

53. A patient is on long-term medication therapy for Parkinson disease. What sign indicates that the patient may be having drug toxicity associated with these drugs?
    a. Acute confusion
    b. Tremors and rigidity
    c. Choreiform movements
    d. Seizure activity

54. A patient has moderate Parkinson disease with an impaired ability to communicate related to psychomotor deficit. Which nursing intervention is the best to use with this patient?
    a. Speaking clearly and slowly
    b. Watching the patient's lips when he speaks
    c. Giving step-by-step instructions to the patient
    d. Providing visual cues when trying to explain

55. The nurse is assessing an older adult patient who was brought to the clinic by her husband after she went out to do some gardening, but several hours later was spotted walking down the street by a neighbor. She is currently "just like herself," but the patient cannot explain what she was doing or where she was going. Which questions does the nurse ask to assess cognitive changes in this patient? *(Select all that apply.)*
    a. "Have you noticed any forgetfulness, for example misplacing your keys?"
    b. "Has there been any memory loss, such as not remembering a recent conversation?"
    c. "Are there any changes in ability to make judgments, such as taking a medication?"
    d. "Have you noticed any weakness; for example, in the arms or legs?"
    e. "Are there any changes in abilities to do a task like balancing your checkbook?"
    f. "Has there been any incontinence; for example, wetting the bed at night?"

56. The nurse observes a patient with Alzheimer's disease pushing at the food on her tray with her eyeglasses. This is documented as an example of what condition?
    a. Apraxia
    b. Aphasia
    c. Agnosia
    d. Anomia

57. The nurse is assessing an older adult patient with Alzheimer's disease using the Mini Mental State Examination (MMSE). What information about the patient does this exam measure?
    a. Level of intelligence
    b. Functional ability
    c. Severity of the patient's dementia
    d. Alterations in ability to communicate

58. A patient has advanced Alzheimer's disease and is staying in a long-term care facility. Which intervention is the best to use with this patient?
    a. Reality orientation
    b. Cognitive training
    c. Memory training
    d. Validation therapy

59. A patient is experiencing mild memory loss and the patient and family are hoping the nurse can offer suggestions to help stimulate and strengthen the patient's current abilities. What is the nurse's first action?
    a. Show the family how to stimulate the memory by repeating what the patient just said.
    b. Discuss with the family and patient any practical memory problems that are occurring.
    c. Suggest that the patient identify and reminisce about pleasant past experiences.
    d. Provide name tags for the patient, family, and friends for use during group gatherings.

60. The daughter of an older adult patient with Alzheimer's disease has heard that there is a genetic disposition for Alzheimer's, and asks the nurse if there are preventive measures she can take. What does the nurse tell her about the current research on Alzheimer's disease?
    a. There is no evidence that first-degree relatives have an increased risk for this disease.
    b. Eating dark-colored fruits and vegetables has been associated with decreased risk.
    c. Use of NSAIDs such as ibuprofen increases the risk for the disease.
    d. Cessation of all tobacco products has been associated with decreased risk.

61. The patient with mild Alzheimer's disease lives at home with her daughter who is the primary caregiver and who works part-time. Which home safety precaution is appropriate for this patient?
    a. Puzzles and board games are provided for the patient.
    b. A geri-chair with a waist belt is in the patient's bedroom.
    c. The patient is wearing an identification bracelet with the daughter's address.
    d. The patient's medications are carefully organized in the bathroom cabinet.

62. The nurse is caring for several patients with Alzheimer's disease in a long-term care facility. Which task is best to delegate to the nursing assistant?
    a. Give hygienic care to the patient who is currently exhibiting sundowning.
    b. Assist the patient who has incontinence with toileting every 2 hours.
    c. Calm the agitated patient by using soft voice tones and distraction.
    d. Follow the patient and observe for hoarding or rummaging.

63. The nurse is assessing a patient with Huntington disease and observes jerky movements of the face, limbs, and trunk. How does the nurse document this assessment finding?
    a. Partial seizure
    b. Chorea
    c. Akinesia
    d. Nuchal rigidity

CASE STUDY: THE SEIZURE PATIENT

Use a separate sheet of paper to answer the questions in this Case Study, or go to the "Prepare for Class" folder on your Evolve website at http://evolve.elsevier.com/Iggy/ to download and complete as a word processing file. Answer guidelines for this Case Study are also available on your Evolve website.

A college student is brought to the emergency department by ambulance. He is alert but confused and uncooperative, and unable to follow simple commands or answer simple questions. His roommate reports, "We were at the library cramming for finals. He just made this really weird sound. Next thing I know he is on the floor shaking and his eyes are rolled back in his head. I turned him on his side. I don't know what is going on with him, but I did call his mother and she said she would meet us here at the hospital." Vital signs are temperature 99° F, pulse 95/min, resp 24/min, BP 140/80.

1. What could the nurse say to the roommate who is most likely to be very stressed by the experience of seeing his friend have a seizure? Why would it be important to calm the roommate and elicit information from him?

2. What should be included in the focused assessment of a patient who has had a seizure?

3. List interventions the nurse would initiate for seizure precautions.

4. Approximately 20 minutes after the patient arrives, he has a repeat seizure. The patient becomes cyanotic and there are copious oral secretions. The tonic-clonic activity lasts approximately 2 minutes. The nurse is at the bedside and immediately intervenes. What interventions does the nurse use?

5. What medications will the physician most likely order for status epilepticus? Describe the nursing implications (administration, side effects, drug level monitoring) for these medications.

6. What are some of the social implications for this young college student who has a new onset of seizures?

7. What should the nurse teach the patient and family about epilepsy?

8. The physician orders 4 mg of Ativan IV push following this second seizure, which the nurse promptly administers. Use the Focus Charting method (also known as the DAR method [data, action, response]) to document this as well as any other interventions carried out.

45 CHAPTER

Care of Patients with Problems of the Central Nervous System: The Spinal Cord

STUDY/REVIEW QUESTIONS

1. The nurse is taking a history on an older adult patient who reports chronic back pain. The nurse seeks to identify factors that are contributing to the pain. Which question is the most useful in eliciting this information?
   a. "Have you had any recent falls or have you been in an accident?"
   b. "Do you have a history of osteoarthritis?"
   c. "Do you have a history of diabetes mellitus?"
   d. "Are you having pain that radiates down your leg or into the buttocks?"

2. The nurse is preparing to physically assess a patient's subjective report of paresthesia in the lower extremities. In order to accomplish this assessment, which assessment technique does the nurse use?
   a. Use a Doppler to locate the pedal pulse, the dorsalis pedis pulse, or the popliteal pulse.
   b. Ask the patient to identify sharp and dull sensation by using a paper clip and cotton ball.
   c. Use a reflex hammer to test for deep tendon patellar or Achilles reflexes.
   d. Ask the patient to walk across the room and observe his gait and equilibrium.

3. Which position is therapeutic and comfortable for a patient with lower back pain?
   a. Semi-Fowler's position with a pillow under the knees to keep them flexed
   b. Supine position with arms and legs in a correct anatomical position
   c. Orthopneic position; sitting with trunk slightly forward; arms supported on a pillow
   d. Modified Sims' position with upper arm and leg supported by pillows

4. A patient has been talking to his physician about drugs that could potentially be used in the treatment of his chronic low back pain. Which statement by the patient indicates a need for additional teaching?
   a. "The doctor may prescribe an antiseizure drug such as oxcarbazepine; therefore, I would need to have blood tests to check my sodium level."
   b. "The doctor may suggest over-the-counter ibuprofen; therefore, I should watch for and report dark or tarry stools."
   c. "The doctor may prescribe an oral steroid such as prednisone; this would be short-term therapy and the dose would gradually taper off."
   d. "The doctor may prescribe hydromorphone and it may cause drowsiness; I should not drive or drink alcohol when I take it."

5. The nurse is assessing a patient who presented to the ED reporting acute onset of numbness and tingling in the right leg. How does the nurse document this subjective finding?
   a. Paraparesis
   b. Paresthesia
   c. Ataxia
   d. Quadriparesis

6. A patient has just undergone a spinal fusion and a laminectomy and has returned from the operating room. Which assessments are done in the first 24 hours? *(Select all that apply.)*
   a. Take vital signs every 4 hours and assess for fever and hypotension.
   b. Perform a neurologic assessment every 4 hours with attention to movement and sensation.
   c. Monitor intake and output and assess for urinary retention.
   d. Assess for ability and independence in ambulating and moving in bed.
   e. Observe for clear fluid on or around the dressing and test for glucose.

7. A patient has a long history of chronic back pain and has undergone several back surgeries in the past. At this point, the surgeon is recommending a surgical procedure for spine stabilization. Which procedure does the nurse anticipate this patient will need?
   a. Laparoscopic diskectomy
   b. Spinal fusion
   c. Laminectomy
   d. Traditional diskectomy

8. A patient has just undergone a laminectomy and returned from surgery at 1300 hours. At 1530 hours, the nurse is performing the change of shift assessment. Which postoperative finding is reported to the surgeon immediately? *(Select all that apply.)*
   a. Minimal serosanguineous drainage in the surgical drain
   b. Pain at the operative site
   c. Swelling or bulging at the operative site
   d. Reluctance or refusal to cough and deep-breathe
   e. Moderate clear drainage on the postoperative dressing

9. A patient has just undergone spinal fusion surgery and returned from the operating room 12 hours ago. Which task is best to delegate to the nursing assistant?
   a. Log-roll the patient every 2 hours.
   b. Help the patient dangle the legs on the evening of surgery.
   c. Assist the patient to put on a brace so he can get out of bed.
   d. Help the patient ambulate to the bathroom as needed.

10. The nurse reviews the discharge and home care instructions with a patient who had back surgery. Which statement by the patient indicates further teaching is needed?
    a. "I will drive myself to my doctor's office next week."
    b. "I will put a piece of plywood under my mattress."
    c. "I will try to increase fruits and vegetables and decrease fat intake."
    d. "I plan to get a new ergonomic chair at work."

11. A patient has had an anterior cervical diskectomy with fusion and has returned from the recovery room. What is the priority assessment?
    a. Assess for the gag reflex and ability to swallow own secretions.
    b. Check for bleeding and drainage at the incision site.
    c. Monitor vital signs and check neurologic status.
    d. Assess for patency of airway and respiratory effort.

12. A patient comes to the emergency department with back pain, but is alert and oriented and is not having any problems breathing. Her husband is very distraught and when the nurse tries to find out what has happened he yells, "Just help her now! Stop asking me these stupid questions!" Why is it important for the nurse to continue trying to obtain information from the husband?
    a. The past medical history and current complaint are part of the legal record.
    b. Engaging the husband will help him to calm down and give him an active role.
    c. Mechanism of injury is important in anticipating potential pathology and damage.
    d. The patient's subjective complaint dictates the focus of the physical examination.

13. Which statements about spinal shock are accurate? *(Select all that apply.)*
    a. It lasts for <48 hours up to a few weeks.
    b. There is temporary loss of motor and sensory function.
    c. There is permanent loss of motor and sensory function.
    d. There is temporary loss of reflex and autonomic function.
    e. There is permanent loss of reflex and autonomic function.

14. The nurse is caring for a patient with a spinal cord injury who is experiencing neurogenic shock. The patient's systolic blood pressure is 88 mm/Hg despite starting a dopamine drip 2 hours earlier. There is a new order to infuse 500 mL of Dextran-40 over 4 hours. At what rate does the nurse set the infusion pump?
    _____ mL/hr

15. A patient involved in a high-speed motor vehicle accident with sustained multiple injuries and active bleeding is transported to the emergency department by ambulance with immobilization devices in place. There is a high probability of cervical spine fracture; the patient has altered mental status and extremities are flaccid. What is the priority assessment for this patient?
    a. Check the mental status using the Glasgow Coma Scale.
    b. Assess the respiratory pattern and ensure a patent airway.
    c. Observe for intra-abdominal bleeding and hemorrhage.
    d. Assess for loss of motor function and sensation.

16. The emergency department nurse is assessing and monitoring a patient with a gunshot wound to the middle of the back. Because the patient is at risk for spinal shock, what does the nurse monitor for?
    a. Decreased blood pressure, bradycardia, and flaccid paralysis
    b. Tachycardia and a change in the level of consciousness
    c. Decreased respiratory rate and loss of sensation to pain and touch
    d. Paralytic ileus and loss of bowel and bladder function

17. Which neurologic assessment technique does the nurse use to test a patient for sensory function?
    a. Touch the skin with a clean paper clip and ask whether it is a sharp or dull sensation.
    b. Ask the patient to elevate both arms off the bed and extend wrists and fingers.
    c. Have the patient close the eyes and move the toes up or down; the patient identifies the positions.
    d. Have the patient sit with the legs dangling; use a reflex hammer to test reflex responses.

18. Assessment of a patient with a lower spinal cord injury confirms that the patient has paralysis of the bilateral lower extremities. How does the nurse document this finding?
    a. Paraparesis
    b. Paraplegia
    c. Quadriparesis
    d. Quadriplegia

Matching. Match each symptom with its corresponding complication.

Complications
a. Spinal shock
b. Autonomic Dysreflexia

Symptoms
_____ 19. Hypertension
_____ 20. Flaccid paralysis
_____ 21. Hypotension
_____ 22. Severe headache
_____ 23. Loss of reflexes below the injury
_____ 24. Blurred vision

25. The nurse is assessing a patient with a spinal cord injury and recognizes that the patient is experiencing Autonomic Dysreflexia. What is the nurse's priority action?
    a. Check for bladder distention.
    b. Raise the head of the bed.
    c. Administer an antihypertensive medication.
    d. Notify the primary health care provider.

26. The nurse is providing discharge teaching for a patient with a spinal cord injury who will be performing intermittent self-catheterizations at home. Which signs and symptoms will the nurse instruct the patient to report immediately to the primary health care provider? *(Select all that apply.)*
    a. Dysuria
    b. Retention
    c. Fever
    d. Urgency
    e. Foul-smelling urine
    f. Back pain

27. The nurse is preparing a quadriplegic patient for discharge and has taught the patient's spouse to assist the patient with a "quad cough" to prevent respiratory complications. Which observation indicates that the spouse has understood what has been taught?
    a. The spouse assists the patient to the side of bed to encourage deep breaths.
    b. The spouse places her hands below the patient's diaphragm and pushes upward as the patient exhales.
    c. The spouse places her hands above the patient's diaphragm and pushes upward as the patient inhales.
    d. The spouse places the patient in an upright sitting position to encourage deep breaths.

28. A patient with an upper spinal cord injury is at risk for Autonomic Dysreflexia. What is the priority problem for this patient?
    a. Decreased cerebral tissue perfusion
    b. Nausea
    c. Headache
    d. Inability to ambulate

29. The nurse is caring for a patient with a recent spinal cord injury (SCI). Which intervention does the nurse use to target and prevent the potential SCI complication of Autonomic Dysreflexia? *(Select all that apply.)*
    a. Frequently perform passive ROM exercises.
    b. Keep the room warm and control environmental stimuli.
    c. Monitor stool output and maintain a bowel program.
    d. Keep the patient immobilized with neck or back braces.
    e. Monitor urinary output and check for bladder distention.

30. What is a potential adverse outcome of Autonomic Dysreflexia in a patient with a spinal cord injury?
    a. Heat stroke
    b. Paralytic ileus
    c. Hypertensive crisis
    d. Aspiration and pneumonia

31. After suffering an SCI, a patient develops autonomic dysfunction, including a neurogenic bladder. What is the priority patient problem for this condition?
    a. Risk for urinary tract infection
    b. Risk for dehydration
    c. Risk for urinary retention
    d. Risk for urinary incontinence

32. The nurse and the nursing student are working together to bathe and reposition a patient who is in a halo fixator device. Which action by the nursing student causes the supervising nurse to intervene?
    a. Uses the log-roll technique to clean the patient's back and buttocks
    b. Turns the patient by pulling on the top of the halo device
    c. Positions the patient with the head and neck in alignment
    d. Supports the head and neck area during the repositioning

33. The nurse is caring for several patients with SCIs. Which task is best to delegate to the nursing assistant?
    a. Encourage use of incentive spirometry; evaluate the patient's ability to use it correctly.
    b. Log-roll the patient; maintain proper body alignment and place a bedpan for toileting.
    c. Check for skin breakdown under the immobilization devices during bathing.
    d. Insert a Foley catheter and report the amount and color of the urine.

34. A patient with an SCI has paraplegia and paraparesis. The nurse has identified a priority patient problem of inability to ambulate. The nurse assesses the calf area of both legs for swelling, tenderness, redness, or possible complaints of pain. This assessment is specific to the patient's increased risk for which condition?
    a. Contractures of joints
    b. Bone fractures
    c. Pressure ulcers
    d. Deep vein thrombosis

35. The nurse is caring for a patient who has been in a long-term care facility for several months following an SCI. The patient has had issues with urinary retention and subsequent overflow incontinence, and a bladder retraining program was recently initiated. Which are expected outcomes of the training program? *(Select all that apply.)*
    a. Demonstrates a predictable pattern of voiding
    b. Is able to independently catheterize himself
    c. Pours warm water over perineum to stimulate voiding
    d. Takes bethanechol chloride (Urecholine) 1 hour before voiding
    e. Is able to empty the bladder completely
    f. Does not experience a urinary tract infection

Matching. *Match each medication with its corresponding indication/effect.*

Medications
a. Methylprednisolone
b. Dextran
c. Atropine
d. Dopamine
e. Dantrolene

Indications/Effects
_____ 36. Increases heart rate
_____ 37. Relieves spasticity
_____ 38. Increases capillary blood flow
_____ 39. Reduces inflammation
_____ 40. Regulates blood pressure

41. What does the nurse do to implement bowel and bladder retraining for a patient with an SCI? *(Select all that apply.)*
    a. Ensure the patient gets a sufficient quantity of fluid each day.
    b. Assist the patient in developing a schedule.
    c. Teach the patient about high-fiber foods.
    d. Teach the patient that continence is dependent upon spinal cord healing.
    e. Teach the patient to stimulate voiding by stroking the inner thigh.
    f. Measure bladder residual with a bladder ultrasound device.

42. The patient is an adolescent who is quadriplegic as a result of a diving accident. The nursing assistant reports that the patient started yelling and spitting at her while she was trying to bathe him. He is angry and hostile, stating "Nobody is going to do anything else to me! I'm going to get out of this place!" What is the priority patient problem?
    a. Noncompliance
    b. Cognitive limitations
    c. Inability to cope with the situation
    d. Feelings of hopelessness

43. The nurse is giving home care instructions to a patient who will be discharged with a halo device. What does the nurse instruct the patient to avoid? *(Select all that apply.)*
    a. Going out in the cold
    b. Swimming or contact sports
    c. Sexual activity
    d. Bathing in the bathtub
    e. Driving

44. During the morning assessment of a patient with a spinal cord tumor, the nurse observes decreased sensation in the lower extremities and the linen is smeared with feces and smells of urine. The patient reports low back pain and appears to be having trouble moving his legs. The nurse suspects the tumor to be in which area of the spine?
    a. Upper cervical
    b. Lower cervical
    c. Thoracic
    d. Lumbosacral

45. A patient is hospitalized for a spinal cord tumor and is receiving medication for pain. The patient is having problems with constipation and urinary retention, and in addition, has limited mobility related to site of the tumor. Which task is best to delegate to the nursing assistant?
    a. Measure and record intake and output.
    b. Check for blanching over reddened skin areas.
    c. Report the patient's relief of pain after using PCA morphine.
    d. Manually disimpact fecaliths.

46. A patient reports increased fatigue and stiffness of the extremities. These symptoms have occurred in the past, but resolved and no medical attention was sought. Which questions does the nurse ask to assess whether the symptoms may be associated with multiple sclerosis? *(Select all that apply.)*
    a. "Do you feel unsteady or unbalanced when you walk?"
    b. "Do you have a persistent sensitivity to cold?"
    c. "Do you ever have slurred speech or trouble swallowing?"
    d. "Do you wake at night and then have trouble getting back to sleep?"
    e. "Has anyone in your family been diagnosed with multiple sclerosis?"

47. A patient with multiple sclerosis is prescribed oral prednisone 60 mg daily for 7 days following a course of IV methylprednisolone (Solu-Medrol). Which laboratory abnormality is a side effect of the medication?
    a. Decrease in hematocrit
    b. Decrease in blood glucose
    c. Decrease in serum potassium
    d. Decrease in serum sodium

48. The patient is a woman in her early 30s who has recently been diagnosed with multiple sclerosis. The nurse has taught the patient's husband about the course of the illness and what problems might occur in the future. Which statement by the husband indicates the need for additional teaching?
    a. "She could fall because she may lose her balance and have poor coordination."
    b. "Eventually she will not be able to drive because of vision problems."
    c. "She will probably have a decreased libido and diminished orgasm."
    d. "Later on she could have intermittent short-term memory loss."

49. The patient and family are referred to the nurse for education about amyotrophic lateral sclerosis (ALS). What information does the nurse include in the educational session? *(Select all that apply.)*
    a. It is a progressive disease involving the motor system.
    b. The cause of ALS is unknown.
    c. Memory loss will occur but it will be very gradual.
    d. Death typically will occur several decades after diagnosis.
    e. There is no known cure for ALS.
    f. Riluzole (Rilutek) is a specific treatment that reverses symptoms.

50. What early symptoms does the nurse expect to observe in a 50-year-old patient recently diagnosed with ALS?
    a. Bowel and bladder incontinence
    b. Tongue atrophy and dysphagia
    c. Blurred vision and headaches
    d. Forgetfulness and decreased attention span

CASE STUDY: THE PATIENT WITH A SPINAL CORD INJURY

Use a separate sheet of paper to answer the questions in this Case Study, or go to the "Prepare for Class" folder on your Evolve website at http://evolve.elsevier.com/Iggy/ to download and complete as a word processing file. Answer guidelines for this Case Study are also available on your Evolve website.

The patient is a 23-year-old man who sustained a C7 fracture during a skiing accident. He is being transferred from the medical-surgical unit to the inpatient rehabilitation unit. He has family in the area and they have been supportive throughout his hospital stay. His mother, in particular, has spent many hours at the bedside and expresses a willingness to take him home and continue his care once his hospital and rehab treatment are completed. The patient has lost approximately 18 lbs. during the hospital stay and demonstrates a weak nonproductive cough. He had been actively participating with physical therapy and occupational therapy, but he is currently discouraged and withdrawn.

1. Identify at least five priority problems for this patient and family.

2. Why is this patient at risk for pneumonia and what nursing interventions could be used to help prevent this complication?

3. What are the major complications of prolonged immobility?

4. Identify the major area of education for the patient with an SCI.

5. What are the expected outcomes of a bladder retraining program?

6. What are the essential elements of a bowel retraining program?

7. The nurse assists the patient with SCI with psychosocial adaptation to successful rehabilitation by doing what kinds of interventions?

8. On the first day in the rehabilitation unit, the physical therapist is working with the patient and observes that the right leg appears larger than the left leg. The nurse is notified, and upon assessment of the bilateral lower extremities, notes that the right lower leg is swollen, a pale pinkish red color, and feels warmer than the left leg. Using the ISBARR format, how would the nurse communicate these findings to the appropriate health care provider?

46 CHAPTER

Care of Patients with Problems of the Peripheral Nervous System

STUDY/REVIEW QUESTIONS

Matching: *Match the terms with the correct definitions.*

Terms

a. Demyelination
b. Paresthesias
c. Hyperesthesia
d. Quadriparesis
e. Ptosis
f. Diplopia
g. Dysphagia
h. Bulbar involvement
i. Eaton-Lambert syndrome
j. Cholinergic crisis
k. Myasthenic crisis
l. Fasciculations
m. Plasmapheresis

Definitions

_____ 1. Overmedication with cholinesterase inhibitors

_____ 2. Weakness in all four extremities

_____ 3. Destruction of myelin between the nodes of Ranvier

_____ 4. Extreme sensitivity to touch

_____ 5. Method to remove antibodies from the plasma to decrease symptoms

_____ 6. Muscles of facial expression, chewing, and speech are affected

_____ 7. Difficulty chewing or swallowing

_____ 8. Double vision

_____ 9. Form of myasthenia; often seen with small cell carcinoma of the lung

_____ 10. Unpleasant sensations such as burning, stinging, and prickly feeling

_____ 11. Undermedication with cholinesterase inhibitors

_____ 12. Muscle twitching

_____ 13. Drooping eyelids

14. The nurse is assessing a patient with a diagnosis of Guillain-Barré syndrome (GBS). Which signs and symptoms are consistent with GBS? *(Select all that apply.)*
    a. Bilateral sluggish pupil response
    b. Sudden onset of weakness in the legs
    c. Muscle atrophy of the legs
    d. Change in level of consciousness
    e. Decreased deep tendon reflexes
    f. Ataxia

15. During shift report, the nurse hears that a patient with GBS has a decrease in vital capacity that is less than two-thirds of normal, and there is a progressive inability to clear and cough up secretions. The physician has been notified and is coming to evaluate the patient. What intervention is the nurse prepared to implement for this patient?
    a. Frequent oral suctioning
    b. Rigorous chest physiotherapy
    c. Elective intubation
    d. Elective tracheostomy

16. A patient with GBS is identified as having poor dietary intake secondary to dysphagia. A feeding tube is prescribed. How does the nurse monitor this patient's nutritional status? *(Select all that apply.)*
    a. Checking the patient's skin turgor and urinary output
    b. Giving the prescribed enteral feedings via feeding tube
    c. Weighing the patient three times a week
    d. Reviewing the patient's potassium and sodium levels
    e. Monitoring weekly serum prealbumin level.

17. A patient with GBS has been intubated for respiratory failure. The nurse must suction the patient. In assessing the risk for vagal nerve stimulation, what does the nurse closely monitor the patient for?
    a. Thick secretions
    b. Atrial fibrillation
    c. Cyanosis
    d. Bradycardia

18. A patient is admitted for a probable diagnosis of GBS, but needs additional diagnostic testing for confirmation. Which tests does the nurse anticipate will be ordered for this patient? *(Select all that apply.)*
    a. Electroencephalography (EEG)
    b. Cerebral blood flow (CBF)
    c. Electrophysiologic studies (EPS)
    d. Electrocardiogram (ECG)
    e. Electromyography (EMG)

19. The nurse is reviewing the cerebral spinal fluid (CSF) results for a patient with probable GBS. Which abnormal finding is common in GBS?
    a. Increase in CSF protein level
    b. Increase in CSF glucose level
    c. Cloudy appearance of CSF fluid
    d. Elevation of lymphocyte count in CSF

20. An ambulatory patient has sought treatment for symptoms of GBS within 2 weeks of symptom onset. Which drug therapy is likely preferred for this patient?
    a. Plasmapheresis and immunoglobulin
    b. Plasmapheresis
    c. Immunoglobulin
    d. Corticosteroids

21. The patient is scheduled to receive immunoglobulin therapy. Before administering the medication, the nurse ensures that which laboratory test has been completed?
    a. Serum IgA
    b. Serum IgE
    c. Serum IgD
    d. Serum IgM

22. Which interventions are appropriate for pain management in an older adult with GBS? *(Select all that apply.)*
    a. IV opiates
    b. Gabapentin (Neurontin)
    c. Tricyclic antidepressants
    d. Massage
    e. Music therapy

23. A patient with GBS is receiving IV immunoglobulin. The nurse monitors for which major potential complication of this drug therapy?
    a. Headache
    b. Itching
    c. Anaphylaxis
    d. Fever

24. The nurse is monitoring a patient with GBS undergoing plasmapheresis. The patient reports dizziness and has a heart rate that has dropped to 48 beats per minute. The nurse notifies the primary care provider. Which order does the nurse anticipate?
    a. Atropine IV push
    b. Epinephrine IV push
    c. Continue to monitor the patient
    d. Defibrillate the patient

25. A patient has been newly diagnosed with GBS. The nurse is teaching the patient and family about the condition. Which statement by the family indicates a need for additional teaching?
    a. "He could recover in 4 to 6 months."
    b. "He'll never be able to walk again."
    c. "He will receive medication for pain."
    d. "It affects men and women equally."

26. Which strategies should be incorporated in the plan of care to provide emotional support for a patient with GBS who has ascending paralysis? *(Select all that apply.)*
    a. Limit information provided to the patient and family.
    b. Encourage the patient to verbalize feelings.
    c. Teach the patient and family about the condition.
    d. Explain all procedures and tests.
    e. Reduce distractions and limit visitors.
    f. Assess previous coping skills.

27. What is the priority expected outcome in a patient with GBS?
    a. Maintain airway patency and gas exchange
    b. Promote communication
    c. Manage pain
    d. Prevent complications of immobility

28. The nurse is reviewing the admission and history notes for a patient admitted for GBS. Which medical condition is most likely to be present before the onset of GBS?
    a. Diabetes mellitus
    b. Recent GI illness
    c. Peripheral vascular disease
    d. Addison's disease

29. The patient with GBS describes a chronological progression of motor weakness that started in the legs and then spread to the arms and the upper body. Which type of GBS do these symptoms indicate?
    a. Ascending
    b. Pure motor
    c. Descending
    d. Miller Fisher variant

30. The patient with GBS is in the plateau period. Which intervention is best for the nurse to delegate to the nursing assistant?
    a. Perform passive range of motion every 2 to 4 hours.
    b. Turn the patient every 2 hours and assess for skin breakdown.
    c. Remove the antiembolism stockings every 24 to 48 hours and perform skin care.
    d. Make a communication board for the patient with a list of common requests.

31. The nurse is assessing a patient with myasthenia gravis (MG). Which manifestations can the nurse expect to observe? *(Select all that apply.)*
    a. Ptosis
    b. Diplopia
    c. Delayed pupillary responses to light
    d. Incomplete eye closure
    e. Decreased pupillary accommodation

32. Which statements about MG are accurate? *(Select all that apply.)*
    a. It is an acquired autoimmune disease.
    b. It has a higher incidence in the U.S. than Guillain-Barré syndrome.
    c. It occurs equally in men and women.
    d. The disease is hereditary.
    e. There is a small familial incidence.
    f. It is characterized by remissions and exacerbations.

33. What is the most common electrodiagnostic test performed to detect MG?
    a. Electromyography (EMG)
    b. Repetitive nerve stimulation (RNS)
    c. Tensilon challenge test
    d. Electrophysiologic studies (EPS)

34. What is the cause of a cholinergic crisis?
    a. Not enough anticholinesterase drugs
    b. Too many anticholinesterase drugs
    c. Some type of infection
    d. Allergic reaction to anticholinesterase drugs

35. What test is used to differentiate a cholinergic crisis from a myasthenic crisis?
    a. Electrophysiologic studies (EPS)
    b. Repetitive nerve stimulation (RNS)
    c. Tensilon testing
    d. CSF protein level

36. What factors are associated with the development of GBS? *(Select all that apply.)*
    a. Recent immunization
    b. Systemic lupus erythematosus
    c. Acute illness
    d. Hyperplasia of the thymus gland
    e. Diabetes mellitus
    f. Trauma

37. The nurse is reviewing the biographic data and history for a patient with MG. What does the nurse expect to see included in the patient's records?
    a. Muscle weakness that increases with exertion or as the day wears on
    b. Difficulty sleeping with early morning waking and restlessness
    c. Confusion and disorientation in the late afternoon
    d. Muscle pain and cramps that interfere with activities of daily living

38. Because the most common symptoms of MG are related to involvement of the levator palpebrae or extraocular muscles, which assessment technique does the nurse use?
    a. Use a penlight and check for pupil size and response.
    b. Observe for protrusion of the eyeballs.
    c. Check accommodation by moving the finger toward the patient's nose.
    d. Face the patient and direct him or her to open and close the eyelids.

39. A patient with MG has "bulbar involvement." What is the nurse's priority assessment for this patient?
    a. Presence of pain in the extremities
    b. Loss of bowel and bladder function
    c. Ability to chew and swallow
    d. Quality and volume of the voice

40. A patient with MG and the nurse are having a long discussion about plans for the future. After an extended conversation, what does the nurse anticipate will occur in this patient?
    a. Speech will be slurred and difficult to understand.
    b. Voice may become weaker or exhibit a nasal twang.
    c. Voice quality will become harsh and strident.
    d. Voice will become toneless and affect will be flat.

41. A patient with MG reports having difficulty climbing stairs, lifting heavy objects, and raising arms over the head. What is the pathophysiology of this patient's symptoms due to?
    a. Limb weakness is more often proximal.
    b. Spinal nerves are affected.
    c. Large muscle atrophy is occurring.
    d. Demyelination of neurons is occurring.

42. The nurse is planning activities for a patient with MG. Which factor does the nurse consider to promote self-care, yet prevent excessive fatigue?
    a. Time of day
    b. Severity of symptoms
    c. Medication times
    d. Sleep schedule

43. A patient is suspected of having MG and a Tensilon test has been ordered. What does the nurse do in order to prepare the patient for the test?
    a. Ensure that the patient has a patent IV access.
    b. Draw a blood sample and send it for baseline analysis.
    c. Keep the patient NPO after midnight.
    d. Have the patient void before the beginning of the test.

44. The nurse is caring for a patient recently diagnosed and admitted with MG. During the morning assessment, the nurse notes some abnormal findings. Which symptom does the nurse report to the physician immediately?
    a. Diarrhea
    b. Fatigue
    c. Inability to swallow
    d. Difficulty opening eyelids

45. What is considered a positive diagnostic finding of a Tensilon test?
    a. After the cholinesterase inhibitor is administered, there are no observable changes in muscle strength or tone.
    b. Within 30 to 60 seconds after receiving the cholinesterase inhibitor, there is increased muscle tone that lasts 4 to 5 minutes.
    c. Within 30 minutes of receiving the cholinesterase inhibitor, there is improved muscle strength that lasts for several weeks.
    d. After the drug cholinesterase inhibitor is first administered, the patient will experience muscle weakness and then return to baseline.

46. Although an adverse reaction to Tensilon is considered rare, which medication should be readily available to give as an antidote in case a patient should experience complications?
    a. Protamine sulfate
    b. Narcan
    c. Atropine sulfate
    d. Regitine

47. The nurse is caring for a patient newly diagnosed with MG. The nurse is vigilant for complications related to both myasthenic crisis and cholinergic crisis. What is the priority nursing assessment for this patient?
    a. Monitor cardiac rate and rhythm.
    b. Assess respiratory status and function.
    c. Monitor fatigue and activity levels.
    d. Perform neurologic checks every 2 to 4 hours.

48. The nurse is performing patient and family teaching about MG medication therapy. What important information does the nurse give during the teaching session? *(Select all that apply.)*
    a. If a dose of cholinesterase is missed, a double dose is taken the next day.
    b. Antibiotics such as kanamycin synergize cholinesterase inhibitors.
    c. Medications must be taken on an empty stomach with a full glass of water.
    d. Administer with a small amount of food to decrease GI upset.
    e. If there is bulbar involvement, eat meals 45 minutes to 1 hour after taking the medication.
    f. Drugs containing morphine or sedatives can increase muscle weakness.

49. A patient with MG develops difficulty coughing. Auscultation of the lungs reveals coarse crackles throughout the lung fields. The nurse identifies that the patient is unable to cough effectively enough to clear the airway of secretions. Which intervention is best for this patient?
    a. Administer oxygen 2 L per nasal cannula.
    b. Perform chest physiotherapy.
    c. Perform endotracheal suction.
    d. Prepare intubation equipment.

50. A patient is experiencing acute respiratory failure secondary to MG crisis. Which alternative to mechanical ventilation may this patient benefit from?
    a. Tracheostomy
    b. Bi-level positive airway pressure (Bi-PAP)
    c. IV immunoglobulin therapy (IVIg)
    d. Bronchodilator treatments

51. A patient with MG has generalized weakness and fatigue and is limited in the ability to perform ADLs. Which nursing action is best to help this patient avoid excessive fatigue?
    a. Schedule activities before medication administration.
    b. Schedule activities during the late afternoon or early evening.
    c. During periods of maximal strength, provide assistance for ambulation.
    d. Assess the patient's motor strength before and after periods of activity.

52. The nurse is reviewing medication orders for a patient with MG. Which order does the nurse question?
    a. Dosage change in pyridostigmine (Mestinon)
    b. PRN order for Milk of Magnesia
    c. Immediate availability of Tensilon in case of MG crisis
    d. Tapering of corticosteroid treatment

53. The nurse is caring for a patient receiving anticholinesterase drugs for MG. Which symptoms does the nurse immediately report to the physician?
    a. Increasing loss of motor function
    b. Ineffective cough
    c. Dyspnea and difficulty swallowing
    d. Gastrointestinal side effects

54. During shift report, the nurse learns that a patient with MG deteriorated toward the end of the shift and the physician was called. A Tensilon test indicated that the patient was having a myasthenic crisis. What is the priority problem for this patient?
    a. Potential for inadequate oxygenation
    b. Potential for decreased ability to perform ADLs
    c. Potential for aspiration
    d. Potential for increase in BP, pulse, and respirations

55. A patient with MG has been referred to a surgeon for a procedure that may improve the patient's symptoms. Which procedure does the nurse anticipate will be recommended for this patient?
    a. Percutaneous stereotactic rhizotomy
    b. Thymectomy
    c. Resecting severed nerve ends
    d. Partial or complete severance of a nerve

56. A patient with MG experienced a cholinergic crisis and is currently being maintained on a ventilator. The patient received several 1-mg doses of atropine. What does the nurse closely monitor this patient for?
    a. Increasing muscle weakness
    b. Increased salivation
    c. Ventricular fibrillation
    d. Development of mucus plugs

57. The nurse is performing patient teaching about plasmapheresis. Which statement by the patient indicates understanding of the material?
    a. "Plasmapheresis causes immunosuppression, so I am at risk for infection."
    b. "I will have to be admitted to the hospital for this procedure."
    c. "Two treatments are given over a 2-month period; then I must follow up on a monthly basis."
    d. "The goal of the treatment is to decrease symptoms, but it is not a cure."

58. The nurse is performing teaching for the family of a patient with MG about fatigue and activities of daily living. Which statement by a family member indicates a need for additional teaching?
    a. "Rest is critical because increased fatigue can precipitate a crisis."
    b. "We should do hygienic care for her to avoid undue frustration and fatigue."
    c. "Activities should be done after we give her the medication."
    d. "The physical therapist will be able to recommend some energy-saving devices."

59. A patient with MG is experiencing impaired communication related to weakness of the facial muscles. Which interventions are best in assisting the patient to communicate with the staff and family? *(Select all that apply.)*
    a. Instruct the patient to speak slowly.
    b. Use short, simple sentences.
    c. Ask "yes" or "no" questions.
    d. Use hand signals.
    e. Have the patient use a picture, letter, or word board.

60. A patient with MG is having difficulty maintaining an adequate intake of food and fluid because of difficulty chewing and swallowing. Which task for this patient is best to delegate to unlicensed assistive personnel (UAP)?
    a. Weigh the patient daily.
    b. Monitor calorie counts.
    c. Ask the patient about food preferences.
    d. Evaluate intake and output.

61. Which interventions are appropriate to protect a patient with MG from corneal abrasions? *(Select all that apply.)*
    a. Instruct the patient to keep the eyes closed.
    b. Apply an eyepatch to both eyes after breakfast.
    c. Administer artificial tears to keep corneas moist.
    d. Place a clean moist washcloth over the patient's eyes.
    e. Apply lubricant gel and shield to the eyes at bedtime.

62. A patient is receiving a cholinesterase (ChE) inhibitor drug for the treatment of MG. What is a nursing implication for the safe administration of this medication?
    a. Monitor for orthostatic hypotension.
    b. Take the patient's apical pulse prior to administration.
    c. Feed meals 45 to 60 minutes after administration.
    d. Drink at least 8 glasses of water each day.

63. A patient with a thymoma had surgery to relieve symptoms of MG. A single chest tube has been inserted into the patient's anterior mediastinum. The nurse notes that the patient is restless with diminished breath sounds and decreased chest wall expansion. What is the nurse's priority action?
    a. Reposition the patient and perform chest physiotherapy.
    b. Activate the Rapid Response Team.
    c. Suction the patient and tell him to breathe deeply.
    d. Provide oxygen and elevate the head of the bed.

64. Following a thymectomy, what postoperative care does the nurse provide for a patient with MG? *(Select all that apply.)*
    a. Use an incentive spirometer once per shift.
    b. Assist the patient to turn, cough, and deep-breathe every 2 hours.
    c. Assess for chest pain, dyspnea, hypotension.
    d. Place the patient supine to encourage rest and sleep.
    e. Assess for diminished or absent breath sounds.
    f. Assist with ambulation every 2 to 3 hours.

65. The nurse is teaching the patient and family about factors that predispose the patient to episodes of exacerbation of MG. Which factors does the nurse mention? *(Select all that apply.)*
    a. Infection
    b. Stress
    c. Change in diet
    d. Any physical exercise
    e. Enemas
    f. Strong cathartics

66. A patient is admitted with a right radial nerve transsection secondary to a knife injury. The nerve distal to the injury will degenerate and retract within how many hours?
    a. 1
    b. 4
    c. 8
    d. 24

67. The nurse has provided discharge teaching for a patient who had a surgical repair for a damaged nerve in the arm. Which statement by the patient requires follow-up by the nurse?
    a. "I will keep my arm in this flexed position."
    b. "I will call the doctor immediately for numbness or coolness in my arm."
    c. "I will use a heating pad on my arm to help with the pain."
    d. "I have a follow-up appointment with the surgeon next week."

68. A patient reports that during a game of football, he was tackled and found himself "at the bottom of a pile-up." He reports weakness in the right arm with a burning and tingling sensation in the hand and fingers. How does the nurse assess for movement?
    a. Put the right arm through the normal range of motion.
    b. Ask the patient to flex and extend the elbow.
    c. Defer the first evaluation of movement to the primary care provider.
    d. Ask the patient how much weight he can lift.

69. The nurse is assessing the skin temperature of a patient's right lower extremity. Which technique does the nurse use?
    a. Place a paper strip thermometer on the patient's skin.
    b. Palpate the extremity using the fingertips.
    c. Compare bilateral extremities using the dorsal surface of the hand.
    d. Ask the patient if the skin feels subjectively hotter or colder than usual.

70. The nurse is caring for a patient with peripheral nerve damage to the lower extremity. What does the postoperative positioning and handling of the extremity include?
    a. ROM exercises for the affected limb to maintain mobility
    b. Joint extension to keep the nerve properly aligned
    c. Joint flexion to keep tension off the suture site
    d. Abduction maintained with a wedge pillow

71. The nurse is assessing the arm of a patient with peripheral nerve damage from incorrect use of crutches which occurred several weeks ago. The nurse observes that the arm is reddish-blue and mottled. What does the nurse interpret this finding as evidence of?
    a. Warm phase
    b. Cold phase
    c. Trophic changes
    d. Plateau period

72. A patient has undergone surgical anastomosis of damaged nerve segments. After suturing and surgery is completed, a cast is placed on the extremity to maintain which position?
    a. Neutral anatomical
    b. Flexed
    c. Partial extension
    d. Abducted

73. The nurse is teaching a patient about postsurgical care after repair of a damaged nerve in the arm. Which information does the nurse include?
    a. "You must protect the nerve sutures for a minimum of 2 weeks."
    b. "Physiotherapy will begin immediately within the first or second day after surgery."
    c. "The cast that is applied after surgery will remain in place for 2 to 3 days."
    d. "Discomfort, tingling, or coolness are considered abnormal and should be reported."

74. Which patient has the highest risk factors for restless leg syndrome (RLS)?
    a. Obese patient with renal failure
    b. 65-year old woman who routinely jogs
    c. 43-year old man with hypertension
    d. Underweight teenager who smokes

75. A patient is diagnosed with RLS. What non-pharmacologic interventions does the nurse suggest for this patient? *(Select all that apply.)*
    a. Limit caffeine intake
    b. Smoking and alcohol cessation
    c. Avoid strenuous activities 2 to 3 hours before bedtime
    d. Avoid taking naps during the day
    e. Apply ice packs and elevate legs
    f. Walk and perform stretching exercises

76. A patient is prescribed ropinirole (Requip) for RLS. What nursing implication is related to this medication?
    a. Teach the patient to take the medication after meals.
    b. Usual dose is between 50 and 200 mg per day.
    c. Medication should be taken at bedtime.
    d. Medication is contraindicated in Parkinson disease.

Matching: Match each statement to the corresponding condition. Answers can be used more than once.

Conditions
a. Trigeminal neuralgia
b. Facial paralysis (Bell's palsy)

Statements

_____ 77. Pain provoked by stimulation of trigger zone

_____ 78. More common in women

_____ 79. Incidence may be higher in diabetic patients

_____ 80. Thought to be related to brainstem activity

_____ 81. Inflammatory in nature

_____ 82. Taste impaired

_____ 83. Requires protection of the cornea

_____ 84. Arterial compression removed by surgery

_____ 85. 30 to 60 mg daily corticosteroids may be prescribed

_____ 86. Soft diet and frequent small meals encouraged

87. What is the priority in caring for a patient with trigeminal neuralgia?
    a. Pain management
    b. Promoting communication
    c. Improving mobility
    d. Providing psychosocial support

88. A patient reports "excruciating, sharp, shooting" unilateral facial pain which lasts from seconds to minutes and describes a reluctance to smile, eat, or talk because of fear of precipitating an attack. This patient's description of symptoms is consistent with the symptoms of which disorder?
    a. Peripheral nerve trauma
    b. Trigeminal neuralgia
    c. Bell's palsy
    d. Eaton-Lambert syndrome

89. A patient is diagnosed with trigeminal neuralgia. Which therapy is the first-line choice for this patient?
    a. Antiepileptic such as carbamazepine (Tegretol)
    b. Muscle relaxant such as baclofen (Lioresal)
    c. Percutaneous stereotactic rhizotomy
    d. Microvascular decompression

90. A patient has had percutaneous stereotactic rhizotomy (PSR) to relieve the pain of trigeminal neuralgia. What is included in the postoperative care of this patient? *(Select all that apply.)*
    a. Apply an ice pack to the operative site on the cheek and jaw for 48 hours.
    b. Perform a focused cranial nerve assessment.
    c. Discourage the patient from chewing on the affected side until paresthesias resolve.
    d. Instruct the patient to avoid rubbing the eye on the affected side.
    e. Teach the patient that he may have enhanced pain sensation during dental procedures.
    f. Teach the patient to inspect the eye daily for redness or irritation.

91. Which statement about Bell's palsy is accurate?
    a. Most patients go into remission in about 1 month.
    b. It is caused by an autoimmune response.
    c. It occurs more frequently in older adults.
    d. It occurs more frequently in young adults.

92. A patient is diagnosed with Bell's palsy and the right side of the face is affected. Related to the patient's right eye, which nursing action is best to implement?
    a. Check the pupil size and reaction using a penlight.
    b. Check the patient's visual acuity in both eyes.
    c. Teach the patient to instill artificial tears four times a day.
    d. Teach the patient to prevent eye strain by resting eyes periodically.

CASE STUDY: THE PATIENT WITH GBS

Use a separate sheet of paper to answer the questions in this Case Study, or go to the "Prepare for Class" folder on your Evolve website at http://evolve.elsevier.com/Iggy/ to download and complete as a word processing file. Answer guidelines for this Case Study are also available on your Evolve website.

The patient is a 45-year-old construction worker who is admitted for diagnostic testing for possible Guillain-Barré syndrome. The patient reports an abrupt weakness in the legs with a crawling sensation, pain, and tingling in the legs. He also reports a burning sensation that started in the lower trunk area. He states, "I feel a little nervous and scared. Am I having a stroke? Sometimes I feel like I am having trouble taking in a deep breath. Is that just my nerves?" There is history of a recent episode of gastroenteritis, but otherwise he reports good general health.

1. List several of the diagnostic tests that this patient is likely to have.
2. Identify and prioritize at least four priority problems for this patient.
3. Discuss the assessment and monitoring associated for adequate respiratory function for a patient with GBS.
4. The physician orders a plasmapheresis treatment for this patient. Explain the purpose and the procedure to the patient.
5. What are the nursing interventions for the patient undergoing plasmapheresis?
6. The preceptor is reviewing the nursing notes documented by Donna Jones, a nursing student. What changes, if any, will the preceptor recommend to the student about her documentation: *0800—Pt is nervous and scared. C/O a burning sensation that started in the lower trunk area.*

47
CHAPTER

Care of Critically Ill Patients with Neurologic Problems

STUDY/REVIEW QUESTIONS

Matching: *Match each symptom of stroke with the hemisphere most often affected by that symptom. Answers can be used more than once.*

Affected Hemispheres
a. Left
b. Right

Symptoms

_____ 1. Loss of depth perception

_____ 2. Aphasia

_____ 3. Loss of hearing

_____ 4. Cannot recognize faces

_____ 5. Impaired sense of humor

_____ 6. Depression

_____ 7. Denies illness

_____ 8. Frustration and anger

_____ 9. Disoriented to person, place, and time

_____ 10. Poor judgment

11. The nurse is performing a neurologic assessment on a patient with a suspected stroke. In addition to the level of consciousness (LOC), what is assessed to evaluate cognitive changes that may be occurring? *(Select all that apply.)*
    a. Denial of illness
    b. Proprioceptive dysfunction
    c. Presence of flaccid paralysis
    d. Impairment of memory
    e. Decreased ability to concentrate

12. Following a left hemisphere stroke, the patient has expressive (Broca's) aphasia. Which intervention is best to use when communicating with this patient?
    a. Repeat the names of objects on a routine basis.
    b. Face the patient and speak slowly and clearly.
    c. Obtain a whiteboard with an erasable marker.
    d. Develop a picture board that has objects and activities.

13. The nurse is caring for a patient with right hemisphere damage. The patient demonstrates disorientation to time and place, he has poor depth perception, and demonstrates neglect of the left visual field. Which task is best delegated to the nursing assistant?
    a. Move the patient's bed so that his affected side faces the door.
    b. Teach the patient to wash both sides of his face.
    c. Ensure a safe environment by removing clutter.
    d. Suggest to the family that they bring familiar family pictures.

14. A patient with a right cerebral hemisphere stroke may have safety issues related to which factor?
    a. Poor impulse control
    b. Alexia and agraphia
    c. Loss of language and analytical skills
    d. Slow and cautious behavior

15. A stroke patient is at risk for increased intracranial pressure (ICP) and is receiving oxygen 2 L via nasal cannula. The nurse is reviewing arterial blood gas (ABG) results. Which ABG value is of greatest concern for this patient?
    a. pH 7.32
    b. $Paco_2$ of 60 mm Hg
    c. Pao_2 of 95 mm Hg
    d. HCO_3^- of 28 mEq/L

16. Which statement is true about motor changes in a patient who has had a stroke?
    a. Motor deficit is ipsilateral to the hemisphere affected.
    b. Motor deficit is contralateral to the hemisphere affected.
    c. Bowel and bladder function remain intact.
    d. Flaccid paralysis is not an expected finding and should be reported promptly.

17. The preferred administration time for recombinant tissue plasminogen activator (rtPA [Retavase]) is within how long of stroke symptom onset?
    a. 30 minutes
    b. 3 hours
    c. 6 hours
    d. 24 hours

18. A priority problem for a patient who was admitted for a brain attack is the potential for aspiration. Which intervention is best to delegate to the nursing assistant?
    a. Monitor the patient for and notify the charge nurse of any occurrence of coughing, choking, or difficulty breathing.
    b. Elevate the head of the bed as appropriate and slowly feed small spoonfuls of pudding, pausing between each spoonful.
    c. Assess the swallow reflex by placing the index finger and thumb on either side of the Adam's apple.
    d. Give the patient a glass of water before feeding solid foods and have oral suction ready at the bedside.

Matching: *Match each deficit with its corresponding definition.*

Deficits
a. Ptosis
b. Hemianopsia
c. Amaurosis fugax
d. Receptive aphasia
e. Agraphia
f. Alexia
g. Photophobia

Definitions
_____ 19. Inability to comprehend language

_____ 20. Sensitivity to light

_____ 21. Difficulty writing

_____ 22. Blindness in half of the visual field

_____ 23. Blindness in one eye

_____ 24. Difficulty reading

_____ 25. Drooping eyelid

26. A patient is diagnosed with an ischemic stroke. The nursing assistant reports that the patient's vital signs are blood pressure 150/100 mm Hg, pulse 78 beats/min, respiratory rate of 20/min, and temperature of 98.7° F. The patient's blood pressure is normally around 120/80. What action does the nurse take?
    a. Report the blood pressure immediately to the physician because there is a danger of rebleeding.
    b. Ask the nursing assistant to repeat the blood pressure measurement in the other extremity with a manual cuff.
    c. Check the physician's orders to see if the blood pressure is within the acceptable parameters.
    d. Nothing; an elevated blood pressure is necessary for cerebral perfusion.

27. A patient with an ischemic stroke is placed on a cardiac monitor. Which cardiac dysrhythmia places the patient at risk for emboli?
    a. Sinus bradycardia
    b. Atrial fibrillation
    c. Sinus tachycardia
    d. First-degree heart block

28. The nurse is caring for a patient receiving medication therapy to prevent a recurrent stroke. Which medication is pharmacologically appropriate for this purpose?
    a. Enteric-coated aspirin (Ecotrin)
    b. Gabapentin (Neurontin)
    c. Recombinant tissue plasminogen activator (Retavase)
    d. Bevacizumab (Avastin)

29. A patient sustained a stroke that affected the right hemisphere of the brain. The patient has visual spatial deficits and deficits of proprioception. After assessing the safety of the patient's home, the home health nurse identifies which environmental feature that represents a potential safety problem for this patient?
    a. The handrail that borders the bathtub is on the left-hand side.
    b. The patient's favorite chair faces the front door of the house.
    c. The patient's bedside table is on the right-hand side of the bed.
    d. Family has relocated the patient to a ground-floor bedroom.

30. A patient with a stroke is having some trouble swallowing. Which interventions does the nurse anticipate the speech-language pathologist to suggest after the swallowing evaluation is completed? *(Select all that apply.)*
    a. Position the patient upright while eating.
    b. Administer orange juice using a straw.
    c. Give small spoonfuls of custard.
    d. Position the head and neck slightly forward and flexed.
    e. Maintain the patient in an upright position for 30 minutes after eating.

31. A patient presents to the emergency department with signs and symptoms of an ischemic stroke. What is the priority factor when considering fibrinolytic therapy?
    a. Age older than 80 years
    b. History of stroke
    c. Recent surgery
    d. Time since onset of symptoms

32. A patient received rtPA for the treatment of ischemic stroke and the physician ordered an IV sodium heparin infusion. In relation to the drug therapy, what does the nurse monitor for?
    a. Elevated prothrombin level
    b. Bleeding gums or bruising
    c. Nausea and vomiting
    d. Elevated hematocrit or hemoglobin

33. The nurse notices that a patient seems to be having trouble swallowing. Which intervention does the nurse employ for this patient?
    a. Limit the diet to clear liquids given through a straw.
    b. Keep the patient on NPO status until swallowing is assessed.
    c. Monitor the patient's weight and compare to baseline.
    d. Sit with the patient while the patient eats and observe for swallowing difficulties.

34. A male patient has sustained a stroke and the nurse is planning interventions to help him re-establish urinary continence. What action does the nurse take?
    a. Obtain an order for a Foley catheter.
    b. Offer the urinal to the patient every 6 hours.
    c. Check post-void residual urine with a bladder ultrasound.
    d. Restrict fluid to 1500 mL/day.

35. A patient with increased intracranial pressure (ICP) is to receive IV mannitol (Osmitrol). Which nursing actions are taken concerning this drug? *(Select all that apply.)*
    a. Draw up the drug through a filtered needle.
    b. Insert a Foley catheter to measure strict urine output.
    c. Monitor serum and urine osmolality on a weekly basis.
    d. Assess for acute renal failure, weakness, or edema.
    e. Administer mannitol through a filter in the IV tubing.
    f. Administer furosemide (Lasix) as an adjunctive therapy.

36. The nurse is talking to the family of a stroke patient about home care measures. Which topics does the nurse include in this discussion? *(Select all that apply.)*
    a. Need for caregivers to plan for routine respite care and protection of own health
    b. Evaluation for potential safety risks such as throw rugs or slippery floors
    c. Awareness of potential patient frustration associated with communication
    d. Avoidance of independent transfers by the patient because of safety issues
    e. Access to health resources such as publications from the American Heart Association
    f. Referral to hospice and encouragement of family discussion of advance directives

37. Which patients are at increased risk for stroke? *(Select all that apply.)*
    a. 66-year-old man with diabetes mellitus
    b. 35-year-old healthy woman who uses oral contraceptives
    c. 47-year-old woman who exercises regularly
    d. 35-year-old man with history of multiple transient ischemic attacks
    e. 25-year-old woman with Bell's palsy
    f. 53-year-old man with chronic alcoholism

38. A patient displays signs of increased ICP, confusion, slurred speech, and unilateral weakness in the upper extremity. Which diagnostic test for this patient does the nurse question?
    a. Lumbar puncture (LP)
    b. Computed tomography (CT)
    c. Positron emission tomography (PET)
    d. Magnetic resonance imaging (MRI)

Matching: *Match each intervention for the stroke patient to the hemisphere most commonly affected. Answers may be used more than once.*

Affected Hemispheres

a.   Right hemisphere
b.   Left hemisphere

Interventions

_____ 39.   Scan side-to-side.

_____ 40.   Place pictures and familiar objects around the patient.

_____ 41.   Approach the patient from the unaffected side.

_____ 42.   Reorient the patient frequently.

_____ 43.   Place objects within the patient's field of vision.

_____ 44.   Establish a structured routine for the patient.

_____ 45.   Teach the patient to wash both sides of body.

_____ 46.   Repeat names of commonly used objects.

47.   The nurse has completed teaching a patient about carotid artery angioplasty with stenting (CAS). Which statement by the patient indicates understanding of the purpose of the procedure?
   a.   "The stent opens the blockage enough to establish blood flow."
   b.   "The stent occludes the abnormal artery to prevent bleeding."
   c.   "The stent bypasses the blockage."
   d.   "The stent catches any clot debris."

48.   The nurse is caring for a patient with an ischemic stroke. Which position is the patient placed in according to current nursing practice?
   a.   Head of the bed is elevated 25 to 30 degrees
   b.   Head of the bed is elevated to 45 degrees
   c.   Supine with hips in flexed position
   d.   Recovery position

49.   The nurse is caring for a patient at risk for increased ICP related to ischemic stroke. For what purpose does the nurse place the patient's head in a midline neutral position?
   a.   Provide comfort for the patient.
   b.   Protect the cervical spine.
   c.   Facilitate venous drainage from brain.
   d.   Decrease pressure from cerebrospinal fluid.

50.   In planning care for a patient with increased ICP, what does the nurse do to minimize ICP?
   a.   Gives the bath, changes the linens, and does passive ROM exercises to hands/fingers, then allows the patient to rest.
   b.   Gives the bath, allows the patient to rest, changes the linens, allows the patient to rest, and then performs passive ROM exercises to hands/fingers.
   c.   Defers the bath, changes the linens, and does passive ROM exercises to extremities until the danger of increased ICP has passed.
   d.   Contacts the physician for specific orders about all activities related to the care of the patient that might cause increased ICP.

51.   The nurse is caring for a patient at risk for increased ICP. Which sign is most likely to be the first indication of increased ICP?
   a.   Decline of level of consciousness
   b.   Increase in systolic blood pressure
   c.   Change in pupil size and response
   d.   Abnormal posturing of extremities

Matching: Match each type of hematoma with its corresponding description.

Types of Hematomas
a. Epidural hematoma
b. Subdural hematoma
c. Intracranial hemorrhage

Descriptions

_____ 52. Caused by tearing of small vessels within brain tissue

_____ 53. Occurs between the skull and the dura

_____ 54. May present as acute, subacute, or chronic

55. The nurse is caring for a patient admitted with the medical diagnosis of probable epidural hematoma and decreased level of consciousness. During the shift, the patient becomes lucid and is alert and talking. The family reports this is her baseline mental status. What is the nurse's next action?
    a. Stay with the patient and have the charge nurse alert the physician because this is an ominous sign for the patient.
    b. Document the patient's exact behaviors, compare to previous nursing entries, and continue the neurologic assessments every 2 hours.
    c. Point out to the family that the dangerous period has passed, but encourage them to leave so the patient does not become overly fatigued.
    d. Monitor the patient for the next 48 hours to 2 weeks because a subacute condition may be slowly developing.

56. Blood flow to the brain remains fairly constant as a result of which process?
    a. Autostasis
    b. Automobilization
    c. Hemodynamic stasis
    d. Autoregulation

57. A patient has been diagnosed with a large lesion of the parietal lobe and demonstrates loss of sensory function. Which nursing intervention is applicable to this patient?
    a. Play music for the patient for at least 30 minutes each day.
    b. Teach the patient to test the water temperature used for bathing.
    c. Position the patient reclining in bed or in a chair for meals.
    d. Use a picture of the patient's spouse and ask the patient to state the spouse's name.

58. A patient has been diagnosed with subarachnoid hemorrhage. Which drug does the nurse anticipate will be ordered to control cerebral vasospasm?
    a. Nimodipine (Nimotop)
    b. Phenytoin (Dilantin)
    c. Dexamethasone (Decadron)
    d. Clopidogrel (Plavix)

Matching: Match each type of trauma with its corresponding definition.

Types of Trauma
a. Laceration
b. Acceleration
c. Concussion
d. Linear fracture
e. Basilar skull fracture
f. Comminuted fracture
g. Depressed fracture
h. Deceleration
i. Open fracture

Definitions
_____ 59. The head hits a stationary object.

_____ 60. There is a simple, clean break in the skull.

_____ 61. Cortical surface is torn.

_____ 62. The head is in motion.

_____ 63. Bone presses inward into brain tissue.

_____ 64. Cerebrospinal fluid leaks from nose or ears.

_____ 65. There is a direct opening to brain tissue.

_____ 66. Fragments of bone are in brain tissue.

_____ 67. There is a brief loss of consciousness.

68. Which determination must be made first in assessing a patient with traumatic brain injury?
a. Presence of spinal injury
b. Whether the patient is hypotensive
c. Presence of a patent airway
d. Level of consciousness using the Glasgow Coma Scale

69. Which statement is true about a patient at risk for increased ICP?
a. The appearance of abnormal posturing occurs only when the patient is not positioned for comfort.
b. Cushing's reflex, an early sign of increased ICP, consists of severe hypertension, widening pulse pressure, and bradycardia.
c. Papilledema, edema, and hyperemia of the optic disk are always signs of increased ICP.
d. Areas of tenderness over the scalp indicate the presence of contrecoup injuries.

70. The nurse is caring for a patient with increased ICP who is on a mechanical ventilator. The patient is awake and agitated, and is attempting to breathe at a different rate than the ventilator setting. Which PRN medication does the nurse administer to the patient?
a. Midazolam (Versed)
b. Promethazine (Phenergan)
c. Naloxone (Narcan)
d. Pentobarbital sodium (Nembutal)

71. A patient has sustained a traumatic brain injury. Which nursing intervention is best for this patient?
a. Assess vital signs every 8 hours.
b. Position to avoid extreme flexion.
c. Increase fluid intake for the first 48 hours.
d. Administer glucocorticoids.

72. The nurse is caring for a patient with a relatively minor head injury after a bump to the head. The nurse has the greatest concern about which symptom?
a. Headache
b. Nausea and vomiting
c. Unequal pupils
d. Dizziness

73. Which statement is true about respiratory problems in a patient with a major head injury?
a. Atelectasis and pneumonia can be prevented by proper pulmonary hygiene.
b. Suctioning should be avoided because of the increase in ICP.
c. Neurologic pulmonary edema occurs frequently.
d. The patient should avoid breathing deeply because of increased ICP.

74. Which Glasgow Coma Scale (GCS) data set indicates the most severe injury for a patient with traumatic brain injury and loss of consciousness (LOC)?
    a. GCS of 13 with LOC of 15 minutes
    b. GCS of 9 with LOC of 30 minutes
    c. GCS of 12 with LOC of 3 hours
    d. GCS of 8 with LOC of 6.5 hours

75. The nurse is assessing a patient who was struck in the head several times with a bat. There is clear fluid that appears to be leaking from the nose. What action does the nurse take?
    a. Hand the patient a tissue and ask him to gently blow the nose; observe the nasal discharge for blood clots.
    b. Immediately report the finding to the physician and document the observation in the nursing notes.
    c. Place a drop of the fluid on a white absorbent background and look for a yellow halo.
    d. Allow the patient to wipe his nose, but no other action is needed; he has most likely been crying.

76. Which statement is true for a patient with a basilar skull fracture?
    a. There is potential for hemorrhage caused by damage to the internal carotid artery.
    b. There is an increased risk for loss of functional abilities such as toileting.
    c. There is an increased risk for cytotoxic or cellular edema with loss of consciousness.
    d. There is potential for decorticate or decerebrate posturing with loss of motor function.

77. A patient is admitted for a closed head injury from a fall down the stairs. The patient has no history of respiratory disease and no apparent respiratory distress, but the physician orders oxygen 2 L via nasal cannula. What does the nurse do next?
    a. Check the pulse oximetry and apply the oxygen if the saturation level drops below 90%.
    b. Call the physician to discontinue the order because it is unnecessary.
    c. Deliver the oxygen as ordered because hypoxemia may precipitate increased ICP.
    d. Apply the nasal cannula as ordered and gradually wean the patient off the oxygen when the LOC improves.

78. The nurse is conducting a presentation to a group of students on the prevention of head injuries. Which statement by a student indicates a need for additional teaching?
    a. "Drinking, driving, and speeding contribute to the risk for injury."
    b. "Males are more likely to sustain head injury compared to females."
    c. "Young people are less likely to get injured because of faster reflexes."
    d. "Following game rules and not 'goofing around' can prevent injuries."

79. The nurse is taking a history on a teenager who was involved in a motor vehicle accident with friends. The patient has an obvious contusion of the forehead, seems confused, and is laughing loudly and yelling, "Stella! Stella!" What is the best question for the nurse to ask the patient's friends?
    a. "Where and why did the accident occur?"
    b. "How can we notify the family for consent for treatment?"
    c. "Was the patient using drugs or alcohol prior to the accident?"
    d. "Who is Stella and why is the patient calling for her?"

80. The provider has prescribed barbiturate coma therapy for a patient with increased ICP. Which complication does the nurse monitor for?
    a. Decreased LOC
    b. Reduced gastric motility
    c. Decreased respiratory rate
    d. Reduced Glasgow Coma Scale score

81. The nurse is performing discharge teaching for the family and patient who has had prolonged hospitalization and rehabilitation therapy for severe craniocerebral trauma after a motorcycle accident. What elements of instruction does the nurse include? *(Select all that apply.)*
    a. Review seizure precautions.
    b. Stimulate the patient with frequent changes in the environment.
    c. Develop a routine of activities with consistency and structure.
    d. Attend follow-up appointments with therapists.
    e. Encourage the family to seek respite care if needed.
    f. Encourage the patient to wear a helmet when riding.

82. A patient has sustained a major head injury and the nurse is assessing the patient's neurologic status every 2 hours. What early sign of increased ICP does the nurse monitor for?
    a. Change in the LOC
    b. Cheyne-Stokes respirations
    c. Severe hypertension with widened pulse pressure (Cushing's reflex)
    d. Dilated and nonreactive pupils

83. The nurse is giving discharge instructions to the mother of a child who bumped her head on a table. Which statement by the mother indicates an understanding of the instructions?
    a. "I should not allow her to fall asleep."
    b. "She may have nausea or headache for the first 24 hours."
    c. "She should gently blow her nose and I'll observe for bleeding."
    d. "She can run and play as she usually does."

84. The nurse is caring for an intubated patient with increased ICP. If the patient needs to be suctioned, which nursing action does the nurse take to avoid further aggravating the increased ICP?
    a. Manually hyperventilate with 100% oxygen before passing the catheter.
    b. Maintain strict sterile technique when performing endotracheal suctioning.
    c. Perform oral suctioning frequently, but do not perform endotracheal suctioning.
    d. Obtain an order for an arterial blood gas before suctioning the patient.

Matching: *Match each key feature of brain tumors with their most likely tumor site. Answers may be used more than once.*

Tumor Sites
a. Cerebral tumor
b. Brainstem tumor

Features of Brain Tumors
_____ 85. Vomiting unrelated to food intake
_____ 86. Hemiparesis
_____ 87. Facial pain or weakness
_____ 88. Nystagmus
_____ 89. Seizures
_____ 90. Headache
_____ 91. Hoarseness
_____ 92. Aphasia
_____ 93. Ataxia
_____ 94. Hearing loss

95. The nurse is caring for a patient with a brain tumor. Which drug therapy does the nurse anticipate this patient will receive?
    a. Glucocorticosteroids for edema
    b. NSAIDs for pain
    c. Insulin for diabetes insipidus
    d. Ticlopidine hydrochloride (Ticlid) for platelet adhesiveness

96. Which statement is true about gamma knife therapy for brain tumors?
    a. It is used for easily reached tumors.
    b. It is noninvasive and has few complications.
    c. It is administered under general anesthesia.
    d. It replaces conventional radiation therapy.

97. A patient is scheduled for a craniotomy. What does the nurse tell the patient and family about the procedure?
    a. The head will not need to be shaved at the surgical site.
    b. There is a coma state for up to several days after surgery.
    c. Drainage of cerebrospinal fluid after surgery is normal; bloody drainage is not.
    d. The family will need to remind the patient of their names and relationships.

98. A patient has had an infratentorial craniotomy. Which position does the nurse use for this patient?
    a. High-Fowler's position, turned to the operative side
    b. Head of bed at 30 degrees, turned to the nonoperative side
    c. Flat in bed, turned to the operative side
    d. Flat in bed, may turn to either side

99. The nurse is performing discharge teaching for a patient who underwent a craniotomy for a brain tumor. What instruction does the nurse include? *(Select all that apply.)*
    a. Suggestions to make the environment safe, such as removing scatter rugs
    b. Reminders that seizures could occur frequently for the first several months
    c. Information about drugs such as dose, administration, and side effects
    d. Directions about how and when to contact emergency services or the physician
    e. Advice about which over-the-counter products are safe to use
    f. Referral to a resource such as the American Brain Tumor Association

100. The nurse is providing education for a patient with a brain tumor. What educational elements does the nurse include?
    a. Instructions to avoid physical activity
    b. Instructions to avoid over-the-counter drugs
    c. Advice that seizures will occur in the immediate postoperative period
    d. Information about dietary changes to prevent recurrence of the tumor

101. A patient who had a craniotomy develops the postoperative complication of syndrome of inappropriate antidiuretic hormone (SIADH). The patient's sodium level is 126 mEq/L and the serum osmolality is decreased. In light of this development, which physician order does the nurse question?
    a. Encourage oral fluids
    b. Normal saline IV at 150 mL/hr
    c. Strict intake and output
    d. Daily weights

102. The nurse is assisting a patient who had a large brain tumor removed to get positioned in bed. Which recommended position does the nurse place the patient in?
    a. Operative side to protect the unaffected side of the brain
    b. Flat and repositioned on either side to decrease tension on the incision
    c. Elevate the head of bed 30 degrees to promote venous drainage
    d. Non-operative side to prevent displacement of the cranial contents by gravity

103. A patient is admitted to the critical care unit after a craniotomy to debulk a grade 3 astrocytoma. What is the priority patient problem?
    a. Risk for Infection
    b. Risk for memory loss
    c. Risk for increased intracranial pressure
    d. Potential for organ ischemia

104. The nurse observes that a patient who had surgery for a benign hemangioblastoma has bilateral periorbital edema and ecchymosis. Because this patient's care is based on the general principles of caring for the patient with a craniotomy, what is the nurse's first action?
    a. Immediately inform the surgeon.
    b. Apply cold compresses.
    c. Check the pupillary response.
    d. Perform a full neurologic assessment.

105. Which statement is true about increased ICP in a surgical patient?
    a. It is a minor postoperative complication.
    b. Diuretics such as furosemide may be given to decrease it.
    c. Cerebral edema usually subsides within 72 hours.
    d. If not contraindicated, the head of bed should be placed at 30 degrees.

106. The nurse is teaching a patient who will receive the disc-shaped Gliadel wafer as part of the treatment for a brain tumor. Which statement by the patient indicates understanding of how the wafer works?
    a. "I'll place the wafer under my tongue and allow it to dissolve."
    b. "The wafer will be taped to my chest and the drug will be absorbed."
    c. "The wafer will be placed directly into the cavity during the surgery."
    d. "The wafer is to be dissolved in water and taken with meals."

107. Which organism is commonly involved in opportunistic central nervous system infections for patients with AIDS?
    a. Streptococcus
    b. Enterobacter
    c. *Haemophilus influenzae*
    d. Toxoplasmosis

108. The nurse who is providing postoperative care for a patient who had a craniotomy immediately notifies the surgeon for which assessment finding?
    a. Drainage in the Jackson Pratt container of 45 mL/8 hours
    b. Intracranial pressure of 15 mm Hg
    c. Pco$_2$ level of 35 mm Hg
    d. Serum sodium of 117 mEq/L

109. What is most likely to be included in the history of a patient with a brain abscess?
    a. Family history of Huntington disease
    b. History of HIV/AIDS
    c. History of osteoarthritis
    d. Vaccination against influenza

110. A patient is admitted for diagnostic testing for probable encapsulated brain abscess and risk for increased ICP. Which statement about diagnostic testing for this patient is true?
    a. WBCs may be normal, even if an infection is present.
    b. Blood cultures are the only cultures likely to grow the causative organism.
    c. MRI is useful late in the course of the disease to identify permanent lesions.
    d. The first test performed is a lumbar puncture to determine if the cerebrospinal fluid is cloudy.

111. A patient has an abscess caused by anaerobic bacteria. Which drug does the nurse expect to be ordered for this patient?
    a. Nafcillin sodium (Nafcil)
    b. Fluconazole (Diflucan)
    c. Metronidazole (Flagyl)
    d. Penicillin G benzathine (Bicillin)

CASE STUDY: THE PATIENT WITH A HEAD INJURY

Use a separate sheet of paper to answer the questions in this Case Study, or go to the "Prepare for Class" folder on your Evolve website at http://evolve.elsevier.com/Iggy/ to download and complete as a word processing file. Answer guidelines for this Case Study are also available on your Evolve website.

The patient is a 68-year-old man who sustained a head injury after falling in the bathroom. He arrives in the emergency department (ED) cheerful, alert, and oriented to person. On physical exam, he has a large hematoma on his left forehead. He reports a headache in the left temporal area, which he rates as an 8/10. His wife was present during the incident. Admission vital signs are blood pressure 170/92 mm Hg, pulse 92 beats/min, respirations 14/min, and temperature 98.7° F. The physician orders a one-time dose of acetaminophen 650 mg orally for the patient's headache, which the nurse promptly administers. The patient reports a pain level of 5/10 one hour after the intervention.

1. Why is it important to determine the circumstances of the fall for this patient?

2. Discuss the importance of obtaining baseline behavior and information from the wife.

3. The ED physician orders computed tomography (CT) of the brain for the patient. What is the purpose of this test and what are the nursing responsibilities in preparing the patient for this procedure?

4. Because the patient is at risk for increased ICP, explain how the patient should be positioned and moved in bed.

5. The CT and other diagnostic results are negative and the patient is diagnosed with a minor head injury and contusion to the right extremity. He is discharged to home. Review the patient teaching instructions that should be given to the patient and his wife.

6. The wife appears unwilling to take her husband home and she states that she doesn't understand the discharge instructions. What can the nurse do in this situation?

7. Use the focus charting method (also known as the DAR method—data, action, response) to document the administration of acetaminophen, including appropriate follow-up.

48 CHAPTER

Assessment of the Eye and Vision

STUDY/REVIEW QUESTIONS

1. Which statement about the optic disk is true?
    a. Nerve fibers and photoreceptor cells are contained in this depressed area on the retina.
    b. It is the clear layer that forms the external coat on the front of the eye.
    c. It is sometimes called the *blind spot*.
    d. It forms a circular, convex structure behind the iris.

2. Light waves pass through each of the eye structures listed below to reach the retina. Place them in sequence using the numbers 1 through 5, with number 1 being the outermost structure, ending at the retina.

    _____ a. Vitreous humor

    _____ b. Aqueous humor

    _____ c. Lens

    _____ d. Cornea

    _____ e. Retina

3. A patient's intraocular pressure (IOP) has increased. Which fluids in the eye does this affect? *(Select all that apply.)*
    a. Blood
    b. Vitreous humor
    c. Vitreous body
    d. Aqueous humor
    e. Fovea centralis
    f. Ciliary body

4. Which muscle is responsible for pulling the eye upward?
    a. Inferior oblique
    b. Lateral rectus
    c. Medial rectus
    d. Superior rectus

Matching. Match each cranial nerve with its function.

Nerves
a. Cranial nerve II (optic)
b. Cranial nerve III (oculomotor)
c. Cranial nerve V (trigeminal)
d. Cranial nerve VII (facial)

Functions

_____ 5. Corneal reflex

_____ 6. Visual acuity

_____ 7. Eyelid closure

_____ 8. Eyelid muscle movements

9. What is astigmatism caused by?
    a. Eye over-refracting light
    b. Eye not refracting enough light
    c. Normal aging process
    d. Unevenly curved surfaces of the eye

Matching. *Match each description with the corresponding name for the eye change associated with aging.*

Eye Changes

a.   Sunken eyes
b.   Decreased ability to accommodate
c.   Astigmatism
d.   Arcus senilis
e.   Loss of night vision

Descriptions

_____ 10.   Opaque, bluish-white ring on the outer aspect of the cornea

_____ 11.   Decreased ability of iris to dilate

_____ 12.   Loss of subcutaneous fat, skin elasticity, and muscle tone

_____ 13.   Flattened cornea, resulting in irregular curvature

_____ 14.   Loss of lens elasticity

15.   A 29-year-old patient has told the nurse that he spends a great deal of time in the sun. In preparing a teaching plan for the patient, what information about protecting vision does the nurse include? *(Select all that apply.)*
a.   Wear sunglasses to filter UV light.
b.   Unprotected UV light exposure increases the risk for cataracts.
c.   Melanoma is the most common eye malignancy in adulthood.
d.   UV light exposure is only a concern with sunlight.
e.   Manifestations of melanoma of the eye will be readily apparent.

16.   The patient is 45 years old with diabetes mellitus. Which information about vision protection does the nurse include in the teaching plan? *(Select all that apply.)*
a.   Wash hands before touching the eyes.
b.   Monitor blood glucose levels closely.
c.   Contact the health care provider immediately if eye infection is suspected.
d.   Do not share eye drops with others.
e.   Twice-yearly eye examinations are recommended for routine care with diabetes mellitus.

17.   Which statement about the pupil of the eye is true?
a.   The patient with myopia has smaller pupils.
b.   Normal pupil size is between 1 and 3 mm.
c.   Pupils are larger in older adults.
d.   Anisocoria is normal in 5% of the population.

18.   A patient reports not being able to see objects in his peripheral vision. Which tests are used to evaluate this symptom? *(Select all that apply.)*
a.   Jaeger card
b.   Visual field testing
c.   Confrontation test
d.   Six cardinal positions of gaze
e.   Cover-uncover test

19.   A patient who works in a machine shop has a suspected metal foreign body in the eye. Which test is contraindicated for this patient?
a.   Corneal staining
b.   CT scan
c.   MRI
d.   Ultrasonography

Matching. *Match each physical finding with the corresponding related technique.*

Techniques
a. Ishihara chart
b. Confrontation
c. Corneal light reflex
d. Snellen chart
e. Six cardinal positions of gaze

Physical Findings
_____ 20. Color blindness

_____ 21. Visual acuity

_____ 22. Peripheral vision

_____ 23. Eye muscle imbalance

_____ 24. Eye muscle weakness, nerve dysfunction

25. When preparing the patient for a fluorescein angiography, which statements are included in the nurse's teaching plan? *(Select all that apply.)*
    a. Intravenous access will be necessary.
    b. Sunlight must be avoided for 2 days.
    c. Urine voided after the test will be bright orange.
    d. Fluids are limited for the first 24 hours after the procedure.
    e. The skin may temporarily have a yellow or green hue for a few hours after the procedure.
    f. Mydriatic drops will be instilled 1 hour before the procedure.

26. Which are correct procedures for instilling ophthalmic drops in a patient's eyes? *(Select all that apply.)*
    a. Check the name, strength, and expiration date of the solution.
    b. Have the patient tilt the head backward and look down.
    c. Release drops into the conjunctival pocket.
    d. Avoid contaminating the tip of the bottle.
    e. After instilling the drop, have the patient close the eyes tightly.

27. Which statement about tonometry is true?
    a. Tonometry readings are indicated for all patients 55 years of age and older.
    b. Tonometry is used to measure IOP.
    c. Adults with a family history of glaucoma should be checked monthly.
    d. IOP stays constant throughout the day.

28. Which procedures are correct for using the ophthalmoscope? *(Select all that apply.)*
    a. The nurse comes toward the patient's eye from 6 inches away.
    b. The nurse comes toward the patient to the side of the patient's line of vision.
    c. When examining the right eye, the nurse holds the ophthalmoscope in the left hand.
    d. The nurse stands on the same side as the eye being examined.
    e. The test should be done in a brightly lit room to enhance visibility.
    f. The nurse should observe for the presence of the red reflex, which should be seen in the pupil.

Matching. Match the assessment findings to the structures observed by ophthalmoscopy. *Answers may be used more than once.*

Structures
a. Red reflex
b. Optic disk
c. Optic blood vessels
d. Fundus
e. Macula

Assessment Findings
_____ 29. Bleeding

_____ 30. Nicking at arteriovenous crossings

_____ 31. Presence or absence

_____ 32. Tears or holes

_____ 33. Margins

_____ 34. Presence of blood vessels

_____ 35. Light reflection

_____ 36. Lesions

_____ 37. Kinks or tangles

38. Which descriptions about the presence of arcus senilis are accurate? *(Select all that apply.)*
    a. It is an opaque, bluish-white ring at the outer edge of the cornea.
    b. It is a gray opacity in the center of the lens nucleus.
    c. It can develop at any age and decreases visual acuity.
    d. It does not affect vision.
    e. It is the result of lipid deposits.

39. Which systemic condition results in exophthalmos?
    a. Overhydration
    b. Sepsis
    c. Thyroid dysfunction
    d. Hypertension

40. A vision acuity of 20/70 means that the patient is able to see at ___ feet what a "healthy eye" can see at ___ feet.

True or False? Read each statement and write T for true or F for false in the blanks provided. If the statement is false, correct the statement to make it true.

_____ 41. The fovea centralis is the point in the macula where the vision is the most acute.

_____ 42. The lacrimal gland is located in the inner canthus and secretes tears over the eye surface.

43. Which assessment findings of the eye are normal? *(Select all that apply.)*
    a. Presbyopia in a 45-year-old woman
    b. Ptosis of the eyelids
    c. Yellow sclera with small pigmented dots in a dark-skinned person
    d. Pupil constriction in response to accommodation
    e. Pupil constriction within 2 seconds in response to light
    f. Nystagmus in the far lateral gaze
    g. Consensual pupil response

44. Computed tomography (CT) is a useful diagnostic tool that can examine which parts pertaining to the eye? *(Select all that apply.)*
    a. Extraocular muscles
    b. Ocular pressure
    c. Bony structures around the eye
    d. Ocular tumors
    e. Retinal circulation

Matching. Match each diagnostic test with its purpose.

Tests
a. Corneal staining
b. Slit-lamp examination
c. Jaeger card
d. Radioisotope scanning
e. MRI

Purpose

_____ 45. Magnifies anterior eye structures, abnormalities of cornea, lens, aqueous humor

_____ 46. Contraindicated with the presence of metal

_____ 47. Topical dye into conjunctival sac, outlines irregularities of cornea

_____ 48. Locates tumors or lesions; patient is not radioactive after procedure

_____ 49. Used to test near vision

50. Which statements about IOP are true? *(Select all that apply.)*
    a. If the IOP is too low, the eyeball can collapse.
    b. IOP is normally low in the eyeball.
    c. If the IOP is too high, pressure is exerted on the blood vessels.
    d. High IOP maintains adequate blood flow to the retina.
    e. High IOP can cause glaucoma.

51. Which medications can adversely affect the eyes and vision? *(Select all that apply.)*
    a. Heparin
    b. Decongestants
    c. Oral contraceptives
    d. Acetaminophen
    e. Corticosteroids

52. Which conditions or diseases can adversely affect a patient's eyes and vision? *(Select all that apply.)*
    a. Pregnancy
    b. Inflammatory bowel disease
    c. Diabetes
    d. Hypertension
    e. Osteoarthritis

53. Change in blood vessels to the eyes as a consequence of diabetes can result in _____ from _____.

CASE STUDY: THE PATIENT WITH EYE AND VISION ALTERATION

Use a separate sheet of paper to answer the questions in this Case Study, or go to the "Prepare for Class" folder on your Evolve website at http://evolve.elsevier.com/Iggy/ to download and complete as a word processing file. Answer guidelines for this Case Study are also available on your Evolve website.

A 71-year-old man is admitted to the hospital for exacerbation of COPD. A history of the patient reveals he has insulin-dependent diabetes mellitus, hypertension, and arthritis. The patient provides a list of home medications that include corticosteroids, beta blockers, enoxaparin, and aspirin. The patient states in the last 6 months that he has noticed some loss of vision in spots of his visual field as well as dryness of his eyes. The nurse notes that the patient lives alone in a basement apartment and his main meal is from Meals-on-Wheels. He admits that his daily diet lacks adequate amounts of vegetables and fruit.

1. What are the top three priority patient problems that need to be documented for this patient?

2. Document a nursing note on the patient. Include any additional notes that may be important.

3. What impact does the patient's nutritional state likely have on his eyes and vision?

4. What impact has IDDM had on this patient?

49 CHAPTER

Care of Patients with Eye and Vision Problems

STUDY/REVIEW QUESTIONS

Matching. *Match the eyelid disorder with its corresponding description. Not all options will be used.*

Disorders
a. Ectropion
b. Blepharitis
c. Hordeolum
d. Chalazion
e. Entropion

Descriptions

_____ 1. Eyelid margin inflammation

_____ 2. Sweat gland infection at the lash/lid margin

_____ 3. Inflammation of a sebaceous gland of the eyelid

4. Entropion may irritate the eye from friction of eye _____.

5. Which descriptions are characteristic of ectropion? *(Select all that apply.)*
    a. Inflammation of the lower lid
    b. Atrophy of elastic tissues
    c. Turning inward of the lower lid
    d. Lower lid turning outward
    e. Atrophy of fibrous tissues

6. Which statements about an entropion are true? *(Select all that apply.)*
    a. Pain and tearing may be present.
    b. The orbicular muscle can be surgically tightened for correction.
    c. Entropion can be caused by eyelid spasms.
    d. The patient lacks sufficient tears to wash adequately over the eye.
    e. Entropion rarely occurs with older adults.

7. Which factors are causes of keratoconjunctivitis sicca? *(Select all that apply.)*
    a. Use of antihistamines
    b. Lacrimal gland malfunction
    c. Rheumatoid arthritis
    d. Cranial nerve VII malfunction
    e. Vision enhancement surgery

8. Which statement about keratoconjunctivitis sicca and its management is true?
    a. Use of antihistamines can stimulate tear production.
    b. Warm, moist compresses help restore moisture to the eye.
    c. Artificial tears can be used as often as necessary.
    d. Care must be taken to avoid transferring contamination from one eye to the other.

9. A patient has been diagnosed with trachoma. Which nursing intervention is the focus of this patient's care?
    a. Pain control
    b. Nutrition
    c. Infection control
    d. Loss of visual function

10. Bacterial conjunctivitis is associated with which signs/symptoms? *(Select all that apply.)*
    a. Ocular discharge
    b. Tearing
    c. Itching
    d. Blurred vision
    e. Mild conjunctival edema
    f. Formation of scales and granulations on the eyelids

11. What are the nursing care priorities for a patient who is a corneal donor? *(Select all that apply.)*
    a. Instill saline solution into the eyes.
    b. Instill antibiotic drops into the eyes.
    c. Raise the head of the bed to 30 degrees.
    d. Close the eyes and apply an ice pack to the eyes.
    e. Contact the patient's family regarding tissue donation.

12. A patient is scheduled for a keratoplasty. What are the possible complications from this procedure? *(Select all that apply.)*
    a. Bleeding
    b. Graft rejection
    c. Infection
    d. Pain
    e. Photosensitivity

13. Which statement about postoperative care for a patient who has had a keratoplasty is true?
    a. The patient should lie on the operative side to reduce intraocular pressure.
    b. The patient's eye will be covered for 1 week with the initial dressing and shield.
    c. The patient should wear the patch at night for the first month after surgery.
    d. The head of the bed must be elevated 15 degrees.

14. A patient who has bilateral cataracts will report which symptoms? *(Select all that apply.)*
    a. Decreased visual acuity
    b. Discomfort caused by light
    c. Slightly blurred vision
    d. Decreased color perception
    e. Decreased depth perception

15. The nurse is using an ophthalmoscope to examine the lens of a patient with bilateral cataracts. Which findings does the nurse expect to see? *(Select all that apply.)*
    a. Dilated pupils
    b. Decreased lens density
    c. Retina that is difficult to see
    d. Clear iris
    e. Opaque lens

16. The deterioration of central vision along with mild blurring is the result of which occurrence?
    a. Wrinkles in the retina
    b. Retinal hole
    c. Deterioration of the macula
    d. Inflammation of the macula

17. A patient reports "floating dark spots" in her vision. What does the nurse suspect is the likely cause of this symptom?
    a. Retinal detachment
    b. Bilateral cataracts
    c. Open-angle glaucoma
    d. Macular degeneration

18. A patient has had cataract surgery and is ready to go home. In the discharge education prepared by the nurse, which activities will the nurse tell the patient to avoid?

19. Which signs and symptoms should a patient who has had cataract surgery report to the physician? *(Select all that apply.)*
    a. Pain with nausea and vomiting
    b. Decreased vision
    c. Significant swelling or bruising
    d. Increasing redness of eyes
    e. Photophobia

20. Drug therapy for glaucoma focuses on reducing increased ocular pressure through what two mechanisms?

    a. 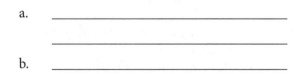 _____
       _____

    b. _____
       _____

21. Which factors may be a cause of blood leakage into the vitreous humor? *(Select all that apply.)*
    a. Hypertension
    b. Aging
    c. Cataract surgery
    d. Glaucoma
    e. Traumatic injury

22. Which statement about uveitis is correct?
    a. Anterior uveitis is also known as *retinitis*.
    b. Posterior uveitis is an inflammation of the iris.
    c. Symptoms include seeing a red haze or series of floaters.
    d. Steroid drops are given hourly to prevent adhesion of the iris to the cornea and lens.

23. Which conditions are associated with posterior uveitis? *(Select all that apply.)*
    a. Tuberculosis
    b. Syphilis
    c. Herpes zoster
    d. Rheumatoid arthritis
    e. Toxoplasmosis
    f. Allergies

24. Which nursing interventions are included for a patient with uveitis?
    a. Patching the affected eye
    b. Offering aspirin and opioids for increased pain
    c. Darkening the room
    d. Instructing the patient to drive only when necessary

25. Which factors are related to dry age-related macular degeneration? *(Select all that apply.)*
    a. Gradual blockage of retinal capillaries
    b. Retinal cells in the macula become ischemic and necrotic
    c. Progresses more rapidly in smokers
    d. Fluid and blood collect under the macula
    e. Eventual loss of all central vision

Matching. *Match the retinal dysfunctions with the correct definitions.*

Retinal Dysfunctions
a. Retinal detachment
b. Retinal tear
c. Retinal hole

Definitions
_____ 26. Separation of the retina from the epithelium

_____ 27. Jagged, irregular break in the retina

_____ 28. Hole in the retina caused by trauma or aging

29. Which statement about retinal detachment is true?
    a. Onset is usually sudden and painful.
    b. Patients may notice loss of peripheral vision.
    c. Patients may suddenly see bright flashes of light.
    d. Hyperopia is directly associated with its occurrence.

30. A patient has a retinal tear that must be closed or sealed. Which procedures may the ophthalmologist use to do this? *(Select all that apply.)*
    a. IV Veteporfin
    b. Laser therapy
    c. Cryotherapy
    d. Patch on the eye and rest
    e. Diathermy

31. After a scleral buckling procedure involving a gas bubble insertion, the patient is placed in which position?
    a. High Fowler's
    b. Supine with head to nonoperative side
    c. Prone with head turned so that the operative eye is facing up
    d. Trendelenburg position

32. What activities should a patient avoid after a scleral buckling procedure?

33. Which sign/symptom is the most common early clinical manifestation of retinitis pigmentosa?
    a. Cataracts
    b. Night blindness
    c. Headache
    d. Vitamin A deficiency

Matching. Match the refractive errors with their definitions. Not all options will be used.

Refractive Errors
a. Myopia
b. Astigmatism
c. Presbyopia
d. Hyperopia

Definitions
_____ 34. Short eye length causes images to be focused behind the retina.

_____ 35. Curve of the cornea is not even.

_____ 36. This condition usually appears in people in their 30s and 40s.

37. Myopia is a refractory error that involves which processes? *(Select all that apply.)*
    a. Farsightedness
    b. Images that are flat and fall in front of the retina
    c. Nearsightedness
    d. Unevenly curved surfaces on or in the eye
    e. Images that are bent and fall in front of the retina

38. A 10-year-old patient was hit in the left eye with a baseball. There is discoloration around the eye. Which treatment does the nurse expect to give for this patient?
    a. Eye patch to rest the eye
    b. Surgical repair of injury
    c. Ice to area
    d. Bedrest in semi-Fowler's position

39. Cycloplegic eye drops may be used with which traumatic disorder of the eye?
    a. Foreign body in eye
    b. Periorbital ecchymosis
    c. Hyphema
    d. Contusion

40. Which traumatic injury of the eye is the most likely to cause loss of vision in the injured eye?
    a. Hyphema
    b. Contusion
    c. Laceration
    d. Penetration injury of eye

41. What is the most common intraocular malignant tumor in adults? _____

42. Which visual acuity test result classifies a person as blind, even if they are wearing corrective lenses?
    a. 20/50
    b. 20/100
    c. 20/150
    d. 20/200

43. What may patients who have lost their sight typically experience? *(Select all that apply.)*
    a. Hopelessness
    b. Grieving
    c. Anger
    d. Immobility
    e. Sense of doom

44. What is the priority intervention to include in the nurse's teaching plan for a patient with impaired vision?
    a. Self-care
    b. Communication
    c. Mobility
    d. Safety

45. The nurse is teaching a patient about self-medication with eyedrops for glaucoma. Which intervention does the nurse suggest the patient do to prevent systemic absorption of the medication?
    a. Wait 10 to 15 minutes between applications of different eye drops
    b. Punctal occlusion
    c. Place all eye medications in one eye, then the other
    d. Blink rapidly after instilling drops

46. What time frame does the nurse use when instilling more than one ophthalmic drug to a patient?
    a. 20 to 30 minutes
    b. 1 hour
    c. 10 to 15 minutes
    d. There is no need to wait to administer subsequent drops

CASE STUDY: THE PATIENT WITH RETINAL DETACHMENT

Use a separate sheet of paper to answer the questions in this Case Study, or go to the "Prepare for Class" folder on your Evolve website at http://evolve.elsevier.com/Iggy/ to download and complete as a word processing file. Answer guidelines for this Case Study are also available on your Evolve website.

A 49-year-old man has come into the ophthalmology office for an urgent eye examination. The patient reports floating dark spots in the vision of his right eye in the last few days.

Examination of the eye reveals right and left pupils 4/2 and 4/2. Pupils are equal, round, and react to light and accommodation. Conjunctiva is clear bilaterally, sclera is white, and the cornea and iris are intact. The right eye has a retinal detachment. The left eye retina background has even color with no hemorrhages or exudates.

Further assessment of the patient reveals that he does drilling as a construction worker. His history includes gastrointestinal reflux disease for which he takes an over-the-counter antacid. He has smoked for 15 years, 1 pack per day.

His lungs are clear anteriorly and posteriorly, with slightly diminished breath sounds in the bases. Heart sounds are clear S_1 and S_2, with no peripheral edema.

1. Document a nursing note for the patient using a body systems format.
2. What type of retinal detachment does the patient have?
3. It is determined that the patient needs surgery. Which surgical procedure will this patient undergo? What will be the patient's preoperative activity orders?

CASE STUDY: THE PATIENT WITH EYE AND VISION PROBLEMS

Use a separate sheet of paper to answer the questions in this Case Study, or go to the "Prepare for Class" folder on your Evolve website at http://evolve.elsevier.com/Iggy/ to download and complete as a word processing file. Answer guidelines for this Case Study are also available on your Evolve website.

A 45-year-old woman has come into the ophthalmology office for an annual eye examination. She has had progressive myopia and astigmatism since age 11 years. In addition to her job as a high school physical education teacher, she also plays in local recreation league volleyball teams and plays tennis with friends. She wears eyeglasses that also correct for beginning presbyopia and has satisfactory correction. This year, the physician notes that she has a very small hole in the retina of her left eye, but no treatment is indicated for now. However, the physician does recommend that she stop playing tennis and volleyball at this time

1. What is the probable cause of this retinal hole? Why did the physician recommend that she stop these activities?

2. Later, the patient works in her yard trimming hedges with an electric clipper. Despite wearing her eyeglasses, a branch whips backward and strikes her in the left eye. She immediately sees bright flashes of light, and at first notes that it seems as if a curtain or shadow is pulled over her eye. What should the patient do?

3. Upon ophthalmoscopic examination, the physician sees gray bulges in the retina that quiver. A tear is seen at the lateral edge of retina. What is the probable diagnosis? Be specific.

4. The patient is scheduled for immediate surgery. Describe the type and purpose of the surgery needed for this condition.

5. Postoperatively, the patient has an eye patch and shield over her left eye. She is now fully awake and wants to use the bathroom. She also is reporting severe nausea. What should the nurse do?

6. The patient tells the nurse that she is looking forward to going home because she wants to be able to work outside in her garden for relaxation. What instructions should the nurse give to the patient about her activity, diet, and postoperative care?

50

CHAPTER

Assessment of the Ear and Hearing

STUDY/REVIEW QUESTIONS

1. Identify the structures in the illustration below.

2. Which is the spiral organ of hearing?
    a. Cochlea
    b. Semicircular canal
    c. Pinna
    d. Stapes

3. Which cranial nerve is stimulated by vibrations, aiding the sense of hearing?
    a. V
    b. VI
    c. VIII
    d. IX

4. A patient who works on the tarmac at a busy airport is being seen for a routine exam. Which appropriate protection measures for hearing does the nurse suggest to the patient? *(Select all that apply.)*
    a. Wear cotton ball ear inserts.
    b. Wear foam ear inserts.
    c. Wear a hat with ear covers.
    d. Wear an over-the-ear headset.
    e. There is no need for ear coverings because exposure time is limited.

5. Which factors can decrease blood supply to the ear in a 77-year-old patient? *(Select all that apply.)*
   a. Chronic obstructive pulmonary disease (COPD)
   b. Diabetes
   c. Smoking
   d. Heart disease
   e. Vitamin B_{12} and folate deficiency

Matching. Match each ear structure with the corresponding locations. Answers may be used more than once.

Locations
a. External ear
b. Middle ear
c. Inner ear

Structures
_____ 6. Mastoid process
_____ 7. Incus
_____ 8. Stapes
_____ 9. Cochlea
_____ 10. Tympanic membrane
_____ 11. Organ of Corti
_____ 12. Malleus

13. Identify the events in sequential order, using the numbers 1 through 6, that lead to the sense of hearing.
    _____ a. Sound waves are transferred to the malleus.
    _____ b. Sound waves are transferred to the incus and the stapes.
    _____ c. Vibrations are transmitted to the cochlea.
    _____ d. Neural impulses are conducted by the auditory nerve.
    _____ e. Sound waves strike the mastoid and the movable tympanic membrane.
    _____ f. Sound is processed and interpreted by the brain.

14. Which are changes in the ear that are related to aging? *(Select all that apply.)*
    a. Tympanic membrane may appear dull and retracted.
    b. Pinna becomes shorter and thickened.
    c. Cerumen is drier and impacts more easily.
    d. Bony ossicles have increased movement.
    e. Hearing of high-frequency sound increases.

15. _____ is the intolerance of sounds that otherwise do not bother other people.

Matching. Match the following terms with their definitions. Not all terms will be used.

Terms
a. Decibel
b. Masking
c. Vestibular hearing loss
d. Otosclerosis
e. Sensorineural

Definitions
_____ 16. A unit of sound for expressing loudness
_____ 17. The process of hiding a specific sound from one ear while the other ear is tested
_____ 18. Hearing loss resulting from neural defects

19. A sensorineural hearing loss results from impairment of which structure?
    a. Fused bony ossicles
    b. First cranial nerve
    c. Seventh cranial nerve
    d. Eighth cranial nerve

20. An adult patient is having problems with hearing. Which of the patient's medications listed are ototoxic? *(Select all that apply.)*
    a. Ibuprofen (Motrin)
    b. Digoxin (Lanoxin)
    c. Furosemide (Lasix)
    d. Levothyroxine (Synthroid)
    e. Aspirin
    f. Cisplatin (Platinol)

21. Which statement about otoscopic assessment is true?
    a. The patient's head should be tilted slightly toward the nurse for support.
    b. The nurse holds the otoscope upside down, like a large pen.
    c. The pinna is pulled down and back.
    d. The internal canal is visualized while the speculum is slowly inserted.

22. In otoscopic assessment, what does a normal tympanic membrane look like? *(Select all that apply.)*
    a. Slightly convex in nature
    b. Pink to deep-red color
    c. Dull red color
    d. Opaque or pearly gray
    e. Always intact

23. Which structure is seen through a normal tympanic membrane?
    a. Utricle
    b. Pars flaccida
    c. Umbo
    d. Cochlea

24. Which is the more sensitive test of hearing, air conduction or bone conduction?

25. Before performing a physical exam, what assessments of a patient's hearing can be done while observing the patient? *(Select all that apply.)*
    a. Noting how the patient is dressed
    b. Observing posture
    c. Checking if the patient replies in brief responses
    d. Seeing if the patient asks for questions to be repeated
    e. Evaluating whether the patient tilts the head toward the examiner

26. The nurse gently taps over the patient's mastoid process and the patient reports tenderness. This finding may indicate which condition?
    a. Excessive cerumen
    b. Hyperacusis
    c. Ruptured eardrum
    d. Inflammatory process

Matching. *Match the hearing test terms with their correct definitions.*

Hearing Tests
a. Voice test
b. Electronystagmography (ENG)
c. Dix-Hallpike test
d. Audiometry
e. Watch test
f. Weber tuning fork test

Definitions
_____ 27. Measurement of hearing acuity
_____ 28. Test for hearing of high-frequency sounds
_____ 29. Used to differentiate between conductive and sensorineural hearing losses
_____ 30. Test for detecting central and peripheral disease of the vestibular system
_____ 31. Tests for vertigo
_____ 32. A simple acuity test

33. Which statement about the Weber tuning fork test is correct?
    a. The preferred site for testing is above the upper lip over the teeth.
    b. Ask the patient in which ear the sound is louder.
    c. Proper handling of the fork includes grasping the upper part of the fork for stability.
    d. Lateralization is a normal result.

34. Which statements are true regarding the Rinne tuning fork test? *(Select all that apply.)*
    a. The test assists in differentiating hearing by air conduction and bone conduction.
    b. The test involves timed responses.
    c. The vibrating fork stem is placed on the patient's mastoid process.
    d. Sound is normally heard longer by bone conduction than by air conduction.
    e. Ask the patient in which ear the sound is heard loudest.

35. What is the measurement of hearing acuity?
    a. Frequency
    b. Audiometry
    c. Threshold
    d. Intensity

36. What is defined as the lowest level of intensity at which pure tones and speech are heard by a patient about 50% of the time?
    a. Frequency
    b. Audiometry
    c. Threshold
    d. Intensity

37. What is defined as the highness or lowness of tones (expressed in Hertz)?
    a. Frequency
    b. Audiometry
    c. Threshold
    d. Intensity

38. Which is a contraindication for a patient having ENG?
    a. Fasting for the past 24 hours
    b. Previous ENG
    c. Prostheses
    d. Pacemaker

39. What does speech discrimination testing determine?
    a. Ability to hear sounds
    b. Ability to understand speech
    c. Ability to receive speech
    d. Ability to hear sounds at varying intensity

40. Tympanometry is helpful in distinguishing which disorder?
    a. Middle ear infections
    b. Outer ear infections
    c. Furuncles
    d. Indurated lesions on the pinna

41. What is the normal response to caloric testing?
    a. Vertigo and nystagmus within 20 to 30 seconds
    b. Vertigo and nystagmus immediately
    c. Vertigo and nystagmus within 5 minutes
    d. Nystagmus with no vertigo

42. What does using a gentle puff of air when examining the external ear canal with an otoscope assess for?
    a. Presence of infection
    b. Pain
    c. Mobility of the eardrum
    d. Eardrum patency

Matching. *Match the type of hearing loss with its definition.*

Types of Loss
a. Sensorineural hearing loss
b. Conductive hearing loss
c. Mixed conductive-sensorineural hearing loss

Definitions
_____ 43. Profound hearing loss

_____ 44. Results from a defect in the cochlea, eighth cranial nerve, or the brain

_____ 45. Results from any physical obstruction of sound wave transmission

CASE STUDY: THE PATIENT WITH HEARING LOSS

Use a separate sheet of paper to answer the questions in this Case Study, or go to the "Prepare for Class" folder on your Evolve website at http://evolve.elsevier.com/Iggy/ to download and complete as a word processing file. Answer guidelines for this Case Study are also available on your Evolve website.

A 47-year-old woman is being seen at the ENT clinic today for reported hearing loss. The patient is alert and answers all questions appropriately. The patient tends to tilt her head to one side and lean slightly forward when asked questions.

The patient's history reveals that 3 months ago she was hospitalized and treated for endocarditis with IV gentamicin (Garamycin). In addition, she takes daily ibuprofen for chronic shoulder pain and lisinopril (Prinivil) for treatment of hypertension. The patient reports that the hearing loss occurred about 1 to 2 weeks after discharge from the hospital. Standing 2 feet away, the nurse asks the patient to alternatively block one external ear canal at a time, and then whispers a statement. The patient is able to repeat back the statement correctly, though she is leaning forward in her chair.

Assessment of the pinna reveals that both are intact and attached to the head at a 10-degree angle. Gentle palpation of the mastoid process elicits no tenderness or pain. Also, bilateral external ear reveals a moderate amount of gray cerumen and the tympanic membrane is transparent. Vital signs are: temperature 37.6° C (99.6° F); heart rate 82/min; respirations 22/min; blood pressure 139/84 mm Hg.

1. What three body systems has the nurse assessed in this patient? Document a nursing note for the above case study using these three body systems.

2. What medication(s) could have contributed to the patient's hearing loss?

3. What hearing assessments have been done so far on this patient?

4. What type of hearing loss might this patient have and what would be the likely cause?

5. What specific hearing test can be done to assess the patient's hearing loss further?

Care of Patients with Ear and Hearing Problems

51
CHAPTER

STUDY/REVIEW QUESTIONS

1. Which treatments are used for external otitis? *(Select all that apply.)*
   a. Application of heat
   b. Oral analgesics
   c. Topical antibiotics
   d. Myringotomy
   e. Bedrest

2. What are the most common organisms associated with external otitis? *(Select all that apply.)*
   a. *E. coli*
   b. Aspergillus
   c. *Pseudomonas aeruginosa*
   d. *Staphylococcus aureus*
   e. Streptococcus

3. Which condition caused by trauma results in the calcification and hardening of the pinna?
   a. Atresia
   b. Furuncle
   c. Hard ear
   d. Boxer's ear

4. Which can be complications from necrotizing or malignant otitis? *(Select all that apply.)*
   a. Extreme pain
   b. Infection of the ear and skull
   c. Brain abscess
   d. Death
   e. Meningitis

5. An adult patient has external otitis. After the inflammation resolves, which actions should the patient *avoid*?
   a. Using earplugs while swimming
   b. Dropping diluted alcohol in the ear to prevent recurrence
   c. Using cotton-tipped applicators to dry the ears thoroughly after bathing
   d. Using analgesics for pain relief

6. Which characteristics pertain to a furuncle? *(Select all that apply.)*
   a. It is a localized infection of a hair follicle.
   b. Permanent hearing loss is a complication.
   c. Most often the infection is caused by Staphylococcus.
   d. No drainage is present unless there is a rupture.
   e. Hearing is impaired if the lesion blocks the canal.

7. Ear irrigation fluid would be *least* likely to stimulate the vestibular sense at what temperature?
   a. 78° F
   b. 98° F
   c. 110° F
   d. 120° F

8. An adult patient has otitis media. What does the nurse expect the patient's chief complaint to be?
   a. Ear pain
   b. Rhinitis
   c. Drainage from the ear canal
   d. Itchiness in the ear canal

9. A patient has been diagnosed with perichondritis. What is the most likely cause of the infection for this patient?
   a. Recent ear piercing
   b. Recent sun exposure
   c. Previous diagnosis of otitis media
   d. Previous treatment of otitis externa

10. An adult patient with a history of otitis media states that his left ear pain is better. Now the patient has noticed some pus with blood in the affected ear. What does the nurse suspect has happened?
    a. Antibiotics have been successful in treating the infection.
    b. The eardrum has perforated.
    c. The condition has worsened.
    d. The ear has been permanently damaged.

11. Which steps are a correct part of the procedure for instilling eardrops? *(Select all that apply.)*
    a. Irrigate the ear if the membrane is not intact.
    b. Place the bottle of eardrops in a bowl of warm water for 5 minutes.
    c. Tilt the patient's head in the opposite direction of the affected ear.
    d. Use sterile gloves during the procedure.
    e. Check medication labels to ensure correct dosage and time.
    f. Pack the opening of the ear with a cotton ball.

12. An adult patient has wax in the left ear. When irrigating his ear, the nurse uses which amount of fluid?
    a. 50 to 70 mL
    b. 90 to 120 mL
    c. 125 to 140 mL
    d. 150 to 170 mL

13. The nurse stops irrigating the ear if the patient reports which symptom?
    a. Persistent pain
    b. Sensation of fullness
    c. Tingling sensation
    d. Fatigue

14. What are the nurse's instructions to a patient after a myringotomy? *(Select all that apply.)*
    a. Report an excessive drainage to your physician.
    b. Restrict hair washing for 1 week.
    c. Use a straw for drinking liquids.
    d. Do not change the ear dressing until the next office visit.
    e. Blow the nose gently, one side at a time, with the mouth open.

15. Mastoiditis is an inflammation of which structure?
    a. Bones in the middle ear
    b. Temporal bone behind the ear
    c. Sixth and seventh cranial nerves
    d. Labyrinth structure

16. Which statements about tinnitus are true? *(Select all that apply.)*
    a. It is one of the most common complaints of patients with hearing disorders.
    b. Diagnostic tests cannot confirm the disorder.
    c. This disorder does not have observable characteristics.
    d. Tinnitus can lead to particularly disturbing emotional consequences.
    e. Treatment may include music during sleeping hours.

17. Tinnitus may be caused by which factors? *(Select all that apply.)*
    a. Repeated otitis media
    b. Otosclerosis
    c. Continuous exposure to loud noise
    d. Medications
    e. Ménière's disease

18. A patient reports an odd sensation of "whirling in space." Based on this description, what is the patient experiencing?

19. Ménière's disease is associated with which condition? *(Select all that apply.)*
    a. Viral or bacterial infection
    b. Allergic reactions
    c. Biochemical disturbances
    d. Genetic and familial traits
    e. Long-term stress

20. An adult patient has been diagnosed with Ménière's disease. Which points does the nurse include in the teaching plan for this patient? *(Select all that apply.)*
    a. Make slow head movements.
    b. Reduce the intake of salt.
    c. Stop smoking.
    d. Take aspirin every 4 hours.
    e. Avoid alcohol and caffeine.

21. Which phrase defines an acoustic neuroma?
    a. Tumor that is benign and rarely causes a problem
    b. Malignant tumor that metastasizes quickly
    c. Benign tumor that can be neurologically damaging
    d. Benign tumor of cranial nerve VI

22. Which factors may be causes of conductive hearing loss? *(Select all that apply.)*
    a. Obstruction of external ear
    b. Obstruction of inner ear
    c. Perforation of eardrum
    d. Otosclerosis from previous middle ear surgery
    e. Prolonged exposure to loud noise

23. Which drug therapies may be used to treat manifestations of Ménière's disease? *(Select all that apply.)*
    a. Mild diuretics
    b. Antiemetics
    c. Angiotensin-converting enzyme (ACE) inhibitors
    d. Beta-blockers
    e. Antihistamines

24. What are causes of presbycusis? *(Select all that apply.)*
    a. Impacted cerumen
    b. Hypertension
    c. Deficiencies of vitamin B_{12} and folic acid
    d. Perforation of the tympanic membrane
    e. Breakdown or atrophy of the nerve cell in the cochlea

25. Ototoxic drugs are used with caution in patients with which conditions or characteristics? *(Select all that apply.)*
    a. Heart failure
    b. Liver disease
    c. Reduced renal function
    d. Young adults
    e. Older adults

26. Presbycusis is the result of what type of hearing loss? _____

27. Which precautions does the nurse instruct a patient to follow after having ear surgery? *(Select all that apply.)*
    a. Avoid air travel for 5 to 7 days.
    b. Stay away from people with colds.
    c. Do not drink through a straw for 2 to 3 weeks.
    d. Keep your ear dry for 6 weeks.
    e. Avoid straining when having a bowel movement.

28. Which action could prevent ear trauma?
    a. Holding the nose when sneezing to reduce pressure.
    b. Not using small objects to clean the external ear canal
    c. Occluding one nostril when blowing the nose
    d. Not washing the external ear and canal

29. Which is a part of the nursing education for a patient beginning hearing aid use? *(Select all that apply.)*
    a. Avoid excessive wetting of the hearing aid.
    b. Turn off the hearing aid when not in use.
    c. Avoid exposing the hearing aid to extreme temperatures.
    d. Adjust volume to the lowest setting that allows hearing.
    e. Avoid hairspray and cosmetics coming in contact with the hearing aid.

30. Which statements are true about tympano-plasty reconstruction of the middle ear? *(Select all that apply.)*
    a. The goal of a tympanoplasty is to improve hearing after conductive hearing loss.
    b. Hearing loss after surgery is usually normal but temporary.
    c. Local anesthesia is preferred over general anesthesia.
    d. Activity is permitted after 6 hours of bedrest.
    e. Postoperative coughing and deep-breathing will be modified to eliminate forceful coughing.

31. Which points are included in the nurse's discharge teaching plan for a patient after ear surgery? *(Select all that apply.)*
    a. Avoid drinking through a straw.
    b. Avoid rapid head movements for 2 months.
    c. Report excessive ear drainage to the physician.
    d. Do not change the ear dressing for 1 to 2 weeks.
    e. Avoid straining with bowel movements.

32. What should a patient who is having a stapedectomy be told about the procedure? *(Select all that apply.)*
    a. Hearing is initially worse after surgery.
    b. Success rate is high.
    c. There is a risk of total hearing loss on the affected side.
    d. Hearing is improved immediately after surgery.
    e. Facial nerve damage is a possible complication of the surgery.

33. Which methods are best for communicating with a hearing-impaired patient? *(Select all that apply.)*
    a. Speak as loudly as possible to the patient.
    b. Assume that the patient is unable to read and do not attempt written messages.
    c. Position yourself directly in front of the patient.
    d. Make sure room is well-lit.
    e. Try not to distract the patient with hand motions.

Matching. *Match each term with its definition.*

Terms
a. Ototoxic
b. Vertigo
c. Cauliflower or boxer's ear
d. Atresia
e. External otitis
f. Dizziness
g. Presbycusis
h. Otitis media
i. Barotrauma

Definitions

_____ 34. Calcification and hardening of the auricle that occurs as a result of trauma and subsequent hematoma

_____ 35. Swimmer's ear

_____ 36. Complete absence of the auditory canal

_____ 37. Damage to the middle ear due to extreme pressure changes

_____ 38. Has three forms: acute, chronic, and serous

_____ 39. Disturbed sense of a person's proper position in space

_____ 40. A sensation of whirling or turning in space

_____ 41. Hearing loss that occurs with aging

_____ 42. Term that describes drugs that damage inner-ear structures

43. Which statements about hearing loss are true? *(Select all that apply.)*
    a. Hearing loss is always gradual.
    b. The ability to hear high-frequency, soft consonants (such as *s, sh, f, th, ch*) sounds is lost first.
    c. Tinnitus rarely accompanies hearing loss.
    d. Vertigo may be present with hearing loss.
    e. Patients often state that they cannot understand specific words.

44. Which therapies are most effective in treating otitis media? *(Select all that apply.)*
    a. Topical ointment moisturizers
    b. Analgesics
    c. Warm irrigations
    d. Systemic antibiotic therapy
    e. Steroids

45. A patient's ear canal is impacted with thick and dry cerumen. Which statements about this condition are true? *(Select all that apply.)*
    a. Cerumen is the most common cause of an impacted canal.
    b. Patients can use a cerumen spoon to remove the cerumen.
    c. Only trained health care professionals may use a cerumen spoon.
    d. Patients can use 50 mL of ear oil to irrigate the canal and remove the cerumen.
    e. Removal of the cerumen will likely improve the patient's hearing.

46. For which ear condition is a myringotomy performed?
    a. Labyrinthitis
    b. Acoustic neuroma
    c. Otitis media
    d. Perichondrium

CASE STUDY: THE PATIENT WITH OTITIS MEDIA

Use a separate sheet of paper to answer the questions in this Case Study, or go to the "Prepare for Class" folder on your Evolve website at http://evolve.elsevier.com/Iggy/ to download and complete as a word processing file. Answer guidelines for this Case Study are also available on your Evolve website.

The 23-year-old patient is being seen in the ENT clinic today for reported right ear pain that started 1 to 2 days ago. The patient is alert, oriented, and cooperative during assessment. She reports having headaches since the ear pain started, a feeling of malaise, and slight dizziness at times. During assessment, it is observed that the patient sits forward in the chair and at times asks for questions to be repeated. The patient tilts her head to the left when she is asked a question or given instructions.

On examination of the external ear, there is no redness or tenderness of the mastoid process or pinna. Otoscope examination reveals a bulging and red tympanic membrane of the right ear. The tympanic membrane of the left ear is transparent and has no redness present.

The patient noticed yesterday that she was asking people to repeat what they said. Patient history includes mild asthma for which she uses as-needed inhalers. She had a cold 2 weeks ago.

1. Document a nursing note for the patient based on the assessment of these categories:
   - Sensory (ear and hearing)
   - Neurologic
   - History

2. What type of mild hearing loss does this patient have?

3. In what stage is this patient's otitis media?

4. What medication will likely be ordered to treat this patient's otitis media?

CASE STUDY: THE PATIENT WITH OTOSCLEROSIS

Use a separate sheet of paper to answer the questions in this Case Study, or go to the "Prepare for Class" folder on your Evolve website at http://evolve.elsevier.com/Iggy/ to download and complete as a word processing file. Answer guidelines for this Case Study are also available on your Evolve website.

The 53-year-old patient is visiting the ENT clinic today. She has had progressive hearing loss since her late 20s. Her ability to hear is better with her right ear, and she has been using bilateral hearing aids for the past 5 years. After being evaluated, it is determined that she has otosclerosis. She discusses options with her physician and the decision is made for her to have a stapedectomy of the left ear.

1. Why is the procedure done on the left ear rather than the right ear?
2. Develop a preoperative teaching-learning plan for this patient. What should the nurse discuss about the hearing aids?
3. Discuss alternative ways for the patient to cope with her reduced hearing ability until the surgery is performed.
4. Postoperatively, the patient is nauseated and states that "things are spinning" when she tries to sit up. Her postoperative orders include meclizine (Antivert) and droperidol (Inapsine). What interventions are implemented for patient safety? What side effects should the nurse monitor for while the patient is receiving these medications?
5. Following removal of the external dressing, the patient becomes upset and begins to cry. She states, "I don't notice any difference; in fact, I think it's worse! Now I can't hear anything with my right ear!" What is the probable cause of her hearing loss? What can the nurse say to the patient to assist her at this time?

52

CHAPTER

Assessment of the Musculoskeletal System

STUDY/REVIEW QUESTIONS

1. Which ethnic group has the *least* risk for developing osteoporosis?
   a. African American
   b. European American
   c. Asian American
   d. Hispanic American

2. The patients with which conditions are most likely to be at risk for osteoporosis related to decreased intake of vitamin D and calcium? *(Select all that apply.)*
   a. Obesity
   b. Bulimia
   c. Anorexia nervosa
   d. Multiple sclerosis
   e. Pancreatitis

Matching. Match each of the following musculoskeletal terms with the corresponding descriptions.

Terms
a. Cancellous
b. Cortex
c. Diaphysis
d. Epiphysis
e. Haversian system
f. Osteoblast
g. Osteoclast
h. Osteocyte
i. Periosteum
j. Trabeculae
k. Volkmann's canal

Descriptions

_____ 3. Living bone cells

_____ 4. Shaft of a long bone

_____ 5. Outer layer of bone tissue

_____ 6. Longitudinal canal network containing microscopic blood vessels

_____ 7. End of a long bone

_____ 8. Spongy inner layer of bone

_____ 9. Network connecting bone marrow vessels to outer bone covering

_____ 10. Bone-forming cells

_____ 11. Bone tissue containing marrow

_____ 12. Highly vascular bone covering

_____ 13. Bone-destroying cells

14. A patient is at risk for a parathyroid hormone (PTH) imbalance related to a recent surgical procedure. Based on this information, which blood level must the nurse monitor in the patient?
    a. Blood glucose
    b. Serum calcium
    c. Serum potassium
    d. Serum magnesium

15. Which vitamin plays a key role in bone health?
    a. Vitamin A
    b. Vitamin B
    c. Vitamin D
    d. Vitamin E

16. The nurse is caring for an adult patient with a recent increase in growth hormone and acromegaly. In assessing this patient, what does the nurse expect to find?
    a. Bone and soft-tissue deformities
    b. Pain that increases when flexing joints
    c. Unusually tall height for ethnic background
    d. Marked lateral curvature of the spine

17. Pivot joints allow for which type of movement?
    a. Flexion
    b. Rotation
    c. Extension
    d. Hinge

18. Condylar joints provide which types of movement? *(Select all that apply.)*
    a. Extension
    b. Hinge
    c. Slight rotation
    d. Gliding
    e. Flexion

19. The knee provides which type of joint movement?
    a. Condylar
    b. Ball-and-joint
    c. Gliding
    d. Hinge

20. The elbow is considered which type of joint?
    a. Gliding
    b. Ball-and-joint
    c. Flexion and extension
    d. Hinge

21. Biaxial joints provide which type of movement?
    a. Hinge
    b. Gliding
    c. Ball-and-joint
    d. Flexion and extension

22. The patient is an athletic young adult man who broke his leg during a sports accident. The cast, which has been in place for several weeks, is being removed for the first time and the patient is stunned by the appearance of his leg. What is the nurse's best response to this patient's surprise?
    a. "Don't worry; it looks crusty and withered, but the strength and function are normal."
    b. "The cast compresses the tissue, but your leg will look normal in a couple of days."
    c. "Let's just wash off the dead skin and you will see that it is not as bad as it seems."
    d. "Without regular exercise muscles atrophy; strength can be restored with use."

23. A 55-year-old woman with a small frame is aware of her increased risk for osteoporosis and loss of bone mass, although she currently reports no pain or loss of function. She asks the nurse to recommend a good type of exercise to counteract the risk. What does the nurse suggest?
    a. Swimming
    b. Deep-breathing and isometric exercise
    c. Walking with arm weights
    d. Golfing

Matching. Match each of the following musculoskeletal terms with their corresponding definitions.

Terms
a.   Atrophy
b.   Bursa
c.   Cartilage
d.   Fascia
e.   Fasciculi
f.   Ligament
g.   Synovium
h.   Synovial fluid
i.   Tendon

Definitions
_____ 24.   Membrane that secretes a lubricating fluid

_____ 25.   Decrease in size and number of muscle fibers

_____ 26.   Small sacs lined with synovial membrane

_____ 27.   Band of tough, fibrous tissue attaching muscle to bone

_____ 28.   Bundles of muscle fibers

_____ 29.   Lubricates joints

_____ 30.   Band of tough, fibrous tissue attaching bone to bone

_____ 31.   Fibrous tissue surrounding muscle

_____ 32.   Collagen fibers at bone ends

33.   Which group has the greatest risk for trauma resulting in injuries to muscles and bones?
a.   Older adult men related to occupational injuries
b.   Young men related to motor vehicle accidents
c.   Young women related to sports injuries
d.   Children who are not supervised during play

34.   The nurse is likely to assess which musculoskeletal findings in the average older adult? *(Select all that apply.)*
a.   Increased bone density
b.   Degenerating synovial joint cartilage
c.   Atrophied muscles
d.   Unchanged strength
e.   Slowed movement

35.   The patient is a construction worker in his early 30s who was treated with oral antibiotics after stepping on a nail. The wound does not appear to be responding to antibiotic treatment as expected, despite the patient's compliance. The nurse suspects the patient may have a family history of which disorder?
a.   Renal disease
b.   Heart disease
c.   Skin or bone cancer
d.   Diabetes mellitus

36.   The concentration of alkaline phosphatase (ALP) (increases or decreases) with bone or liver damage.

37.   A patient has had an arthroscopy in the right leg. In assessing the patient's neurovascular status of the extremity, what does the nurse evaluate? *(Select all that apply.)*
a.   Presence of pain
b.   Hair pattern on skin
c.   Movement
d.   Capillary refill
e.   Sensation

38.   Which instrument is used to assess joint ROM?
a.   Odometer
b.   Ergometer
c.   Goniometer
d.   Spectrometer

39.   Which assessment finding of the musculoskeletal system indicates an abnormality?
a.   Symmetry in the upper extremities and equal muscle mass
b.   Gait balance and a smooth and regular stride
c.   Flexion, extension, and rotation of the neck
d.   Opposition of three of four fingers to the thumb

40. Which factor is primarily responsible for regulating serum calcium levels?
    a. Calcitonin
    b. Vitamin D
    c. Glucocorticoids
    d. Growth hormone

41. The nurse is reviewing the laboratory results for a patient with severe diarrhea and hypocalcemia. What does the nurse find is present in bone and serum in inverse proportion to calcium?
    a. Estrogen
    b. Phosphorus
    c. Thyroxine
    d. Insulin

42. Which hormones affect bone growth? *(Select all that apply.)*
    a. Glucocorticoids
    b. Renin
    c. Thyroxine
    d. Estrogens
    e. Androgens
    f. Catecholamines

43. Which laboratory result may indicate bone or liver damage, such as metastatic cancer of the bone?
    a. Serum calcium 9.5 mg/dL
    b. Serum calcium 8.2 mg/dL
    c. Lactate dehydrogenase (LDH) 185 units/L
    d. Alkaline phosphatase 140 units/L

44. Which minerals affect bone growth? *(Select all that apply.)*
    a. Chloride
    b. Calcium
    c. Vitamin C
    d. Phosphorus
    e. Vitamin D

45. A patient reports pain in the left lower ankle. Which questions does the nurse ask to elicit relevant information about this patient's musculoskeletal problem? *(Select all that apply.)*
    a. "Do you have adequate calcium and vitamin D intake?"
    b. "What seems to make the pain worse?"
    c. "What measures seem to help alleviate the symptoms?"
    d. "What did your family doctor tell you?"
    e. "When did your pain start?"
    f. "Do you have a history of diabetes mellitus?"

46. The nurse is assessing a patient's posture and gait, and notes that the patient shifts his shoulders from side to side while walking. How is this finding considered?
    a. Abnormality in the swing phase, called a *lurch*
    b. Abnormality in the stance phase, called an *antalgic gait*
    c. Normal and automatic gait
    d. Limp or other type of asymmetric body movement

47. In assessing a patient's functional ability and ROM, the patient is unable to actively move a joint through the expected ROM. Which technique does the nurse use to assess joint mobility?
    a. The patient relaxes the muscles in the extremity, then moves the joint through the fullest motion possible.
    b. The nurse holds the part with one hand above and one hand below the joint to be evaluated, and allows passive ROM to evaluate joint mobility.
    c. The patient moves the joints while the nurse applies gentle resistance.
    d. The patient moves the joint to the best of ability while the nurse palpates for crepitus.

48. The nurse is assessing a patient who is obese, especially in the abdominal area. What is the most common musculoskeletal assessment finding in this patient?
    a. Scoliosis
    b. Crepitus
    c. Lordosis
    d. Kyphosis

49. What activity does the nurse ask a patient to perform when assessing ROM in the patient's hands?
    a. Wave the hand as though waving good-bye.
    b. Grip the nurse's hand as hard as possible.
    c. Rapidly move the hands into the palm-up and palm-down positions.
    d. Make a fist and then appose each finger to the thumb.

50. A patient has an effusion of the right knee. Which assessment finding does the nurse expect to see in this patient?
    a. Limitations in movement and accompanying pain
    b. Obvious appearance of genu valgum
    c. Crepitus and difficulty bearing weight
    d. Obvious redness and skin breakdown

51. Which orthopedic conditions will require a patient to have a neurovascular assessment performed at least every 4 hours? *(Select all that apply.)*
    a. Presence of a cast
    b. Crush injury to the forearm
    c. Multiple rib fractures
    d. Femoral angiogram assessment
    e. Recent hip surgery

52. The nurse is reviewing laboratory results for a patient who was involved in an accident. There is no evidence of fracture or bone damage, but multiple soft tissue injuries were sustained. Which muscle enzymes are expected to be elevated because of the injuries? *(Select all that apply.)*
    a. Creatine kinase (CK)
    b. Aspartate aminotransferase (AST)
    c. Alkaline phosphatase (ALP)
    d. Lactic dehydrogenase (LDH)
    e. Aldolase (ALD)

53. A patient who is currently on anticoagulant therapy is advised to undergo diagnostic testing for musculoskeletal weakness. Which diagnostic test is contraindicated because of the therapy?
    a. Electromyography
    b. Computed tomography
    c. Xeroradiography
    d. Magnetic resonance imaging

54. The _____ hormone is responsible for increasing bone length.

55. The primary function of which substance is to regulate protein metabolism?
    a. Parathyroid hormone
    b. Growth hormone
    c. Glucocorticoid
    d. Calcitonin

56. How does parathyroid hormone respond when serum calcium levels are lowered in the body? *(Select all that apply.)*
    a. Secretion increases.
    b. It stimulates bone to promote osteoclastic activity.
    c. Secretion decreases.
    d. Secretion raises serum calcium levels back up.
    e. Secretion further decreases serum calcium levels.

Matching. *Match the substances related to the musculoskeletal system with their functions. Not all substances will be used.*

Substances

a.   Glucocorticoids
b.   Calcitonin
c.   Vitamin D
d.   Parathyroid hormone
e.   Growth hormone

Functions

_____ 57.   Promotes absorption of calcium and phosphorus from the small intestine

_____ 58.   If serum calcium levels are increased above normal, this hormone decreases serum calcium levels by inhibiting bone resorption and increasing renal excretion of calcium and phosphorus

True or False? *Read each statement and write T for true or F for false in the blanks provided. If a statement is false, correct the statement to make it true.*

_____ 59.   African-American women have denser bones than African-American men.

_____ 60.   Caucasian women are more likely, out of all groups, to have osteoporosis and fractures.

_____ 61.   Lactose-intolerant people need to obtain calcium from other sources, such as yogurt and cheese.

62.   **Crossword Puzzle.** Complete the puzzle by answering the questions related to physical assessment of the musculoskeletal system.

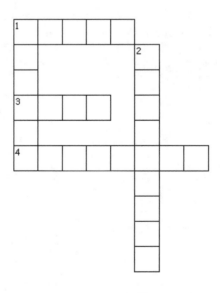

Across

1.   Genu _____, also called *bowlegged*
3.   Assess the stance phase and the swing phase
4.   Assess by asking the patient to perform activities of daily living

Down

1.   Genu _____, also called *knock-kneed*
2.   A lateral curve in the spine found upon inspection when the patient flexes forward from the hips

Matching. *Match each of the following radiographic examinations and diagnostic tests with the corresponding definitions.*

Radiographic Examinations

a. Tomography
b. Xeroradiography
c. Myelography
d. Arthrography
e. Computed tomography (CT)
f. Bone biopsy
g. Muscle biopsy
h. Electromyography (EMG)
i. Arthroscopy
j. Bone scan
k. Gallium/thallium scan
l. Ultrasonography

Definitions

_____ 63. A more sensitive and specific isotope scan used to detect bone problems. Can be used to examine the brain, liver, and breast tissue when disease is suspected.

_____ 64. Used to detect musculoskeletal problems, particularly in the vertebral column. Can produce three-dimensional images. Can be done with or without contrast.

_____ 65. Helpful in detailing the musculoskeletal system because it produces planes, or slices, for focus and blurs the images of other structures.

_____ 66. Invasive test that may confirm the presence of infection or neoplasm of the bone.

_____ 67. Margins and edges are clearly seen because this test highlights the contrast between structures.

_____ 68. A contrast medium or dye is injected into the subarachnoid space of the spine. The vertebral column, intervertebral disks, spinal nerve roots, and blood vessels all can be visualized.

_____ 69. Used for the diagnosis of atrophy (as in muscular dystrophy) and inflammation (as in polymyositis).

_____ 70. A fiberoptic tube is inserted into a joint (usually the knee or shoulder) for direct visualization. Procedures such as synovial biopsy or repair of traumatic injury may also be done.

_____ 71. Radioactive material is injected for visualization of the entire skeletal system. This test is used to detect tumors, arthritis, osteomyelitis, vertebral compression fractures, osteoporosis, and unexplained bone pain.

_____ 72. A test that uses sound waves to produce an image of the tissue. This test may be used to visualize osteomyelitis, soft-tissue disorders (such as masses and fluid accumulation), and traumatic injuries.

_____ 73. An x-ray study of a joint after contrast medium (air or solution) is injected to enhance visualization. Most commonly done on the knee and shoulder joints.

_____ 74. Used to determine the electrical potential of an individual muscle, and usually accompanied by nerve conduction studies. Used to diagnose neuromuscular, lower motor neuron, and peripheral nerve disorders.

75. Magnetic resonance imaging (MRI) is a diagnostic test used mostly to visualize which of the following? *(Select all that apply.)*
    a. Joints
    b. Fluid accumulation
    c. Soft tissue
    d. Vertebrae
    e. Bony tumors

CASE STUDY: THE PATIENT WITH MUSCULOSKELETAL INJURY

Use a separate sheet of paper to answer the questions in this Case Study, or go to the "Prepare for Class" folder on your Evolve website at http://evolve.elsevier.com/Iggy/ to download and complete as a word processing file. Answer guidelines for this Case Study are also available on your Evolve website.

The patient with a 5-year history of osteoarthritis comes to the clinic with severe intermittent left knee pain. She describes the pain as starting yesterday in her left foot and moving up her shin to her knee. The patient reports that when she was gardening in her yard and was walking to the curb to put out the trash, the pain suddenly stopped her. She says that the pain is a burning pain "like nothing I've ever had before," and rates it as between an 8 or 9 on a 10-point scale. She says that she hobbled up to her house, put an ice pack on her knee, and rested for the remainder of the evening after taking Tylenol. The ice helped at first, but her knee throbbed all night; this morning the pain has resumed even though she has tried to stay off of her leg. On assessment, the left knee appears slightly swollen, pain increases with movement, and she is unable to fully bear weight on it. Skin is intact, no redness, warm to the touch; capillary refill in bilateral toes less than 3 seconds.

1. From the scenario above, find the answers to these questions:
   a. When did the pain start?
   b. What factors caused the pain or made it worse?
   c. What has been the course of the pain?
   d. What are the clinical manifestations?
   e. What was the description of the pain?
   f. Were there any functional problems?
   g. What measures were tried to reduce pain? Were those methods successful?

2. Describe the physical assessment that should be conducted for this patient.

3. The physician orders an arthroscopy for surgical repair. Explain the procedure in terms that the patient will understand.

4. Document a nursing note for this patient using the body systems approach.

Care of Patients with Musculoskeletal Problems

53

CHAPTER

STUDY/REVIEW QUESTIONS

Matching. *Match each musculoskeletal disorder with its corresponding risk factor.*

Musculoskeletal Disorder
a. Osteoporosis
b. Osteomalacia
c. Osteomyelitis

Risk Factor
_____ 1. Older adults, vitamin D deficiency, insufficient exposure to sunlight

_____ 2. Possibly a result of latent viral infection

_____ 3. Female, white, menopausal, thin, lean, immobilization

Matching. *Match the objective patient data with the musculoskeletal disorders they are primarily associated with. Answers may be used more than once.*

Musculoskeletal Disorders
a. Osteoporosis
b. Osteomalacia
c. Paget's disease

Objective Patient Data
_____ 4. Unsteady gait
_____ 5. Hip flexion contractures
_____ 6. Flushed, warm skin
_____ 7. Vertebral fracture
_____ 8. Bone tenderness over rib cage
_____ 9. Kyphosis
_____ 10. Long bone bowing
_____ 11. Discomfort on vertebral palpation
_____ 12. Soft skull

13. The nurse is conducting an assessment on a patient with osteoporosis. Which factors and/or patient data may be associated with this disorder? *(Select all that apply.)*
a. Muscle cramps
b. Sedentary lifestyle
c. Back pain relieved by rest
d. Fracture
e. Urinary or renal stones

14. Which factors and/or patient data may be associated with osteomalacia? *(Select all that apply.)*
a. Vitamin D deficiency
b. Drinks 8 cups of coffee per day
c. Muscle weakness in the pelvic girdle area
d. Bone pain worsened by walking
e. Muscle weakness in legs

15. Which factors may be associated with Paget's disease? *(Select all that apply.)*
    a. Loss of height
    b. Apathy or lethargy
    c. Urinary or renal stones
    d. Cigarette smoker
    e. Muscle cramps

16. The nurse is reviewing T-scores for a 68-year-old woman. The patient has a T-score of –2.5. How does the nurse interpret this data?
    a. The patient has osteopenia.
    b. The patient has osteoporosis.
    c. This is a normal score for the patient's age.
    d. There is osteoblastic activity.

17. Which patient is at risk for regional osteoporosis?
    a. Patient who has been in a long leg cast for 10 weeks
    b. Patient on long-term corticosteroid therapy
    c. Patient with a history of hyperparathyroidism
    d. Menopausal patient

18. Which patients are at risk for osteoporosis because of nutritional issues? *(Select all that apply.)*
    a. Older adult female patient who likes to drink a lot of coffee
    b. Patient who has had gastric bypass surgery for obesity
    c. Patient who is on the high-protein Atkins diet
    d. Patient who prefers to drink diluted powdered milk
    e. Patient who drinks two diet sodas per day
    f. Patient with chronic alcoholism

19. The nurse is assessing an older adult patient at risk for osteoporosis. Which task can be delegated to the unlicensed assistive personnel (UAP)?
    a. Inspect the vertebral column.
    b. Take height and weight measurements.
    c. Compare observations to previous findings.
    d. Ask if the patient is shorter or has gained or lost weight.

20. A patient with osteoporosis moves slowly and carefully with voluntarily restriction of movement. The lower thoracic area is tender on palpation. How does the nurse interpret this assessment data?
    a. Vertebral compression fracture
    b. Kyphosis of the dorsal spine
    c. Osteopenia related to immobility
    d. Increased osteoblastic activity

21. The home health nurse is visiting an older adult patient with osteoporosis and severe kyphosis. When the nurse asks about activities she has been doing, the patient replies, "I used to be very active and beautiful when I was younger." What is the nurse's best response?
    a. "You are still very beautiful."
    b. "Activity can help to prevent fractures and complications."
    c. "Tell me what you used to do."
    d. "Do you need information about age-appropriate exercises?"

22. A patient is scheduled to have a dual x-ray absorptiometry (DXA). What information does the nurse give to the patient about preparing for the test?
    a. "Leave metallic objects such as jewelry, coins, and belt buckles at home."
    b. "Have someone come with you to drive you home after the test."
    c. "You will be asked to give a urine specimen prior to the test."
    d. "Bring a comfortable loose nightgown without buttons or snaps."

23. A patient is lactose intolerant and would like suggestions about food sources that supply adequate calcium and vitamin D. In addition to a generally well-balanced diet, what foods does the nurse suggest?
    a. Fresh apples and pears
    b. Whole-wheat bread
    c. Fortified soy or rice products
    d. Prune or cranberry juice

24. The nurse wishes to provide additional diet information for the patient in question #23. What other resources does the nurse suggest? *(Select all that apply.)*
    a. Physician consultation
    b. Registered dietitian consultation
    c. Handouts from the clinic
    d. Internet websites
    e. Social worker consultation

25. A patient has been advised by the health care provider that exercising may help prevent osteoporosis. Which exercise does the nurse recommend to the patient?
    a. Swimming 10 to 15 laps three to five times a week
    b. Running for 20 minutes four times a week
    c. Bowling for 60 minutes three times a week
    d. Walking for 30 minutes three to five times a week

26. Calcitonin (Calcimar) has been prescribed to a patient. What instructions does the nurse provide about this medication? *(Select all that apply.)*
    a. It is a parathyroid hormone that will increase bone density.
    b. It will help prevent bone loss.
    c. It will stimulate the production of bone cells.
    d. Flushing, headache, nausea, and vomiting may be side effects.
    e. Nasal mucosa irritation may occur if taken intranasally.

27. Which drug should not be given to women with a history of venous thromboembolism?

28. Which are potential adverse reactions of alendronate (Fosamax)? *(Select all that apply.)*
    a. Difficulty swallowing
    b. Drowsiness
    c. Esophagitis
    d. Constipation
    e. Esophageal ulcers

29. _____ is a side effect of taking calcium and can cause serious damage to the urinary system.

30. Men develop osteoporosis after the age of 50 because their _____ levels decrease.

31. Peripheral quantitative ultrasound (pQUS) is an effective and low-cost screening tool that can detect osteoporosis and predict risk for _____ fracture.

32. The nurse is reviewing the prescriptions for a patient receiving drug therapy for the prevention of osteoporosis. The patient also has hypertension. Which prescription order does the nurse question?
    a. Calcium supplements
    b. Hormone replacement therapy
    c. Alendronate (Fosamax)
    d. Raloxifene (Evista)

33. Standards for the diagnosis of osteoporosis are based on bone mineral density (BMD) testing that provides a _____ for the patient.

34. A patient is prescribed calcitonin for treatment of Paget's disease. What does the nurse advise the patient to do?
    a. Avoid eating salmon because calcitonin is derived from salmon.
    b. Alternate nares to prevent nasal mucosal irritation.
    c. Take a drug holiday after 1 year of therapy.
    d. Store the drug in a cool, dry, dark place.

35. A patient reports pain in the lower legs and pelvis which is aggravated by activity and worse at night. The nurse observes muscle weakness which appears to be causing a waddling and unsteady gait. What additional information supports the likelihood of osteomalacia in this patient?
    a. Recent immigration from a country where famine is common
    b. Taking hormone replacement therapy for a prolonged time
    c. Unable to perform a prescribed exercise regimen
    d. History of recent vertebroplasty for osteoporosis

36. An x-ray shows the presence of radiolucent bands (Looser's lines or zones) in a patient. What is this diagnostic finding specific for?
    a. Osteoporosis
    b. Osteomalacia
    c. Paget's disease
    d. Osteomyelitis

37. The nurse is assessing a patient who reports moderate bone pain in the hip and has a family history of Paget's disease. In performing a musculoskeletal assessment, the nurse pays particular attention to which element?
    a. Size and shape of the skull
    b. Long-bone bowing in the legs
    c. Asymmetrical deformity of the extremities
    d. Loose teeth and difficulty chewing

38. A patient with Paget's disease has complications related to bony enlargements of the skull. Which complication is potentially the most serious and life-threatening?
    a. Basilar complications with compression on the cranial nerves
    b. Platybasia, or basilar invagination with brainstem manifestations
    c. Blockage of cerebrospinal fluid (CSF), resulting in hydrocephalus
    d. Pressure from an enlarged temporal bone leading to deafness and vertigo

39. A patient with Paget's disease comes to the clinic for evaluation. Which symptom reported by the patient alerts the nurse to the possibility of osteogenic sarcoma?
    a. Change in hearing
    b. Warmth and redness of the joints
    c. Changes in balance and gait
    d. Severe bone pain

40. A patient with Paget's disease has a kidney problem associated with an increased serum calcium. What is the nursing priority for this patient?
    a. Encourage the patient to increase fluids, unless contraindicated.
    b. Encourage moderate consumption of milk and dairy products.
    c. Assist the patient to problem-solve incontinence issues.
    d. Direct the UAP to measure and record all urine output.

41. A patient is having diagnostic testing to determine the probability of Paget's disease. If the disease is present, which laboratory result does the nurse expect to see?
    a. Slightly decreased serum calcium level
    b. Increased serum alkaline phosphatase (ALP)
    c. Decreased pyridinium (PYD)
    d. Absence of osteocalcin

42. A patient with Paget's disease has been prescribed drug therapy. The nurse prepares patient teaching information for which medication as a first-line therapy?
    a. Calcitonin
    b. Ibuprofen (Motrin)
    c. Plicamycin (Mithracin)
    d. Risedronate (Actonel)

43. A patient is admitted for acute osteomyelitis of the left lower leg. What does the nurse expect to find documented in the patient's admitting assessment?
    a. Temperature greater than 101° F; swelling, tenderness, erythema, and warmth of area
    b. Ulceration resulting with sinus tract formation, localized pain, and drainage
    c. Pain is aching, poorly described, deep, and worsened by pressure and weight bearing
    d. Shortening of the extremity with pain during weight bearing or palpation

44. The nurse is caring for a patient with osteomyelitis. Which laboratory results are of primary concern for this disorder?
    a. Bone-specific alkaline phosphatase and osteocalcin
    b. Serum calcium level and alkaline phosphatase
    c. White blood cell count and erythrocyte sedimentation rate
    d. Thyroid function tests and uric acid levels

45. Which patient is mostly likely to be a candidate for hyperbaric oxygen therapy?
    a. Patient with chronic, unremitting osteomyelitis
    b. Patient with an advanced case of Paget's disease
    c. Patient with osteomalacia related to poverty
    d. Patient with osteoporosis and recurrent fractures

46. A patient comes to the emergency department (ED) after accidentally puncturing his hand with an automatic nail gun. Which disorder is this patient primarily at risk for?
    a. Osteoporosis
    b. Osteomyelitis
    c. Osteomalacia
    d. Dupuytren's contracture

47. The nurse is caring for a patient with acute osteomyelitis. What assessment findings typically accompany this medical diagnosis? *(Select all that apply.)*
    a. Fever; temperature usually above 101° F
    b. Sinus tract formation
    c. Erythema of the affected area
    d. Swelling around the affected area
    e. Decreased peripheral pulses

48. The nurse is teaching a patient about antibiotic therapy for osteomyelitis. What information does the nurse give to the patient?
    a. Single-agent therapy is the most effective treatment for acute infections.
    b. Chronic osteomyelitis may require 1 month of antibiotic therapy.
    c. Patients usually remain hospitalized to complete the full course of antibiotic therapy.
    d. The infected wound may be irrigated with one or more types of antibiotic solutions.

49. A patient is diagnosed with Ewing's sarcoma. Which characteristics are specific to this type of bone cancer? *(Select all that apply.)*
    a. Low-grade fever is present.
    b. Leukocytosis is present.
    c. In 50% of cases, the tumor is found in a distal femur.
    d. Death usually results from metastasis to lungs and other bones.
    e. Ribs and upper extremities are most affected.

50. A patient is being seen in the clinic for dull pain and swelling of the proximal femur over 2-3 months. Which malignant bone tumor might this be?
    a. Ewing's sarcoma
    b. Chondrosarcoma
    c. Fibrosarcoma
    d. Osteosarcoma

51. The nurse is seeing a 49-year-old man in the clinic for left mid-tibia tenderness for the past 3 months. What type of malignant bone tumor might this patient have?
    a. Chondrosarcoma
    b. Ewing's sarcoma
    c. Fibrosarcoma
    d. Osteosarcoma

52. Which radiographic findings are associated with a malignant bone tumor growth? *(Select all that apply.)*
    a. Sharp margins
    b. Irregular new periosteal bone
    c. Intact cortices
    d. Bone destruction
    e. Poor margination

53. Which radiographic findings are associated with benign bone tumor growth? *(Select all that apply.)*
    a. Intact cortices
    b. Cortical breakthrough
    c. Smooth uniform periosteal bone
    d. Sharp margins
    e. Irregular new periosteal bone

54. _____ cancerous bone tumors occur most frequently in patients who are between 10 and 30 years of age.

55. What is the most common type of malignant bone tumor?
    a. Ewing's sarcoma
    b. Chondrosarcoma
    c. Fibrosarcoma
    d. Osteosarcoma

56. Which assessment finding in a patient who has undergone a bone graft for a tumor does the nurse report to the health care provider immediately?
    a. Extremity distal to the operative site is warm and pink.
    b. Cast over the operative site is cool to the touch.
    c. Delayed capillary refill presents in digits distal to the site.
    d. Pain is present in the operative extremity.

57. A patient with a bone tumor is grieving and anxious. The nurse includes which psychosocial interventions? *(Select all that apply.)*
    a. Allow the patient to verbalize feelings.
    b. Offer to call the patient's spiritual or religious adviser.
    c. Prepare the patient for death.
    d. Share stories of personal losses.
    e. Redirect the patient to more cheerful topics.
    f. Listen attentively while the patient talks.

58. A patient being evaluated for bone pain has an x-ray report that includes poor demonstration of bone margins, bone destruction, irregular periosteal new bone, and breakthrough of the cortical layer. What do these findings indicate?
    a. Malignant bone tumor such as osteosarcoma
    b. Benign bone tumor such as osteochondroma
    c. Advanced Paget's disease
    d. Osteomalacia with osteoporosis

59. A patient with bone sarcoma had surgery to salvage an upper limb. The nurse has identified the patient has impaired physical mobility related to musculoskeletal impairment. Which intervention does the nurse perform in the early postoperative period?
    a. Encourage the patient to use the opposite hand to achieve forward flexion and abduction of the affected shoulder.
    b. Encourage the patient to emphasize strengthening the quadriceps muscles by using passive and active motion.
    c. Instruct the UAP to completely perform hygiene for the patient until the patient expresses readiness to do self-care.
    d. Evaluate the patient's and family's readiness to use the continuous passive motion machine in the home setting.

60. A patient with bone cancer has had the right lower leg surgically removed. The patient has been brave and uncomplaining, but the nurse recognizes that the patient is likely to experience grieving. What is the nurse's most important role?
    a. Act as a patient advocate to promote the physician-patient relationship.
    b. Encourage the patient to talk to the family and complete an advance directive.
    c. Be an active listener and encourage the patient and family to verbalize feelings.
    d. Help the patient and family cope with and resolve grief and loss issues.

Matching. Match each term related to bone tumors with its corresponding definition.

Bone Tumors
a. Chondrogenic
b. Fibrogenic
c. Osteogenic
d. Sarcoma
e. Secondary tumor

Definitions
_____ 61. Tumor arising from bone.
_____ 62. Malignant tumor metastasizing to bone.
_____ 63. Tumor arising from cartilage.
_____ 64. Tumor arising from fibrous tissue.
_____ 65. Malignant bone tumor arising from underlying tissue.

Matching. Match each type of benign tumor with its most common location.

Types of Benign Tumors
a. Chondroma
b. Giant cell tumor
c. Osteochondroma

Most Common Locations
_____ 66. Hands and feet
_____ 67. Femur and tibia
_____ 68. Often spreads to lungs

Matching. Match each type of malignant bone tumor with the associated signs and symptoms.

Types of Malignant Bone Tumors
a. Chondrosarcoma
b. Ewing's sarcoma
c. Fibrosarcoma
d. Osteosarcoma

Signs and Symptoms
_____ 69. Local tenderness in lower extremity long bones
_____ 70. Short-term pain and swelling in distal femur
_____ 71. Long-term dull pain near proximal femur
_____ 72. Pain and swelling in lower pelvis

73. A patient who is a long-distance runner reports severe pain in the arch of the foot, especially when getting out of bed and with weight bearing. What does the nurse suspect in this patient?
    a. Morton's neuroma
    b. Plantar fasciitis
    c. Hammertoe
    d. Hallux valgus deformity

74. The nurse is assessing an older Caucasian man and notes there are flexion contractures of the fourth or and fifth fingers. The patient reports that he had a similar problem on the other hand and had a fasciectomy which improved the function. What is this condition known as?
    a. Dupuytren's contracture
    b. Ganglion cyst
    c. Bunion
    d. Plantar digital neuritis

75. A patient is diagnosed with plantar fasciitis. What instruction does the nurse give to the patient about self-care for this condition?
    a. Use rest, elevation, and warm packs.
    b. Perform gentle jogging exercises.
    c. Strap the foot to maintain the arch.
    d. Wear loose or open shoes, such as sandals.

Matching. Match the characteristics to the hand disorders they are primarily associated with. Answers may be used more than once.

Hand Disorders

a. Ganglion
b. Dupuytren's contracture

Characteristics

_____ 76. Usually occurs in older Caucasian men

_____ 77. Round, cyst-like lesion

_____ 78. Can be bilateral

_____ 79. Progressive palmar flexion deformity

_____ 80. Joint discomfort after strain

_____ 81. Cause unknown

_____ 82. Fourth and fifth digits affected

_____ 83. Painless on palpation

_____ 84. Familial tendency common

_____ 85. Function becomes impaired; surgical release is required

_____ 86. Most likely to develop in people between 15 and 50 years of age

Matching. Match each characteristic to the foot disorder it is primarily associated with. Answers may be used more than once.

Foot Disorders

a. Hallux valgus
b. Hammertoe
c. Morton's neuroma
d. Bunion
e. Plantar fasciitis

Characteristics

_____ 87. Dorsiflexion of any metatarsophalangeal joint with plantar flexion of the adjacent proximal interphalangeal joint

_____ 88. Small tumor in a digital nerve of the foot

_____ 89. Great toe deviates laterally

_____ 90. Acute pain; burning sensation in the web space

_____ 91. First metatarsal head becomes enlarged

_____ 92. Pain in the arch of the foot, especially when getting out of bed

_____ 93. Can occur as a result of poorly fitted shoes

_____ 94. Corns may develop on the dorsal side of the toe

_____ 95. Insertion of wires or screws for fixation

_____ 96. Removal of the bony overgrowth and bursa

_____ 97. May be seen in athletes, especially runners

_____ 98. Inflammation of the plantar fascia

99. The nurse is assessing a patient with a spinal deformity. Which technique does the nurse use to accomplish inspection of the spine?
   a. Observe the patient from the front and back while standing and during forward flexion from the hips.
   b. Observe the patient in a sitting and standing position and ask the patient to walk around the room.
   c. Ask the patient to remove the clothes from the waist up and then view the visible curvature of the spine.
   d. Look at the patient's back while the patient moves in different positions: touching toes, lateral bending, twisting.

100. Which clinical findings does the nurse assess in the affected area of a patient with osteomyelitis? *(Select all that apply.)*
   a. Erythema
   b. Tenderness
   c. Numbness and tingling
   d. Swelling
   e. Constant bone pain

101. The nurse is caring for a patient with muscular dystrophy. Although all body systems can be affected, the nurse is alert and carefully assesses for which major problem?
   a. Renal failure
   b. Cardiac failure
   c. Muscle weakness
   d. Respiratory failure

102. Which statements about scoliosis are true? *(Select all that apply.)*
   a. Scoliosis screening is best done during middle-school years.
   b. Scoliosis is characterized by a C- or S-shaped lateral curvature of the vertebral spine.
   c. Scoliosis screening is best done during preschool years.
   d. A curvature greater than 50 degrees results in an unstable spine.
   e. The forward-bend test is used to determine scoliosis.

CASE STUDY: THE PATIENT WITH OSTEOPOROSIS

Use a separate sheet of paper to answer the questions in this Case Study, or go to the "Prepare for Class" folder on your Evolve website at http://evolve.elsevier.com/Iggy/ to download and complete as a word processing file. Answer guidelines for this Case Study are also available on your Evolve website.

A 67-year-old postmenopausal woman has come to the clinic reporting moderate and, at times, severe backache. She states that this pain is interfering with her sleep. She works 4 days per week, and gets together weekly with her friends to play golf and tennis, but lately has had to cancel her golf outings. She says she is afraid her back will give out on her and she will fall. She states that the pain is interfering with her social life and other daily activities and that the episodes are becoming unbearable so she has decided to seek treatment. The patient rates her pain as a 7 on a scale of 0 to 10, 0 being pain-free, and 10 being the worst pain imaginable.

Nutritionally, the patient says she eats 2 to 3 meals a day, but does not like milk and rarely drinks it. She admits to drinking alcohol 3-4 times a week. In addition, the patient reports that she has started wearing mostly slip-on shoes to avoid bending (to tie shoes). Aside from playing golf, her daily routine does not involve much time outside, and she avoids yard work, which she used to enjoy. Vital signs are: temp 37.8° C (100° F); heart rate 82/min; respirations 22/min; and blood pressure 140/87 mm Hg. Medical history includes hypertension; the patient reports taking lisinopril 10 mg orally daily. She has no known drug allergies.

The patient is to be admitted to the hospital for diagnostic tests of her spine and pain management.

1. Identify six questions that the nurse would ask the patient while performing the assessment.
2. The patient says that she does not like milk and rarely drinks it. How could she increase her calcium intake?
3. The health care provider suspects osteoporosis. What test is most likely to be ordered and what should the nurse tell the patient about the test?
4. The patient is given a prescription for alendronate (Fosamax). What should the nurse tell her before she begins therapy with this drug?
5. Determine appropriate measures to relieve this patient's back pain.
6. Using the SBAR format, outline how the nurse should communicate this patient's case to the floor nurse who will be admitting the patient.

54 CHAPTER

Care of Patients with Musculoskeletal Trauma

STUDY/REVIEW QUESTIONS

Matching. *Match each of the following terms related to the fracture healing process with its definition.*

Terms
a. Callus
b. Granulation
c. Hematoma
d. Remodeling

Definitions
_____ 1. Mass of clotted blood at fracture site
_____ 2. Process of bone building and resorption
_____ 3. Vascular and cellular proliferation
_____ 4. Nonbony union at fracture site

5. The nurse is caring for several patients on an orthopedic trauma unit. Which conditions have a high risk for development of acute compartment syndrome? *(Select all that apply.)*
   a. Lower legs caught between the bumpers of two cars
   b. Massive infiltration of IV fluid into forearm
   c. Bivalve cast on the lower leg
   d. Multiple insect bites to lower legs
   e. Daily use of oral contraceptives
   f. Severe burns to the upper extremities

6. A patient has a fracture of the right wrist. What is an early sign that indicates this patient may be having a complication?
   a. Patient loses ability to wiggle fingers without pain.
   b. Fingers are cold and pale; capillary refill is sluggish.
   c. Pain is severe and seems out of proportion to injury.
   d. Patient reports a subjective numbness and tingling.

7. The nurse is assessing a patient for severe pain in the right wrist after falling off a step stool. How does the nurse assess this patient's motor function?
   a. Performing passive range of motion for the wrist
   b. Asking the patient to move the fingers
   c. Having the patient flex and extend the elbow
   d. Instructing the patient to rotate the wrist

8. A patient in traction reports severe pain from a muscle spasm. What is the nurse's priority action?
   a. Assess the patient's body alignment.
   b. Give the patient a PRN pain medication.
   c. Notify the health care provider.
   d. Remove some of the weights.

9. The nurse is reviewing the orders for a patient who was admitted for 24-hour observation of a leg fracture. A cast is in place. Which order does the nurse question?
   a. Elevate lower leg above the level of the heart.
   b. Perform neuro-circ checks every 8 hours.
   c. Apply ice pack for 24 hours.
   d. Provide regular diet as tolerated.

10. A patient with a leg cast denies pain; toes are pink; capillary refill is brisk and toes move freely; the leg is elevated with an ice pack. Six hours later, the patient reports worsening pain unrelieved by medication. The patient's toes are cool and capillary refill is sluggish. What does the nurse suspect is occurring with this patient?
    a. Crush syndrome
    b. Fat embolism syndrome
    c. Acute compartment syndrome
    d. Fasciitis

11. An older adult sustained injury to the lower legs after being trapped underneath a fallen bookcase. Because this patient is at high risk for crush syndrome, which laboratory values will the nurse specifically monitor?
    a. Serum potassium level and myoglobin in urine
    b. White cell count and red cells in the urine
    c. Prothrombin level and serum lipase level
    d. Platelet count and serum calcium level

12. An older adult has been admitted with a hip fracture. Approximately 20 hours post-injury, the patient develops a symptom recognized as an early sign of fat embolism syndrome. Which symptom is the patient displaying?
    a. Severe respiratory distress
    b. Significantly increased pulse rate
    c. Change in mental status
    d. Petechiae rash over the neck

13. Indicate the numeric sequence of bone healing from the beginning using the numbers 1 through 5.

    _____ a. Callus formation

    _____ b. Bone remodeling

    _____ c. Hematoma formation

    _____ d. Osteoblastic proliferation

    _____ e. Hematoma to granulation tissue

14. The student nurse is assessing a patient with a probable fractured tibia-fibula. What assessment technique used by the student nurse causes the supervising nurse to intervene?
    a. Inspects the fracture site for swelling or deformity.
    b. Instructs the patient to wiggle the toes.
    c. Assesses the bilateral dorsalis pedis pulse.
    d. Pushes on the leg to elicit pain response.

15. The nurse is caring for several orthopedic patients who are in different types of traction. What should the nurse do in assessing the traction equipment? *(Select all that apply.)*
    a. Inspect all ropes, knots, and pulleys once every 24 hours.
    b. Inspect ropes and knots for fraying or loosening every 8 to 12 hours.
    c. Check the amount of weight being used against the prescribed weight.
    d. Observe the traction equipment for proper functioning.
    e. Check if the ropes have been changed or cleaned within the past 48 hours.

16. A patient was put into traction at 0800 hours. Hourly neuro-circ checks were ordered for the first 24 hours and then every 4 hours thereafter. At what time can the nursing staff start performing the every-4-hour checks?
    a. 2000 hours same day
    b. 0000 hours next day
    c. 0800 hours next day
    d. 1200 hours next day

17. The nurse is educating a patient who will have external fixation for treatment of a compound tibial fracture. What information does the nurse include in the teaching session?
    a. "The device allows for early ambulation."
    b. "There is some danger of blood loss, but no danger of infection."
    c. "The device is a substitute therapy for a cast."
    d. "The advantage of the device is rapid bone healing."

18. The nurse is helping to evaluate several patients to determine candidacy for the Ilizaroz external fixation device. Which patient is the best candidate?
    a. Older woman who lives alone with a fracture of nonunion
    b. Child with a congenital bone deformity whose mother is a licensed practical nurse
    c. Teenager with an open fracture and bone loss of the left lower leg
    d. Middle-aged man with a new comminuted fracture of the dominant forearm

19. An older adult patient has a fractured humerus. The physician is considering the use of electrical bone stimulation and asks the nurse to take a medical history on the patient. Which specific condition, which is a contraindication for this therapy, does the nurse ask the patient about?
    a. Seizures
    b. Cardiac pacemaker
    c. Stroke
    d. Peripheral nerve damage

20. A patient is prescribed low-intensity pulsed ultrasound treatments for a very slow-healing fracture of the right lower leg. What instructions does the nurse give this patient related to the treatment?
    a. Test for pregnancy before the therapy and use birth control until treatment is complete.
    b. The treatment is experimental, but there are no known adverse effects.
    c. The device is implanted directly into the fracture site and there is no external apparatus.
    d. Expect to dedicate approximately 20 minutes a day for one treatment.

21. The nursing student is assisting with the care of a patient with musculoskeletal pain related to soft tissue injury and bone disruption. The student sees that the patient has a PRN order for pain medication. What does the student do first in order to decide when to give the pain medication?
    a. Ask the physician to clarify the order for specific parameters.
    b. Check with the primary nurse or the charge nurse for advice.
    c. Ask the patient about types of activities that increase the pain.
    d. Ask the instructor for help in interpreting the order.

22. A patient is receiving scheduled and PRN narcotics for severe pain related to a musculoskeletal injury. The nurse finds that the patient's abdomen is distended and bowel sounds are hypoactive. Because the nurse suspects that the patient is having a medication side effect, which question does the nurse ask the patient?
    a. "Are you having nausea and vomiting?"
    b. "When was your last bowel movement?"
    c. "Does your abdomen hurt?"
    d. "Are you having diarrhea or loose stool?"

23. A patient comes into the ED after falling off his four-wheeler. His lower leg is obviously broken; it is bleeding and bone fragments are protruding from the skin. What type of fracture does this patient likely have?
    a. Impacted
    b. Open (compound)
    c. Comminuted (fragmented)
    d. Displaced

24. A patient comes to the ED after slipping on some chalk in her classroom. She did not fall far and was able to walk with the assistance of one of her students. What type of fracture does this patient likely have?
    a. Closed, nondisplaced
    b. Oblique
    c. Impacted
    d. Incomplete

25. A female patient with osteoporosis comes to the ED after falling suddenly while opening her car door. She said it felt as though her "leg gave way" and caused her to fall. What type of fracture does this patient likely have?
    a. Pathologic (spontaneous)
    b. Spiral
    c. Impacted
    d. Incomplete

Fill in the blank.

26. The _____ technique is used to treat nonunion or malunion fractures.

27. An external _____ bone stimulator system is directed at nonhealed fracture sites.

28. Low-intensity _____ _____ is used for slow-healing fractures.

29. The nurse is caring for a patient with an open fracture. Which intervention does the nurse perform in order to prevent infection of the fracture?
    a. Use strict aseptic technique for dressing changes and wound irrigations.
    b. Use clean techniques for dressing changes and wound irrigations.
    c. Place the patient in contact isolation and wear sterile gloves.
    d. Place the patient in reverse isolation and perform scrupulous hand hygiene.

30. The nurse must adjust a pair of crutches to properly fit a patient. Which description illustrates correct crutch adjustment?
    a. Axilla rests lightly on the top of the crutch when the crutch is moved forward.
    b. Patient can easily use the crutch without subjective complaints.
    c. Elbow is flexed no more than 30 degrees when the palm is on the handle.
    d. Adult patient is of average height and the crutches are medium-sized.

31. An older patient's family is trying to find an appropriate cane for the patient to use because of chronic pain in the right ankle. The nurse instructs the family to purchase which type of cane?
    a. One with the top being parallel to the greater trochanter of the femur
    b. One that creates about 45 degrees of flexion of the elbow
    c. One that is based on the patient's weight to provide adequate support
    d. One that has padding on the handle grip to ensure safety

32. What members of the health care team will be consulted to teach the patient in question #31 about proper use of the cane? *(Select all that apply.)*
    a. Occupational therapist
    b. Physical therapist
    c. Registered nurse
    d. Unlicensed assistive personnel
    e. Medical social worker

33. The nurse is caring for a patient with an external fixation of a bone fracture. What are the advantages of this type of treatment? *(Select all that apply.)*
    a. It is less painful than other treatments.
    b. It allows for earlier ambulation.
    c. It decreases the risk for infection.
    d. It maintains bone alignment.
    e. It stabilizes commuted fractures that require bone grafting.

34. An older patient with a lower leg fracture is having difficulty performing the weight-bearing exercises. Based on fracture pathophysiology and the patient's abilities, which condition could the patient develop?
    a. Osteomyelitis
    b. Internal derangement
    c. Neuroma
    d. Pulmonary embolism

35. The nurse case manager is making a home visit to assist an older patient with a hip fracture. During the home visit, the nurse reviews home environment safety. Which observation indicates a need for additional teaching?
    a. Patient's bed has been moved to the ground floor level.
    b. There are handle bars around the toilet and tub.
    c. Floors are clean and shiny and covered with throw rugs.
    d. Patient's walker is close to the patient's bedside.

36. Which is a potentially fatal complication of acute compartment syndrome?
    a. Myoglobinuric renal failure
    b. Ischemic heart failure
    c. Acute liver failure
    d. Hypovolemic shock

37. A patient comes to the ED with crush syndrome from a crush injury to his right upper extremity and right lower extremity when heavy equipment fell on him at a construction site. The patient has signs and symptoms of hypovolemia, hyperkalemia, and compartment syndrome. Management of care for this patient will focus on preventing which complications? *(Select all that apply.)*
    a. Sepsis
    b. Cardiac dysrhythmias
    c. Respiratory failure
    d. Acute tubular necrosis
    e. Fluid overload

38. A chronic complication of bone healing is called *avascular necrosis*. Which statements about this complication are true? *(Select all that apply.)*
    a. It involves disrupting the blood supply to the bone.
    b. It occurs when fat globules disrupt the blood supply to the bone.
    c. It involves disrupting the nerve supply to the bone.
    d. It results in the death of bone tissue.
    e. It is most often a complication of hip fractures.

39. A 30-year-old patient who is hospitalized for repair of a fractured tibia and fibula reports shortness of breath. Which complication related to the injury might the patient be experiencing?
    a. Hypovolemic shock
    b. Fat embolism
    c. Acute compartment syndrome
    d. Pneumonia

Matching. *Match the fracture complication with its corresponding description. Not all complications will be used.*

Fracture Complications
a. Malunion
b. Fat embolism
c. Crush syndrome
d. Osteomyelitis
e. Avascular necrosis
f. Nonunion

Descriptions
_____ 40. Disrupted blood supply to the bone, resulting in the death of bone tissue

_____ 41. Fat globules released from the yellow bone marrow into the bloodstream

_____ 42. Incorrect fracture healing

_____ 43. Lack of fracture healing

44. A patient who tripped and fell down several stairs reports having heard a popping sound and fears that she has broken her ankle. How does the nurse initially assess for fracture in this patient?
   a. Measuring the circumference of the distal leg
   b. Gently moving the ankle through the full range of motion
   c. Inspecting for crepitus and skin color
   d. Observing for deformity or misalignment

45. The nurse is assessing a patient with an injury to the shoulder and upper arm after being thrown from a horse. What is the best position for this patient's assessment?
   a. Supine so that the extremity can be elevated
   b. Low Fowler's on an exam table for patient comfort
   c. Sitting to observe for shoulder droop
   d. Slow ambulation to observe for natural arm movement

46. The nurse is caring for a patient with skeletal pins that have been placed for traction. What does the nurse expect to see in the first 48 hours?
   a. Clear fluid drainage weeping from the pin insertion site
   b. Some bloody drainage, but very minimal
   c. Swelling at the site with tenderness to gentle touch
   d. Dressings around the pin sites to be dry and intact

47. The pathophysiologic changes with increased compartment pressure are described as the _____-_____ cycle.

48. What potential adverse effect prevents meperidine (Demerol) from being used in older adults?
   a. Hypertension
   b. Angina
   c. Kidney failure
   d. Seizures

49. The unlicensed assistive personnel (UAP) is assisting the orthopedic physician to cut a window in a patient's cast. What does the nurse instruct the UAP to do?
   a. Check the pulse that is accessed after the window is cut.
   b. Clean up and dispose of all casting debris.
   c. Inform the patient that the procedure is painless.
   d. Save the plaster piece that was cut so it can be taped in place.

50. The nurse is caring for a patient in Buck's traction. Which task is best to delegate to the UAP (with supervision)?
   a. Turning and repositioning
   b. Inspecting heels and sacral area
   c. Asking the patient about muscle spasms
   d. Adjusting the weights on the apparatus

51. The nurse is instructing a teenage patient with a tibia-fibula fracture that was treated with internal fixation and a long leg cast. He is anxious to know when the cast will be removed so that he can resume football practice. Which statement by the patient indicates a need for additional teaching?
   a. "There's a possibility that the cast could be removed in 4 weeks."
   b. "The plates and screws reduce the length of time I'll be in the cast."
   c. "The cast could remain in place as long as 6 weeks."
   d. "I'll use crutches for 2 weeks and then the cast will be removed."

52. The patient was an unrestrained driver involved in a motor vehicle accident who sustained a 5th rib fracture. As the patient is being assessed, what is the nurse's major concern?
    a. Pain that increases with inspiration
    b. Muffled heart sounds
    c. Widespread bruising over the chest
    d. Crepitus over the 5th rib

53. Place the steps in the correct order for emergency care of the patient with fracture using the numbers 1 through 6.

    _____ a. Cover the affected area with a dressing (preferably sterile).

    _____ b. Check the neurovascular status of the area distal to the extremity: temperature, color, sensation, movement, and capillary refill. Compare affected and unaffected limbs.

    _____ c. Remove the patient's clothing (cut if necessary) to inspect the affected area while supporting the injured area above and below the injury. Do not remove shoes because this can cause increased trauma.

    _____ d. Apply direct pressure on the area if there is bleeding and pressure over the proximal artery nearest the fracture.

    _____ e. Immobilize the extremity by splinting; include joints above and below the fracture site. Recheck circulation after splinting.

    _____ f. Put the patient in a supine position; keep patient warm.

54. According to the patient's chart, there is a family history of osteoporosis. In order to plan interventions related to this finding, what action does the nurse take?
    a. Ask the patient's age and assess for weight loss.
    b. Review the patient's dietary intake of calcium.
    c. Assess the patient for kyphoscoliosis or other deformities.
    d. Assess the patient for occult fractures of the long bones.

55. The nurse's neighbor comes running over because her husband "cut his finger off with a power saw." After calling for help, what is the priority action when the nurse gets to the neighbor's house?
    a. Examine the amputation site.
    b. Assess for airway or breathing problems.
    c. Elevate the hand above the heart.
    d. Assess the severed finger.

56. An excited group of teenagers brings a friend to the ED who severed a finger while playing sports. The bleeding from the site is well controlled and the patient is alert and stable. What does the nurse do with the severed finger?
    a. Place it directly into a bag of ice and then put the bag into a refrigerator.
    b. Wrap it in moist sterile gauze and ensure that it stays with the patient.
    c. Wrap it in a dry gauze, place it in a waterproof bag, and put the bag in ice water.
    d. Carefully clean it with sterile saline, then place it in a sterile container.

57. Which nursing intervention is best to prevent increased pain in a patient experiencing phantom limb pain?
    a. Handle the residual limb carefully when assessing the site or changing the dressing.
    b. Advise the patient that the sensation is temporary and will diminish over time.
    c. Remind the patient that the part is not really there, so the pain is not real.
    d. Encourage the patient to mourn the loss of the body part and express grief.

58. A young patient had a great toe amputated because of severe injury. The patient is depressed and withdrawn after the physician tells him that the amputation will affect balance and gait. What is the nurse's best response?
    a. "The physical therapy department can help you with exercises for balance and gait."
    b. "Let me get your parents and we can talk about rehabilitation programs."
    c. "When the doctor was explaining things to you, what were you thinking about?"
    d. "How have you usually handled stressful situations in the past?"

59. The patient is a middle-aged man with a history of uncontrolled diabetes. His right foot is a dark brownish-purple color and there is no palpable dorsalis pedis or posterior tibial pulse. The nurse prepares the patient for which diagnostic test?
   a. X-ray of the foot and ankle
   b. Doppler ultrasound
   c. Electromyelogram
   d. Arthrogram

60. The pain a patient experiences from a bone fracture results from which processes? *(Select all that apply.)*
   a. Loss of muscle tone
   b. Edema
   c. Neuropathy
   d. Bone healing
   e. Muscle spasms

61. A patient injured a lower extremity and has been placed in a running traction. What instructions does the nurse give to the UAP?
   a. Support the weights when turning the patient every 2 hours.
   b. Apply countertraction before moving the patient.
   c. Defer hygienic care and moving the patient until traction is removed.
   d. Moving the patient or the bed during care can alter the countertraction.

62. The nurse is caring for a patient with an above-the-knee amputation (AKA). In order to prevent hip flexion contractures, how does the nurse position the patient?
   a. Supine position with the residual limb elevated on a pillow
   b. Prone position every 3 to 4 hours for 20- to 30-minute periods
   c. Supine position with an abduction pillow placed between the legs
   d. Head of the bed elevated 30 degrees with assurance that the bandage is wrapped around the limb

63. The nurse applies bandages to a patient's residual limb in order to help shape and shrink the limb for a prosthesis. What is the proper technique for the nurse to use?
   a. Reapply the bandages every 8 hours or more often if they become loose.
   b. Use a proximal to distal direction when wrapping.
   c. Use a soft and flexible bandage material and pad the area with gauze.
   d. Use a figure-eight wrapping method to prevent restriction of blood flow.

Matching. *Match each definition to its corresponding type of traction.*

Types of Traction
a. Plaster traction
b. Skin traction
c. Skeletal traction

Definitions

_____ 64. Involves the use of a fabric fastener boot (Buck's), belt, or halter, which is secured around a body part

_____ 65. Pins, wires, tongs, or screws surgically inserted directly into bone

_____ 66. Combines skeletal traction and a plaster cast

67. An older patient is discharged to home following an orthopedic injury. Which mobilization device is usually preferred for older patients?
    a. Crutches
    b. Cane
    c. Walker
    d. Wheelchair

68. The nurse is interviewing an older adult with a history of osteoporosis who reports falling and catching her weight on her outstretched dominant hand. This patient is most likely to have sustained what type of fracture?
    a. Carpal scaphoid bone
    b. Phalanges fracture
    c. Humeral fracture
    d. Colles' wrist fracture

69. Which factor carries the greatest risk for hip fracture?
    a. Decreased visual acuity
    b. Joint stiffness
    c. Osteoporosis
    d. Cardiac drug regimen

70. An older adult patient has skin traction in place for a hip fracture. What is the main purpose for this type of traction?
    a. It decreases painful muscle spasms.
    b. It helps heal the fracture.
    c. It prevents extension of the fracture.
    d. It prevents compression syndrome.

71. The nurse is caring for a patient with open reduction and internal fixation (ORIF) for a hip fracture. Because the patient is at risk for hip dislocation, the nurse ensures that the hip is maintained in which position?
    a. Adduction
    b. Anatomically neutral
    c. Abduction
    d. Extended

72. A patient reports dramatic changes in color and temperature of the skin over the left foot with intense burning pain, sensitive skin, excessive sweating, and edema. The physician makes a preliminary medical diagnosis of complex regional pain syndrome. What is the priority for nursing care?
    a. Patient education
    b. Care of the skin to prevent skin breakdown
    c. Management of pain
    d. Assessment of circulation

73. A patient is admitted to the same-day surgery unit following a meniscectomy. What does postoperative care for this patient include? *(Select all that apply.)*
    a. Perform neurovascular checks every hour for the first few hours and then every 4 hours.
    b. Check the surgical dressing for bleeding
    c. Monitor vital signs
    d. Strict I&O
    e. Teach about signs and symptoms of infection
    f. NPO until fully awake

74. Following a meniscectomy, the nurse assists a patient to immediately start performing which exercises?
    a. Range-of-motion exercises to both legs
    b. Straight leg raises on both legs
    c. Flexion and extension of knees
    d. Flexion and extension of ankles

75. A patient arrives in the ED reporting pain and immobility of the right shoulder. The patient reports a history of recurrent dislocations of the same shoulder. The nurse observes for which other signs and symptoms that are associated with a dislocation injury? *(Select all that apply.)*
    a. Alteration in contour of the joint
    b. Deviation in length of the extremity
    c. Muscle atrophy
    d. Mottled skin discoloration
    e. Rotation of the extremity

76. Which descriptions are true about sprains? (*Select all that apply.*)
    a. They involve an injury to a ligament.
    b. Second- and third-degree sprains require immobilization.
    c. Sprains are usually precipitated by twisting motions from a sports injury.
    d. They are caused by excessive stretching of a muscle or tendon.
    e. Surgical repair is required for second- and third-degree sprains.

77. Which statements are true about dislocations? (*Select all that apply.*)
    a. Surgical repair is usually performed to re-align a dislocated joint.
    b. Dislocation of a joint occurs when two bones are moved away from each other.
    c. Partial dislocation of a joint is referred to as "subluxed."
    d. A health care provider performs closed reductions on dislocated joints.
    e. Joint dislocation is most common in the hip, spine, and fingers.

True or False? *Read each statement and write T for true or F for false in the blanks provided. If the statement is false, correct the statement to make it true.*

_____ 78. The lateral meniscus is more likely to tear than the medial meniscus.

_____ 79. When the anterior cruciate ligament (ACL) is torn, the person may feel a "snap."

_____ 80. Complete healing of knee ligaments after surgery only takes 3 to 4 weeks.

_____ 81. Rupture of the Achilles tendon is common in older adults.

_____ 82. A strain is excessive stretching of a ligament.

_____ 83. Management of a strain usually involves cold and heat applications.

_____ 84. Patients with a torn rotator cuff have shoulder pain and cannot initiate or maintain adduction of the arm at the shoulder (drop arm test).

85. The health care provider tells a patient that she has a mild first-degree sprain to the ankle. What instructions does the nurse give to the patient about the treatment for the injury? (*Select all that apply.*)
    a. Rest.
    b. Apply ice for the first 4 to 6 hours.
    c. Apply a compression bandage for a few days to reduce swelling and provide joint support.
    d. Elevate the foot.
    e. Perform range-of-motion exercises every 4 hours.

86. A patient is informed by the physician that he must have a plaster cast applied to the lower extremity. What does the nurse teach the patient about the procedure before the cast is applied?
    a. "Plaster will be applied directly to the skin surface."
    b. "The cast material will feel hot at first, but will quickly become cool."
    c. "The cast will be dry within 2 to 3 hours after application."
    d. "The plaster is a durable, waterproof material that protects the skin."

87. The nurse is caring for a patient with a plaster splint applied to the ankle. The patient received oral pain medication at 0900. At 1100, the patient reports that the pain is getting worse, not better. What is the nurse's priority action?
    a. Give the patient IV pain medication.
    b. Reposition the extremity on a pillow and place an ice pack.
    c. Assess the pulses and skin temperature distal to the splint.
    d. Call the physician to report the patient's increasing pain.

88. Which factors affect bone healing after a fracture has occurred? *(Select all that apply.)*
    a. Patient's age
    b. Patient's occupation
    c. Type of bone injured
    d. How the fracture is managed
    e. Presence of infection at the fracture site

89. The nurse is providing teaching for a patient with a forearm cast. What information does the nurse give to the patient?
    a. "The hand should be elevated above the shoulder when resting."
    b. "Use an ice pack for the first 6 to 8 hours, and cover the pack with a towel to absorb condensation."
    c. "The sling should distribute the weight over a large area of the shoulders and trunk."
    d. "Limit movement of the fingers or wrist joints to prevent pain."

90. The nurse and nursing student are assisting a patient with a new hip spica cast to transfer from the stretcher to the bed. What does the nurse advise the student to do?
    a. Delay the transfer until the cast is dry.
    b. Assist the patient to log-roll from the stretcher to the bed.
    c. Keep the affected leg elevated during the transfer.
    d. Handle the cast with the flat palmar surface of the hand.

Matching. Match each term related to musculoskeletal injuries with its corresponding definition.

Types of Injury
a. Dislocation
b. Sprain
c. Strain
d. Subluxation

Definitions
_____ 91. Partial joint surface separation

_____ 92. Injury to ligament

_____ 93. Joint surfaces not approximated

_____ 94. Excessive stretching of muscle or tendon

95. A patient with a lower extremity injury is being treated by external fixation. What nursing assessment is of particular concern in the care of this patient with this type of system?
    a. Maintaining a 30-degree flexed position of the knee
    b. Measuring the weights used for counter-traction
    c. Observing the patient's abilities to adjust the clickers
    d. Observing the points of entry of the pins and wires

96. The nurse's older neighbor has slipped and fallen and reports pain to the left forearm. There is also a small abrasion over the area. Place the steps for first responder care in the correct order using the numbers 1 through 6.

    _____ a. Applies a splint that extends below the wrist and above the elbow

    _____ b. Inspects the extremity for swelling and deformity

    _____ c. Palpates for pulse and questions about sensation

    _____ d. Places a sterile gauze loosely over the abrasion to protect from further contamination

    _____ e. Assesses for motor function

    _____ f. Reevaluates neurovascular function after immobilization

97. The nurse is caring for a patient who had a kyphoplasty. What does postoperative care for this patient include? *(Select all that apply.)*
    a. Place the patient in a flat supine position for 8 hours.
    b. Monitor and record vital signs.
    c. Perform frequent neurologic assessments.
    d. Apply a warm pack to the puncture site if needed to relieve pain.
    e. Assess the patient's pain level and compare it to the preoperative level.
    f. Give opioid analgesics as needed.
    g. Monitor for bleeding at the puncture site.

98. A patient in a body cast reports nausea, vomiting, and epigastric pain. The nurse notifies the physician for orders. Which intervention is the most conservative, and therefore the first thing to try, to address this patient's symptoms?
    a. Insert a nasogastric tube and attach to low wall suction.
    b. Cut a window over the abdominal area of the cast.
    c. Obtain an order for an x-ray to diagnose a paralytic ileus.
    d. Administer PRN antiemetic and PRN pain medication.

99. A patient with a long leg cast that was applied in the ED is being admitted to the orthopedic unit. Which task is best for the nurse to delegate to the UAP?
    a. Obtain a fracture pan and use caution to prevent spillage on the cast.
    b. Obtain several plastic-covered pillows for elevation of the leg.
    c. Check flexion/extension and color of the toes.
    d. Turn the patient every 4 to 6 hours to allow the cast to dry.

100. A patient who has sustained a traumatic amputation of the left leg expresses concern about working and taking care of his family after his injury. What resources does the nurse recommend to help the patient adjust to his lost limb? *(Select all that apply.)*
    a. Chaplain
    b. Medical social worker
    c. Physical therapist
    d. Physician
    e. National Amputation Foundation

CASE STUDY: THE PATIENT WITH AN AMPUTATION

Use a separate sheet of paper to answer the questions in this Case Study, or go to the "Prepare for Class" folder on your Evolve website at http://evolve.elsevier.com/Iggy/ to download and complete as a word processing file. Answer guidelines for this Case Study are also available on your Evolve website.

A 35-year-old carpenter is brought into the ED by paramedics with a blood-saturated shirt wrapped over his right hand. The patient was working on a house when the saw slipped and sawed off his right index and third finger. A paramedic hands the nurse a plastic bag containing the fingers. The nurse puts on gloves, applies pressure with sterile gauze to the amputated site, and places the closed bag in ice water. The patient has a history of hypertension for which he takes amlodipine (Norvasc). Further assessment reveals 2+ bilateral radial pulses.

The nurse helps to transfer the patient to an examining table where vital signs are taken by UAP and the nurse starts a peripheral IV of normal saline 0.9% at 100 mL/hr. Vital signs are: temp 37.9° C (100.2° F); heart rate 102/min with rhythm of sinus tachycardia; respirations 32/min. He has no known allergies. The patient rates his pain a 10 on a 0-10 scale, with 0 being pain-free and 10 being the worst pain imaginable.

The nurse is given an order to medicate the patient with 4 mg of IV morphine. The surgeon concurrently examines the patient and requests that the patient be taken to surgery immediately.

1. Using the SBAR format, outline the conversation the ED nurse will have with the surgical intake nurse in the handoff of the patient.
2. Identify the two top nursing priorities in providing care to this patient in the ED.
3. What type of shock is this patient at risk for?
4. What type of amputation has this patient sustained?

CASE STUDY: THE PATIENT WITH FRACTURE

Use a separate sheet of paper to answer the questions in this Case Study, or go to the "Prepare for Class" folder on your Evolve website at http://evolve.elsevier.com/Iggy/ to download and complete as a word processing file. Answer guidelines for this Case Study are also available on your Evolve website.

The 20-year-old patient was admitted with fractures of the right tibia and fibula after a fall. She has a long leg cast that was applied this morning. The physician has ordered bedrest for now until her condition stabilizes.

1. What is the priority for assessment during this time?

2. Later that evening, as the nurse performs an assessment, the patient states that the cast seems "too tight." It was difficult, but not impossible, for the nurse to insert one finger between the top of the cast and the patient's skin. Is this a concern, and what actions, if any, should the nurse take at this time?

3. A few days later, the patient is allowed to get out of bed with crutches. The crutches have been delivered, but the physical therapist has not yet been in to see the patient. The patient states, "I can't wait any longer. Let me try walking with those crutches—I'm sure I can do it because I've played with my brother's crutches before." Should the nurse let her walk with the crutches? Why or why not?

4. What type of gait will she be taught to use while crutch-walking?

5. The patient has been discharged, and has received instructions for cast care. One week later, she calls the office and asks, "Can I get a new cast? This one smells moldy or musty, and it's getting uncomfortable." What does the nurse suspect? When she comes to the office to have it checked, what further assessments should be done?

6. The patient is fearful when she sees the cast saw. What should the nurse tell her?

Assessment of the Gastrointestinal System

STUDY/REVIEW QUESTIONS

Matching. *Match the terms associated with the GI system with their corresponding definitions. Not all terms will be used.*

Terms

a. Bile
b. Chyme
c. Duodenum
d. Elimination
e. Esophagus
f. Gallbladder
g. Kupffer cells
h. Jejunum
i. Sphincter of Oddi
j. Liver
k. Mouth
l. Mastication
m. Saliva
n. Secretin
o. Stomach
p. Submucosa
q. Villi

Definitions

_____ 1. Muscle that surrounds the ampulla of Vater

_____ 2. Finger-like projections into the small intestine

_____ 3. Oral secretion that softens food

_____ 4. Thick, liquid mass of partially digested food

_____ 5. Temporary reservoir for food

_____ 6. Intestinal hormone that inhibits acid secretion and decreases gastric motility

_____ 7. Epithelial cell layer lining the GI tract

_____ 8   Process of expelling feces

_____ 9. Central part of small intestine

_____ 10. Chewing

_____ 11. Conduit for food from mouth to stomach

_____ 12. First 10 inches of small intestine

_____ 13. Liver secretion essential to fat emulsification

_____ 14. Largest abdominal organ with numerous functions

_____ 15. Organ that concentrates and stores bile

_____ 16. Beginning pathway for digestion

17. The pancreas performs which functions? *(Select all that apply.)*
    a. Breaks down amino acids
    b. Secretes enzymes for digestion from the exocrine part of the organ
    c. Breaks down fatty acids and triglycerides
    d. Produces glucagon from the endocrine part of the organ
    e. Produces enzymes that digest carbohydrates, fats, and proteins

18. Which statements about intrinsic factor are correct? *(Select all that apply.)*
    a. It is produced by the parietal cells.
    b. It is essential to fat emulsification.
    c. It aids in the absorption of vitamin B_{12}.
    d. It forms and secretes bile.
    e. Its absence causes pernicious anemia.

19. Which statements about Kupffer cells are true? *(Select all that apply.)*
    a. They are located in the epithelial cell layer lining in the GI tract.
    b. They are cells found in the liver.
    c. They are cells found in the wall of the stomach.
    d. They are part of the substance that aids in the absorption of vitamin B_{12}.
    e. They are part of the body's reticuloendothelial system.

20. Which drugs predispose a patient to peptic ulcer disease and GI bleeding? *(Select all that apply.)*
    a. Nonsteroidal anti-inflammatory drugs
    b. Steroids
    c. Aspirin
    d. Lasix
    e. Digitalis

21. Which gastrointestinal problem is related to anorexia?
    a. Heartburn
    b. Constipation
    c. Steatorrhea
    d. Loss of appetite

22. Dyspepsia is characterized by which factors? *(Select all that apply.)*
    a. Indigestion associated with eating
    b. Loss of appetite for food
    c. Heartburn associated with eating
    d. Vomiting that occurs after eating
    e. Malabsorption

23. The nurse is caring for a patient with abdominal pain. While assessing the patient, which questions will the nurse ask the patient? *(Select all that apply.)*
    a. "Is the pain burning, gnawing, or stabbing?"
    b. "Can you point to where you feel the pain?"
    c. "Does your skin feel itchy?"
    d. "When did you first notice the pain?"
    e. "Does the pain spread anywhere?"

24. Indicate the usual sequence that the abdominal examination occurs using the numbers 1 through 4.

    _____ a. Right lower quadrant (RLQ)

    _____ b. Left lower quadrant (LLQ)

    _____ c. Left upper quadrant (LUQ)

    _____ d. Right upper quadrant (RUQ)

25. Indicate the correct sequence of examination techniques for abdominal assessment using the numbers 1 through 4.

    _____ a. Inspection

    _____ b. Percussion

    _____ c. Palpation

    _____ d. Auscultation

26. The nurse is performing an abdominal assessment on a patient. For which finding does the nurse alert the physician?
    a. Cullen's sign
    b. Borborygmus
    c. Blumberg's sign
    d. Bulging, pulsating mass

Matching. *Match the terms with the correct descriptions.*

Terms
a.   Cullen's sign
b.   Bruits
c.   Tympanic
d.   Blumberg's sign

Descriptions

_____ 27.   Areas of pain that also show rebound tenderness

_____ 28.   High pitched, loud, musical sound of an air-filled intestine

_____ 29.   "Swooshing" sounds

_____ 30.   The presence of ecchymoses around the umbilicus

31.   What will laboratory values for a patient with liver disease most likely show? *(Select all that apply.)*
a.   Increased prothrombin time
b.   Increased AST and ALT
c.   Increased albumin levels
d.   Decreased ammonia levels
e.   Increased unconjugated bilirubin

32.   Laboratory values for a patient with acute pancreatitis may show which abnormal findings? *(Select all that apply.)*
a.   Increased hemoglobin
b.   Decreased serum amylase
c.   Increased serum lipase
d.   Decreased urine nitrates
e.   Increased serum amylase

33.   A patient being seen the ED has been vomiting blood for the past 12 hours. What test will likely be ordered for the patient?
a.   Endoscopic retrograde cholangiopancreatography (ERCP)
b.   Upper GI radiographic series
c.   Esophagogastroduodenoscopy (EGD)
d.   Barium enema

Matching. *Match the diagnostic studies with their corresponding descriptions. Not all diagnostic studies will be used.*

Diagnostic Studies

a.   Esophagogastroduodenoscopy (EGD)
b.   Upper GI radiographic series
c.   Small bowel series follow through (SBFT)
d.   Barium enema
e.   Acute abdomen series
f.   Gallbladder radiographic series
g.   Liver-spleen scan
h.   Endoscopic retrograde cholangiopancreatography (ERCP)
i.   Small bowel capsule endoscopy
j.   Percutaneous transhepatic cholangiography (PTC)

Descriptions

_____ 34.   A small bowel enteroscopy that visualizes the entire small bowel, including the distal ileum.

_____ 35.   Visual radiographic examination of the liver, gallbladder, bile ducts, and pancreas to identify the cause and location of an obstruction.

_____ 36.   A radiographic visualization of the large intestine; usually ordered for the patient with blood or mucus in the stool or a change in bowel habits.

_____ 37.   Visualization of the gallbladder after oral ingestion of radiopaque, iodine-based contrast medium. The day before the test, the patient eats a fat-free or low-fat meal and takes six radiopaque iodine tablets approximately 2 hours after the meal. Patient is NPO from midnight on the night before the test.

_____ 38.   A scan that uses IV injection of a radioactive material that is taken up primarily by the liver and secondarily by the spleen.

_____ 39.   An x-ray study of the biliary duct system using an iodinated dye instilled via a percutaneous needle inserted through the liver into the intrahepatic ducts.

40.   A noninvasive imaging procedure to obtain multidimensional views of the entire colon is called a _____ _____ _____, or more popularly known as the *virtual colonoscopy*.

41.   Mild gas pain and flatulence may be experienced as a result of air instilled into the rectum during the examination, and if a biopsy specimen is obtained, a small amount of bleeding may be observed. For which endoscopic procedure is this follow-up care describing?
       a.   Colonoscopy
       b.   Proctosigmoidoscopy
       c.   Enteroscopy
       d.   ERCP

42. A feeling of fullness, cramping, and passage of flatus can be expected for several hours after the test, and a small amount of blood may be in the first stool after the test if a biopsy specimen is taken or a polypectomy is performed. Vital signs should be checked every 15 minutes, the patient should be monitored for signs of perforation or hemorrhage, and excessive bleeding should be reported immediately. For which procedure is this follow-up care describing?
    a. EGD
    b. Enteroscopy
    c. Small bowel series
    d. Colonoscopy

43. The patient should be observed for cholangitis, perforation, sepsis, and pancreatitis, and the patient should report abdominal pain, fever, nausea, or vomiting that fails to resolve. The patient is on NPO status until the gag reflex returns. For which procedure is this follow-up care describing?
    a. Enteroscopy
    b. EGD
    c. ERCP
    d. PTC

44. The patient should be monitored for signs of perforation such as pain, bleeding, or fever, and the patient is instructed not to drive for 12 hours after the test. A hoarse voice and sore throat may persist for several days; throat lozenges may be used to relieve the discomfort. For which procedure is this follow-up care describing?
    a. EGD
    b. ERCP
    c. Enteroscopy
    d. Small bowel series

Matching. *Match the abdominal quadrant to the appropriate body structures in which they are located. Not all body quadrants will be used.*

Body Quadrants
a. Right upper quadrant
b. Right lower quadrant
c. Midline
d. Left upper quadrant
e. Left lower quadrant

Location of Body Structures

_____ 45. Abdominal aorta

_____ 46. Sigmoid colon

_____ 47. Appendix

_____ 48. Gallbladder

CASE STUDY: THE PATIENT WITH UPPER GI PAIN

Use a separate sheet of paper to answer the questions in this Case Study, or go to the "Prepare for Class" folder on your Evolve website at http://evolve.elsevier.com/Iggy/ to download and complete as a word processing file. Answer guidelines for this Case Study are also available on your Evolve website.

The patient is an 87-year-old woman who is admitted to a medical nursing unit from a local nursing home. She had surgery for abdominal adhesions 4 weeks ago and is now passing blood-streaked stools. She also reports that her stomach hurts, especially during the night. "It feels like someone is burning a hole inside me." Last week, a close friend and neighbor visited her at the nursing home and reported news of deaths of two mutual friends who were residents of the apartment building where she used to live.

1. Document a nursing note using the following format:
   • Subjective
   • Objective
   • Note

2. What additional data should the nurse collect for a thorough GI system assessment of the patient?

3. The patient is scheduled to have an upper GI and small bowel series the next day. What does the nurse do to prepare her for these diagnostic studies?

4. The patient is unable to tolerate the barium solution, becomes nauseated, and vomits. Her physician orders that an EGD be done. What additional preparation is needed before this procedure can be performed on the patient?

5. Following the EGD, the patient is returned to her room by stretcher. The nurse assists her to transfer to bed. What position should the patient be assisted to assume? What assessments should the nurse initially perform? Why?

6. While the nurse is assessing her, the patient asks for some water to drink. What should the nurse do?

56

CHAPTER

Care of Patients with Oral Cavity Problems

STUDY/REVIEW QUESTIONS

1. What statement is true about the *Candida albicans* form of stomatitis?
   a. It is common type of primary stomatitis.
   b. *Candida albicans* is a bacterial infection.
   c. This infection is uncommon in patients who are immunocompromised.
   d. Patients on steroid therapy often experience this infection.

2. The nurse has provided teaching to a patient on ways to prevent the recurrence of aphthous ulcers. Which statement by the patient indicates teaching has been effective?
   a. "I will avoid gluten in my diet."
   b. "Potatoes have nothing to do with the development of the ulcers."
   c. "I will continue to eat peanut butter and jelly sandwiches."
   d. "It doesn't matter what types of foods I eat as long as I brush my teeth after every meal."

3. When caring for a patient with stomatitis, what is it most important for the nurse to assess?
   a. Nutritional status
   b. Level of pain
   c. Self-care abilities
   d. Airway status

4. The nurse is performing an oral assessment on a patient and notes white plaque-like lesions on the tongue, palate, pharynx, and buccal mucosa. When the patches are wiped away, the underlying surface is red and sore. What disorder does the nurse suspect the patient has?
   a. Leukoplakia
   b. *Candida albicans*
   c. Erythroplakia
   d. Kaposi's sarcoma

5. The nurse's aide is providing care to a patient with stomatitis. Which intervention by the nurse's aide illustrates correct care for this patient?
   a. Using a hard-bristled toothbrush to thoroughly clean the oral cavity
   b. Rinsing the mouth with a commercial mouthwash
   c. Using a warm saline, hydrogen peroxide, or sodium bicarbonate solution to rinse the mouth
   d. Rinsing the mouth frequently with cold tap water and vinegar solution

6. What is the drug of choice for the treatment of a fungal mouth infection?
   a. Nystatin (Mycostatin)
   b. Acyclovir (Zovirax)
   c. Minocycline
   d. Benzocaine (Kenalog in Orabase)

7. Which statement by the student nurse indicates the need for a better understanding of the care of patients with oral cavity problems?
   a. "I will use lemon-glycerin swabs to clean the patient's mouth."
   b. "The patient should eat a soft, bland diet."
   c. "Dentures should be removed."
   d. "Gauze may be used for oral care."

8. A patient is in the clinic for a non-healing sore on the lower left corner of her bottom lip and right side of her tongue. The lesions are red, raised, and have erosions. After taking a history, the nurse suspects the patient may have which type of oral cancer?
   a. Basal cell carcinoma
   b. Kaposi's sarcoma
   c. Squamous cell carcinoma
   d. Erythroplakia

9. A patient has a Kaposi's sarcoma lesion on his hard palate. How is this lesion described? *(Select all that apply.)*
   a. Small raised lesion
   b. Dark-yellow nodule
   c. Lesions are painful
   d. Purplish-brown nodule
   e. Usually not painful

Matching. *Match the types of oral cavity tumors with their corresponding descriptions. Not all oral cavity tumors will be used.*

Oral Cavity Tumors
a. Leukoplakia
b. Erythroplakia
c. Squamous cell carcinoma
d. Basal cell carcinoma
e. Kaposi's sarcoma

Descriptions
_____ 10. Thickened, white, firmly attached patches in the oral mucosa, lips, or tongue

_____ 11. Raised scab, primarily on the lips; evolves to an ulcer with a raised pearly border

_____ 12. Red, velvety lesion on the tongue, palate, floor of the mouth, or mandibular mucosa

13. A patient is scheduled for multiple tests to evaluate an oral tumor. The patient asks the nurse which of the tests is the best to determine if the tumor is cancerous. How does the nurse respond?
    a. "All of the tests need to be looked at together because no one test can tell if you have cancer."
    b. "Magnetic resonance imaging is the only diagnostic test that will need to be done."
    c. "Biopsy is the definitive method for diagnosing oral cancer."
    d. "An aqueous solution of toluidine blue 1% can be applied to the oral lesion. If the lesion is malignant it will not absorb the solution; however, the preparation stains the normal tissue."

14. During an assessment of a patient with an oral tumor, the nurse notes that the patient develops stridor. What functional assessment is the *least* important for the nurse to complete?
    a. Ability to speak
    b. Gag reflex
    c. Quality of respirations
    d. Pain rating

Matching. *Match the operative procedures with their correct descriptions.*

Procedures

a. Radical neck dissection
b. Glossectomy
c. Mandibulectomy
d. Commando procedure

Descriptions

_____ 15. Excision of a segment of the mandible with the oral lesion, and radical neck dissection

_____ 16. Tongue removal

_____ 17. Jaw removal

_____ 18. Removal of all cervical lymph nodes on the affected side, along with cranial nerve XI, the internal jugular vein, and the sternocleidomastoid muscle

19. After a patient has undergone a radical neck dissection, what is the priority nursing intervention?
    a. Manage the patient's pain.
    b. Maintain fluid and electrolyte balance.
    c. Maintain the patient's airway.
    d. Enhance the patient's ability to communicate.

20. Which interventions prevent or minimize the risk factors in patients at risk for aspiration? *(Select all that apply.)*
    a. Requesting medications in pill form
    b. Avoiding liquids or using a thickening agent
    c. Positioning the patient upright at 30 degrees
    d. Keeping the head of bed elevated 10 to 15 minutes after eating
    e. Keeping suction equipment nearby

21. How is xerostomia characterized?
    a. Reduction of taste sensation
    b. Inflammation of a salivary gland
    c. Excessive mouth dryness
    d. Inflammation of the mouth

22. Which are considered acute effects of radiation therapy? *(Select all that apply.)*
    a. Excessive drooling
    b. Stomatitis
    c. Herpes simplex
    d. Treatment-related mucositis
    e. Alteration in taste

23. _____ is a common side effect of radiation therapy.

24. _____ production is greatly reduced as a consequence of radiation.

25. The nurse's aide is caring for a patient undergoing radiation therapy to the neck. Which action by the nurse's aide requires intervention by the supervising nurse?
    a. Using powder on the patient's neck
    b. Shaving the patient with an electric razor
    c. Avoiding use of alcohol-based aftershave lotion
    d. Using gentle nondeodorant soap to wash the patient

26. A patient with which condition or disorder is at lowest risk for the development of acute sialoadenitis?
    a. Sjögren's syndrome
    b. HIV infection
    c. Anemia
    d. Phenothiazine use

27. When assessing a patient with a salivary gland tumor, the nurse pays particular attention to the facial nerve. Which request by the nurse is *least* likely to determine if the tumor has affected the facial nerve?
    a. "Puff out your cheeks."
    b. "Wrinkle your nose."
    c. "Cough."
    d. "Raise your eyebrows."

28. The nurse has taught a patient with acute sialoadenitis to use sialagogues to stimulate saliva. The patient demonstrates teaching has been effective when the patient states he will eat which food?
    a. Lemon slices
    b. Apple slices
    c. Bananas
    d. Bread

CASE STUDY: THE PATIENT WITH AN ORAL TUMOR

Use a separate sheet of paper to answer the questions in this Case Study, or go to the "Prepare for Class" folder on your Evolve website at http://evolve.elsevier.com/Iggy/ to download and complete as a word processing file. Answer guidelines for this Case Study are also available on your Evolve website.

The patient is admitted to the surgical unit for a radical neck dissection. He has a painless raised purple nodule on the hard palate. The lesion is large and the patient states, "I feel like there is something back there that makes it hard for me to breathe." His vital signs are: temp 102.2° F; pulse 98; blood pressure 138/90 mm Hg; respiratory rate 22. The patient has a CBC which indicates an Hgb of 18 g/dL, Hct 47%, and a WBC count of 18,000/mm^3. When reviewing the notes, the nurse reads that he had testing with an aqueous solution of toluidine blue 1% before his admission.

1. Based on the description, what kind of tumor does the nurse identify the tumor as most likely being?

2. What effect does the nurse expect for the toluidine solution if the tumor is malignant?

3. The patient is diagnosed with Kaposi's sarcoma. After this diagnosis, the nurse anticipates that the patient will most likely be tested for what other disease?

4. Based on the patient's assessment and laboratory results, what should the nurse anticipate as priority nursing interventions for the patient at this time?

5. The patient undergoes a radical neck dissection. Describe the nursing care for patients after this procedure.

6. Document a nursing note for the patient using the following systems:
   • Oral cavity
   • Hematologic

57
CHAPTER

Care of Patients with Esophageal Problems

STUDY/REVIEW QUESTIONS

1. Which physiologic factor contributes to gastroesophageal reflux disease (GERD)?
   a. Accelerated gastric emptying
   b. Irritation from refluxate
   c. Competent lower esophageal sphincter
   d. Increased esophageal clearance

2. Which statement is true about Barrett's epithelium in the patient with GERD?
   a. While the body heals, a different type of cell forms on the lower part of the esophagus.
   b. This new tissue is less resistant to acid so it must be taken care of.
   c. Barrett's epithelium is resistant to the development of cancer.
   d. Esophageal strictures are less likely to occur with this type of epithelium.

3. Which statements about GERD are correct? *(Select all that apply.)*
   a. Overweight and obese patients are at an increased risk.
   b. Thin and underweight patients are at an increased risk.
   c. It is a common disorder in the Asian and Hispanic populations.
   d. There is a high incidence in patients who eat mostly hot and spicy foods.
   e. It is a common upper gastrointestinal disorder in the United States.

Matching. Match each of the following GERD-associated conditions with their corresponding definitions.

GERD-Associated Conditions
a. Dyspepsia
b. Regurgitation
c. Water brash
d. Dysphagia
e. Odynophagia
f. Flatulence
g. Globus
h. Eructation
i. Pyrosis

Definitions
_____ 4. Pain described as a substernal or retrosternal burning sensation that tends to move up and down the chest in a wavelike fashion
_____ 5. Difficulty swallowing
_____ 6. Occurrence of warm fluid traveling up the throat with a sour or bitter taste
_____ 7. Painful swallowing
_____ 8. Reflex salivary hypersecretion in response to reflux
_____ 9. Gas
_____ 10. Belching
_____ 11. Feeling of something in the back of the throat
_____ 12. Retrosternal burning

13. A patient is scheduled to have several diagnostic tests to verify the medical diagnosis of GERD. Which diagnostic test is the most accurate method of diagnosing this disorder?
    a. Esophagogastroduodenoscopy (EGD)
    b. 24-hour ambulatory pH monitoring
    c. Esophageal manometry
    d. Motility testing

14. The nurse has provided teaching to a patient with GERD. Which statement by the patient indicates the teaching has been effective?
    a. "I will eat three meals a day."
    b. "I won't snack for 1 hour before I go to bed."
    c. "I won't nap for 30 minutes after eating dinner."
    d. "I won't lift heavy objects."

15. A patient is on nizatidine (Axid) therapy for the treatment of GERD. Which sign indicates that the patient may be having an adverse effect associated with this drug?
    a. Dysrhythmia
    b. Constipation
    c. Diarrhea
    d. Headache

16. A patient who has been prescribed metoclopramide (Reglan) is being discharged home. Which statement by the patient indicates a need for further discharge teaching by the nurse?
    a. "I will take the drug after meals."
    b. "I am using this drug to increase the rate at which my stomach empties."
    c. "I will call the health care provider if I have any ataxia."
    d. "I will inform the doctor if I start to have any hallucinations."

17. Which statement is true about the drug rabeprazole (Aciphex) for treatment of GERD?
    a. It is rapidly released into the body after it is administered.
    b. The tablets are large and may be crushed if the patient has difficulty swallowing them.
    c. It is a histamine receptor antagonist.
    d. Patients who use this drug should be instructed to wear sunscreen.

18. A patient has returned to the unit after a Stretta procedure for GERD. Which action by the student nurse requires the supervising nurse to intervene?
    a. The patient is offered clear liquids in the early postprocedure period.
    b. The patient's routine 81 mg of aspirin is held.
    c. A proton pump inhibitor is administered.
    d. A nasogastric tube is prepared for insertion.

19. Which lifestyle adjustment may a patient have to make to best control GERD?
    a. Sleep in the Trendelenburg position.
    b. Attain and maintain ideal body weight.
    c. Wear snug-fitting belts and waistbands.
    d. Engage in strenuous exercise such as weightlifting.

20. Which statements will the nurse include when providing health teaching for a patient with hiatal hernia? *(Select all that apply.)*
    a. "Elevate the head of your bed at least 6 inches for sleeping at night."
    b. "Remain in the upright position for several hours after eating."
    c. "Avoid straining or excessive vigorous exercise."
    d. "Avoid wearing clothing that is tight around the abdomen."
    e. "Avoid eating in the late evening."

21. Hiatal hernias are also called _____ hernias.

22. What diagnostic test best identifies a hiatal hernia?
    a. EGD
    b. 24-hour ambulatory pH monitoring
    c. Esophageal manometry
    d. Barium swallow study with fluoroscopy

23. Barrett's epithelium is considered _____ even though it is new epithelium.

24. The nurse has provided postoperative teaching for a patient who underwent a laparoscopic Nissen fundoplication (LNF). Which statement by the patient indicates a need for additional teaching?
    a. "I will walk every day."
    b. "I'll discontinue the antireflux drugs."
    c. "I will report a fever above 101° F."
    d. "I'll remove the gauze dressing 2 days after surgery and shower."

25. What is the primary focus of care after conventional surgery for hiatal hernia?
    a. Prevention of respiratory complications
    b. Pain management
    c. Management of fluid balance
    d. Teaching the patient self-care activities

26. GERD can be a cause of which adult onset disorders? *(Select all that apply.)*
    a. Dental caries
    b. Ileus
    c. Laryngitis
    d. Diverticulitis
    e. Asthma

27. The nurse is assessing a patient's nasogastric drainage following a fundoplication procedure. How does the nurse expect to find the drainage to appear the first 8 hours after surgery?
    a. Dark brown
    b. Bright red mixed with brown
    c. Yellowish to green
    d. Green to clear

28. The nurse is giving discharge instructions to a patient after a fundoplication procedure. Which activities is the patient instructed to *avoid*? *(Select all that apply.)*
    a. Drinking more than 8 oz of water at one time
    b. Chewing gum
    c. Drinking with a straw
    d. Eating gas-producing foods
    e. Drinking noncarbonated beverages

29. A patient is prescribed pantoprazole (Protonix). What does the nurse tell the patient is the major action of this medication?
    a. It produces a coating on the stomach lining.
    b. It neutralizes gastric acid.
    c. It heals esophageal irritation.
    d. It inhibits gastric acid secretion.

30. A patient is undergoing a workup for squamous cell carcinoma of the esophagus. What are the two primary risk factors associated with the development of this carcinoma?
    a. High-fat, low-fiber diet and tobacco use
    b. Tobacco use and heavy alcohol intake
    c. Sedentary lifestyle and family history of squamous cell carcinoma
    d. Heavy alcohol intake and high-fat, low-fiber diet

31. The definitive diagnosis for esophageal cancer is made with which procedure?
    a. Barium swallow
    b. Esophageal manometry
    c. Esophageal ultrasound with fine needle aspiration
    d. EGD

32. Nonsurgical treatment options for cancer of the esophagus can include which therapies? *(Select all that apply.)*
    a. Swallowing therapy
    b. Chemoradiation
    c. Targeted therapies
    d. Photodynamic therapy
    e. Endoscopic therapies

CASE STUDY: THE PATIENT WITH AN ESOPHAGEAL PROBLEM

Use a separate sheet of paper to answer the questions in this Case Study, or go to the "Prepare for Class" folder on your Evolve website at http://evolve.elsevier.com/Iggy/ to download and complete as a word processing file. Answer guidelines for this Case Study are also available on your Evolve website.

The 53-year-old man comes to the clinic for an appointment reporting heartburn, chest pain, and frequent belching. He describes the pain as a substernal burning sensation that tends to move up and down the chest in a wavelike fashion. He reports that the symptoms are impacting his ability to concentrate at work and to sleep through the night, even though he sleeps with his head elevated at least 6 inches.

1. What other questions should the nurse ask the patient at this time? What are the possible causes of this substernal burning?

History reveals that the patient eats 3 meals a day. His diet previously consisted of mostly fatty foods, 4 to 5 cups of coffee daily, and 3 to 4 colas daily. He reports that in the past 2 to 3 weeks he has eliminated most of the fatty foods in his diet, drinks less than half the amount of coffee, and drinks no colas. The patient smokes 1 to 2 packs of cigarettes per day for the past 30 years.

2. The patient is ordered to have 24-hour ambulatory pH monitoring. What patient teaching concerning this test should the nurse provide?

3. The patient is diagnosed with GERD. What patient and family health promotion modifications to control reflux should the nurse include in the teaching?

The patient is prescribed medication that includes omeprazole (Prilosec) 20 mg orally daily; metoclopramide (Reglan) 10 mg orally 3 times daily; and Gaviscon one tablet after each meal and at bedtime. However, the patient returns to the clinic 3 weeks later to report that these medications are not helping him.

One week later, a barium swallow with fluoroscopy is performed and a rolling hiatal hernia is diagnosed. The patient is here today to discuss his test results and treatment with a laparoscopic Nissen fundoplication (LNF). He agrees to the surgery.

4. Using the SBAR format, outline the discussion that the nurse will have with the person responsible in handing off the patient to the surgical department.

58 CHAPTER

Care of Patients with Stomach Disorders

STUDY/REVIEW QUESTIONS

1. Which are pathologic changes associated with acute gastritis? *(Select all that apply.)*
   a. Vascular congestion
   b. Severe mucosal damage and ruptured vessels
   c. Edema
   d. Acute inflammatory cell infiltration
   e. Increased cell production in the superficial epithelium of the stomach lining

2. Which are possible complications of chronic gastritis? *(Select all that apply.)*
   a. Pernicious anemia
   b. Thickening of the stomach lining
   c. Gastric cancer
   d. Decreased gastric acid secretion
   e. Peptic ulcer disease

True or False? *Read each statement and write T for true or F for false in the blanks provided. If the statement is false, correct the statement to make it true.*

_____ 3. The diagnosis of gastritis is made solely on clinical symptoms.

_____ 4. The onset of infection with *Helicobacter pylori* can result in acute gastritis.

_____ 5. Long-term use of acetaminophen (Tylenol) creates a high risk for acute gastritis.

_____ 6. Atrophic gastritis is a type of chronic gastritis that is seen most often in older adults.

7. The nurse is teaching a patient about health promotion and maintenance to prevent gastritis. Which information does the nurse include? *(Select all that apply.)*
   a. "A balanced diet can help prevent gastritis."
   b. "To prevent gastritis, you should limit your intake of salt."
   c. "If you stop smoking, there is less of a chance that you will develop gastritis."
   d. "Yoga has been found to be effective in preventing gastritis."
   e. "Although regular exercise is good for you, it has not been found to have an effect on the prevention of gastritis."

8. A patient with chronic gastritis is being admitted. Which sign/symptom does the nurse identify as being associated with this patient's condition?
   a. Pernicious anemia
   b. Gastric hemorrhage
   c. Hematemesis
   d. Dyspepsia

9. When teaching a patient about pernicious anemia, which statement does the nurse include?
   a. "Patients with pernicious anemia are not able to digest fats."
   b. "Pernicious anemia results in a deficiency of vitamin B_{12}."
   c. "All patients with gastrointestinal bleeding will eventually develop pernicious anemia."
   d. "Oral iron supplements are an effective treatment for pernicious anemia."

10. A patient comes to the emergency department (ED) reporting rapid onset of epigastric pain with nausea and vomiting. The patient says the pain is worse than any heartburn he has had, and that he has not had an appetite for the past day. What does the nurse suspect this patient has?
    a. Peritonitis
    b. *H. pylori* infection
    c. Duodenal ulcer
    d. Acute gastritis

11. Which diagnostic test is the gold standard for diagnosing gastritis?
    a. Esophagogastroduodenoscopy (EGD)
    b. CT scan
    c. Upper GI series
    d. Cholangiogram

12. The nurse is teaching a patient about ranitidine (Zantac) prescribed for gastritis. Which statement by the patient indicates effective teaching by the nurse?
    a. "The drug will heal the areas of my stomach that are sore."
    b. "This drug will block the secretions of my stomach."
    c. "Zantac will make the inside of my stomach not as acidy as it is now."
    d. "This pill kills the bacterial infection I have in my stomach."

13. A patient with acute gastritis is receiving treatment to block and buffer gastric acid secretions to relieve pain. Which drug does the nurse identify as an antisecretory agent (proton-pump inhibitor)?
    a. Sucralfate (Carafate)
    b. Ranitidine (Zantac)
    c. Mylanta
    d. Omeprazole (Prilosec)

14. The nursing student caring for a patient with a duodenal ulcer is about to administer a proton pump inhibitor (PPI). Which statement about this medication is true?
    a. These drugs should not be used for a prolonged period of time because they may contribute to osteoporotic-related fractures.
    b. PPIs may not be given via feeding tube.
    c. These drugs help prevent stress-induced ulcers.
    d. PPIs work by coating the stomach with a protective barrier.

15. The nurse is teaching a patient being discharged home about taking prescribed medications that include sucralfate (Carafate). Which statement by the patient indicates teaching has been effective?
    a. "The main side effect of sucralfate is diarrhea."
    b. "I will take sucralfate with meals."
    c. "I will take sucralfate along with the antacid medication I take."
    d. "Sucralfate works to heal my ulcer."

True or False? *Read each statement and write T for true or F for false in the blanks provided. If the statement is false, correct the statement to make it true.*

_____ 16. *Peptic ulcer* is the term used to describe both gastric and duodenal ulcers.

_____ 17. Prostaglandins increase the stomach's resistance to ulceration.

_____ 18. Cushing's ulcer is a type of stress ulcer commonly seen in patients with extensive burns.

_____ 19. IV famotidine (Pepcid) or pantoprazole (Protonix) are often prescribed to prevent stress ulcers.

_____ 20. Hematemesis usually indicates bleeding at or below the duodenojejunal junction.

_____ 21. COX-2 inhibitors such as celecoxib (Celebrex) are less likely to cause mucosal damage to the stomach as compared to nonsteroidal anti-inflammatory drugs (NSAIDs).

22. Drug therapy for peptic ulcer disease is implemented for which purposes? *(Select all that apply.)*
   a. Pain relief
   b. Rebuild the mucosal lining of the stomach
   c. Eliminate *H. pylori* infection
   d. Heal ulcerations
   e. Prevent recurrence

Matching. *Match the drugs used to treat peptic ulcer disease with their corresponding nursing interventions.*

Drugs
a. Magnesium hydroxide (Maalox)
b. Omeprazole (Prilosec)
c. Esomeprazole (Nexium)
d. Misoprostol (Cytotec)

Interventions

_____ 23. Assess the patient for hepatic problems because he or she will need to take a lower dose of this drug.

_____ 24. Observe the patient for the side effect of diarrhea.

_____ 25. Useful for patients to protect against NSAID-induced ulcers.

_____ 26. Caution patients taking clopidogrel (Plavix) that this drug may reduce its effectiveness.

27. Which statement about the use of antacids in the treatment of gastric ulcers is true?
   a. Antacids should be administered with meals.
   b. The patient should take calcium carbonate (Tums) if they still have pain after taking their usual antacid.
   c. The patient should take antacid on an empty stomach.
   d. Avoid using antacids with phenytoin (Dilantin).

28. A patient with peptic ulcer disease is receiving Maalox. Which actions does the nurse take in regards to administering this medication? *(Select all that apply.)*
   a. Give the medication 2 hours after the patient's meal.
   b. Do not give other drugs within 1 to 2 hours of antacids.
   c. Assess the patient for a history of renal disease before giving Maalox.
   d. Assess the patient for a history of heart failure before giving Maalox.
   e. Observe the patient for the side effect of diarrhea.

29. The nurse has provided instruction for a patient prescribed sucralfate (Carafate) to treat a gastric ulcer. Which statement by the patient indicates that teaching has been effective?
    a. "This drug will stop the secretion of acid in my stomach."
    b. "I will take this drug on an empty stomach."
    c. "I will not be able to take ranitidine (Zantac) with this drug."
    d. "The main side effect of this drug that I can expect is diarrhea."

30. A patient is admitted with an upper GI bleed. Which finding does the nurse expect to assess in the patient?
    a. Decreased pulse
    b. Increased hemoglobin and hematocrit
    c. Syncope
    d. Increased blood pressure

31. A patient develops an active upper GI bleed. Which are the priority actions the nurse takes in caring for this patient? *(Select all that apply.)*
    a. Provide oxygen.
    b. Start 1 or 2 large-bore IV lines.
    c. Prepare to infuse 0.9% normal saline solution or lactated Ringer's solution.
    d. Monitor serum electrolytes.
    e. Prepare for nasogastric (NG) tube insertion.

32. When performing an assessment on a patient with an active upper GI bleed, which conditions does the nurse identify as common causes of upper GI bleeding? *(Select all that apply.)*
    a. Esophageal cancer
    b. Esophageal varices
    c. Duodenal ulcer
    d. Gastritis
    e. Gastric cancer

33. The licensed practical nurse (LPN) is caring for a patient with an NG tube. The supervising nurse intervenes when the LPN attempts to perform which action?
    a. Lubricate the tube with a petroleum-based product.
    b. Measure the length of the tube to be passed from the bridge of the nose to the earlobe to the xiphoid process.
    c. Ask the patient to swallow while the tube is being passed.
    d. Obtain a sample of gastric contents by aspirating with a 50 mL catheter-tipped syringe.

34. The student nurse is performing a gastric lavage on a patient with an active upper GI bleed. Which action by the student requires intervention by the supervising nurse?
    a. Using an ice-cold solution to lavage the stomach.
    b. Instilling the lavage solution in volumes of 200 to 300 mL.
    c. Continuing the lavage until the solution returned is clear or light pink without clots.
    d. Positioning the patient on his left side during the procedure.

35. Which drug is the drug of choice for aggressive acid suppression to prevent rebleeding in a patient with a gastric bleed?
    a. Ranitidine (Zantac)
    b. Omeprazole (Prilosec)
    c. Ocetreotide (Sandostatin)
    d. Pantoprazole (Protonix)

36. Which are findings in a patient who has Zollinger-Ellison syndrome? *(Select all that apply.)*
    a. Gastrinomas
    b. Steatorrhea
    c. Increased amounts of gastric acids
    d. *H. pylori* infection
    e. Immediate relief of symptoms with traditional ulcer therapy

37. The nurse is caring for several patients with gastric and duodenal ulcers. Which differential features of gastric ulcers compared to duodenal ulcers does the nurse identify? *(Select all that apply.)*
    a. Normal secretion or hyposecretion
    b. Relieved by ingestion of food
    c. Hematemesis more common
    d. No gastritis present
    e. Most often, the patient has type O blood

38. The nurse is performing a physical assessment on a patient admitted to the unit with gastric cancer. Which findings indicate signs of distant metastasis? *(Select all that apply.)*
    a. Cullen's sign
    b. Virchow's nodes
    c. Blumer's shelf
    d. "Sister Mary Joseph nodes"
    e. Krukenberg's tumor

39. The nurse is assessing a patient who has had a total gastrectomy and notes bright red blood in the NG and abdominal distention. What does the nurse do next?
    a. Irrigate the NG tube.
    b. Reposition the NG tube.
    c. Inform the surgeon of these findings.
    d. Remove the NG tube.

True or False? *Read each statement and write T for true or F for false in the blanks provided. If the statement is false, correct the statement to make it true.*

_____ 40. *Dumping syndrome* is a term that refers to a group of vasomotor symptoms that occur after eating.

_____ 41. Late dumping syndrome is caused by a release of an excessive amount of insulin.

_____ 42. To manage dumping syndrome, the patient needs to eliminate liquid ingested with meals.

_____ 43. Patients with dumping syndrome are instructed to eat a diet that is high in carbohydrates and low in fat and protein.

_____ 44. After gastric resection, patients should be assessed for the development of atrophic glossitis which occurs secondary to vitamin B_{12} deficiency.

45. The nurse is teaching a patient with dumping syndrome about diet. Which statement by the patient indicates that teaching has been effective?
    a. "I will use sugar-free gelatin with caution."
    b. "I will avoid rice in my diet."
    c. "Meat in my diet will consist of a total of 4 ounces a day."
    d. "I will limit fluids with my meals to 8 ounces."

46. Which statement about general principles of diet therapy for patients with dumping syndrome is true?
    a. Patients with dumping syndrome should have liquids between meals only.
    b. Patients with dumping syndrome should be encouraged to eat a diet high in roughage.
    c. Patients with dumping syndrome should eat a high-carbohydrate diet.
    d. The diet for a patient with dumping syndrome must be low in fat and protein.

CASE STUDY: THE PATIENT WITH A GASTRIC ULCER

Use a separate sheet of paper to answer the questions in this Case Study, or go to the "Prepare for Class" folder on your Evolve website at http://evolve.elsevier.com/Iggy/ to download and complete as a word processing file. Answer guidelines for this Case Study are also available on your Evolve website.

A 45-year-old woman with a history of arthritis has been admitted with a possible diagnosis of peptic ulcer disease. The patient states that she takes ibuprofen to treat the arthritis pain instead of the medication that was prescribed for her. The patient says, "I told my doctor I wasn't going to take expensive drugs that will do more harm to me than good. The ibuprofen works just fine." After a diagnosis of peptic ulcer disease is confirmed, the health care provider prescribes misoprostol (Cytotec). On the day of discharge, the nurse enters the patient's room and finds her in bed spitting bright red blood. After the bleeding is controlled, the patient is discharged home.

1. The patient asks, "Why do people keep talking about an infection that I might have in my stomach?" What patient teaching should the nurse provide? Document your answer in a nursing note.

2. What role did ibuprofen play in the development of the peptic ulcer?

3. Why has misoprostol (Cytotec) been prescribed for this patient?

4. What complication is likely happening to the patient and what actions should the nurse take?

5. The patient is to be followed-up by a home health care agency. Using the SBAR format, document the report that would be given to the home care agency by the nurse.

59 CHAPTER

Care of Patients with Noninflammatory Intestinal Disorders

STUDY/REVIEW QUESTIONS

True or False? *Read each statement and write T for true or F for false in the blanks provided. If the statement is false, correct the statement to make it true.*

_____ 1. Irritable bowel syndrome (IBS) is a functional GI disorder characterized by chronic or recurrent diarrhea, constipation, and/or abdominal pain and bloating.

_____ 2. No actual pathophysiologic changes occur in IBS.

_____ 3. Symptoms of IBS typically begin in late adulthood.

_____ 4. IBS is the most common digestive disorder seen in clinical practice.

_____ 5. The most common symptom of IBS is pain in the right lower quadrant of the abdomen.

_____ 6. A hydrogen breath test may be used in the diagnostic phase of the disease.

_____ 7. A newer group of drugs used to manage IBS are the muscarinic (M3) receptor antagonists which act by inhibiting intestinal motility.

8. Which drug is the drug of choice for the treatment of IBS when pain is the predominant symptom?
   a. Amitriptyline (Elavil)
   b. Muscarinic (M3) receptor antagonists
   c. Loperamide (Imodium)
   d. Psyllium hydrophilic mucilloid (Metamucil)

9. The nurse is teaching a patient with IBS about complementary and alternative therapies for the disease. Which patient statements indicate that teaching has been effective? *(Select all that apply.)*
   a. "Hydrotherapy may help decrease symptoms."
   b. "I should exercise regularly to help manage the disease."
   c. "Peppermint oil has been used to expel gas and relax spastic intestinal muscles."
   d. "Fish oil can be used to ease constipation."
   e. "Ginkgo can be used for abdominal discomfort and to expel gas."

Matching. *Match each type of hernia with its appropriate description.*

Hernia Types

a. Femoral
b. Incarcerated
c. Indirect inguinal
d. Reducible
e. Strangulated
f. Umbilical
g. Incisional

Descriptions

_____ 10. Contents of the sac can be replaced into the abdominal cavity by gentle pressure.

_____ 11. A plug of fat in the femoral canal enlarges and eventually pulls the peritoneum and often the urinary bladder into the sac.

_____ 12. Acquired as a result of increased intra-abdominal pressure.

_____ 13. Sac formed from the peritoneum that contains a portion of the intestine omentum. Hernia pushes downward at an angle into the inguinal canal.

_____ 14. Cannot be replaced back into the abdominal cavity.

_____ 15. Blood supply to the herniated bowel segment is cut off.

_____ 16. Occurs at the site of a previous surgical incision.

17. The nurse is performing an abdominal assessment on a patient suspected of having an abdominal hernia. The nurse auscultates the abdomen and determines the absence of bowel sounds. What does the nurse suspect in this patient?
    a. Peritonitis
    b. IBS
    c. Obstruction and strangulation
    d. Low intra-abdominal pressure

18. Which are true statements about caring for a patient with a truss? *(Select all that apply.)*
    a. A surgical binder holds the truss in place.
    b. The truss is removed only for bathing.
    c. The truss is only used after the hernia has been reduced by the physician.
    d. The truss is applied before the hernia is reduced to decrease pain.
    e. Powder should be applied to the skin under the truss daily.

19. Which activity does the nurse tell the patient to *avoid* after surgery for a hernia repair?
    a. Ambulating
    b. Turning
    c. Coughing
    d. Deep-breathing

20. What do postoperative measures for a male patient who has had an inguinal herniorrhaphy include?
    a. Applying a warm pack to the scrotum
    b. Elevating the scrotum on a pillow
    c. Encouraging use of a bedpan to void
    d. Decreasing fluid intake to decrease bladder emptying

True or False? *Read each statement about colorectal cancer (CRC) and write T for true or F for false in the blanks provided. If the statement is false, correct the statement to make it true.*

_____ 21. CRC is one of the most prevalent malignancies in the United States.

_____ 22. To reduce the risk of CRC, diets should be low in fat, low in refined carbohydrates, and high in fiber.

_____ 23. The most common signs of CRC are rectal bleeding, anemia, and a change in stool.

_____ 24. Hematochezia is the passage of red blood via the rectum.

_____ 25. Hemoglobin and hematocrit values are usually increased as a result of the intermittent bleeding associated with the tumor.

_____ 26. A negative test result for occult blood in the stool confirms bleeding in the GI tract.

_____ 27. Colonoscopy with biopsy is the definitive test for the diagnosis of CRC.

_____ 28. Carcinoembryonic antigen (CEA), an oncofetal antigen, is elevated in many people with CRC.

29. After colostomy surgery, which intervention does the nurse employ?
   a. Cover the stoma with a dry, sterile dressing.
   b. Apply a pouch system as soon as possible.
   c. Make a hole in the pouch for gas to escape.
   d. Watch for the colostomy to start functioning on day 1.

30. Which discharge instruction does the nurse include for a patient after abdominoperitoneal (AP) resection?
   a. "Use a soft pillow to sit on whenever you sit down."
   b. "Lie on your back when you are resting in bed."
   c. "Use a rubber doughnut device for sitting on when in the car."
   d. "Sit in a chair for at least 4 consecutive hours a day."

31. The nurse immediately reports to the surgeon all but which sign/symptom related to a colostomy?
   a. Liquid stool immediately postoperatively
   b. Unusual bleeding
   c. Signs of ischemia and necrosis
   d. Mucocutaneous separation

32. Which statement about the care of a patient with a colostomy is correct?
   a. A healthy stoma should be dry.
   b. The stoma should protrude about 2 inches from the abdominal wall.
   c. When palpating the stoma, it should feel firm.
   d. A slight amount of edema is normal in the initial postoperative period.

33. The nurse is teaching a patient about what to expect after a descending colon colostomy. The nurse tells the patient to expect the stool to have what kind of form?
   a. Similar to that of stool expelled from the rectum
   b. Thick and paste-like
   c. Thin and gelatin-like
   d. Watery

34. Which sign/symptom is a patient who had an AP resection instructed to report to the health care provider immediately?
    a. Serosanguineous drainage from the wound
    b. Sensations of having a bowel movement
    c. Constant perineal odor and pain
    d. Occasional perineal pain and itching

35. The nurse is teaching a patient about colostomy care. Which information does the nurse include in the teaching plan?
    a. The stoma will enlarge within 6 to 8 weeks of surgery.
    b. Use a moisturizing soap to cleanse the area around the stoma.
    c. Place the colostomy bag on the skin when the skin sealant is still damp.
    d. An antifungal cream or powder can be used if a fungal rash develops.

36. A patient with a colostomy may safely include which food item in the diet?
    a. Burritos
    b. Chicken noodle soup
    c. Cabbage
    d. Carbonated beverages

37. The nurse is teaching a patient about how to control gas and odor from a colostomy. Which information does the nurse include?
    a. Do not chew gum.
    b. Place an aspirin in the colostomy.
    c. Do not consume buttermilk.
    d. Do not eat parsley.

True or False? *Read each statement and write T for true and F for false in the blanks provided. If the statement is false, correct the statement to make it true.*

_____ 38. Crohn's disease can cause a mechanical obstruction.

_____ 39. Nonmechanical obstruction is also known as *paralytic ileus* or *adynamic ileus*.

_____ 40. Hypovolemia is a common complication of intestinal obstruction.

_____ 41. An obstruction high in the small intestine often results in metabolic acidosis.

_____ 42. Intussusception is twisting of the intestine.

_____ 43. Volvulus is telescoping of a segment of the intestine within itself.

_____ 44. Hypokalemia is the most common electrolyte disturbance that predisposes the patient to intestinal obstruction.

_____ 45. *Obstipation* is the term which refers to no passage of stool.

46. Which key feature does the nurse most likely find when performing a physical assessment on a patient with a small-bowel obstruction?
    a. Visible peristaltic waves in the upper and middle abdomen
    b. Minimal or no vomiting
    c. No major fluid and electrolyte imbalances
    d. Metabolic acidosis

47. What does care of a patient with an nasogastric (NG) tube require? *(Select all that apply.)*
    a. Assessment of proper placement at least every 4 hours
    b. Cleansing of the nose with the same type of skin protectant used for ostomy skin care before applying the NG tube securing device
    c. Confirmation of NG tube placement by x-ray if it is repositioned
    d. Aspiration of contents of the NG tube and irrigation of the tube with 30 mL of normal saline every 4 hours
    e. Questioning the patient about the passage of flatus

48. What does nursing care of a patient with intestinal obstruction who reports discomfort in the early diagnostic period consist of?
    a. Administration of opioid analgesics
    b. Placing the patient in a semi-Fowler's position
    c. Providing the patient with fluids
    d. Offering the patient semi-soft foods

49. Which NG tubes can be connected to low intermittent suction? *(Select all that apply.)*
    a. Salem sump
    b. Levin
    c. Anderson
    d. Carney
    e. Jones

50. Which interventions apply to patients with hypovolemia related to an intestinal obstruction?
    a. Provide frequent mouth care with lemon-glycerin swabs.
    b. Offer ice chips to suck on before surgery.
    c. Offer a small glass of water.
    d. Assess for edema from third-spacing.

51. Which observation of a patient with an intestinal obstruction does the nurse report immediately?
    a. Urinary output of 1000 mL in an 8-hour period
    b. The patient's request for something to drink
    c. Abdominal pain changing from colicky to constant discomfort
    d. The patient who is changing positions frequently

52. Which discharge information does the nurse include for the patient who has had an intestinal obstruction caused by fecal impaction?
    a. Encourage the patient to report abdominal distention, nausea or vomiting, and constipation.
    b. Provide the patient a written description of a low-fiber diet.
    c. Remind the patient to limit activity.
    d. Remind the patient to decrease fluid intake.

True or False? Read each statement and write T for true or F for false in the blanks provided. If the statement is false, correct the statement to make it true.

_____ 53. The spleen is the most commonly injured organ in blunt abdominal trauma.

_____ 54. The liver is the most commonly injured organ in blunt and penetrating trauma.

_____ 55. Once the ABCs of the patient with abdominal trauma have been stabilized, the nurse focuses on risks of hemorrhage, shock, and peritonitis.

_____ 56. Ecchymoses in the distribution of a lap seat belt should be reported to the health care provider immediately because the bowel may be injured.

57. A patient with abdominal trauma has a positive Ballance's sign. What does the nurse suspect in the patient?
    a. Ruptured spleen
    b. Lacerated liver
    c. Infarcted bowel
    d. Pelvic fracture

58. Emergency care of a patient with abdominal trauma includes which interventions? *(Select all that apply.)*
    a. Insertion of at least two large-bore IV catheters in the lower extremities
    b. Type and cross-matching of four to eight units of blood
    c. Measurement of arterial blood gases
    d. Continuous hemodynamic monitoring
    e. Insertion of a Foley catheter

59. Which statement about intra-abdominal pressure (IAP) monitoring is correct?
    a. The normal IAP for adults is 15 to 20 mm Hg.
    b. Patients with high IAP have bradycardia.
    c. High IAP leads to increased afterload and decreased preload.
    d. Patients with high IAP are hypertensive.

60. Which information does the nurse include when teaching a patient with new onset hemorrhoids about prevention of hemorrhoid flare-up? *(Select all that apply.)*
    a. Increase the fiber in your diet to prevent constipation.
    b. Do not participate in any physical exercise.
    c. Maintain a healthy weight.
    d. Increase your amount of fluid intake.
    e. Prolonged sitting or standing will not affect the development of hemorrhoids.

61. Which intervention is contraindicated in the nonsurgical management of hemorrhoids?
    a. Diets low in fiber and fluids
    b. Dibucaine (Nupercainal) ointment
    c. Warm sitz baths three or four times a day
    d. Cleansing the anal area with moistened cleaning tissues

62. Which statement by a patient indicates an understanding of surgical management of hemorrhoids?
    a. "It will take 10 to 14 days for the rubber band used on the hemorrhoid to fall off."
    b. "Urinary retention is a complication of surgical resection of the hemorrhoid."
    c. "After surgery, I will need to eat a low-fiber, low-fluid diet."
    d. "Stool softeners and laxatives are avoided after hemorrhoid surgery."

True or False? Read each statement and write T for true or F for false in the blanks provided. If the statement is false, correct the statement to make it true.

_____ 63. Deficiencies of bile salts can lead to malabsorption of fats and fat-soluble vitamins.

_____ 64. Pancreatic enzymes are necessary for absorption of vitamin B_{12}.

_____ 65. Gastric surgery is one of the most common causes of malabsorption and maldigestion.

_____ 66. Constipation is a classic symptom of malabsorption.

_____ 67. The Schilling test measures urinary excretion of vitamin B_{12} for diagnosis of pernicious anemia and a variety of other malabsorption syndromes.

68. Which drug is used to treat tropical sprue?
    a. Bentyl
    b. Lomotil
    c. Steroids
    d. Bactrim

CASE STUDY: THE PATIENT WITH A BOWEL OBSTRUCTION

Use a separate sheet of paper to answer the questions in this Case Study, or go to the "Prepare for Class" folder on your Evolve website at http://evolve.elsevier.com/Iggy/ to download and complete as a word processing file. Answer guidelines for this Case Study are also available on your Evolve website.

An 80-year-old man comes to the ED reporting acute upper to mid-abdominal, sporadic pain and cramping. Upon assessment, the nurse observes abdominal distention and high-pitched bowel sounds. The physician has ordered flat plate and upright abdominal x-rays that show distention of loops of intestine, with fluid and gas in the small intestine in conjunction with absence of gas in the colon. The physician has diagnosed a bowel obstruction.

1. Based on the findings, identify which type of bowel obstruction this patient most likely has.

2. What other signs and symptoms would the nurse observe for in this patient?

3. Identify the most likely interventions for this patient based on his type of bowel obstruction.

4. It is found that the patient has a small fecal impaction. Document the preventive care that the nurse would include in patient/family teaching for this patient.

60
CHAPTER

Care of Patients with Inflammatory Intestinal Disorders

STUDY/REVIEW QUESTIONS

True or False? *Read each statement and write T for true or F for false in the blanks provided. If the statement is false, correct the statement to make it true.*

_____ 1. Appendicitis is the most common cause of right lower quadrant pain.

_____ 2. The initial obstruction of the appendix is usually a result of fecaliths.

_____ 3. The diagnosis of appendicitis is difficult to establish in the older adult because symptoms of pain and tenderness may not be as pronounced in this age group, resulting in increased risk for perforation, peritonitis, and mortality.

_____ 4. Classically, appendicitis presents with cramp-like pain in the right lower quadrant.

_____ 5. McBurney's point is the area in the left lower quadrant between the anterior iliac crest and the umbilicus.

_____ 6. Laboratory findings do not establish the diagnosis of appendicitis.

7. The nurse is caring for the patient with acute appendicitis. Which interventions will the nurse perform? *(Select all that apply.)*
   a. Maintain the patient on NPO status.
   b. Administer IV fluids as prescribed.
   c. Apply warm compresses to the right lower abdominal quadrant.
   d. Maintain the patient in the supine position.
   e. Administer laxatives.

8. The patient has been diagnosed with acute appendicitis. Based on this diagnosis, which intervention does the nurse perform?
   a. Start a bowel cleansing program.
   b. Prepare the patient for surgery.
   c. Apply a heating pad to the lower abdomen.
   d. Assess the patient's knowledge about dietary modifications.

9. The nurse on the surgical unit is expecting to admit the patient who has had an appendectomy with abscess. What does the nurse anticipate care for this patient will include? *(Select all that apply.)*
   a. Clear liquids
   b. Wound drains
   c. IV antibiotics
   d. Nonsteroidal anti-inflammatory drugs (NSAIDs) for pain control
   e. Bedrest for 24 hours

10. Which statements about peritonitis are true? *(Select all that apply.)*
    a. Peritonitis is caused by contamination of the peritoneal cavity by bacteria or chemicals.
    b. Continuous ambulatory peritoneal dialysis (CAPD) can cause peritonitis.
    c. White blood cell counts are often decreased with peritonitis.
    d. Abdominal wall rigidity is a classic finding in patients with peritonitis.
    e. Chemical peritonitis is caused by leakage of pancreatic and liver enzymes or gastric acids.

11. The fluid shift that occurs in peritonitis may result in which of the following?
    a. Intracellular fluid moving into the peritoneal cavity
    b. Significant increase in circulatory volume
    c. Eventual renal failure and electrolyte imbalance
    d. Increased bowel motility caused by increased fluid volume

12. The respiratory problems that may accompany peritonitis are a result of which factor?
    a. Associated pain interfering with ventilation
    b. Decreased pressure against the diaphragm
    c. Fluid shifts to the thoracic cavity
    d. Decreased oxygen demands related to the infectious process

13. Which nursing intervention is part of nonsurgical management for a patient with peritonitis?
    a. Monitor weekly weight and intake and output.
    b. Insert a nasogastric tube to decompress the stomach.
    c. Order a breakfast tray when the patient is hungry.
    d. Administer NSAIDs for pain.

14. What are the cardinal signs of peritonitis?
    a. Fever and headache
    b. Dizziness and vomiting
    c. Abdominal pain and tenderness
    d. Nausea and loss of appetite

15. The nurse is instructing a patient about home care after an exploratory laparotomy for peritonitis. Which statement by the patient indicates that teaching has been effective?
    a. "It is normal for the incision site to be warm."
    b. "I will stop taking the antibiotics if diarrhea develops."
    c. "I will call the health care provider for a temperature greater than 101° F."
    d. "I will resume activity with my bowling league this week for exercise."

True or False? *Read each statement and write T for true or F for false in the blanks provided. If the statement is false, correct the statement to make it true.*

_____ 16. Gastroenteritis is an increase in the frequency and water content of stools or vomiting as a result of inflammation of the mucous membranes of the stomach and intestinal tract.

_____ 17. *E. coli* can release enterotoxin which results in diarrhea.

_____ 18. *Shigella* and *Campylobacter* will attach themselves to the mucosal epithelium and penetrate it, resulting in destruction of the intestinal villi and malabsorption.

_____ 19. The Norwalk virus infection can occur year-round and affects adults and children.

20. The nurse is assessing a patient with viral gastroenteritis. Which symptom is the nurse most concerned about?
    a. Orthostatic blood pressure changes
    b. Poor skin turgor
    c. Dry mucous membranes
    d. Rebound tenderness

21. What is the priority nursing concern for a patient with gastroenteritis?
    a. Nutrition therapy
    b. Fluid replacement
    c. Skin care
    d. Drug therapy

22. As part of the routine treatment plan for a patient with bacterial gastroenteritis, which drugs does the nurse anticipate the patient will be prescribed? *(Select all that apply.)*
    a. Anticholinergics
    b. Antiemetics
    c. Antiperistaltic drugs
    d. Antibiotics
    e. Bismuth subsalicylate (Pepto-Bismol)

23. The nurse is caring for a patient with gastroenteritis who has frequent stools. Which task is best to delegate to the nursing assistant?
    a. Teach the patient to avoid toilet paper and harsh soaps.
    b. Instruct the patient on how to take a sitz bath.
    c. Use a warm washcloth to remove stool from the skin.
    d. Dry the skin with absorbent cotton.

24. Identify whether each characteristic pertains to Crohn's disease (CD) or ulcerative colitis (UC).

    _____ a. Begins in the rectum and proceeds in a continuous manner toward the cecum

    _____ b. Fistulas commonly develop

    _____ c. Infrequent need for surgery

    _____ d. Five to six soft, loose stools per day that are non-bloody

    _____ e. Increased risk of colon cancer

    _____ f. Some patients experience extraintestinal manifestations such as migratory polyarthritis, ankylosing spondylitis, and erythema nodosum

    _____ g. Cobblestone appearance of the internal intestine

25. A patient is suspected to have UC. Which definitive diagnostic test does the nurse expect the patient to undergo in order to confirm the diagnosis?
    a. Colonoscopy
    b. C-reactive protein
    c. Albumin levels
    d. Erythrocyte sedimentation rate

26. A patient is prescribed sulfasalazine (Azulfidine) for the treatment of UC. Which patient statement indicates the patient is experiencing a side effect of this drug?
    a. "My skin is turning a yellow color."
    b. "My knees hurt."
    c. "My stomach hurts when I take this pill."
    d. "I wake up at night sweating sometimes."

27. Which statement is true about the medical treatment of UC?
    a. Infliximab (Remicade) is approved as a first-line therapy.
    b. Immunomodulators are not thought to be effective; however, in combination with steroids, they may offer a synergistic effect.
    c. When a therapeutic level of glucocorticoids is reached, the dosage of the drug stays the same to maintain the therapeutic effect.
    d. The method of action for the aminosalicylates is interruption of the pain pathway.

28. A patient with UC who has had an ileostomy is being discharged home. The nurse has provided discharge teaching. Which statements by the patient indicate the teaching has been effective? *(Select all that apply.)*
    a. "I will avoid foods that cause gas."
    b. "I will call the health care provider if I have a fever over 101° F."
    c. "I will change the adhesive for the appliance daily."
    d. "I know the pouch needs emptying when I feel pain in that area."
    e. "I will call the health care provider if I feel like my heart is beating fast."

Matching. Match each type of surgical procedure with its description.

Procedures

a. Restorative proctolectomy with ileo pouch–anal anastomosis (RPC-IPAA)
b. Ileoanal reservoir
c. Ileostomy
d. Total proctocolectomy with a permanent ileostomy
e. Sigmoid colostomy
f. Natural orifice transluminal endoscopic surgery (NOTES)

Descriptions

_____ 29. Procedure in which a loop of the ileum is placed through the abdominal wall

_____ 30. Performed because the sigmoid colon is the most common site of diverticulitis

_____ 31. Removal of the colon, rectum, and anus with surgical closure of the anus

_____ 32. Can be performed via the anus or vagina for select patients

_____ 33. The gold standard for patients with UC

_____ 34. "J pouch"

35. Which statement is true about drug therapy for CD?
    a. Budesonide (Entocort EC) is a rapid-release compound that delivers low local glucocorticoid concentrations to the terminal ileum for patients with CD.
    b. Methotrexate (Rheumatrex) is contraindicated in the treatment of CD.
    c. Metronidazole (Flagyl) has been helpful in patients with fistulas and CD.
    d. Adalimumab (Humira) is a glucocorticoid approved for the treatment of CD.

36. A patient with CD has a fistula. Which assessment finding indicates possible dehydration?
    a. Weight gain of 2 pounds in one day
    b. Abdominal pain
    c. Foul-smelling urine
    d. Decreased urinary output

37. In caring for a patient with CD, the nurse observes for which complications? *(Select all that apply.)*
    a. Peritonitis
    b. Small bowel obstruction
    c. Nutritional and fluid imbalances
    d. Presence of fistulas
    e. Appendicitis
    f. Severe nausea and vomiting

True or False? Read each statement and write T for true or F for false in the blanks provided. If the statement is false, correct the statement to make it true.

_____ 38. Diverticulitis is the inflammation of one or more diverticula.

_____ 39. Diverticulosis is the presence of many abnormal pouch-like herniations in the wall of the intestine.

_____ 40. Diets high in cereal fiber that cause more bulky stool have been implicated in the formation of diverticula.

_____ 41. The patient with diverticulosis usually has no symptoms.

_____ 42. Diverticulosis is found in one-half of adults over age 60 years.

_____ 43. The patient with diverticulitis usually undergoes a barium enema procedure in the acute phase of the illness to confirm the diagnosis.

44. Which drug is often used in older patients for pain management of moderate to severe diverticulitis?
    a. Meperidine hydrochloride (Demerol)
    b. Acetaminophen (Tylenol)
    c. ASA (aspirin)
    d. MSO4 (morphine)

45. Which statement about diverticular disease is true?
    a. Most diverticula occur in the sigmoid colon.
    b. Diverticula are uncomfortable even when not inflamed.
    c. High-fiber diets contribute to diverticula occurrence.
    d. Diverticula form where intestinal wall muscles are weak.

46. Which is a preventive measure for diverticular disease?
    a. Excluding whole-grain breads from the diet
    b. Avoiding fresh apples, broccoli, and lettuce
    c. Taking bulk agents such as psyllium hydrophilic mucilloid
    d. Taking routine anticholinergics to reduce bowel spasms

47. Which type of stoma will a patient with diverticulitis most likely have postoperatively?
    a. Ileostomy
    b. Jejunostomy
    c. Colostomy
    d. Cecostomy

Matching. *Match each anorectal problem with its corresponding description.*

Anorectal Problem
a. Anal fissure
b. Anal fistula
c. Anorectal abscess

Description
_____ 48. Duct obstruction and infection
_____ 49. Perianal laceration, superficial erosion
_____ 50. Communicating tract

51. The nurse is providing teaching for a patient with an anal fissure as a complication of CD. Which statement by the patient indicates the need for further teaching?
    a. "I will use warm sitz baths."
    b. "A diet that is low in bulk-producing agents is best for me."
    c. "I will use opiate suppositories if spasms are severe."
    d. "Topical anti-inflammatory agents will help if I am uncomfortable."

Matching. *Match the parasitic infection with its appropriate description.*

Parasitic Infections
a. *Entamoeba histolytica*
b. *Cryptosporidium*
c. *Giardia lamblia*

Descriptions
_____ 52. A protozoal parasite that causes superficial invasion, destruction, and inflammation of the mucosa in the small intestine. It is a well-recognized problem in travelers, campers, and immunosuppressed patients.
_____ 53. This condition is also known as *amebiasis*.
_____ 54. This infection is manifested by diarrhea and occurs most commonly in immunosuppressed patients, particularly those with human immunodeficiency virus (HIV).

55. Which statements does the nurse include while providing discharge instructions for a patient with giardiasis? *(Select all that apply.)*
   a. "Avoid contact with stool from dogs and beavers."
   b. "All household and sexual partners should have stool examinations for parasites."
   c. "Treatment will most likely consist of metronidazole."
   d. "The infection can be transmitted to others until the amebicides kill the parasites."
   e. "Stools are examined 6 days after treatment to assess for eradication."

True or False? *Read each statement and write T for true or F for false in the blanks provided. If the statement is false, correct the statement to make it true.*

_____ 56. Food poisoning is communicable from person to person.

_____ 57. The incubation period for food poisoning is shorter than gastroenteritis.

_____ 58. Food poisoning can be differentiated from gastroenteritis by obtaining a thorough history of common food intake in patients who have common symptoms of acute diarrhea, nausea, and vomiting.

_____ 59. Patients may be carriers of the salmonellosis bacterium for up to 1 year.

_____ 60. Botulism is a paralytic disease resulting from an ingestion of toxin in a food contaminated with *Clostridium botulinum*. Botulism occurs most often with home-canned foods.

_____ 61. Staphylococcal infections occur most commonly with the slow cooling of food after it is cooked.

CASE STUDY: THE PATIENT WITH DIVERTICULITIS

Use a separate sheet of paper to answer the questions in this Case Study, or go to the "Prepare for Class" folder on your Evolve website at http://evolve.elsevier.com/Iggy/ to download and complete as a word processing file. Answer guidelines for this Case Study are also available on your Evolve website.

An 18-year-old body-builder has just come into the office reporting left lower quadrant abdominal pain, temperature of 100.8° F, constipation, and blood-streaked stool. On examination of the abdomen, the nurse observes slight distention and tenderness on palpation, especially in the left lower quadrant. This patient has an elevated white blood cell count and his stool for occult blood is positive. Diverticulitis is diagnosed.

1. Document key findings in your assessment using the focus charting method (otherwise known as the Data, Action, Response [DAR] method). How are these findings significant?

2. The patient says, "Oh, I'll just go home and take a laxative or an enema and I'll be fine." Explain why these should be avoided.

3. Nonsurgical management has been selected for this patient, and he may return home after receiving special instructions. Identify a key factor, based on your assessment, on which the nurse would need to instruct him.

4. What community-based care will the nurse incorporate for the care of this patient?

Care of Patients with Liver Problems

STUDY/REVIEW QUESTIONS

True or False? Read each statement and write T for true or F for false in the blanks provided. If the statement is false, correct the statement to make it true.

_____ 1. Cirrhosis is extensive, irreversible scarring of the liver, usually caused by a chronic reaction to hepatic inflammation and necrosis.

_____ 2. The most common causes for cirrhosis in the United States are alcoholic liver disease and hepatitis C.

_____ 3. Laennec's cirrhosis is caused by viral hepatitis and exposure to drugs or chemicals.

_____ 4. Ascites is the accumulation of free fluid within the peritoneal cavity caused by increased hydrostatic pressure from portal hypertension.

_____ 5. Massive ascites may cause renal vasoconstriction, triggering the renin-angiotensin system resulting in sodium and water loss.

_____ 6. Esophageal varices occur when fragile, thin-walled esophageal veins become distended from increased pressure.

_____ 7. *Melena* is the term that refers to black, tarry stools.

_____ 8. Patients with cirrhosis are susceptible to bleeding and easy bruising because they are lacking in factors II, VII, IX, and X.

_____ 9. Hepatorenal syndrome is often the cause of death in patients with cirrhosis.

_____ 10. Cirrhosis has a rapid onset with severe and specific early manifestations.

11. When admitting the patient with cirrhosis, the nurse assesses for which conditions as possible complications of the disease? *(Select all that apply.)*
    a. Ascites
    b. Bleeding esophageal varices
    c. Hepatorenal syndrome
    d. Coagulation defects
    e. Portal hypertensive gastropathy

12. Patients with cirrhosis are susceptible to bleeding and easy bruising because there is a decrease in the production of bile in the liver preventing the absorption of which vitamin?
    a. A
    b. D
    c. E
    d. K

13. The nurse identifies which laboratory value as the usual indication of hepatic encephalopathy?
    a. Elevated sodium level
    b. Elevated ammonia level
    c. Increased blood urea nitrogen (BUN)
    d. Increased clotting time

Matching. Match the terms to their correct definitions.

Terms
a. Pruritus
b. Petechiae
c. Gynecomastia
d. Icterus
e. Spider angiomas
f. Palmar erythema
g. Melena
h. Ecchymosis
i. Fetor hepaticus
j. Asterixis

Definitions
_____ 14. Nonrhythmic extensions and flexions in the wrists and fingers
_____ 15. Itching
_____ 16. Warm, bright red palms
_____ 17. Fruity or musty breath odor
_____ 18. Enlarged breasts
_____ 19. Blood in the stool
_____ 20. Vascular lesions with a red center and radiating branches
_____ 21. Large purple, blue, or yellow bruises
_____ 22. Yellowing of the sclera
_____ 23. Round, pinpoint, red-purple lesions

24. Which elevated laboratory test results indicate hepatic cell destruction? *(Select all that apply.)*
    a. Serum aspartate aminotransferase (AST)
    b. Serum alanine aminotransferase (ALT)
    c. Lactate dehydrogenase (LDH)
    d. Serum total bilirubin
    e. Urine urobilinogen
    f. International Normalized Ratio (INR)

25. A patient is scheduled for a procedure to place a stent in the biliary tract. For which procedure does the nurse provide patient teaching?
    a. Esophagogastroduodenoscopy (EGD)
    b. Endoscopic retrograde cholangiopancreatography (ERCP)
    c. Upper GI series
    d. Cholangiogram

26. When caring for a patient with cirrhosis who has pruritus, the nurse delegates which task to the unlicensed assistive personnel (UAP)?
    a. Assessment of open skin areas from scratching
    b. Use of warm water for bathing
    c. Use of lotion to soothe the skin
    d. Temperature control of the room to maintain a warm environment

27. The nurse is teaching a patient with cirrhosis about nutrition therapy. Which statement by the patient indicates teaching has been effective?
    a. "I will only use table salt with my dinner meal."
    b. "I will read the sodium content labels on all food and beverages."
    c. "I will avoid the use of vinegar."
    d. "I will not take vitamin supplements."

28. When preparing a patient for paracentesis, what does the nurse do? *(Select all that apply.)*
    a. Ask the patient to void before the procedure.
    b. Place the patient in the supine position.
    c. Weigh the patient before the procedure.
    d. Obtain the patient's heart rate.
    e. Assess the patient's respiratory rate.
    f. Obtain the patient's blood pressure.

29. A patient will undergo an abdominal paracentesis. Which factor provides an additional safety measure?
    a. The procedure is performed using ultrasound.
    b. The procedure is performed at the bedside.
    c. A trocar is inserted into the peritoneal cavity.
    d. General anesthesia is administered.

30. The student nurse is caring for a patient with cirrhosis. Which action by the student nurse causes the supervising nurse to intervene?
    a. Uses a straight-edge razor to shave the patient
    b. Monitors for orthostatic changes of blood pressure
    c. Avoids intramuscular injections
    d. Uses a toothette for oral care

31. The nurse who is assessing a patient with portal-systemic encephalopathy finds that the patient has fetor hepaticus, a positive Babinski's sign, and seizures, but no asterixis. The nurse identifies the patient as being in which stage of portal-systemic encephalopathy?
    a. Stage I prodromal
    b. Stage II impending
    c. Stage III stuporous
    d. Stage IV comatose

True or False? *Read each statement about esophageal varices and write T for true or F for false in the blanks provided. If the statement is false, correct the statement to make it true.*

_____ 32. All patients with cirrhosis should be screened for esophageal varices by endoscopy to detect them early before they bleed.

_____ 33. Bleeding esophageal varices are a medical emergency.

_____ 34. A nonselective beta blocking agent such as propranolol (Inderal) is usually prescribed to prevent esophageal varices from bleeding.

_____ 35. IV octreotide is the mainstay for acute hemorrhage due to esophageal varices in the United States.

_____ 36. Esophagogastric balloon tamponade is rarely used today because it is difficult to use, uncomfortable for the patient, and prone to dangerous complications.

37. The nurse is teaching a patient with cirrhosis about lactulose therapy. Which statement by the patient indicates the teaching has been effective?
    a. "This therapy will promote the removal of ammonia in my stool."
    b. "Constipation is a frequent side effect of this therapy."
    c. "I will know the therapy is working when I am less itchy."
    d. "The drug tastes bitter and is watery."

38. How is neomycin sulfate (Mycifradin) used to treat patients with cirrhosis?
    a. It treats the current infection the patient has.
    b. It prevents future infections of the liver.
    c. It restores normal function to the liver cells.
    d. It destroys the normal flora of the bowel, diminishing protein breakdown and decreasing the rate of ammonia production.

True or False? *Read the statements about the different types of hepatitis and write T for true or F for false in the blanks provided. If the statement is false, correct the statement to make it true.*

_____ 39. Hepatitis D is the leading cause of cirrhosis and liver failure in the United States.

_____ 40. Hepatitis A is spread via the fecal-oral route.

_____ 41. Hepatitis B can be transmitted by unprotected sexual intercourse with an infected partner.

_____ 42. Hepatitis carriers have chronic obvious signs of hepatitis B.

_____ 43. Hepatitis C is transmitted by casual contact or intimate household contact.

_____ 44. Hepatitis D only occurs with hepatitis B to cause viral replication.

_____ 45. Hepatitis E is transmitted via the fecal-oral route.

46. When teaching a group of adult patients measures for preventing hepatitis A (HAV), which information does the nurse include? *(Select all that apply.)*
   a. Perform proper handwashing, especially after handling shellfish.
   b. Receive immune globulin within 14 days if exposed to the virus.
   c. Receive the HAV vaccine before traveling to Mexico or the Caribbean.
   d. Receive the vaccine if living in a college dormitory.
   e. Receive the vaccine if working in a long-term care facility.

47. Which people are in need for immunization against hepatitis B (HBV)? *(Select all that apply.)*
   a. People who have unprotected sex with more than one partner
   b. Men who have sex with men
   c. People with any chronic liver disease
   d. Firefighters
   e. Police officers

True or False? *Read each statement about hepatitis and write T for true or F for false in the blanks provided. If the statement is false, correct the statement to make it true.*

_____ 48. Needle sticks are the major source of hepatitis B transmission in health care workers.

_____ 49. The hepatitis B vaccine is administered in a series of two injections.

_____ 50. Hepatitis B vaccine also prevents hepatitis E.

_____ 51. If a health care worker is exposed to hepatitis A, immunoglobulin (Ig) should be administered immediately.

_____ 52. All cases of hepatitis should be reported to the health department.

_____ 53. A person who has a history of being infected with hepatitis may never donate blood, body organs, or other body tissue.

_____ 54. A person with viral hepatitis can no longer transmit the disease once the jaundice is resolved.

_____ 55. Patients with hepatitis should eat small frequent meals with a high-carbohydrate, moderate-fat, and moderate-protein content.

_____ 56. People who have been vaccinated against HBV have a positive HBsAb because they also have immunity to the disease.

57. Which laboratory test result indicates permanent immunity to hepatitis A?
    a. Immunoglobulin G (IgG) antibodies
    b. Immunoglobulin M (IgM) antibodies
    c. A positive enzyme-linked immunosorbent assay (ELISA)
    d. The presence of anti-HAV antibodies

58. Which antiviral drugs are given to patients with hepatitis B virus? *(Select all that apply.)*
    a. Lamivudine (Epivir-HBV)
    b. Entecavir (Baraclude)
    c. Telbivudine (Tyzeka)
    d. Pegylated interferon alpha-2b (Peg-Intron)
    e. Oral ribavirin (Rebetol)

59. Which conditions place a patient at high risk for the development of fatty liver (steatosis)? *(Select all that apply.)*
    a. Hypertension
    b. Diabetes mellitus
    c. Obesity
    d. Elevated lipid profile
    e. Alcohol abuse

60. In performing an assessment on a patient with liver trauma, what does the nurse expect to find? *(Select all that apply.)*
    a. Positive Kehr's sign
    b. Guarding of the abdomen
    c. Abdominal distention
    d. Bradypnea
    e. Dry skin

True or False? *Read each statement and write T for true or F for false in the blanks provided. If the statement is false, correct the statement to make it true.*

_____ 61. Liver cancer is most often seen in regions of Asia and the Mediterranean.

_____ 62. Risk factors for the development of liver cancer include use of anabolic steroids, androgens, or estrogens.

_____ 63. Alpha-fetoprotein (AFP) is a tumor marker for cancers of the liver.

_____ 64. Chemotherapy is the treatment of choice for cancer of the liver.

_____ 65. Liver transplantation may be used for the patient with a primary liver tumor.

_____ 66. Patients with advanced cardiac disease are not considered candidates for liver transplantation.

_____ 67. The success of all transplantation has greatly improved since the introduction of cyclosporin, an immunosuppressant drug.

_____ 68. Transplant rejection is treated aggressively with immunosuppressive medication.

_____ 69. Clinical manifestations of organ rejection may include tachycardia, fever, right upper quadrant or flank pain, decreased bile pigment and volume, and increasing jaundice.

CASE STUDY: THE PATIENT WITH CIRRHOSIS AND ESOPHAGEAL BLEEDING

Use a separate sheet of paper to answer the questions in this Case Study, or go to the "Prepare for Class" folder on your Evolve website at http://evolve.elsevier.com/Iggy/ to download and complete as a word processing file. Answer guidelines for this Case Study are also available on your Evolve website.

A recently retired locomotive engineer is looking forward to his retirement so he and his wife "can finally enjoy" their lives together. He states he feels he has maintained sobriety quite well, but occasionally "sneaks a little drink now and then." Unfortunately, his cirrhotic liver has never fully recovered from 25 years of fairly heavy drinking. Although he has been diagnosed with Laennec's cirrhosis, the patient has not been compliant with follow-up visits to his health care provider. Periodically, and through the years, he still has symptoms of residual effects. For the past several days, he states he has been coughing on and off. His wife states that this morning he coughed up "bright red blood" and that is why she made him come to the hospital. As for now, he is not coughing or bleeding but has been admitted for observation. The nurse notes that he is jaundiced, has gynecomastia, and has multiple ecchymotic areas on his body. The site for the maintenance IV has fresh bloodstains noted on the dressing. As the nurse is doing rounds, his wife comes out of his room hysterical; the nurse enters his room and observes blood all over his gown and bed linens. He appears terrified.

1. What does the nurse suspect has happened? How could this have been prevented?

2. The nurse notifies the physician using the SBAR method of communication. What will the nurse's side of the conversation be?

3. What is an older treatment for bleeding esophageal varices and why is it rarely used today?

4. The patient is discharged back to the unit after some time in the intensive care unit where his bleeding esophageal varices were controlled. The patient is ordered neomycin sulfate (Mycifradin) and lactulose. The patient asks the nurse, "Why is my body so changed? I have yellow skin, my chest looks like a woman's, and everywhere I look there are bruises. Even my IV seems to be leaking." Document the patient teaching that the nurse will provide.

5. The patient's wife asks the nurse if her husband has an infection. She says, "The other nurse told me my husband is getting neomycin. I took that once for an infection I had. Where is my husband's infection?" How should the nurse respond?

6. What are the nursing interventions associated with lactulose therapy?

62 CHAPTER

Care of Patients with Problems of the Biliary System and Pancreas

STUDY/REVIEW QUESTIONS

1. A patient is admitted to the unit with obstructive jaundice. Which sign/symptom does the nurse expect to find upon assessment of the patient?
   a. Pruritus
   b. Pale urine in increased amounts
   c. Pink discoloration of sclera
   d. Dark, tarry stools

2. The daughter of a patient with cholelithiasis has heard that there is a genetic disposition for cholelithiasis. The daughter asks the nurse about the risk factors. How does the nurse respond?
   a. "There is no evidence that first-degree relatives have an increased risk for this disease."
   b. "Cholecystitis is seen more frequently in patients who are underweight."
   c. "Hormone replacement therapy has been associated with increased risk for cholecystitis."
   d. "Patients with diabetes mellitus are at increased risk for cholecystitis."

3. Which patient is at low risk for the development of gallbladder disorders?
   a. Patient with sickle cell anemia
   b. Patient who is Mexican American
   c. Patient who is 20 years old and male
   d. Patient with a history of prolonged parenteral nutrition

4. The nurse on a medical-surgical unit is caring for several patients with acute cholecystitis. Which task is best to delegate to the nursing assistant?
   a. Obtain the patients' vital signs.
   b. Determine if any foods are not tolerated.
   c. Assess what measures relieve the abdominal pain.
   d. Ask the patients to describe their daily activity or exercise routines.

Matching. *Match each term with its correct definition.*

Terms
a. Flatulence
b. Dyspepsia
c. Eructation
d. Biliary colic
e. Prostration
f. Blumberg's sign
g. Steatorrhea

Definitions
_____ 5. Belching
_____ 6. Gas
_____ 7. Severe pain that is produced by obstruction of the cystic duct of the gallbladder
_____ 8. Indigestion
_____ 9. Extreme exhaustion
_____ 10. Assessment for rebound tenderness on deep palpation
_____ 11. Fatty stools

12. A patient is scheduled for tests to verify the medical diagnosis of cholecystitis. For which diagnostic test does the nurse provide patient teaching?
    a. Extracorporeal shock wave lithotripsy (ESWL)
    b. Ultrasonography of the right upper quadrant
    c. Endoscopic retrograde cholangiopancreatography (ERCP)
    d. Serum level of aspartate aminotransferase (AST)

13. Which type of drug is used to treat acute biliary pain?
    a. Acetaminophen (Tylenol)
    b. NSAIDs (Ibuprofen)
    c. Meperidine (Demerol)
    d. Opioids (Morphine)

14. The nurse is administering meperidine (Demerol) to a 78-year-old patient for pain management. Which assessment finding indicates the patient is experiencing a side effect of this drug?
    a. Seizure
    b. Cardiac dysrhythmia
    c. Low urinary output
    d. Jaundice

15. The nurse is caring for an older adult patient with acute biliary pain. Which drug order does the nurse question?
    a. Ketorolac (Toradol, Acular)
    b. Erlotinib (Tarceva)
    c. Morphine
    d. Hydromorphone (Dilaudid)

16. Which factor renders a patient the *least* likely to benefit from ESWL for the treatment of gallstones?
    a. Height 5 feet 10 inches, 250 lbs.
    b. Cholesterol-based stones
    c. Good gallbladder function
    d. Small gallstones

17. Which statements are true regarding laparoscopic cholecystectomy? *(Select all that apply.)*
    a. Laparoscopic cholecystectomy is considered the "gold standard" and is performed far more often than the traditional open approach.
    b. Patients who have chronic lung disease or heart failure unable to tolerate the oxygen used in the laparoscopic procedure are examples of patients who have the open surgical approach (abdominal laparotomy).
    c. Removing the gallbladder with the laparoscopic technique reduces the risk of wound complications.
    d. Patients who have their gallbladder removed by the laparoscopic technique should be taught the importance of early ambulation to promote absorption of carbon dioxide.
    e. Use of open surgical approach (abdominal laparotomy) has greatly declined during past 15 years.

18. Which statement about the care of a patient with a T-tube after a cholecystectomy is true?
    a. The patient is maintained in the prone position.
    b. When the patient is allowed to eat, the T-tube is clamped continuously.
    c. The T-tube is irrigated every hour for the first 72 hours.
    d. Avoid raising the drainage system above the level of the gallbladder.

Matching. Match each definition with the associated procedure.

Procedures

a. Cholecystectomy
b. Natural orifice transluminal endoscopic surgery (NOTES)
c. Percutaneous transhepatic biliary catheter
d. Post-cholecystectomy syndrome
e. ESWL

Definitions

_____ 19. Powerful shock waves shatter gallstones

_____ 20. Used to open blocked bile ducts alleviating blockage

_____ 21. Removal of gallbladder

_____ 22. Complications of cholecystitis evidenced by abdominal pain with vomiting several weeks to months after surgery

_____ 23. Removal of the gallbladder via the vagina

24. The nurse is evaluating electrolyte values for a patient with acute pancreatitis and notes that the serum calcium is 6.8 mEq/L. How does the nurse interpret this finding?

   a. Within normal limits considering the diagnosis of acute pancreatitis
   b. The result of the body not being able to use bound calcium
   c. A protective measure that will reduce the risk of complications
   d. Full compensation of the parathyroid gland

Matching. Match each complication of pancreatitis with its pathophysiology.

Complications

a. Acute kidney failure
b. Paralytic (adynamic) ileus
c. Acute respiratory distress syndrome (ARDS)
d. Disseminated intravascular coagulation (DIC)

Pathophysiology

_____ 25. Disruption of alveolar-capillary membrane results in edema

_____ 26. Hypovolemia

_____ 27. Consumption of clotting factors and microthrombi formation

_____ 28. Peritoneal irritation and seepage of pancreatic enzymes into the abdominal cavity

True or False? Read each statement about acute pancreatitis and write T for true or F for false in the blanks provided. If the statement is false, correct the statement to make it true.

_____ 29. Patients with pancreatitis often have a gray-blue discoloration of the abdomen and periumbilical area.

_____ 30. The pain of acute pancreatitis is often described as intense, boring, and continuous.

_____ 31. Typically, a patient is diagnosed with acute pancreatitis after presenting with severe abdominal pain in the mid-epigastric area or left upper quadrant.

_____ 32. Abdominal pain is the prominent symptom of pancreatitis.

_____ 33. Pain management for acute pancreatitis should begin with IV opioids by means of patient-controlled analgesia (PCA).

_____ 34. Helping the patient to assume a supine position decreases the abdominal pain of pancreatitis.

_____ 35. Surgical intervention for acute pancreatitis is usually not indicated.

_____ 36. Patients in the early stages of acute pancreatitis are usually maintained on NPO status.

37. Which diagnostic test is the most accurate in verifying a diagnosis of acute pancreatitis?
   a. Trypsin
   b. Lipase
   c. Alkaline phosphatase
   d. Alanine aminotransferase

38. A patient with acute pancreatitis is at risk for the development of paralytic (adynamic) ileus. Which action provides the nurse with the best indication of bowel function?
   a. Observing contents of the nasogastric drainage
   b. Auscultation of bowel sounds
   c. Asking the patient if he or she has passed flatus or had a stool
   d. Obtaining a computed tomography (CT) scan of the abdomen with contrast medium

39. Which condition is most likely to be treated with antibiotics?
   a. Cancer of the gallbladder
   b. Acute cholelithiasis
   c. Chronic pancreatitis
   d. Acute necrotizing pancreatitis

40. The nurse has instructed a patient in the recovery phase of acute pancreatitis about diet therapy. Which statement by the patient indicates that teaching has been successful?
   a. "I will eat the usual three meals a day that I am used to."
   b. "I am eating tacos for my first meal back home."
   c. "I will avoid eating chocolate."
   d. "I will limit the amount of protein in my diet."

41. The nursing student is caring for a patient with chronic pancreatitis who is receiving pancreatic enzyme replacement therapy. Which statement by the student indicates the need for further study concerning this therapy?
   a. "The enzymes will be administered with meals."
   b. "The patient will take the drugs with a glass of water."
   c. "If the patient has difficulty swallowing the enzyme preparation, I will mix it with foods containing protein."
   d. "The effectiveness of pancreatic enzyme treatment is monitored by the frequency and fat content of stools."

True or False? *Read each statement about pancreatic cancer and write T for true or F for false in the blanks provided. If the statement is false, correct the statement to make it true.*

_____ 42.   Venous thromboembolism is a common complication of pancreatic cancer.

_____ 43.   Pancreatic cancer often presents in a slow and vague manner.

_____ 44.   The most common concern of the patient with pancreatic cancer is pain.

_____ 45.   There are no specific blood tests to diagnose pancreatic cancer.

_____ 46.   Chemotherapy is the treatment of choice for pancreatic cancer.

_____ 47.   The position of choice for the patient after a Whipple procedure is semi-Fowler's.

CASE STUDY: THE PATIENT WITH PANCREATIC CANCER

Use a separate sheet of paper to answer the questions in this Case Study, or go to the "Prepare for Class" folder on your Evolve website at http://evolve.elsevier.com/Iggy/ to download and complete as a word processing file. Answer guidelines for this Case Study are also available on your Evolve website.

A patient is admitted to the medical-surgical unit with jaundice, abdominal pain, and reports fatigue over the past several weeks. The patient states that he has been losing weight but didn't think too much of it because he hadn't had much of an appetite due to some nausea and vomiting as well as some dull abdominal pain. On physical assessment the nurse's findings include splenomegaly, ascites, and a tender, warm, enlarged right calf. The patient rates his pain at this time as an 8 on a scale of 0 to 10. The patient's family is very concerned. His adult daughter states, "The doctor doesn't even know what is wrong with Dad. Why don't they just do an x-ray of his stomach to find out the problem?" Pancreatic cancer is suspected.

1. What is the most likely cause of the patient's tender, warm, and enlarged right calf?

2. What is the most likely cause of the patient's jaundice, ascites, and splenomegaly?

3. Document the patient/family teaching that the nurse would perform regarding the diagnostic tests for pancreatic cancer.

4. A diagnosis of pancreatic cancer is confirmed. The patient is scheduled to undergo a Whipple procedure. Document the patient/family preoperative teaching that the nurse would perform.

5. When caring for the patient postoperatively, what should nursing care include?

6. The patient's daughter wishes to care for her father at home. She works full-time as a waitress and is a single parent of two small children. The physician has told the patient and his daughter that he has a short time to live because of the advanced state of the disease. What should nursing care for this family include?

63

CHAPTER

Care of Patients with Malnutrition and Obesity

STUDY/REVIEW QUESTIONS

1. The nurse is assisting a patient who follows a lacto-vegetarian diet to fill out a menu. Based on this diet, which foods does the patient select for breakfast? *(Select all that apply.)*
   a. Milk
   b. Scrambled eggs
   c. Toast
   d. Sausage
   e. Cereal

2. The nurse is assisting a patient who follows a lacto-ovo-vegetarian diet to fill out a menu. Based on this diet, which foods does the patient select for breakfast? *(Select all that apply.)*
   a. Milk
   b. Scrambled eggs
   c. Toast
   d. Sausage
   e. Cereal

3. When caloric energy is inadequate, what does the body use for energy?
   a. Carbohydrates
   b. Proteins
   c. Glucose
   d. Fats

4. Which statement by the new graduate nurse about nutritional assessment requires clarification by the student's mentor?
   a. "A complete nutritional assessment must be completed on every patient admitted to the hospital."
   b. "A nutritional screening must be completed on every patient admitted to the hospital."
   c. "An unintentional weight loss of 10% within a 6-month period should be evaluated."
   d. "Measurement of height and weight are part of the nutritional assessment."

5. Which activity of a nutritional assessment can be delegated to the unlicensed assistive personnel (UAP)?
   a. Review of the patient's nutritional history
   b. Review of the patient's laboratory data
   c. Obtaining the patient's height and weight
   d. Psychosocial assessment of the patient

6. Which signs/symptoms in an older adult can be an indication of "failure to thrive?" *(Select all that apply.)*
   a. Weakness
   b. Slow walking speed
   c. Low physical activity
   d. Unintentional weight loss
   e. Exhaustion

7. The nurse is providing teaching about the risk factors for malnutrition for a group of older adults. What factors does the nurse emphasize in the teaching plan? *(Select all that apply.)*
   a. Poor dental health
   b. Hypersecretion of saliva
   c. Depression
   d. Fatigue
   e. Lack of transportation

8. A patient is malnourished. What is the priority nursing intervention?
   a. Determine the patient's food preferences.
   b. Provide the patient with high-calorie, high-protein food.
   c. Weigh the patient.
   d. Offer the patient snacks.

9. The nurse is caring for three patients who have undergone bariatric surgery. Which activity is most appropriate for the nurse to delegate to the unlicensed assistive personnel (UAP)?
   a. Give analgesics about 1 hour before mealtimes.
   b. Document the percentage of food eaten at mealtimes.
   c. Assess the patient's food preferences.
   d. Teach the patient about portion control.

10. After the UAP tells the nurse that an older patient will not eat her dinner, the nurse enters the patient's room to assess the situation. Which factors likely contribute to the patient's lack of desire to eat? *(Select all that apply.)*
    a. An emesis basin is on the bedside table.
    b. The volume of the television is loud.
    c. The food is cold.
    d. The cleaning lady is in the room disinfecting the bathroom.
    e. The patient's roommate has two adults and three children visiting.

11. The nurse is teaching a male patient about the 2010 Dietary Guidelines for Americans. Which statement by the patient indicates a need for additional teaching?
    a. "I'll limit consumption of alcohol to two drinks a day."
    b. "I'll consume at least 6 cups of milk products a day."
    c. "I'll consume 3 or more ounce-equivalents of whole-grain products per day."
    d. "I'll limit added sugar and salt in my diet."

Matching. Match each nutritional deficiency with its appropriate sign/symptom.

Nutritional Deficiency
a. Zinc
b. Vitamin A
c. Riboflavin
d. Vitamin C
e. Niacin
f. Protein
g. Vitamin D
h. Thiamine
i. Selenium

Signs/Symptoms
_____ 12. Hepatomegaly

_____ 13. Osteomalacia, bone pain, rickets

_____ 14. Xerosis of conjunctiva

_____ 15. Alopecia

_____ 16. Swollen, bleeding gums

_____ 17. Fissured tongue

_____ 18. Magenta tongue

_____ 19. Confabulation

_____ 20. Cardiomyopathy

21. What is the most reliable indicator of fluid status?
    a. Intake and output
    b. Trends in weight
    c. Skin turgor
    d. Edema

22. The nurse hears the UAP instructing a new UAP about obtaining patients' weights. Which statements by the UAP indicate a need for clarification? *(Select all that apply.)*
    a. "It is best to weigh the patients before breakfast."
    b. "Just ask the patients how much they weigh."
    c. "You can weigh the patients whenever you have time during your shift."
    d. "Weigh the patients while they are in minimal clothing and no shoes."
    e. "Ambulatory patients can be weighed on the upright scales."

23. Which is the most accurate way to obtain a height measurement for a patient who cannot stand?
    a. Review the patient's old chart.
    b. Ask the patient's family member.
    c. Estimate height based on the patient's position in bed.
    d. Use a sliding blade knee height caliper.

24. Which statements about body mass index (BMI) measurements are accurate? *(Select all that apply.)*
    a. It is a measure of nutritional status that varies according to frame size.
    b. It is based on a formula using height and weight.
    c. Health risks are associated with BMIs >25.
    d. It indirectly estimates total fat scores.
    e. There are no health risks associated with a low BMI.

25. The nurse is providing discharge instructions to the family of an older female patient who was admitted for failure to thrive. The patient has a history of osteoarthritis, stroke, and dementia. What information does the nurse include to promote nutritional intake? *(Select all that apply.)*
    a. Do not allow her to get out of bed while eating.
    b. Withhold analgesics prior to meals.
    c. Provide analgesics as needed 1 hour before meals.
    d. Encourage self-feeding as much as possible.
    e. Keep environmental noise to a minimum.

26. The nurse observes that a patient has been eating only small portions of meals. When discussing this concern with the patient, the nurse learns that the patient is Muslim. Which interventions are appropriate to promote nutritional intake for this patient? *(Select all that apply.)*
    a. Ensure that fruit is available.
    b. Allow the family to bring food.
    c. Offer only pork for dinner.
    d. Offer a vegetarian diet.
    e. Consult with the registered dietitian.

27. The nurse is assessing a patient with acquired immune deficiency syndrome (AIDS) who has muscle wasting related to poor nutrition. How does the nurse interpret this finding?
    a. Cachexia
    b. Candidiasis
    c. Protein catabolism
    d. Positive nitrogen balance

28. Which characteristics are consistent with bulimia nervosa? *(Select all that apply.)*
    a. It is a self-induced starvation.
    b. There are episodes of binge eating.
    c. Binge eating is followed by purging.
    d. It is most often seen in older adults.
    e. It is most often seen in teens and young adults.

29. The nurse assesses for which potential complications in a patient who is malnourished? *(Select all that apply.)*
    a. Poor wound healing
    b. Intolerance to heat
    c. Infection
    d. Lethargy
    e. Edema

Matching. *Match the laboratory test values with their indications of nutritional status.*

Laboratory Tests
a.   Cholesterol
b.   Total lymphocyte count (TLC)
c.   Serum albumin
d.   Prealbumin
e.   Hemoglobin
f.   Hematocrit

Indications

_____ 30.   Low levels may indicate anemia, recent hemorrhage, or hemodilution caused by fluid retention.

_____ 31.   Low levels may reflect anemia, hemorrhage, excessive fluid, kidney disease, or cirrhosis.

_____ 32.   Reflects nutritional status a few weeks before testing.

_____ 33.   More sensitive indicator of protein deficiency because of its short half-life of 2 days.

_____ 34.   Values are typically low with malabsorption, liver disease, pernicious anemia, terminal stages of cancer, or sepsis.

_____ 35.   Used to assess immune function.

36.   The nurse is providing discharge instructions to a patient who is malnourished and will be taking iron supplements at home. Which statement by the patient indicates a correct understanding of the instructions?
a.   "These supplements may cause me to have diarrhea."
b.   "I will take these supplements with my meals."
c.   "I will limit my fiber intake from now on."
d.   "I will limit my fluid intake from now on."

37.   Total enteral nutrition (TEN) is contraindicated for which patient?
a.   Older adult receiving chemotherapy
b.   Patient who has had a stroke and has dysphagia
c.   Patient who has had extensive jaw and mouth surgery
d.   Patient with intestinal obstruction that has progressed to diffuse peritonitis

Matching. *Match the types of feedings to their descriptions.*

Types of Feeding
a.   Bolus feeding tube
b.   Continuous feeding tube
c.   Cycle feeding tube

Descriptions

_____ 38.   Small amounts are continually infused over a specified time.

_____ 39.   Infusion is stopped for a specified time.

_____ 40.   Intermittent feeding of a specified amount at specified times.

41. What is the most reliable method to confirm initial placement of nasoduodenal or nasogastric tube placement?
    a. Auscultation
    b. X-ray
    c. Capnometry
    d. Testing pH of gastric contents

42. After initial placement of nasoduodenal and nasogastric tubes is confirmed, how often must placement be checked? *(Select all that apply.)*
    a. Before intermittent feeding
    b. Before medication administration
    c. Every 4 to 8 hours during feeding
    d. It is not necessary to recheck placement
    e. According to facility policy

43. The nurse is using capnometry testing to check nasogastric (NG) tube placement prior to medication administration and the capnometry test is positive for carbon dioxide. What action does the nurse take?
    a. Administer the medication orally.
    b. Remove the NG tube.
    c. Administer the medication through the NG tube.
    d. Verify placement by auscultation.

44. The nurse is caring for a patient receiving a continuous feeding through an NG tube. Which position is best to prevent aspiration?
    a. Semi-Fowler's
    b. Trendelenburg
    c. Supine
    d. Sims'

45. Which interventions are necessary to provide safe, quality care to a patient receiving enteral tube feeding? *(Select all that apply.)*
    a. Check the residual volume every 4 to 6 hours.
    b. Change the feeding bag and tubing every 12 hours.
    c. Keep the head of the bed elevated at least 30 degrees.
    d. Use clean technique when changing the feeding system.
    e. Allow closed system containers to hang for 24 hours.

46. A patient is receiving a tube feeding. Which action by the UAP requires intervention by the supervising nurse?
    a. Weighing the patient
    b. Placing food coloring in the tube feeding to assess for aspiration
    c. Discarding any unused open cans of feeding solution after 24 hours
    d. Monitoring the patient for the development of diarrhea

47. Which statement about a patient with a tube feeding indicates best practice for patient safety and quality care?
    a. If the tube becomes clogged, use 30 mL of water for flushing, while applying gentle pressure with a 50 mL piston syringe.
    b. Use cranberry juice to flush the tube if it is clogged.
    c. When administering medications, use cold water to dissolve the drug before administering it.
    d. Administer drugs down the feeding tube without flushing first, but flush the feeding tube after the drug is given.

48. A patient in a starvation state has been started on enteral feedings. The nurse assesses the patient and finds shallow respirations, weakness, acute confusion, and oozing from the IV site. What does the nurse suspect is happening in this patient?
    a. Septicemia
    b. Hypoglycemia
    c. Aspiration
    d. Refeeding syndrome

49. Which statement describes the correct method of testing the pH of GI contents at the bedside?
    a. The tube is in the stomach if the pH reading is 8.0.
    b. Before aspirating the GI contents, flush the tube with 10 mL of air.
    c. If the patient takes certain medications such as H_2 blockers, the pH of the stomach is usually 2.0.
    d. Wait at least 1 hour after drug administration before assessing the pH of GI contents.

50. A patient receiving intravenous fat emulsions should be monitored closely for which manifestations of fat overload syndrome? *(Select all that apply.)*
    a. Increased triglycerides
    b. Clotting problems
    c. Fever
    d. Multi-system organ failure
    e. Excessive weight gain
    f. Infection

51. The nurse is assessing a patient receiving TPN at 100 mL/hour. The TPN solution has 50 mL left in the bag. The nurse looks for the next bag of TPN but it is not on the unit. When the pharmacy is called, the nurse is told it will take at least 1 hour for the next bag of TPN solution to be delivered. What does the nurse do?
    a. Call the health care provider.
    b. Administer 10% dextrose/water (D/W) until the TPN is available.
    c. Prepare to treat the patient for hyperglycemia.
    d. Cap the TPN line until the next TPN solution is available.

Matching. *Match the terms related to obesity with their definitions.*

Terms
a. Obesity
b. Overweight
c. Morbid obesity

Definitions
_____ 52. Weight that has a severely negative effect on health.

_____ 53. Excessive amount of body fat when compared to lean body mass.

_____ 54. Increase in body weight for height as compared to a standard.

55. Which statements about obesity are accurate? *(Select all that apply.)*
    a. Waist to hip ratio (WHR) is a strong predictor of colon cancer.
    b. Obesity is the second-leading cause of preventable deaths in the United States.
    c. Genetics have been found to have no role in obesity.
    d. Drug therapy is the first-line treatment for obesity.
    e. Waist circumference is a stronger predictor of coronary artery disease than is body mass index (BMI).

56. The nurse is performing an admission assessment on a morbidly obese patient. Which common complications of obesity does the nurse assess for? *(Select all that apply.)*
    a. Type 1 diabetes mellitus
    b. Metabolic syndrome
    c. Urinary incontinence
    d. Gout
    e. Early osteoarthritis

57. Which prescribed drugs can contribute to weight gain when they are taken on a long-term basis? *(Select all that apply.)*
    a. Estrogens
    b. Acetaminophen
    c. Corticosteroids
    d. NSAIDs
    e. Antiepileptics

58. Which drug is the only drug available for long-term treatment of obesity?
    a. Phentermine (Adipex-p)
    b. Diethylpropion (Tenuate)
    c. Sibutramine (Meridia)
    d. Orlistat (Xenical)

59. The nurse is caring for a patient after bariatric surgery. What is the nursing priority for this patient?
    a. Nutritional intake
    b. Pain management
    c. Prevention of infection
    d. Airway management

60. A patient comes to the clinic after having bariatric surgery and says, "After I eat, I feel really funny. My heart races, I feel nauseated, and my abdomen cramps up. I even have diarrhea." What does the nurse suspect is happening with this patient?
    a. Hyperglycemia
    b. Intestinal obstruction
    c. Peritonitis
    d. Dumping syndrome

CASE STUDY: THE PATIENT WITH OBESITY

Use a separate sheet of paper to answer the questions in this Case Study, or go to the "Prepare for Class" folder on your Evolve website at http://evolve.elsevier.com/Iggy/ to download and complete as a word processing file. Answer guidelines for this Case Study are also available on your Evolve website.

A patient is 100% above ideal body weight and has been diagnosed with morbid obesity. The patient tells the nurse, "I've always been big; my family is big and so am I. What's so wrong about being a plus size? Can being overweight really cause problems for me?" The patient has tried to lose weight by following fad diets such as the Hollywood diet. The patient did initially lose some weight, but gained it back plus more. The patient has also tried an over-the-counter medication called orlistat (Xenical) to help with weight loss. The patient stopped taking the drug because he had loose stools, abdominal cramps, and nausea while taking it. The patient decides to undergo gastric bypass surgery.

1. The patient asks the nurse, "What is wrong with me that I am this heavy?" How should the nurse explain the pathophysiology of obesity?

2. How should the nurse respond to the patient's question about complications of obesity?

3. Why has dieting by the patient not been effective?

4. Why did the patient have side effects while using orlistat (Xenical)?

5. Describe preoperative nursing care for the patient undergoing gastric bypass surgery.

6. What is the most common complication that the nurse must assess the patient for postoperatively?

7. The nurse is caring for the patient on postoperative day one after gastric bypass surgery. The patient is receiving dilaudid 0.2 mg bolus every 5 minutes prn (demand dose) via patient-controlled analgesia (PCA). The patient is consistently rating his pain as 9/10 despite trying nonpharmacologic interventions. Abdominal assessment reveals that dressings are dry/intact, abdomen is obese, soft, and tender with hypoactive bowel sounds. Using the ISBARR format, how would the nurse communicate these findings to the appropriate health care provider?

64 CHAPTER

Assessment of the Endocrine System

STUDY/REVIEW QUESTIONS

1. Which glands are part of the endocrine system? *(Select all that apply.)*
   a. Thyroid
   b. Occipital
   c. Parathyroid
   d. Adrenal
   e. Pituitary

2. Which is the name of the substance secreted by the glands in question #1 above?
   a. Vasoactive amines
   b. Chemotaxins
   c. Hormones
   d. Cytotoxins

3. Which mechanism is used to transport the substance produced by the endocrine glands to their target tissue?
   a. Lymph system
   b. Bloodstream
   c. Direct seeding
   d. Gastrointestinal system

Matching. *Match each hormone with its corresponding gland. Answers may be used more than once.*

Glands

a. Anterior pituitary
b. Posterior pituitary
c. Adrenal cortex
d. Adrenal medulla
e. Thyroid gland
f. Alpha cells—islets of Langerhans
g. Beta cells—islets of Langerhans
h. Delta cells—islets of Langerhans
i. Parathyroid
j. Ovaries
k. Testes
l. Hypothalamus

Hormones

_____ 4. Somatostatin
_____ 5. Thyrocalcitonin (calcitonin)
_____ 6. Cortisol
_____ 7. Epinephrine and norepinephrine
_____ 8. Corticotropin-releasing hormone (CRH)
_____ 9. Growth hormone
_____ 10. Glucagon
_____ 11. Parathyroid hormone (PTH)
_____ 12. Aldosterone
_____ 13. Triiodothyronine (T_3)
_____ 14. Estrogen
_____ 15. Insulin
_____ 16. Testosterone
_____ 17. Antidiuretic hormone (ADH)
_____ 18. Oxytocin
_____ 19. Thyroxin (T_4)
_____ 20. Thyroid-stimulating hormone (TSH)
_____ 21. Adrenocorticotropic hormone (ACTH)

22. The target tissue for ADH is which organ?
    a. Hypothalamus
    b. Thyroid
    c. Ovary
    d. Kidney

23. Which statements about hormones and the endocrine system are accurate? *(Select all that apply.)*
    a. There are specific normal blood levels of each hormone.
    b. Hormones exert their effects on specific target tissues.
    c. Each hormone can bind with multiple receptor sites.
    d. The endocrine system works independently to regulate homeostasis.
    e. More than one hormone can be stimulated before the target tissue is affected.

24. The binding of a hormone to a specific receptor site is an example of which endocrine process?
    a. "Lock and key" manner
    b. Negative feedback mechanism
    c. Neuroendocrine regulation
    d. "Fight-or-flight" response

25. What are tropic hormones?
    a. Hormones that trigger female and male sex characteristics.
    b. Hormones that have a direct effect on final target tissues.
    c. Hormones produced by the anterior pituitary gland that stimulates other endocrine glands.
    d. Hormones that are synthesized in the hypothalamus and stored in the posterior pituitary gland.

26. Which hormone is directly suppressed when circulating levels of cortisol are above normal?
    a. CRH
    b. ADH
    c. ACTH
    d. Growth hormone–releasing hormone (GH-RH)

27. The maintenance of internal body temperature at approximately 98.6° F (37° C) is an example of which endocrine process?
    a. "Lock and key" manner
    b. Neuroendocrine regulation
    c. Positive feedback mechanism
    d. Stimulus-response theory

28. Which statements about the pituitary glands are correct? *(Select all that apply.)*
    a. The main role of the anterior pituitary is to secrete tropic hormones.
    b. The posterior pituitary gland stores hormones produced by the hypothalamus.
    c. The anterior pituitary is connected to the thalamus gland.
    d. The anterior pituitary releases stored hormones produced by the hypothalamus.
    e. The anterior pituitary gland secretes gonadotropins.

29. The anterior pituitary gland secretes tropic hormones in response to which hormones from the hypothalamus?
    a. Releasing hormones
    b. Target tissue hormones
    c. Growth hormones
    d. Demand hormones

30. Which statement about pituitary hormones is correct?
    a. ACTH acts on the adrenal medulla.
    b. Follicle-stimulating hormone (FSH) stimulates sperm production in men.
    c. Growth hormone promotes protein catabolism.
    d. Vasopressin decreases systolic blood pressure.

31. Which statement about the gonads is correct?
    a. Gonads are reproductive glands found in males only.
    b. The function of the hormones begins at birth in low, undetectable levels.
    c. The placenta secretes testosterone for the development of male external genitalia.
    d. External genitalia maturation is stimulated by gonadotropins during puberty.

32. Which statements about the adrenal glands are correct? *(Select all that apply.)*
    a. The cortex secretes androgens in men and women.
    b. Catecholamines are secreted from the cortex.
    c. Glucocorticoids are secreted by the medulla.
    d. The medulla secretes hormones essential for life.
    e. The cortex secretes aldosterone that maintains extracellular fluid volume.

33. Which is the major function of the hormones produced by the adrenal cortex?
    a. "Fight-or-flight" response
    b. Control of glucose, sodium, and water
    c. Regulation of cell growth
    d. Calcium and stress regulation

34. Which statements about the hormone cortisol being secreted by the adrenal cortex are accurate? *(Select all that apply.)*
    a. Cortisol peaks occur late in the day, with lowest points 12 hours after each peak.
    b. Cortisol has an effect on the body's immune function.
    c. Stress causes an increase in the production of cortisol.
    d. Blood levels of cortisol have no effect on its secretion.
    e. Cortisol affects carbohydrate, protein, and fat metabolism.

35. Which assessment findings does the nurse monitor in response to catecholamines released by the adrenal medulla? *(Select all that apply.)*
    a. Increased heart rate related to vasoconstriction
    b. Increased blood pressure related to vasoconstriction
    c. Increased perspiration
    d. Constriction of pupils
    e. Increased blood glucose in response to glycogenolysis

36. Which statements about the thyroid gland and its hormones are correct? *(Select all that apply.)*
    a. The gland is located in the posterior neck below the cricoid cartilage.
    b. The gland has two lobes joined by a thin tissue called the *isthmus*.
    c. Thyroxine (T_4) and triiodothyronine (T_3) are two thyroid hormones.
    d. Thyroid hormones increase red blood cell production.
    e. Thyroid hormone production depends on dietary intake of iodine and potassium.

37. Which hormone responds to a low serum calcium blood level by increasing bone resorption?
    a. PTH
    b. T_4
    c. T_3
    d. Calcitonin

38. Which hormone responds to elevated serum calcium blood level by decreasing bone resorption?
    a. PTH
    b. T_4
    c. T_3
    d. Calcitonin

39. Which statements about T_3 and T_4 hormones are correct? *(Select all that apply.)*
    a. The basal metabolic rate is affected.
    b. Hypothalamus is stimulated by cold and stress to secrete thyrotropin-releasing hormone (TRH).
    c. These hormones need intake of protein and iodine for production.
    d. Circulating hormone in the blood directly affects the production of TSH.
    e. T_3 and T_4 increase oxygen use in tissues.

40. Which are the target organs of PTH in the regulation of calcium and phosphorus? *(Select all that apply.)*
    a. Stomach
    b. Kidney
    c. Bone
    d. Intestinal tract
    e. Thyroid gland

41. Which statement about the pancreas is correct?
    a. Endocrine functions of the pancreas include secretion of digestive enzymes.
    b. Exocrine functions of the pancreas include secretion of glucagon and insulin.
    c. The islets of Langerhans are the only source of somatostatin secretion.
    d. Somatostatin inhibits pancreatic secretion of glucagon and insulin.

42. Which statement about glucagon secretion is correct?
    a. It is stimulated by an increase in blood glucose levels.
    b. It is stimulated by a decrease in amino acid levels.
    c. It exerts its primary effect on the pancreas.
    d. It acts to increase blood glucose levels.

43. Which statements about insulin secretion are correct? *(Select all that apply.)*
    a. Insulin levels increase following the ingestion of a meal.
    b. Insulin is stimulated primarily by fat ingestion.
    c. Basal levels are secreted continuously.
    d. Insulin promotes glycogenolysis and gluconeogenesis.
    e. Carbohydrate intake is the main trigger for insulin secretion.

44. In addition to the pancreas that secretes insulin, which gland secretes hormones that affect protein, carbohydrate, and fat metabolism?
    a. Posterior pituitary
    b. Thyroid
    c. Ovaries
    d. Parathyroid

45. The bloodstream delivers glucose to the cells for energy production. Which hormone controls the cells' use of glucose?
    a. T_4
    b. Growth hormone
    c. Adrenal steroids
    d. Insulin

46. Which disease involves a disorder of the islets of Langerhans?
    a. Diabetes insipidus
    b. Diabetes mellitus
    c. Addison's disease
    d. Cushing's disease

47. Which endocrine tissues are most commonly found to have reduced function as a result of aging? *(Select all that apply.)*
    a. Hypothalamus
    b. Ovaries
    c. Testes
    d. Pancreas
    e. Thyroid gland

48. Which statement about age-related changes in older adults and the endocrine system is true?
    a. All hormone levels are elevated.
    b. Thyroid hormone levels decrease.
    c. Adrenal glands enlarge.
    d. The thyroid gland enlarges.

Matching. *Match the physiologic changes noted with the decreased function of glands due to aging.*

Glands
a. Thyroid
b. Pancreas
c. Ovary
d. Posterior pituitary gland

Physiologic Changes

_____ 49. Osteoporosis, decreased production of estrogen

_____ 50. Decreased sensitivity of peripheral tissues to the effects of insulin

_____ 51. Decreased concentrating ability of the kidneys

_____ 52. Decreased metabolic rate

53. An older adult reports a lack of energy and not being able to do the usual daily activities without several naps during the day. Which problem may these symptoms indicate that is often seen in the older adult?
    a. Hypothyroidism
    b. Hyperparathyroidism
    c. Overproduction of cortisol
    d. Underproduction of glucagon

54. The nurse is performing a physical assessment of a patient's endocrine system. Which gland can be palpated?
    a. Pancreas
    b. Thyroid
    c. Adrenal glands
    d. Parathyroid

55. Which statement about performing a physical assessment of the thyroid gland is correct?
    a. The thyroid gland is easily palpated in all patients.
    b. The patient is instructed to swallow to aid palpation.
    c. The anterior approach is preferred for thyroid palpation.
    d. The thumbs are used to palpate the thyroid lobes.

56. Which are diagnostic methods to measure patient hormone levels? *(Select all that apply.)*
    a. Stimulation testing
    b. Suppression testing
    c. 24-hour urine testing
    d. Chromatographic assay
    e. Needle biopsy

57. What is the correct nursing action before beginning a 24-hour urine collection for endocrine studies?
    a. Place each voided specimen in a separate collection container.
    b. Check whether any preservatives are needed in the collection container.
    c. Start the collection with the first voided urine.
    d. Weigh the patient before beginning the collection.

58. Which instructions are included when teaching a patient about urine collection for endocrine studies? *(Select all that apply.)*
    a. Fast before starting the urine collection.
    b. Measure the urine in mL rather than ounces.
    c. Empty the bladder completely, then start timing.
    d. Time the test for exactly the instructed number of hours.
    e. Notify the laboratory of all medications you are taking.
    f. Empty the bladder at the end of the time period and keep that specimen.

59. Which are the types of radiographic tests that may be used for an endocrine assessment? *(Select all that apply.)*
    a. Ultrasonography
    b. Skull x-ray
    c. Chest x-ray
    d. Magnetic resonance imaging (MRI)
    e. Computed tomography (CT)

60. A patient is suspected of having a pituitary tumor. Which radiographic test aids in determining this diagnosis?
    a. Skull x-rays
    b. CT/MRI
    c. Angiography
    d. Ultrasound

61. After an ultrasound of the thyroid gland, which diagnostic tests determine the need for surgical intervention?
    a. CT scan
    b. MRI
    c. Angiography
    d. Needle biopsy

62. A patient is at risk for falling related to the effect of pathologic fractures as a result of bone demineralization. Which endocrine problem is this pertinent to?
    a. Underproduction of PTH
    b. Overproduction of PTH
    c. Underproduction of thyroid hormone
    d. Overproduction of thyroid hormone

65 CHAPTER

Care of Patients with Pituitary and Adrenal Gland Problems

STUDY/REVIEW QUESTIONS

1. Problems in the hypothalamus that change the function of the anterior pituitary gland result in which condition?
   a. Adenohypophysis
   b. Panhypopituitarism
   c. Primary pituitary dysfunction
   d. Secondary pituitary dysfunction

2. Which are hormones produced and secreted by the anterior pituitary gland? *(Select all that apply.)*
   a. Growth hormone (GH; somatotropin)
   b. Prolactin (PRL)
   c. Thyrotropin (thyroid-stimulating hormone [TSH])
   d. Serotonin (5-HT)
   e. Gonadotropins (follicle-stimulating hormone [FSH] and luteinizing hormone [LH])
   f. Epinephrine (EPI)

3. A malfunctioning posterior pituitary gland can result in which disorders? *(Select all that apply.)*
   a. Hypothyroidism
   b. Altered sexual function
   c. Diabetes insipidus
   d. Growth retardation
   e. Syndrome of inappropriate antidiuretic hormone (SIADH)

4. A malfunctioning anterior pituitary gland can result in which disorders? *(Select all that apply.)*
   a. Pituitary hypofunction
   b. Pituitary hyperfunction
   c. Diabetes insipidus
   d. Hypothyroidism
   e. Osteoporosis

5. The assessment findings of a male patient with anterior pituitary tumor include reports of changes in secondary sex characteristics, such as episodes of impotence and decreased libido. The nurse explains to the patient that these findings are a result of overproduction of which hormone?
   a. Gonadotropins inhibiting PRL
   b. Thyroid hormone inhibiting PRL
   c. PRL inhibiting secretion of gonadotropins
   d. Steroids inhibiting production of sex hormones

6. A patient with PRL-secreting tumor is likely to be treated with which medication?
   a. Dopamine agonists
   b. Vasopressin
   c. Steroids
   d. Growth hormone

7. A patient is prescribed bromocriptine mesylate (Parlodel). Which information does the nurse teach the patient? *(Select all that apply.)*
   a. Get up slowly from a lying position.
   b. Take medication on an empty stomach.
   c. Take daily for purposes of raising GH levels to reduce symptom of acromegaly.
   d. Begin therapy with a maintenance level dose.
   e. Report watery nasal discharge to the health care provider immediately.

8. Patients diagnosed with an anterior pituitary tumor can have symptoms of acromegaly or gigantism. These symptoms are a result of overproduction of which hormone?
   a. ACTH
   b. PRL
   c. Gonadotropins
   d. GH

9. The nurse is performing an assessment of an adult patient with new-onset acromegaly. What does the nurse expect to find?
   a. Extremely long arms and legs
   b. Thickened lips
   c. Changes in menses with infertility
   d. Rough, extremely dry skin

10. When analyzing laboratory values, the nurse expects to find which value as a direct result of overproduction of GH?
    a. Hyperglycemia
    b. Hyperphosphatemia
    c. Hypocalcemia
    d. Hypercalcemia

11. In caring for a patient with hyperpituitarism, which symptoms does the nurse expect the patient to report? *(Select all that apply.)*
    a. Joint pain
    b. Visual disturbances
    c. Changes in menstruation
    d. Decreased libido
    e. Headache

12. A deficiency of which anterior pituitary hormones is considered life-threatening? *(Select all that apply.)*
    a. GH
    b. Melanocyte-stimulating hormone (MSH)
    c. PRL
    d. TSH
    e. ACTH

13. Which statements about the etiology of hypopituitarism are correct? *(Select all that apply.)*
    a. Dysfunction can result from radiation treatment to the head or brain.
    b. Dysfunction can result from infection or a brain tumor.
    c. Infarction following systemic shock can result in hypopituitarism.
    d. Severe malnutrition and body fat depletion can depress pituitary gland function.
    e. There is always an underlying cause of hypopituitarism.

14. Which statement about hormone replacement therapy for hypopituitarism is correct?
    a. Once manifestations of hypofunction are corrected, treatment is no longer needed.
    b. The most effective route of androgen replacement is the oral route.
    c. Testosterone replacement therapy is contraindicated in men with prostate cancer.
    d. Clomiphene citrate (Clomid) is used to suppress ovulation in women.

15. A female patient has been prescribed hormone replacement therapy. What does the nurse instruct the patient to do regarding this therapy?
    a. Report any recurrence of symptoms, such as decreased libido, between injections.
    b. Monitor blood pressure at least weekly for potential hypotension.
    c. Treat leg pain, especially in the calves, with gentle muscle stretching.
    d. Take measures to reduce risk for hypertension and thrombosis.

16. A patient requires 100 g of oral glucose for suppression testing and GH levels are measured serially for 120 minutes. The results of the suppression testing are abnormal. The nurse assesses for the signs and symptoms of which endocrine disorder?
    a. Adrenal insufficiency
    b. Diabetes insipidus
    c. Hyperpituitarism
    d. Hypothyroidism

17. A patient is recovering from a transsphenoidal hypophysectomy. What postoperative nursing interventions apply to this patient? *(Select all that apply.)*
    a. Vigorous coughing and deep-breathing exercises
    b. Instructing on the use of a soft-bristled toothbrush for brushing the teeth
    c. Strict monitoring of fluid balance
    d. Hourly neurologic checks for first 24 hours
    e. Instructing the patient to alert the nurse regarding postnasal drip

18. Following a hypophysectomy, the patient requires instruction on hormone replacement for which hormones? *(Select all that apply.)*
    a. Cortisol
    b. Thyroid
    c. Gonadal
    d. Vasopressin
    e. PRL

19. After a hypophysectomy, home care monitoring by the nurse includes assessing which factors? *(Select all that apply.)*
    a. Hypoglycemia
    b. Bowel habits
    c. Possible leakage of cerebrospinal fluid (CSF)
    d. 24-hour intake of fluids and urine output
    e. 24-hour diet recall
    f. Activity level

20. Postoperative care for a patient who has had a transsphenoidal hypophysectomy includes which intervention?
    a. Encouraging coughing and deep-breathing to decrease pulmonary complications
    b. Testing nasal drainage for glucose to determine whether it contains CSF
    c. Keeping the bed flat to decrease central CSF leakage
    d. Assisting the patient with brushing the teeth to reduce risk of infection

21. While caring for a postoperative patient following a transsphenoidal hypophysectomy, the nurse observes nasal drainage that is clear with yellow color at the edge. This "halo sign" is indicative of which condition?
    a. Worsening neurologic status of the patient
    b. Drainage of CSF from the patient's nose
    c. Onset of postoperative infection
    d. An expected finding following this surgery

22. A patient with a hypophysectomy can postoperatively experience transient diabetes insipidus. Which manifestation alerts the nurse to this problem?
    a. Output much greater than intake
    b. Change in mental status indicating confusion
    c. Laboratory results indicating hyponatremia
    d. Nonpitting edema

23. The action of ADH influences normal kidney function by stimulating which mechanism?
    a. Glomerulus to control the filtration rate
    b. Proximal nephron tubules to reabsorb water
    c. Distal nephron tubules and collecting ducts to reabsorb water
    d. Constriction of glomerular capillaries to prevent loss of protein in urine

24. What is the disorder that results from a deficiency of vasopressin (ADH) from the posterior pituitary gland called?
    a. SIADH
    b. Diabetes insipidus
    c. Cushing's syndrome
    d. Addison's disease

25. Which statements about diabetes insipidus (DI) are accurate? *(Select all that apply.)*
    a. It is caused by antidiuretic hormone (ADH) deficiency.
    b. It is characterized by a decrease in urination.
    c. Urine output of greater than 4 L/24 hours is the first diagnostic indication.
    d. The water loss increases plasma osmolarity.
    e. Nephrogenic DI can be caused by lithium (Eskalith).

26. What does the nurse instruct patients with permanent DI to do? *(Select all that apply.)*
    a. Continue vasopressin therapy until symptoms disappear.
    b. Monitor for recurrence of polydipsia and polyuria.
    c. Monitor and record weight daily.
    d. Check urine specific gravity three times a week.
    e. Wear a medical alert bracelet.

27. A patient uses desmopressin acetate metered dose spray as a replacement hormone for ADH. Which is an indication for another dose? *(Select all that apply.)*
    a. Excessive urination
    b. Specific gravity of 1.003
    c. Dark, concentrated urine
    d. Edema in the legs
    e. Decreased urination

28. The nurse is caring for a patient with DI. What is the priority goal of collaborative care?
    a. Correct the water metabolism problem.
    b. Control blood sugar and blood pH.
    c. Measure urine output, specific gravity, and osmolality hourly.
    d. Monitor closely for respiratory distress.

29. Which medications are used to treat DI? *(Select all that apply.)*
    a. Chlorpropamide (Diabinese)
    b. Desmopressin acetate (DDAVP)
    c. Lithium (Eskalith)
    d. Vasopressin (Pitressin)
    e. Demeclocycline (Declomycin)

30. Which patient's history puts him or her at risk for developing SIADH?
    a. 27-year-old patient on high-dose steroids
    b. 47-year-old hospitalized adult patient with acute renal failure
    c. 58-year-old with metastatic lung or breast cancer
    d. Older adult with history of a stroke within the last year

31. Which statement about the pathophysiology of SIADH is correct?
    a. ADH secretion is inhibited in the presence of low plasma osmolality.
    b. Water retention results in dilutional hyponatremia and expanded extracellular fluid (ECF) volume.
    c. The glomerulus is unable to increase its filtration rate to reduce the excess plasma volume.
    d. Renin and aldosterone are released and help to decrease the loss of urinary sodium.

32. Which statement about the etiology and incidence of SIADH is correct?
    a. Malignant cells act on the posterior pituitary gland to decrease ADH release.
    b. Demeclocycline may be used to treat SIADH.
    c. Ectopic ADH production can result from benign gastrointestinal polyps.
    d. SIADH that results from vasopressin overdose in DI is irreversible.

33. The effect of increased ADH in the blood results in which effect on the kidney?
    a. Urine concentration tends to decrease.
    b. Glomerular filtration tends to decrease.
    c. Tubular reabsorption of water increases.
    d. Tubular reabsorption of sodium increases.

34. In SIADH as a result of water retention from excess ADH, which laboratory value does the nurse expect to find? *(Select all that apply.)*
    a. Increased urine osmolality (increased sodium in urine)
    b. Elevated serum sodium level
    c. Increased specific gravity (concentrated urine)
    d. Decreased serum osmolarity
    e. Decreased urine specific gravity

35. Which nursing intervention is the priority for a patient with SIADH?
    a. Restrict fluid intake.
    b. Monitor neurologic status at least every 2 hours.
    c. Offer ice chips frequently to ease discomfort of dry mouth.
    d. Monitor urine tests for decreased sodium levels and low specific gravity.

36. Which type of IV fluid does the nurse use to treat a patient with SIADH when the serum sodium level is very low?
    a. D_5 1/2 normal saline
    b. D_5W
    c. 3% normal saline
    d. Normal saline

37. In addition to IV fluids, a patient with SIADH is on a fluid restriction as low as 500 to 600 mL/24 hours. Indicate the serum and urine results that demonstrate effectiveness of this treatment by writing *increases* or *decreases* for each item below.
    a. Urine specific gravity results

    b. Serum sodium results

    c. Urine output

38. Which medications are used in SIADH to promote water excretion without causing sodium loss? *(Select all that apply.)*
    a. Tolvaptan (Samsca)
    b. Demeclocycline (Declomycin)
    c. Furosemide (Lasix)
    d. Conivaptan (Vaprisol)
    e. Spironolactone (Aldactone)

39. Which statement about pheochromocytoma is correct?
    a. It is most often malignant.
    b. It is a catecholamine-producing tumor.
    c. It is found only in the adrenal medulla.
    d. It is manifested by hypotension.

40. A patient in the emergency department is diagnosed with possible pheochromocytoma. What is the priority nursing intervention for this patient?
    a. Monitor the patient's intake and output and urine specific gravity.
    b. Monitor blood pressure for severe hypertension.
    c. Monitor blood pressure for severe hypotension.
    d. Administer medication to increase cardiac output.

41. The nurse expects to perform which diagnostic test for pheochromocytoma?
    a. 24-hour urine collection for sodium, potassium, and glucose
    b. Catecholamine stimulation test
    c. Administration of beta-adrenergic blocking agent and monitor results
    d. 24-hour urine collection for vanillylmandelic acid (VMA)

42. Which intervention applies to a patient with pheochromocytoma?
    a. Assist to sit in a chair for blood pressure monitoring.
    b. Instruct not to smoke or drink coffee.
    c. Encourage to maintain an active exercise schedule including activity such as running.
    d. Encourage one glass of red wine nightly to promote rest.

43. Which intervention is contraindicated for a patient with pheochromocytoma?
    a. Monitoring blood pressure
    b. Palpating the abdomen
    c. Collecting 24-hour urine specimens
    d. Instructing the patient to limit activity

44. Which diuretic is ordered by the health care provider to treat hyperaldosteronism?
    a. Furosemide (Lasix)
    b. Ethacrynic acid (Edecrin)
    c. Bumetanide (Bumex)
    d. Spironolactone (Aldactone)

45. Which statement about hyperaldosteronism is correct?
    a. Painful "charley horses" are common from hyperkalemia.
    b. It occurs more often in men than in women.
    c. It is a common cause of hypertension in the population.
    d. Hypokalemia and hypertension are the main issues.

46. When diagnosed with Cushing's syndrome, the manifestations are most likely related to an excess production of which hormone?
    a. Insulin from the pancreas
    b. ADH from posterior pituitary gland
    c. PRL from anterior pituitary gland
    d. Cortisol from the adrenal cortex

47. What is the most common cause of endogenous hypercortisolism, or Cushing's syndrome?
    a. Pituitary hypoplasia
    b. Insufficient ACTH production
    c. Adrenocortical hormone deficiency
    d. Hyperplasia of the adrenal cortex

48. Which are physical findings of Cushing's syndrome? *(Select all that apply.)*
    a. "Moon-faced" appearance
    b. Decreased amount of body hair
    c. Barrel chest
    d. Truncal obesity
    e. Coarse facial features
    f. Thin, easily damaged skin
    g. Excessive sweating
    h. Extremity muscle wasting

49. When assessing a patient with Cushing's syndrome, what does the nurse expect to find?
    a. Signs of dehydration
    b. Facial flushing
    c. Hypertension
    d. Muscle hypertrophy

50. Which laboratory findings does the nurse expect to find with Cushing's syndrome? *(Select all that apply.)*
    a. Decreased serum sodium
    b. Increased serum glucose
    c. Increased serum sodium
    d. Increased serum potassium
    e. Decreased serum potassium

51. The nurse determines a priority patient problem of altered self-concept in a female patient with Cushing's syndrome who expresses concern about the changes in her general appearance. What is the expected outcome for this patient?
    a. To verbalize an understanding that treatment will reverse many of the problems
    b. To ventilate about the frustration of these lifelong physical changes
    c. To verbalize ways to cope with the changes such as joining a support group or changing style of dress
    d. To achieve a personal desired level of sexual functioning

Matching. *Match each drug with its corresponding clinical use for hypercortisolism.*

Drugs
a. Mitotane (Lysodren)
b. Aminoglutethimide (Cytadren)
c. Cyproheptadine (Periactin)

Clinical Uses
_____ 52. Adrenal cytotoxic agent used for inoperable adrenal tumors

_____ 53. Interferes with ACTH production

_____ 54. Adrenal enzyme inhibitor that decreases cortisol production

55. A patient is scheduled for bilateral adrenalectomy. Before surgery, steroids are to be given. Which is the reasoning behind the administration of this drug?
    a. To promote glycogen storage by the liver for body energy reserves
    b. To compensate for sudden lack of adrenal hormones following surgery
    c. To increase the body's inflammatory response to promote scar formation
    d. To enhance urinary excretion of salt and water following surgery

56. The nurse is teaching a patient being discharged after bilateral adrenalectomy. What medication information does the nurse emphasize in the teaching plan?
    a. The dosage of steroid replacement drugs will be consistent throughout the patient's lifetime.
    b. The steroid drugs should be taken in the evening so as not to interfere with sleep.
    c. The patient should take the drugs on an empty stomach.
    d. The patient should learn how to give himself an intramuscular injection of hydrocortisone.

57. Which statement about a patient with hyperaldosteronism after a successful unilateral adrenalectomy is correct?
    a. The low-sodium diet must be continued postoperatively.
    b. Glucocorticoid replacement therapy is temporary.
    c. Spironolactone (Aldactone) must be taken for life.
    d. Additional measures are needed to control hypertension.

58. Which are causes for decreased production of adrenocortical steroids? *(Select all that apply.)*
    a. Inadequate secretion of ACTH
    b. Dysfunction of hypothalamic-pituitary control mechanism
    c. Adrenal gland dysfunction
    d. Cancer
    e. AIDS

59. Which patient is at risk for developing secondary adrenal insufficiency?
    a. Patient who suddenly stops taking high-dose steroid therapy
    b. Patient who tapers the dosages of steroid therapy
    c. Patient deficient in ADH
    d. Patient with an adrenal tumor causing excessive secretion of ACTH

60. An ACTH stimulation test is the most definitive test for which disorder?
    a. Adrenal insufficiency
    b. Cushing's syndrome
    c. Pheochromocytoma
    d. Acromegaly

61. Which interventions are necessary for a patient with acute adrenal insufficiency (Addisonian crisis)? *(Select all that apply.)*
    a. IV infusion of normal saline
    b. IV infusion of 3% saline
    c. Hourly glucose monitoring
    d. Insulin administration
    e. IV potassium therapy

62. A patient in the emergency department who reports lethargy, muscle weakness, nausea, vomiting, and weight loss over the past weeks is diagnosed with Addisonian crisis (acute adrenal insufficiency). Which drugs does the nurse expect to administer to this patient?
    a. Beta blocker to control the hypertension and dysrhythmias
    b. Solu-Cortef IV along with IM injections of hydrocortisone
    c. IV fluids of D_5NS with KCl added for dehydration
    d. Spironolactone (Aldactone) to promote diuresis

63. The nurse determines that the administration of hydrocortisone for Addisonian crisis is effective when which assessment is made?
    a. Increased urine output
    b. No signs of pitting edema
    c. Weight gain
    d. Lethargy improving; patient alert and oriented

64. Which nursing intervention is a preventive measure for adrenocortical insufficiency?
    a. Maintaining diuretic therapy
    b. Instructing the patient on salt restriction
    c. Reducing high-dose glucocorticoid therapy quickly
    d. Reducing high-dose glucocorticoid doses gradually

65. The nurse should instruct a patient who is taking hydrocortisone to report which symptoms to the health care provider for possible dose adjustment? *(Select all that apply.)*
    a. Rapid weight gain
    b. Round face
    c. Fluid retention
    d. GI irritation
    e. Urinary incontinence

CASE STUDY: THE PATIENT WITH DIABETES INSIPIDUS

Use a separate sheet of paper to answer the questions in this Case Study, or go to the "Prepare for Class" folder on your Evolve website at http://evolve.elsevier.com/Iggy/ to download and complete as a word processing file. Answer guidelines for this Case Study are also available on your Evolve website.

A 22-year-old man has been admitted to the emergency department after his girlfriend found him lying on the floor of their apartment. He had fallen off a ladder 2 days ago but "seemed fine," according to the girlfriend, even though he had hit his head slightly when he fell. He never lost consciousness. He has a few abrasions on his arms, face, and legs, and is drowsy but arousable. His girlfriend states that yesterday he started "going to the bathroom nonstop" and he drank "everything in sight" because he was so thirsty. A magnetic resonance imaging (MRI) scan reveals a small intracerebral hemorrhage, and he is admitted to the intensive care unit with the diagnosis of head trauma and diabetes insipidus.

1. What physical and laboratory findings led to the diagnosis of diabetes insipidus?

2. The health care provider is considering whether this patient is a candidate for the fluid deprivation and hypertonic saline tests to confirm the diagnosis of diabetes insipidus. How is this determined?

3. Identify potential priority problems for this patient based on the above data.

4. Identify nursing measures that would assist the patient to maintain an adequate fluid balance. State the rationale for these measures.

5. The health care provider initially orders aqueous vasopressin (Pitressin) 10 units IM every 3 to 4 hours as indicated. How does the nurse determine when to give the medication?

6. The patient is on strict intake and output (I&O). The patient's intake for the 7-3 shift includes the following:
   - Breakfast: 8 oz coffee; 4 oz orange juice
   - Lunch: 12 oz tea
   - Patient reports drinking 6 cups of water (8 oz each) during the day.
   - IV has been running at 150 mL/hr
   - Foley was emptied at 1500 for 1.5 L of urine
   - Record the I&O on the documentation chart below for your shift. (Remember that this is recorded in milliliters.)

Intake	07-1500	1500-2300	2300-0700
IV			
IVPB			
PO			

Output	07-1500	1500-2300	2300-0700
Urine Void			
Foley			
Incontinent			

66 CHAPTER

Care of Patients with Problems of the Thyroid and Parathyroid Glands

STUDY/REVIEW QUESTIONS

1. The nurse is performing a physical examination of a patient's thyroid gland. Precautions are taken in performing the correct technique because palpation can result in which occurrence?
    a. Damage to the esophagus causing gastric reflux
    b. Obstruction of the carotid arteries causing a stroke
    c. Pressure on the trachea and laryngeal nerve causing hoarseness
    d. Exacerbation of symptoms by releasing additional thyroid hormone

Matching. *Differentiate the general assessment findings by matching them with the corresponding type of thyroid deficiency. Answers will be used more than once.*

Thyroid Deficiencies
a. Hyperthyroidism
b. Hypothyroidism

Assessment Findings
_____ 2. Weight loss with increased appetite
_____ 3. Constipation
_____ 4. Increased heart rate, palpitations
_____ 5. Photophobia
_____ 6. Manic behavior
_____ 7. Decreased libido
_____ 8. Dyspnea with or without exertion
_____ 9. Insomnia
_____ 10. Cold intolerance
_____ 11. Increased stools
_____ 12. Corneal ulcers
_____ 13. Fatigue, increased sleeping
_____ 14. Irritability
_____ 15. Impaired memory
_____ 16. Fine, soft, silky body hair
_____ 17. Facial puffiness
_____ 18. Increased libido
_____ 19. Heat intolerance, warm skin
_____ 20. Weight gain
_____ 21. Dry, coarse, brittle hair
_____ 22. Diaphoresis
_____ 23. Tremors

24. Which factor is a hallmark assessment finding that signifies hyperthyroidism?
    a. Weight loss
    b. Increased libido
    c. Heat intolerance
    d. Diarrhea

25. Which factor is a main assessment finding that signifies hypothyroidism?
    a. Irritability
    b. Cold intolerance
    c. Diarrhea
    d. Fatigue

26. Which sign/symptom is one of the first indicators of hyperthyroidism that is often noticed by the patient?
    a. Eyelid or globe lag
    b. Vision changes or tiring of the eyes
    c. Protruding eyes
    d. Photophobia

27. Which laboratory result is consistent with a diagnosis of hyperthyroidism?
    a. Decreased serum triiodothyronine (T_3) and thyroxine (T_4) levels
    b. Elevated serum thyrotropin-releasing hormone (TRH) level
    c. Decreased radioactive iodine uptake
    d. Increased serum T_3 and T_4

28. The laboratory results for a 53-year-old patient indicate a low T_3 level and elevated TSH. What do these results indicate?
    a. Hyperthyroidism
    b. Hypothyroidism
    c. Malfunctioning pituitary gland
    d. Normal laboratory values for this age

29. The clinical manifestations of hyperthyroidism are known as which condition?
    a. Thyrotoxicosis
    b. Euthyroid function
    c. Graves' disease
    d. Hypermetabolism

30. What is the most common cause of hyperthyroidism?
    a. Radiation to thyroid
    b. Graves' disease
    c. Thyroid cancer
    d. Thyroiditis

31. The nurse assessing a patient palpates enlargement of the thyroid gland, along with noticeable swelling of the neck. How does the nurse interpret this finding?
    a. Globe lag
    b. Myxedema
    c. Exophthalmos
    d. Goiter

32. The nurse is assessing a patient diagnosed with hyperthyroidism and observes dry, waxy swelling of the front surfaces of the lower legs. How does the nurse interpret this finding?
    a. Globe lag
    b. Pretibial myxedema
    c. Exophthalmos
    d. Goiter

33. Which statement best describes globe lag in a patient with hyperthyroidism?
    a. Abnormal protrusion of the eyes
    b. Upper eyelid fails to descend when the patient gazes downward
    c. Upper eyelid pulls back faster than the eyeball when the patient gazes upward
    d. Inability of both eyes to focus on an object simultaneously

34. The nurse is assessing a patient with Graves' disease and observes an abnormal protrusion of both eyeballs. How does the nurse document this assessment finding?
    a. Globe lag
    b. Pretibial myxedema
    c. Exophthalmos
    d. Goiter

35. Which statements about hyperthyroidism are accurate? *(Select all that apply.)*
    a. It is most commonly caused by Graves' disease.
    b. It can be caused by overuse of thyroid replacement medication.
    c. It occurs more often in men between the ages of 20-40.
    d. Weight gain is a common manifestation.
    e. Serum T_3 and T_4 results will be elevated.

36. The nurse is providing instructions to a patient taking levothyroxine (Synthroid). When does the nurse tell the patient to take this medication?
    a. With breakfast
    b. At lunchtime
    c. On an empty stomach
    d. At dinnertime

37. The nurse is providing instructions to a patient who is taking the antithyroid medication propylthiouracil (PTU). The nurse instructs the patient to notify the health care provider immediately if which sign/symptom occurs?
    a. Weight gain
    b. Dark-colored urine
    c. Cold intolerance
    d. Headache

38. A patient who has been diagnosed with Graves' disease is going to receive radioactive iodine (RAI) in the oral form of ^{131}I. What does the nurse teach the patient about how this drug works?
    a. It destroys the hormones T_3 and T_4.
    b. It destroys the tissue that produces thyroid hormones.
    c. It blocks thyroid hormone production.
    d. It prevents T_4 from being converted to T_3.

39. A patient who has been diagnosed with Graves' disease is to receive radioactive iodine (RAI) in the oral form of ^{131}I as a treatment. What instructions does the nurse include in the teaching plan about preventing radiation exposure to others? *(Select all that apply.)*
    a. Do not share a toilet with others for 2 weeks after treatment.
    b. Flush the toilet three times after each use.
    c. Wash clothing separately from others in the household.
    d. Limit contact with pregnant women, infants, and children.
    e. Do not use a laxative within 2 weeks of having the treatment.

40. Which statements about hypothyroidism are accurate? *(Select all that apply.)*
    a. It occurs more often in women.
    b. It can be caused by iodine deficiency.
    c. Weight loss is a common manifestation.
    d. It can be caused by autoimmune thyroid destruction.
    e. Myxedema coma is a rare but serious complication.

41. The nurse is assessing a patient with a diagnosis of Hashimoto's disease. What are the primary manifestations of this disease? *(Select all that apply.)*
    a. Dysphagia
    b. Painless enlargement of the thyroid gland
    c. Painful enlargement of the thyroid gland
    d. Weight loss
    e. Intolerance to heat

42. Laboratory findings of elevated T_3 and T_4, decreased TSH, and high thyrotropin receptor antibody titer indicate which condition?
    a. Multinodular goiter
    b. Hyperthyroidism related to overmedication
    c. Pituitary tumor suppressing TSH
    d. Graves' disease

Matching. *Match the cause of hyperthyroidism with its mechanism.*

Causes

a. Thyroid carcinoma
b. Thyroiditis (radiation-induced)
c. Graves' disease
d. Toxic multinodular goiter
e. Pituitary hyperthyroidism

Mechanisms

_____ 43. Autoimmune disease; antibodies bind to TSH receptors and keep them activated, increasing the size of the gland and increasing the production of thyroid hormones.

_____ 44. Uncommon; usually occurs with large follicular carcinomas.

_____ 45. T_3 and T_4 secretion increased before destruction of gland. Hyperthyroid state usually transient.

_____ 46. Multiple thyroid nodules resulting in thyroid hyperfunction.

_____ 47. Pituitary adenoma resulting in excessive TSH secretion.

48. After a visit to the health care provider's office, a patient is diagnosed with general thyroid enlargement and elevated thyroid hormone level. This is an indication of which condition?
    a. Hyperthyroidism and goiter
    b. Hypothyroidism and goiter
    c. Nodules on the parathyroid gland
    d. Thyroid or parathyroid cancer

49. Which condition is a life-threatening emergency and serious complication of untreated or poorly treated hypothyroidism?
    a. Endemic goiter
    b. Myxedema coma
    c. Toxic multinodular goiter
    d. Thyroiditis

50. A patient with exophthalmos from hyperthyroidism reports dry eyes, especially in the morning. The nurse teaches the patient to perform which intervention to help correct this problem?
    a. Wear sunglasses at all times when outside in the bright sun.
    b. Use cool compresses to the eye four times a day.
    c. Tape the eyes closed with nonallergenic tape.
    d. There is nothing that can be done to relieve this problem.

51. Which factors are considered to be triggers for thyroid storm? *(Select all that apply.)*
    a. Infection
    b. Cold temperatures
    c. Vigorous palpation of a goiter
    d. Pregnancy
    e. Extremely warm temperatures

52. A patient has the following assessment findings: elevated TSH level, low T_3 and T_4 level, difficulty with memory, lethargy, and muscle stiffness. These are clinical manifestations of which disorder?
    a. Hypothyroidism
    b. Hyperthyroidism
    c. Hypoparathyroidism
    d. Hyperparathyroidism

53. A patient has been prescribed thyroid hormone for treatment of hypothyroidism. Within what time frame does the patient expect improvement in mental awareness with this treatment?
    a. A few days
    b. 2 weeks
    c. 1 month
    d. 3 months

54. Which signs and symptoms are assessment findings indicative of thyroid storm? *(Select all that apply.)*
    a. Abdominal pain and nausea
    b. Hypothermia
    c. Fever
    d. Tachycardia
    e. Elevated systolic blood pressure
    f. Bradycardia

55. Management of the patient with hyperthyroidism focuses on which goals? *(Select all that apply.)*
    a. Blocking the effects of excessive thyroid secretion
    b. Treating the signs and symptoms the patient experiences
    c. Establishing euthyroid function
    d. Preventing spread of the disease
    e. Maintaining an environment of reduced stimulation

56. Which are preoperative instructions for a patient having thyroid surgery? *(Select all that apply.)*
    a. Teach postoperative restrictions such as no coughing and deep-breathing exercises to prevent strain on the suture line.
    b. Teach the moving and turning technique of manually supporting the head and avoiding neck extension to minimize strain on the suture line.
    c. Inform the patient that hoarseness for a few days after surgery is usually the result of a breathing tube (endotracheal tube) used during surgery.
    d. Humidification of air may be helpful to promote expectoration of secretions. Suctioning may also be used.
    e. Clarify any questions regarding placement of incision, complications, and postoperative care.
    f. A supine position and lying flat will be maintained postoperatively to avoid strain on suture line.
    g. Teach the patient to report immediately any respiratory difficulty, tingling around the lips or fingers, or muscular twitching.
    h. A drain may be present in the incision. All drainage and dressings will be monitored closely for 24 hours.

57. The nurse is preparing for a patient to return from thyroid surgery. What priority equipment does the nurse ensure is immediately available? *(Select all that apply.)*
    a. Tracheostomy equipment
    b. Calcium gluconate or calcium chloride for IV administration
    c. Humidified oxygen
    d. Suction equipment
    e. Sandbags

58. After a thyroidectomy, a patient reports tingling around the mouth and muscle twitching. Which complication do these assessment findings indicate to the nurse?
    a. Hemorrhage
    b. Respiratory distress
    c. Thyroid storm
    d. Hypocalcemia

59. The nurse assesses a patient post-thyroidectomy for laryngeal nerve damage. Which findings indicate this complication? *(Select all that apply.)*
    a. Dyspnea
    b. Sore throat
    c. Hoarseness
    d. Weak voice
    e. Dry cough

60. After hospitalization for myxedema, a patient is prescribed thyroid replacement medication. Which statement by the patient demonstrates a correct understanding of this therapy?
    a. "I'll be taking this medication until my symptoms are completely resolved."
    b. "I'll be taking thyroid medication for the rest of my life."
    c. "Now that I'm feeling better, no changes in my medication will be necessary."
    d. "I'm taking this medication to prevent symptoms of an overactive thyroid gland."

61. Which statements about thyroiditis are accurate? *(Select all that apply.)*
    a. It is an inflammation of the thyroid gland.
    b. Hashimoto's disease is the most common type.
    c. It always resolves with antibiotic therapy.
    d. There are three types: acute, subacute, and chronic.
    e. The patient must take thyroid hormones.

62. Which statements about acute thyroiditis are accurate? *(Select all that apply.)*
    a. It is caused by a bacterial infection of the thyroid gland.
    b. It is treated with antibiotic therapy.
    c. It results from a viral infection of the thyroid gland.
    d. Subtotal thyroidectomy is a form of treatment.
    e. Manifestations include neck tenderness, fever, and dysphagia.

63. Serum calcium levels are maintained by which hormone?
    a. Cortisol
    b. Calcium
    c. Antidiuretic hormone (ADH)
    d. Parathyroid hormone (PTH)

Matching. *Match each hormone with its corresponding effect on serum calcium levels.*

Effects
a. Raises levels
b. Lowers levels

Hormones
_____ 64. PTH production

_____ 65. Calcitonin production

66. Bone changes in the older adult are often seen with endocrine dysfunction and increased secretion of which substance?
    a. PTH
    b. Calcitonin
    c. Insulin
    d. Testosterone

67. In addition to regulation of calcium levels, PTH and calcitonin regulate the circulating blood levels of which substance?
    a. Potassium
    b. Sodium
    c. Phosphate
    d. Chloride

68. A patient has a positive Trousseau's or Chvostek's sign resulting from hypoparathyroidism. What condition does this assessment finding indicate?
    a. Hypercalcemia
    b. Hypocalcemia
    c. Hyperphosphatemia
    d. Hypophosphatemia

69. Which food does the nurse instruct a patient with hypoparathyroidism to avoid?
    a. Canned vegetables
    b. Fresh fruit
    c. Red meat
    d. Milk

70. A patient with continuous spasms of the muscles is diagnosed with hypoparathyroidism. The muscle spasms are a clinical manifestation of which condition?
    a. Nerve damage
    b. Seizures
    c. Tetany
    d. Decreased potassium

Matching. *Match the parathyroid disorders with their causes. Answers will be used more than once.*

Parathyroid Disorders
a. Hypoparathyroidism
b. Hyperparathyroidism

Causes

_____ 71. Chronic kidney disease

_____ 72. Vitamin D deficiency

_____ 73. Removal of the thyroid gland

_____ 74. Neck trauma

_____ 75. Carcinoma of the lung, kidney, or GI tract producing PTH-like substance

_____ 76. Parathyroidectomy

77. A patient has hyperparathyroidism and high levels of serum calcium. Which initial treatment does the nurse prepare to administer to the patient?
    a. Force fluids (intravenous or oral) and administer Lasix
    b. Calcitonin
    c. Oral phosphates
    d. Mithramycin

78. Which are assessment findings of hypocalcemia? *(Select all that apply.)*
    a. Numbness and tingling around the mouth
    b. Muscle cramping
    c. Mental status changes including irritability
    d. Fever
    e. Tachycardia

79. Which medication therapies does the nurse expect patients with hypoparathyroidism to receive? *(Select all that apply.)*
    a. Calcium chloride
    b. Calcium gluconate
    c. Calcitrol
    d. Magnesium sulfate
    e. Ergocalciferol

80. Discharge planning for a patient with chronic hypoparathyroidism include which instructions? *(Select all that apply.)*
    a. Prescribed medications must be taken for the patient's entire life.
    b. Eat foods low in vitamin D and high in phosphorus.
    c. Eat foods high in calcium but low in phosphorus.
    d. After several weeks, medications can be discontinued.
    e. Kidney stones are no longer a risk to the patient.

81. In older adults, assessment findings of fatigue, altered thought processes, dry skin, and constipation are often mistaken for signs of aging rather than assessment findings for which endocrine disorder?
    a. Hyperthyroidism
    b. Hypothyroidism
    c. Hyperparathyroidism
    d. Hypoparathyroidism

82. Which conditions may precipitate myxedema coma? *(Select all that apply.)*
    a. Rapid withdrawal of thyroid medication
    b. Vitamin D deficiency
    c. Untreated hypothyroidism
    d. Surgery
    e. Excessive exposure to iodine

CASE STUDY: THE PATIENT WITH ENDOCRINE PROBLEMS

Use a separate sheet of paper to answer the questions in this Case Study, or go to the "Prepare for Class" folder on your Evolve website at http://evolve.elsevier.com/Iggy/ to download and complete as a word processing file. Answer guidelines for this Case Study are also available on your Evolve website.

The nurse is caring for a 41-year-old woman who is the mother of two small children. She states that she has felt "nervous and tired" for approximately 1 month. Today she has had a sudden onset of breathlessness with cardiac palpitations. She states, "I have not been feeling well for about a month, but when I felt breathless I thought I should be checked out." Upon further questioning the nurse finds that the woman also has had an unexplained loss of weight of approximately 30 lbs. over 3 months, frequent loose stools, loss of hair on the scalp, and a feeling of "burning up."

1. What findings would the nurse expect to see on physical examination of this patient?

2. What laboratory tests would the nurse expect to be ordered for this patient? What abnormalities could be expected for these laboratory tests?

3. What nonsurgical interventions would the nurse expect to be ordered for this patient?

4. If surgical intervention is necessary, what preoperative care would the nurse anticipate?

5. If surgical intervention is employed, identify the appropriate postoperative care for this patient.

6. Identify complications of the surgical procedure that the nurse should remain alert for.

7. At 8 PM, the health care provider orders 1 mg of propranol (Inderal) IV push for the patient's heart rate of 124 bpm and the patient's subjective reports of "feeling like my heart is beating fast." The nurse promptly administers the medication at 8:05 PM. Fifteen minutes after administration, the patient's heart rate has decreased to 98 bpm and the patient states she can no longer feel her heart beating fast. Using the focus charting method (also known as the DAR method—data, action, response), document this information in the patient's chart.

67 CHAPTER

Care of Patients with Diabetes Mellitus

STUDY/REVIEW QUESTIONS

Matching. Match the descriptions with the corresponding type of diabetes. Answers may be used more than once.

Types of Diabetes
a. Type 1
b. Type 2
c. Gestational

Descriptions

_____ 1. Diagnosis based on results of 100 g glucose tolerance test.

_____ 2. Cells have a reduced ability to respond to insulin.

_____ 3. Autoimmune process is causing beta cell destruction.

_____ 4. Carbohydrate intolerance is first recognized during pregnancy.

_____ 5. Most who suffer with this type of diabetes are obese adults.

_____ 6. Usually abrupt onset of thirst and weight loss.

7. Which statement is true about insulin?
    a. It is secreted by alpha cells in the islets of Langerhans.
    b. It is a catabolic hormone that builds up glucagon reserves.
    c. It is necessary for glucose transport across cell membranes.
    d. It is stored in muscles and converted to fat for storage.

8. Why is glucose vital to the body's cells?
    a. It is used to build cell membranes.
    b. It is used by cells to produce energy.
    c. It affects the process of protein metabolism.
    d. It provides nutrients for genetic material.

9. A patient with diabetes presents to the emergency department with a blood sugar of 640 mg/dL and reports being constantly thirsty and having to urinate "all of the time." How does the nurse document this subjective finding?
    a. Polydipsia and polyphagia
    b. Polydipsia and polyuria
    c. Polycoria and polyuria
    d. Polyphagia and polyesthesia

10. Which cultures tend to have a higher incidence of diabetes mellitus (DM)? *(Select all that apply.)*
    a. Mexican American
    b. African American
    c. Caucasian
    d. American Indian
    e. Eastern European

11. Which individual is at greatest risk for developing type 2 DM?
    a. 25-year-old African-American woman
    b. 36-year-old African-American man
    c. 56-year-old Hispanic woman
    d. 40-year-old Hispanic man

12. According to the American Diabetes Association (ADA), which laboratory finding is most indicative of DM?
    a. Fasting blood glucose = 80 mg/dL
    b. 2-hour postprandial blood glucose = 110 mg/dL
    c. 1-hour glucose tolerance blood glucose = 110 mg/dL
    d. 2-hour glucose tolerance blood glucose = 210 mg/dL

13. Untreated hyperglycemia results in which condition?
    a. Respiratory acidosis
    b. Metabolic alkalosis
    c. Respiratory alkalosis
    d. Metabolic acidosis

14. In a patient with hyperglycemia, the respiratory center is triggered in an attempt to excrete more carbon dioxide and acid, thus causing a rapid and deep respiratory pattern. What is the term for this respiratory pattern?
    a. Tachypnea
    b. Cheyne-Stokes respiration
    c. Kussmaul respiration
    d. Biot respiration

15. Which electrolyte is most affected by hyperglycemia?
    a. Sodium
    b. Chloride
    c. Potassium
    d. Magnesium

16. Which complications of DM are considered emergencies? *(Select all that apply.)*
    a. Diabetic ketoacidosis (DKA)
    b. Hypoglycemia
    c. Diabetic retinopathy
    d. Hyperglycemic-hyperosmolar state (HHS)
    e. Diabetic neuropathy

17. In determining if a patient is hypoglycemic, the nurse looks for which characteristics in addition to checking the patient's blood glucose? *(Select all that apply.)*
    a. Nausea
    b. Hunger
    c. Irritability
    d. Palpitations
    e. Profuse perspiration
    f. Rapid, deep respirations

18. Which factors differentiate DKA from HHS? *(Select all that apply.)*
    a. Level of hyperglycemia
    b. Amount of ketones produced
    c. Serum bicarbonate levels
    d. Amount of volume depletion
    e. Dosage of insulin needed

19. A patient is admitted with a blood glucose level of 900 mg/dL. IV fluids and insulin are administered. Two hours after treatment is initiated, the blood glucose level is 400 mg/dL. Which complication is the patient most at risk for developing?
    a. Hypoglycemia
    b. Pulmonary embolus
    c. Renal shutdown
    d. Pulmonary edema

20. What type of insulin is used in the emergency treatment of DKA and hyperglycemic-hyperosmolar nonketotic syndrome (HHNS)?
    a. NPH
    b. Lente
    c. Regular
    d. Protamine zinc

21. Early treatment of DKA and HHNS includes IV administration of which fluid?
    a. Glucagon
    b. Potassium
    c. Bicarbonate
    d. Normal saline

22. Glucagon is used primarily to treat the patient with which disorder?
    a. DKA
    b. Idiosyncratic reaction to insulin
    c. Severe hypoglycemia
    d. HHNS

23. Why is glucagon given in a dextrose solution?
    a. Dextrose promotes more storage of glucose in the liver.
    b. Dextrose stimulates the pancreas to produce more insulin.
    c. Dextrose increases blood sugar levels at a controlled rate.
    d. Dextrose inhibits glycogenesis, gluconeogenesis, and lipolysis.

24. When glucagon is administered, what does it do?
    a. Competes for insulin at the receptor sites
    b. Frees glucose from hepatic stores of glycogen
    c. Supplies glycogen directly to the vital tissues
    d. Provides a glucose substitute for rapid replacement

25. Which statements about type 1 DM are accurate? *(Select all that apply.)*
    a. It is an autoimmune disorder.
    b. Most people with type 1 DM are obese.
    c. Age of onset is typically younger than 30.
    d. Etiology can be attributed to viral infections.
    e. It can be treated with oral antidiabetic medications and insulin.

26. Which statements about type 2 DM are accurate? *(Select all that apply.)*
    a. It peaks at about the age of 50.
    b. Most people with type 2 DM are obese.
    c. It typically has an abrupt onset.
    d. People with type 2 DM have insulin resistance.
    e. It can be treated with oral antidiabetic medications and insulin.

27. Which are modifiable risk factors for type 2 diabetes mellitus? *(Select all that apply.)*
    a. Age
    b. Family history
    c. Working in a low-stress environment
    d. Maintaining ideal body weight
    e. Maintaining adequate physical activity

28. A diabetic patient is scheduled to have a blood glucose test the next morning. What does the nurse tell the patient to do before coming in for the test?
    a. Eat the usual diet but have nothing after midnight.
    b. Take the usual oral hypoglycemic tablet in the morning.
    c. Eat a clear liquid breakfast in the morning.
    d. Follow the usual diet and medication regimen.

29. The nurse is providing discharge teaching to a patient about self-monitoring of blood glucose (SMBG). What information does the nurse include? *(Select all that apply.)*
    a. Only perform SMBG before breakfast.
    b. Wash hands before using the meter.
    c. Do a retest if the results seem unusual.
    d. It is okay to reuse lancets in the home setting.
    e. Do not share the meter.

30. Which is considered the earliest sign of diabetic nephropathy?
    a. Positive urine RBCs
    b. Microalbuminuria
    c. Positive urine glucose
    d. Positive urine WBCs

31. Which class of antidiabetic medication should be taken with the first bite of a meal to be fully effective?
    a. Alpha-glucosidase inhibitors, which include miglitol (Glyset)
    b. Biguanides, which include metformin (Glucophage)
    c. Meglitinides, which include nateglinide (Starlix)
    d. Sulfonylureas, which include chlorpromadine (Diabinese)

32. Which class of antidiabetic medication must be held for 48 hours if the patient is having an x-ray with iodinated contrast materials?
    a. Alpha-glucosidase inhibitors, which include miglitol (Glyset)
    b. Biguanides, which include metformin (Glucophage)
    c. Meglitinides, which include nateglinide (Starlix)
    d. Sulfonylureas, which include chlorpromadine (Diabinese)

33. Which class of antidiabetic medication is most likely to cause a hypoglycemic episode because of the long duration of action?
    a. Alpha-glucosidase inhibitors, which include miglitol (Glyset)
    b. Biguanides, which include metformin (Glucophage)
    c. Meglitinides, which include nateglinide (Starlix)
    d. Sulfonylureas, which include chlorpromadine (Diabinese)

34. Which class of antidiabetic medication should be given 1-30 minutes before meals?
    a. Alpha-glucosidase inhibitors, which include miglitol (Glyset)
    b. Biguanides, which include metformin (Glucophage)
    c. Meglitinides, which include nateglinide (Starlix)
    d. Sulfonylureas, which include chlorpromadine (Diabinese)

35. Which oral agent may cause lactic acidosis?
    a. Nateglinide
    b. Repaglinide
    c. Metformin
    d. Miglitol

36. Which statement about insulin is true?
    a. Exogenous insulin is necessary for management of all cases of type 2 DM.
    b. Insulin's effectiveness depends on the individual patient's absorption of the drug.
    c. Insulin doses should be regulated according to self-monitoring urine glucose levels.
    d. Insulin administered in multiple doses per day decreases the flexibility of a patient's lifestyle.

37. Which statement about insulin administration is correct?
    a. Insulin may be given orally, intravenously, or subcutaneously.
    b. Insulin injections should be spaced no closer than one-half inch apart.
    c. Rotating injection sites improves absorption and prevents lipohypertrophy.
    d. In a mixed-dose protocol, the longer-acting insulin should be withdrawn first.

38. A diabetic patient is on a mixed-dose insulin protocol of 8 units regular insulin and 12 units NPH insulin at 7 AM. At 10:30 AM, the patient reports feeling uneasy, shaky, and has a headache. Which is the probable explanation for this?
    a. The NPH insulin's action is peaking, and there is an insufficient blood glucose level.
    b. The regular insulin's action is peaking, and there is an insufficient blood glucose level.
    c. The patient consumed too many calories at breakfast and now has an elevated blood glucose level.
    d. The symptoms are unrelated to the insulin administered in the early morning or diet taken in at lunchtime.

39. A patient will be using an external insulin pump. What does the nurse tell the patient about the pump?
    a. Self-monitoring of blood glucose levels can be done only twice a day.
    b. The insulin supply must be replaced every 2 to 4 weeks.
    c. The pump's battery should be checked on a regular weekly schedule.
    d. The needle site must be changed every 1 to 3 days.

40. A 47-year-old patient with a history of type 2 DM and emphysema that reports smoking three packs of cigarettes per day is admitted to the hospital with a diagnosis of acute pneumonia. The patient is placed on the regular oral antidiabetic agents, sliding scale insulin, and antibiotic medications. On day 2 of hospitalization, the health care provider orders prednisone therapy. What does the nurse expect the blood glucose to do?
    a. Decrease
    b. Stay the same
    c. Increase
    d. Return to normal

41. Which laboratory test is the best indicator of a patient's average blood glucose level and/or compliance with the DM regimen over the last 3 months?
    a. Postprandial blood glucose test
    b. Oral glucose tolerance test (OGTT)
    c. Casual blood glucose test
    d. Glycosylated hemoglobin (HbA$_{1c}$)

42. A patient with diabetic ketoacidosis is on an insulin drip of 50 units of regular insulin in 250 mL of normal saline. The current blood glucose level is 549 mg/dL. According to insulin protocol, the insulin drip needs to be changed to 8 units per hour. At what rate does the nurse set the pump? _____ mL/hr

43. Which insulins are considered to have a rapid onset of action? (Select all that apply.)
    a. Novolin 70/30
    b. Glulisine
    c. Humulin N
    d. Aspart
    e. Lispro

44. A diabetic patient has just returned from surgery with stable blood glucose levels between 120 and 180 mg/dL. Which IV solution will promote adequate hydration and stable blood glucose levels?
    a. D$_5$1/2 NS at 125 mL/hr
    b. D$_5$W at 125 mL/hr
    c. 0.45% NSS at 100 mL/hr
    d. 0.9% NSS at 100 mL/hr

45. A patient with type 2 DM, usually controlled with a sulfonylurea, develops a urinary tract infection. Due to the stress of the infection, the patient must be treated with insulin. What additional information about this treatment does the nurse relay to the patient?
    a. The sulfonylurea must be discontinued and insulin taken until the infection clears.
    b. Insulin will now be necessary to control the patient's diabetes for life.
    c. The sulfonylurea dose must be reduced until the infection clears.
    d. The insulin is necessary to supplement the sulfonylurea until the infection clears.

Matching. Match each diabetic complication with its corresponding pathophysiology. Answers may be used more than once.

Pathophysiology
a. Nephropathy
b. Neuropathy
c. Retinopathy

Complications
_____ 46. Neovascularization

_____ 47. End-stage kidney disease

_____ 48. Muscle weakness

_____ 49. Proteinuria

_____ 50. Hemorrhage into the eye

_____ 51. Pain or numbness

_____ 52. Hard exudate deposits

_____ 53. Permanent blindness

54. Which statements about sensory alteration in patients with diabetes are accurate? *(Select all that apply.)*
    a. Healing of foot wounds is reduced because of impaired sensation.
    b. Very few patients with diabetic foot ulcers have peripheral sensory neuropathy.
    c. Loss of pain, pressure, and temperature sensation in the foot increases the risk for injury.
    d. Sensory neuropathy causes loss of normal sweating and skin temperature regulation.
    e. It can be delayed by keeping the blood glucose level as close to normal as possible.

55. According to the Diabetes Control and Complication Trial (DCCT) study of type 1 DM patients, intensive therapy with good glucose control resulted in delays in which complications? *(Select all that apply.)*
    a. Macrovascular disease
    b. Cardiovascular disease
    c. Retinopathy
    d. Nephropathy
    e. Neuropathy

Matching. Match the definition with its corresponding foot condition.

Foot Conditions
a. Hallux valgus
b. Claw toe deformity
c. Charcot foot

Definitions
_____ 56. Hyperextended toes causing increased pressure on the ball of the foot

_____ 57. Deformity where the foot is warm, swollen, painful, and walking causes the arch to collapse, giving the foot a "rocker bottom" shape

_____ 58. Turning of the great toe

59. In developing an individualized meal plan for a patient with diabetes, which goals are the focus of the plan? *(Select all that apply.)*
    a. Maintaining blood glucose levels at or as close to the normal range as possible
    b. Patient food preferences
    c. Allowing patients to eat as much as they desire
    d. Patient cultural preferences
    e. Limiting food choices only when guided by scientific evidence

60. What is the basic principle of meal planning for a patient with type 1 DM?
    a. Five small meals per day plus a bedtime snack
    b. Taking extra insulin when planning to eat sweet foods
    c. High-protein, low-carbohydrate, and low-fiber foods
    d. Considering the effects and peak action times of the patient's insulin

61. Which statement about dietary concepts for a patient with diabetes is true?
    a. Alcoholic beverage consumption is unrestricted.
    b. Carbohydrate counting is emphasized when adjusting dietary intake of nutrients.
    c. Sweeteners should be avoided because of the side effects.
    d. Both soluble and insoluble fiber foods should be limited.

62. What is the recommended protocol for patients with type 2 DM who must lose weight?
    a. Participate in an aerobic program twice a week for 20 minutes each session.
    b. Slowly increase insulin dosage until mild hypoglycemia occurs.
    c. Reduce calorie intake moderately and increase exercise.
    d. Reduce daily calorie intake to 1000 calories and monitor urine for ketones.

63. What is the recommended calorie reduction for a patient with diabetes who must lose weight?
    a. 500 calories/week
    b. 1500 calories/week
    c. 2500 calories/week
    d. 3500 calories/week

64. A patient with diabetes who swims for exercise is taught to administer insulin in which area of the body?
    a. Abdomen
    b. Thighs
    c. Arms
    d. Hips

65. The nurse is teaching a patient with diabetes about proper foot care. Which instructions does the nurse include? *(Select all that apply.)*
    a. Use rubbing alcohol to toughen the skin on the soles of the feet.
    b. Wear open-toed shoes or sandals in warm weather to prevent perspiration.
    c. Apply moisturizing cream to the feet after bathing, but not between the toes.
    d. Use cold water for bathing the feet to prevent inadvertent thermal injury.
    e. Do not go barefoot.
    f. Inspect your feet daily.

66. A 25-year-old female patient with type 1 diabetes tells the nurse, "I have two kidneys and I'm still young. I expect to be around for a long time, so why should I worry about my blood sugar?" What is the nurse's best response?
    a. "You have little to worry about as long as your kidneys keep making urine."
    b. "You should discuss this with your physician because you are being unrealistic."
    c. "You would be right if your diabetes was managed with insulin."
    d. "Keeping your blood sugar under control now can help to prevent damage to both kidneys."

67. Self-monitoring of blood glucose levels is most important in which patients? *(Select all that apply.)*
    a. Patients taking multiple daily insulin injections
    b. Patients with mild type 2 diabetes
    c. Patients with hypoglycemic unawareness
    d. Patients using a portable infusion device for insulin administration
    e. Ill patients
    f. Pregnant patients

68. Which statement about sexual intercourse for patients with diabetes is true?
    a. The incidence of sexual dysfunction is lower in men than women.
    b. Retrograde ejaculation does not interfere with male fertility.
    c. Impotence is associated with DM in male patients.
    d. Sexual dysfunction in female patients includes inability to achieve pregnancy.

69. A patient with insulin-dependent diabetes is planning to travel by air and asks the nurse about preparations for the trip. What does the nurse tell the patient to do?
    a. Pack insulin and syringes in a labeled, crushproof kit in the checked luggage.
    b. Carry all necessary diabetes supplies in a clearly identified pack aboard the plane.
    c. Ask the flight attendant to put the insulin in the galley refrigerator once on the plane.
    d. Take only minimal supplies and get the prescription filled at his or her destination.

70. Which statement by a patient with diabetes indicates an understanding of the principles of self-care?
    a. "I don't like the idea of sticking myself so often to measure my sugar."
    b. "I plan to measure the sugar in my urine at least four times a day."
    c. "I plan to get my spouse to exercise with me to keep me company."
    d. "If I get a cold, I can take my regular cough medication until I feel better."

71. After a 2-hour glucose challenge, which result demonstrates impaired glucose tolerance?
    a. Less than 100 mg/dL
    b. Less than 140 mg/dL
    c. Greater than 140 mg/dL
    d. Greater than 250 mg/dL

72. A 50-year-old patient seen in the emergency department (ED) reported nausea, vomiting, and dehydration. When admitted to the hospital, the patient's fasting blood glucose was over 500 mg/dL, and a blood gas showed a pH of 7.38. The patient was diagnosed with diabetes and treated with insulin and fluids. What do these events tell the nurse about the patient?
    a. The diabetes is temporary.
    b. The patient will only require insulin when stressed or ill; the diabetes is temporary.
    c. The pancreas is producing enough insulin to prevent ketoacidosis.
    d. The pancreas is not producing enough insulin to prevent ketoacidosis.

73. A patient with type 2 diabetes often has which laboratory value?
    a. Elevated thyroid studies
    b. Elevated triglycerides
    c. Ketones in the urine
    d. Low hemoglobin

74. A patient has been diagnosed with diabetes. Which aspects does the nurse consider in formulating the teaching plan for this patient? (Select all that apply.)
    a. Covering all needed information in one teaching session
    b. Assessing visual impairment regarding insulin labels and markings on syringes
    c. Assessing manual dexterity to determine if the patient is able to draw insulin into a syringe
    d. Assessing patient motivation to learn and comprehend instructions
    e. Assessing the patient's ability to read printed material

75. Which are signs and symptoms of *mild* hypoglycemia? (Select all that apply.)
    a. Headache
    b. Weakness
    c. Cold, clammy skin
    d. Irritability
    e. Pallor
    f. Tachycardia

76. A patient with type 1 diabetes is taking a mixture of NPH and regular insulin at home. The patient has been NPO for surgery since midnight. What action does the nurse take regarding the patient's morning dose of insulin?
    a. Administer the dose that is routinely prescribed at home because the patient has type 1 diabetes and needs the insulin.
    b. Administer half the dose because the patient is NPO.
    c. Hold the insulin with all the other medications because the patient is NPO and there is no need for insulin.
    d. Contact the health care provider for an order regarding the insulin.

77. The nurse is preparing to administer 20 units of NPH insulin (Humulin N) along with 6 units of regular insulin (Humulin R) to a patient with diabetes. How does the nurse prepare the injection? (Place the steps in order using the numbers 1 through 7.)

    _____ a. Gently roll the NPH insulin vial in the hands.

    _____ b. Wash hands.

    _____ c. Wipe off the tops of the insulin vials with an alcohol pad.

    _____ d. Inject 20 units of air into the NPH insulin vial.

    _____ e. Invert the regular insulin vial and withdraw 8 units of insulin.

    _____ f. Invert the NPH insulin vial and withdraw 20 units of insulin.

    _____ g. Inject 8 units of air into the regular insulin vial.

78. A patient with diabetes has signs and symptoms of hypoglycemia. The patient is alert and oriented with a blood glucose of 56 mg/dL. What does the nurse do next?
    a. Give a glass of orange juice with two packets of sugar and continue to monitor the patient.
    b. Give 8 oz of skim milk and then a carbohydrate and protein snack.
    c. Give a complex carbohydrate and continue to monitor the patient.
    d. Administer D50 IV push and give the patient something to eat.

79. A patient with diabetes has signs and symptoms of hypoglycemia. The patient has a blood glucose of 56 mg/dL, is not alert but responds to voice, and is confused and is unable to swallow fluids. What does the nurse do next?
    a. Give a glass of orange juice with two packets of sugar and continue to monitor the patient.
    b. Give a glass of orange or other type of juice and continue to monitor the patient.
    c. Give a complex carbohydrate and continue to monitor the patient.
    d. Administer D50 IV push.

80. A patient has been receiving insulin in the abdomen for 3 days. On day 4, where does the nurse give the insulin injection?
    a. Deltoid
    b. Thigh
    c. Abdomen, near the navel
    d. Abdomen, but in an area different from the previous day's injection
    e. Abdomen, in the same area as the previous day's injection

81. Place the injection sites in order of speed of absorption using the numbers 1 through 4, with 1 having the fastest absorption and 4 having the slowest absorption.

    _____ a. Buttocks

    _____ b. Abdomen

    _____ c. Deltoid

    _____ d. Thigh

Matching. Match the insulin characteristics with the corresponding types of insulin. Answers may be used more than once.

Types of Insulin
a. Insulin glargine (Lantus)
b. Regular insulin
c. NPH insulin

Insulin Characteristics

_____ 82. This type of insulin does not have a peak time.

_____ 83. This type of insulin is a long-acting insulin analogue given once daily for basal insulin coverage.

_____ 84. When mixing insulins, this type is always drawn up first.

_____ 85. This type of insulin should be given 30 minutes before meals.

_____ 86. This type of insulin should not be diluted or mixed with any other insulin or solution.

CASE STUDY: THE PATIENT WITH DIABETES MELLITUS

Use a separate sheet of paper to answer the questions in this Case Study, or go to the "Prepare for Class" folder on your Evolve website at http://evolve.elsevier.com/Iggy/ to download and complete as a word processing file. Answer guidelines for this Case Study are also available on your Evolve website.

The patient is a 48-year-old unconscious woman admitted to the ED. She has a known history of type 1 diabetes mellitus. Her daughter accompanies her and tells the staff that her mother has had the "flu" and has been unable to eat or drink very much. The daughter is uncertain whether her mother has taken her insulin in the past 24 hours. The patient's vital signs are temperature 101.8° F; pulse 120, weak and irregular; respiration 22, deep, and fruity odor; and blood pressure 80/42 mm Hg. Blood specimens and arterial blood gases are drawn and an IV infusion begun.

1. Based on this patient's history, give the probable changes in laboratory results for serum glucose, serum osmolarity, serum acetone, BUN, arterial pH, and arterial Pco_2. What medical emergency do these data indicate?
2. What type of IV solutions should the nurse be prepared to administer to this patient? What drugs should the nurse be prepared to give? Explain your answers.
3. The patient is placed on continuous cardiac monitoring. What is the rationale for this intervention?
4. During the first 24 hours, what complications should the nurse monitor for in this patient? Why?
5. The patient eventually becomes normoglycemic, regains consciousness, and begins a 1500-calorie diabetic diet. Develop a teaching-learning plan for her about this diet.
6. Before this emergency, this patient had been monitoring urine glucose and ketones for self-care and insulin administration. Her physician prescribes blood glucose monitoring instead of urine testing. What is the rationale for this change?
7. Which aspect of diabetic self-care should the nurse discuss with this patient before her discharge?
8. The patient is to be discharged on a mixed-dose regimen for insulin. She is to receive 10 units regular insulin and 18 units NPH insulin before breakfast and another 5 units regular insulin and 12 units NPH at dinnertime. Develop a teaching-learning plan for these medications.
9. Considering the patient's insulin protocol, the patient should keep in mind what principles about the actions of the insulins she is taking?
10. What should the nurse discuss with this patient about diabetes, insulin, and illness? What can this patient do to prevent future emergency episodes? Consider "Instructions for Sick Day" rules.
11. At 4 PM, the initial finger stick blood glucose result is 642 mg/dL. An insulin drip is ordered to be started at 10 units/hr. The drip is started at 4:20 PM. One hour after initiating the insulin drip the patient's blood glucose level is 502 mg/dL. The drip is left at 10 units/hr per insulin protocol. Use the focus charting method (also known as the DAR method—data, action, response) to document this information.

68 CHAPTER

Assessment of the Renal/Urinary System

STUDY/REVIEW QUESTIONS

Matching. Match the terms with their correct definitions. Not all terms will be used.

Terms
a. Nephron
b. Glomerulus
c. Renin
d. Aldosterone
e. Antidiuretic hormone (ADH)
f. Prostaglandin E_2 (PGE_2)
g. Bradykinin
h. Erythropoietin
i. Vitamin D
j. Glomerular filtration

Definitions
_____ 1. Also known as vasopressin

_____ 2. Series of specialized capillary loops

_____ 3. Acts on distal tubule and collecting duct to increase sodium and water excretion

_____ 4. Needed to absorb calcium in the intestinal tract and to regulate calcium balance

_____ 5. Small hormone that dilates the afferent arteriole and increases capillary membrane permeability to some solutes

6. A patient has sustained a minor kidney injury. Which structure must remain functional in order for urine to be removed from the blood?
   a. Medulla
   b. Nephron
   c. Calyx
   d. Capsule

7. Blood flows into the _____, and through these specialized capillaries, water and small particles are filtered from the blood to make urine.

8. Renin is a hormone that helps regulate which functions? *(Select all that apply.)*
   a. Blood flow
   b. Production of platelets
   c. Glomerular filtration rate (GFR)
   d. Heart rate
   e. Blood pressure

9. Which substance increases kidney reabsorption of sodium and water?
   a. Bradykinins
   b. Aldosterone
   c. Antidiuretic hormone
   d. Renin

10. _____ is a hormone produced in the kidney parenchyma that stimulates the bone marrow to make red blood cells.

11. Which hormone is released from the posterior pituitary and makes the distal convoluted tubule and the collecting duct permeable to water to maximize reabsorption and produce a concentrated urine?
    a. Aldosterone
    b. Vasopressin
    c. Bradykinins
    d. Natriuretic

12. Based on knowledge of the normal function of the kidney, which large particles are not found in the urine because they are too large to filter through the glomerular capillary walls? *(Select all that apply.)*
    a. Blood cells
    b. Albumin
    c. Other proteins
    d. Electrolytes
    e. Water

13. What is the average urine output of a healthy adult for a 24-hour period?
    a. 500 mL to 1000 mL per day
    b. 1500 mL to 2000 mL per day
    c. 3000 mL to 5000 mL per day
    d. 5000 mL to 7000 mL per day

14. Kidney function, in particular the GFR, is compromised when the systolic blood pressure drops below what reading?
    a. 50 mm Hg
    b. 70 mm Hg
    c. 80 mm Hg
    d. 100 mm Hg

15. Damage to which renal structure or tissues can change the actual production of urine?
    a. Kidney parenchyma
    b. Convoluted tubules
    c. Calyces
    d. Ureters

16. A patient has been immobilized for several days after a motor vehicle accident. The nurse encourages ambulation to stimulate the movement of urine through the ureter by what phenomenon?
    a. Peristalsis
    b. Gravity
    c. Pelvic pressure
    d. Backflow

17. Which renal change associated with aging does the nurse expect an older adult patient to report?
    a. Nocturnal polyuria
    b. Micturition
    c. Hematuria
    d. Dysuria

18. An older adult male patient has a history of an enlarged prostate. The patient is most likely to report which symptom associated with this condition?
    a. Inability to sense the urge to void
    b. Difficulty starting the urine stream
    c. Excreting large amounts of very dilute urine
    d. Frequent leakage of small amounts of urine

19. Impairment in the thirst mechanism associated with aging makes an older adult patient more vulnerable to which disorder?
    a. Hypovolemia
    b. Hypocalcemia
    c. Hypokalemia
    d. Hyponatremia

20. The nurse is talking to a group of older women about changes in the urinary system related to aging. What symptom is likely to be the common concern for this group?
    a. Incontinence
    b. Hematuria
    c. Retention
    d. Dysuria

Fill in the blanks.

21. The most important roles of the kidneys are to maintain body fluid _____ and _____, and to filter _____ products for elimination.

22. The kidneys help regulate blood pressure and _____ balance.

23. The kidneys have a rich blood supply and receive _____% to _____% of the total cardiac output.

24. Normal GFR averages _____ mL/min.

25. GFR is controlled by blood _____ and blood _____.

26. _____ increases tubular permeability to water, allowing water to leave the tube and be reabsorbed into the capillaries.

27. Where sodium goes, _____ follows.

28. During water reabsorption, the membrane of
the distal convoluted tubule is more permeable
to water due to the influence of _____
_____.

29. The primary function of the proximal convoluted tubule is _____ of water
and electrolytes.

30. The nurse is taking a history on a 55-year-old
patient who denies any serious chronic health
problems. Which sudden-onset sign/symptom
suggests possible kidney disease in this patient?
   a. Weakness
   b. Hypertension
   c. Confusion
   d. Dysrhythmia

31. Which patient narrative describes the symptom of dysuria?
   a. "I have to pee all the time."
   b. "I have to wait before the pee starts."
   c. "It burns when I pee."
   d. "It feels like I am going to pee in my pants."

32. The nurse and nutritionist are evaluating the
diet and nutritional therapies for a patient with
kidney problems. Blood urea nitrogen (BUN)
levels for this patient are tracked because of the
direct relationship to the intake and metabolism of which substance?
   a. Lipids
   b. Carbohydrates
   c. Protein
   d. Fluids

33. The nurse is taking a history on a patient with
a change in urinary patterns. In addition to
the medical and surgical history, what does the
nurse ask the patient about to complete the assessment? *(Select all that apply.)*
   a. Occupational exposure to toxins
   b. Use of illicit substances, such as cocaine
   c. Financial resources for payment of treatments
   d. Religious beliefs about urination
   e. Potential exposure to sexually transmitted
disease

34. The nurse is determining whether a patient has
a history of hypertension because of the potential for kidney problems. Which question is
best to elicit this information?
   a. "Do you have high blood pressure?"
   b. "Do you take any blood pressure medications?"
   c. "Have you ever been told that your blood
pressure was high?"
   d. "When was the last time you had your
blood pressure checked?"

35. A patient appears very uncomfortable with the
nurse's questions about urinary functions and
patterns. What is the best technique for the
nurse to use to elicit relevant information and
decrease the patient's discomfort?
   a. Defer the questions until a later time.
   b. Direct the questions toward a family member.
   c. Use anatomic or medical terminology.
   d. Use the patient's own terminology.

36. The nurse is taking a nutritional history on a
patient. The patient states, "I really don't drink
as much water as I should." What is the nurse's
best response?
   a. "We should probably all drink more water
than we do."
   b. "It's an easy thing to forget; just try to remember to drink more."
   c. "What would encourage you to drink the
recommended 3 liters per day?"
   d. "I'd like you to read this brochure about
kidney health and fluids."

37. When patients have problems with the kidneys
or urinary tract, what is the most common
symptom that prompts them to seek medical
attention?
   a. Change in the frequency or amount of urination
   b. Pain in flank or abdomen or pain when
urinating
   c. Noticing a change in the color or odor of
the urine
   d. Exposure to a nephrotoxic substance

38. Which ethnic group has the highest risk for end-stage kidney disease secondary to diabetes mellitus and hypertension?
    a. Caucasian Americans
    b. African Americans
    c. Asian Americans
    d. Native Americans

39. Which over-the-counter product used by a patient does the nurse explore further for potential impact on kidney function?
    a. Peroxide-containing mouthwash
    b. Milk of magnesia laxative
    c. Vitamin C
    d. NSAIDs

40. The nurse is performing an assessment of the renal system. What is the first step in the assessment process?
    a. Percuss the lower abdomen; continue toward the umbilicus.
    b. Observe the flank region for asymmetry or discoloration.
    c. Listen for a bruit over each renal artery.
    d. Lightly palpate the abdomen in all quadrants.

41. The nurse is auscultating the renal artery and hears a bruit. What does this finding indicate?
    a. Acute kidney injury
    b. Renal artery stenosis
    c. Renal artery aneurysm
    d. Renal tumor

42. A patient has anorexia, nausea and vomiting, muscle cramping, and pruritus. How does the nurse interpret these findings?
    a. Oliguria
    b. Azotemia
    c. Anuria
    d. Uremia

43. A patient is diagnosed with renal artery stenosis. Which sound does the nurse expect to hear by auscultation when a bruit is present in a renal artery?
    a. Quiet, pulsating sound
    b. Swishing sound
    c. Faint wheezing
    d. No sound at all

44. Which volume of urine does the nurse expect to find documented for a patient who is oliguric?
    a. Between 100 and 400 mL in 24 hours
    b. Greater than 2000 mL in 24 hours
    c. Less than 100 mL in 24 hours
    d. Greater than 400 mL during the night

45. The nurse is assessing a patient for bladder distention. What technique does the nurse use?
    a. Gently palpate for the outline of the bladder, percuss the lower abdomen, continue toward the umbilicus until dull sounds are no longer produced.
    b. Gently palpate for the outline of the bladder, auscultate for sounds in the lower abdomen.
    c. Place one hand under the back and palpate with the other hand over the bladder, percuss the lower abdomen until tympanic sounds are no longer produced.
    d. Use the hand to depress the bladder as the patient takes a deep breath, then percuss.

46. A patient reports flank pain or tenderness. What technique does the nurse use to assess for costovertebral tenderness?
    a. Percuss the nontender flank and assess for rebound.
    b. Thump the CVA area with the flat surface of the hand.
    c. Thump the CVA area with a clenched fist.
    d. Place one hand flat over the CVA area, thump with the other fist.

47. The nurse is preparing to assess a female patient's urethra prior to the insertion of a Foley catheter. In addition to sterile gloves, which equipment does the nurse obtain to perform the initial assessment?
    a. Glass slide
    b. Good light source
    c. Speculum
    d. Cotton swab

48. A female patient who has been running 3 to 4 miles four times a week for the past 2 weeks is being seen for a routine physical. Urinalysis results reveal a protein level of >0.8 mg/dL and a white blood cell count of 4 per high-powered field. What might be the cause of these findings?
   a. Urinary tract infection
   b. Hepatic or biliary disease
   c. Kidney infection
   d. Strenuous exercise

49. Ketones in the urine may indicate which occurrence or process? *(Select all that apply.)*
   a. Incomplete metabolism of fatty acids
   b. Increased glomerular membrane permeability
   c. Kidney disease
   d. Body's use of fat instead of glucose for cellular energy
   e. Urinary tract infection

Matching. *Match each urine specimen finding with its corresponding characteristic.*

Findings
a. Color
b. Odor
c. Turbidity
d. Specific gravity
e. pH
f. Glucose
g. Protein
h. Microalbuminuria
i. Sediment
j. Cells
k. Cast
l. Crystals
m. Bacteria

Characteristics
_____ 50. Less than 7 acidic, greater than 7 alkaline

_____ 51. Only identified by microscopic examination for protein

_____ 52. Structure found around cell, bacteria, protein, and clumps

_____ 53. Urine is normally sterile; these multiply and grow

_____ 54. Urochrome pigment

_____ 55. 1.005 to 1.030

_____ 56. Not normally in the urine

_____ 57. Cells, casts, crystals, and bacteria

_____ 58. Various salts

_____ 59. Epithelial cells, RBC, WBC, tubular cells

_____ 60. Not seen in urine until blood sugar above 220 mg/dL

_____ 61. Cloudiness or haziness

_____ 62. Faint ammonia

63. The nurse is caring for a patient with dehydration. Which laboratory test results does the nurse anticipate to see for this patient?
   a. BUN and creatinine ratio stay the same.
   b. BUN rises faster than creatinine level.
   c. Creatinine rises faster than BUN.
   d. BUN and creatinine have a direct relationship.

64. What does the BUN test measure?
   a. Kidney excretion of urea nitrogen
   b. GFR
   c. Creatinine clearance
   d. Urine output

65. Which patient is most likely to have a decreased calcium level?
    a. Patient with nephritis
    b. Patient with cystitis
    c. Patient with a Foley catheter
    d. Patient with urinary retention

66. The nurse performs a dipstick urine test for a patient being evaluated for kidney problems. Glucose is present in the urine. How does the nurse interpret this result?
    a. Blood glucose level is greater than 220 mg/dL.
    b. The kidneys are failing to filter any glucose.
    c. The patient is at risk for hypoglycemia.
    d. The renal threshold has not been exceeded.

67. In addition to kidney disease, which patient condition causes the BUN to rise above the normal range?
    a. Anemia
    b. Asthma
    c. Infection
    d. Malnutrition

68. The community health nurse is talking to a group of African-American adults about renal health. The nurse encourages the participants to have which type of yearly examination to screen for kidney problems?
    a. Kidney ultrasound
    b. Serum creatinine and blood urea nitrogen
    c. Urinalysis and microalbuminuria
    d. 24-hour urine collection

69. Which test is the best indicator of kidney function?
    a. Urine osmolarity
    b. Serum creatinine
    c. Urine pH
    d. Color of urine

70. In relation to kidney problems, what does an increase in the ratio of BUN to serum creatinine indicate?
    a. Highly suggestive of kidney dysfunction
    b. Definitive for kidney dysfunction
    c. Suggests nonkidney factors causing an elevation in BUN
    d. Suggests nonkidney factors causing an elevation in serum creatinine

71. Which urine characteristic listed on a urinalysis report arouses the nurse's suspicion of a problem in the urinary tract?
    a. Cloudiness
    b. Straw color
    c. Ammonia odor
    d. One cast per high-powered field

72. A patient has a urinalysis ordered. When is the best time for the nurse to collect the specimen?
    a. In the evening
    b. After a meal
    c. In the morning
    d. After a fluid bolus

73. During the day, the nursing student is measuring urine output and observing for urine characteristics in a patient. Which abnormal finding in the urine is the most urgent finding that must be reported to the supervising nurse?
    a. Specific gravity is decreased.
    b. Output is decreased.
    c. pH is decreased.
    d. Color has changed.

74. A 24-hour urine specimen is required from a patient. Which strategy is best to ensure that all the urine is collected for the full 24-hour period?
    a. Instruct the unlicensed assistive personnel (UAP) to collect all the urine.
    b. Put a bedpan or commode next to the bed as a reminder.
    c. Place a sign in the bathroom reminding the patient to save the urine.
    d. Verbally remind the patient about the test.

75. Place the steps of using a bedside bladder scanner in the correct order using the numbers 1 through 8.

_____ a. Select the male or female icon on the bladder scanner.

_____ b. Aim the scan head towards the expected location of the bladder.

_____ c. Place the probe midline about 1.5 inches (4 cm) above the pubic bone.

_____ d. Explain the purpose and what sensations to expect.

_____ e. Listen for the sound of a beep and a volume display.

_____ f. Place the ultrasound probe with gel right above the symphysis pubis.

_____ g. Press and release the scan button.

_____ h. Repeat for best accuracy.

76. A patient is scheduled for an IV urography. Which medication is discontinued at the time of the procedure and for at least 48 hours until kidney function has been re-evaluated?
    a. Glucophage (Metformin)
    b. Diphenhydramine (Benadryl)
    c. Prednisone (Deltasone)
    d. Acetylcysteine (Mucomyst)

77. Several patients are scheduled for testing to diagnose potential kidney problems. Which test requires a patient to have a urinary catheter inserted before the test?
    a. IV urography
    b. Computed tomography
    c. Cystography
    d. Kidney scan

78. A patient has had an IV urography. What is included in the postprocedural care for this patient?
    a. Bowel cleansing with laxatives
    b. IV or oral fluid hydration
    c. Administration of captopril (Capoten)
    d. Insertion of a urinary catheter

79. Which diagnostic test incorporates contrast dye, but does not place a patient at risk for nephrotoxicity?
    a. IV urography
    b. Renal angiography
    c. Voiding cystourethrogram
    d. Computed tomography

80. The nurse is reviewing the results of a patient's ultrasound of the kidney. The report reveals an enlarged kidney which suggests which possible problem?
    a. Polycystic kidney
    b. Kidney infection
    c. Renal carcinoma
    d. Chronic kidney disease

81. A patient returns to the unit after a kidney scan. Which instruction about the patient's urine does the nurse give to the UAP caring for the patient?
    a. It is radioactive, so it should be handled with special biohazard precautions.
    b. It does not place anyone at risk because of the small amount of radioactive material.
    c. Its radioactivity is dangerous only to those who are pregnant.
    d. It is potentially dangerous if allowed to sit for prolonged periods in the commode.

82. The nurse is alerted by the radiology department that a patient had a "captopril renal scan." What does the nurse monitor for when the patient returns from the procedure?
    a. Cardiac dysrhythmias
    b. Urine discoloration
    c. Signs of dehydration
    d. Orthostatic hypotension

83. The nurse is teaching a patient scheduled for an ultrasonography. What preprocedural instruction does the nurse give the patient?
    a. Void just before the test begins.
    b. Drink a of lot water.
    c. Stop routine medications.
    d. Complete a bowel preparation.

84. A patient had a cystoscopy. After the procedure, what does the nurse expect to see in this patient?
    a. Pink-tinged urine
    b. Bloody urine
    c. Very dilute urine
    d. Decreased urine output

85. A patient is scheduled for retrograde urethrography. Postprocedural care is similar to postprocedural care given for which test?
    a. Ultrasonography
    b. Computed tomography
    c. IV urography
    d. Cystoscopy

86. A patient has undergone a kidney biopsy. What does the nurse monitor for in the patient related to this procedure?
    a. Nephrotoxicity
    b. Hemorrhage
    c. Urinary retention
    d. Hypertension

87. A patient has undergone a kidney biopsy. In the immediate postprocedural period, the nurse notifies the health care provider about which findings? *(Select all that apply.)*
    a. Hematuria
    b. Localized pain at the site
    c. "Tamponade effect"
    d. Decreasing urine output
    e. Flank pain
    f. Decreasing blood pressure

CASE STUDY: ASSESSING THE RENAL/URINARY SYSTEM IN THE OLDER ADULT

Use a separate sheet of paper to answer the questions in this Case Study, or go to the "Prepare for Class" folder on your Evolve website at http://evolve.elsevier.com/Iggy/ to download and complete as a word processing file. Answer guidelines for this Case Study are also available on your Evolve website.

A 74-year-old man comes to the clinic for changes in urinary patterns. He reports, "I am pretty healthy for my age. I do have some of the typical problems that all old folks have, but nothing serious." The patient describes having difficulty starting his urine stream and has to get up two times during the night to void. The patient denies having any burning on urination. His urine specimen is clear, yellow, and without any foul odor.

1. What types of questions would the nurse ask using Gordon's functional assessment?

2. Identify changes related to aging and appropriate nursing interventions for older adults with regard to the renal system.

3. The patient is scheduled to have a series of urologic studies for diagnostic purposes. The physician orders the following: urinalysis, urine for culture and sensitivity, BUN, serum creatine, and 24-hour urine for creatinine clearance. The tests will be conducted on an outpatient basis. Describe what the nurse should do to instruct the patient in the collection of these laboratory specimens.

4. Which specimens should be collected first?

5. The patient returns the collection container with a 24-hour urine specimen to the physician's office. As he gives it to the nurse, he comments, "I had a hard time remembering to save it all. Actually, I think I missed some when I forgot and used a bathroom at the shopping mall yesterday." What should the nurse do?

6. Further tests are ordered for the patient, including a kidney ultrasound and IV pyelography (IVP). These are scheduled at an outpatient radiology clinic. Design a teaching-learning plan for the patient to prepare him for these studies.

7. Following the ultrasound and IVP, what assessments should be made for the patient?

8. Document a nursing note for the patient using the SBAR format.

Care of Patients with Urinary Problems

STUDY/REVIEW QUESTIONS

Matching. *Match the terms with their correct definitions.*

Terms

a. Cystitis
b. Bacteriuria
c. Colonization
d. *Escherichia coli*
e. Urosepsis
f. Frequency
g. Dysuria
h. Urgency
i. Trabeculation
j. Hunner's ulcers
k. Pyuria
l. Cystocele

Definitions

_____ 1. Bacteria in the urine

_____ 2. Urge to urinate frequently in small amounts

_____ 3. Inflammation of the bladder

_____ 4. Feeling that urination will occur immediately

_____ 5. Bacteriuria is without symptoms of infection

_____ 6. White blood cells (WBCs) in the urine

_____ 7. Causes about 90% of urinary tract infections (UTIs)

_____ 8. Type of bladder lesion

_____ 9. Pain or burning with urination

_____ 10. Abnormal thickening of the bladder wall caused by urinary retention and obstruction

_____ 11. Herniation of the bladder into the vagina

_____ 12. Spread of the infection from the urinary tract to the bloodstream

13. The nurse is caring for a patient with an indwelling catheter. What interventions does the nurse use to minimize catheter-related infections? *(Select all that apply.)*
    a. Consider appropriate alternatives to an indwelling catheter.
    b. Use sterile technique for daily routine handling of equipment.
    c. Select the largest catheter available.
    d. Apply antiseptic solutions or antibiotic ointments to the perineal area.
    e. Maintain a closed system irrigation by ensuring connections are sealed securely.
    f. Irrigate the catheter daily.
    g. Keep urine collection bags below the level of the bladder at all times.

14. The most common prevalence of UTIs is seen in which patient group?
    a. Young men
    b. Older women
    c. Older men
    d. School-aged girls

15. Noninfectious _____ is caused by irritation from chemicals or radiation.

16. About _____% of patients with indwelling catheters become infected within 1 week of insertion.

17. Patients who have central nervous system lesions from stroke, multiple sclerosis, or parasacral spinal cord lesions may have which type of urinary incontinence?
    a. Detrusor hyperreflexia
    b. Mixed
    c. Stress
    d. Functional

18. A patient reports intense urgency, frequency, and bladder pain. Urinalysis results show WBCs and RBCs and urine culture results are negative for infection. How does the nurse interpret these findings?
    a. Interstitial cystitis
    b. Urethritis
    c. Bacteriuria
    d. Infectious cystitis

19. The nurse is teaching a patient about bladder and urinary health. What information does the nurse include? *(Select all that apply.)*
    a. Have a minimal fluid intake of 3 L daily, unless contraindicated.
    b. Drink more water rather than sugar-containing drinks.
    c. Avoid urinary stasis by urinating every 6 to 8 hours.
    d. Bathe daily or thoroughly wash the perineal and urethral areas.
    e. Avoid straining or pushing when expelling urine.

20. A patient has been started on oxybutynin (Ditropan) for urinary incontinence. What is the major action of this medication?
    a. Increases blood flow to and tone of the urethra
    b. Blocks acetylcholine receptors
    c. Causes slight numbing of the bladder
    d. Relaxes bladder muscles

21. A young female patient reports experiencing burning with urination. What question does the nurse ask to differentiate between a vaginal infection and a urinary infection?
    a. "Have you noticed any blood in the urine?"
    b. "Have you had recent sexual intercourse?"
    c. "Have you noticed any vaginal discharge?"
    d. "Have you been voiding less frequently?"

22. A patient reports symptoms indicating a UTI. The nurse obtains an order for which diagnostic test to verify a UTI?
    a. Urine culture and sensitivity
    b. Urinalysis for white and red blood cells
    c. Complete blood count
    d. Voiding cystourethrography

23. A patient is diagnosed with a fungal UTI. Which drug does the nurse anticipate the patient will be treated with?
    a. Sulfa drugs
    b. Cephalosporins
    c. Ketoconazole
    d. Quinolones

24. The nurse is teaching a patient about self-care measures to prevent UTIs. Which daily fluid intake does the nurse recommend to the patient to prevent a bladder infection?
    a. 2 to 3 L of water
    b. 3 to 6 glasses of iced tea
    c. 4 to 6 cups of electrolyte fluid
    d. 3 to 4 glasses of juice

25. The nursing student sees an order for a urinalysis for a patient with frequency, urgency, and dysuria. In order to collect the specimen, what does the student do?
    a. Use sterile technique to insert a small-diameter (6 Fr) catheter.
    b. Instruct the patient on how to collect a clean-catch specimen.
    c. Tell the patient to urinate approximately 10 mL into a specimen cup.
    d. Take the urine from a bedpan and transfer it into a specimen cup.

26. The nurse is reviewing the laboratory results for an older adult patient with an indwelling catheter. The urine culture is pending, but the urinalysis shows greater than 10^5 colony-forming units, and the differential WBC count shows a "left shift." How does the nurse interpret these findings?
    a. Interstitial cystitis
    b. Urosepsis
    c. Complicated cystitis
    d. Radiation-induced cystitis

27. A patient has UTI symptoms but there are no bacteria in the urine. The physician suspects interstitial cystitis. The nurse prepares patient teaching material for which diagnostic test?
    a. Urography
    b. Abdominal sonography
    c. Computed tomography (CT)
    d. Cystoscopy

28. The cystoscopy results for a patient include a small-capacity bladder, the presence of Hunner's ulcers, and small hemorrhages after bladder distention. How does the nurse interpret this report?
    a. Urosepsis
    b. Complicated infection cystitis
    c. Interstitial cystitis
    d. Urethritis

29. Several patients at the clinic have just been diagnosed with UTIs. Which patients may need to be hospitalized? *(Select all that apply.)*
    a. Postmenopausal patient
    b. Patient with a long-term indwelling catheter
    c. Diabetic patient
    d. Immunosuppressed patient
    e. Pregnant patient

30. The nurse is counseling a patient with recurrent cystitis about dietary therapy. What information does the nurse give to the patient?
    a. Drink 50 mL of concentrated cranberry juice every day.
    b. Limit calorie intake during peaks of infection.
    c. Caffeine, carbonated beverages, and tomato products cause cystitis.
    d. Cranberry tablets are more effective than juice or fluids.

31. A patient received an antibiotic prescription several hours ago and has started the medication, but states needing "some relief from the burning." What comfort measures does the nurse suggest to the patient?
    a. Take over-the-counter acetaminophen.
    b. Sit in a sitz bath and urinate into the warm water.
    c. Place a cold pack over the perineal area.
    d. Rest in a recumbent position with legs elevated.

32. A patient's recurrent cystitis appears to be related to sexual intercourse. The patient seems uncomfortable talking about the situation. What communication technique does the nurse use to assist the patient?
    a. Have a frank and sensitive discussion with the patient.
    b. Give the patient reading material with instructions to call with any questions.
    c. Call the patient's partner and invite the partner to discuss the problem.
    d. Talk about other topics until the patient feels more comfortable disclosing.

33. A male college student comes to the clinic reporting burning or difficulty with urination and a discharge from the urethral meatus. Based on the patient's chief complaint, what is the most logical question for the nurse to ask about the patient's past medical history?
    a. "Do you have a history of a narrow urethra or a stricture?"
    b. "Could you have been exposed to a sexually transmitted disease (STD)?"
    c. "Do you have a history of kidney stones?"
    d. "Have you been drinking an adequate amount of fluids?"

34. A patient is diagnosed with urethral stricture. What findings does the nurse expect to see documented in the patient's chart for this condition?
    a. Pain on urination
    b. Pain on ejaculation
    c. Overflow incontinence
    d. Hematuria and pyuria

35. A patient is diagnosed with a urethral stricture. The nurse prepares the patient for which temporary treatment?
    a. Dilation of the urethra
    b. Antibiotic therapy
    c. Fluid restriction
    d. Urinary diversion

36. A patient reports the loss of small amounts of urine during coughing, sneezing, jogging, or lifting. Which type of incontinence do these symptoms describe?
    a. Urge
    b. Overflow
    c. Functional
    d. Stress

37. The nurse is caring for an obese older adult patient with dementia. The patient is alert and ambulatory, but has functional incontinence. Which nursing intervention is best for this patient?
    a. Help the patient to lose weight.
    b. Help the patient apply an estrogen cream.
    c. Offer assistance with toileting every 2 hours.
    d. Intermittently catheterize the patient.

38. Which patient is mostly likely to have mixed incontinence?
    a. Older woman who had four full-term pregnancies
    b. Patient with a stroke who has neurologic deficits
    c. Patient with benign prostatic hyperplasia
    d. Patient with a pelvic fracture

39. The nurse is caring for an older adult patient with urinary incontinence. The patient is alert and oriented, but refuses to use the call bell and has fallen several times while trying to get to the bathroom. What is the nurse's priority concern for this patient?
    a. Managing severe confusion
    b. Accurately measuring urinary output
    c. Providing fall prevention measures
    d. Managing urinary incontinence

40. The nurse is performing an assessment on a patient with probable stress incontinence. Which assessment technique does the nurse use to validate stress incontinence?
    a. Assess the abdomen to estimate bladder fullness.
    b. Check for residual urine using a portable ultrasound.
    c. Catheterize the patient immediately after voiding.
    d. Ask the patient to cough while wearing a perineal pad.

41. The advanced-practice nurse is performing a digital rectal examination (DRE) and notes that the rectal sphincter contracts on digital insertion. How does the nurse interpret this finding?
    a. Nerve supply to the bladder is most likely intact.
    b. Adequate strength in the pelvic floor.
    c. A rectocele is placing pressure on the bladder.
    d. Normal function for the bowel and bladder.

42. A middle-aged patient has urinary stress incontinence related to weak pelvic muscles. The patient is highly motivated to participate in self-care. Which interventions does the nurse include in the treatment plan? *(Select all that apply.)*
    a. Keep a detailed diary of urine leakage, activities, and foods eaten.
    b. Wear absorbent pads and undergarments during the assessment process.
    c. Teach pelvic floor (Kegel) exercise therapy.
    d. Teach about vaginal cone therapy.
    e. Drink orange juice every day for 4 to 6 weeks.
    f. Refer to a nutritionist for diet therapy for weight reduction.

43. A patient has been performing Kegel exercises for 2 months. How does the nurse know whether the exercises are working?
    a. Incontinence is still present, but the patient states that it is less.
    b. The patient is able to stop the urinary stream.
    c. There are no complaints of urgency from the patient.
    d. The patient is using absorbent undergarments for protection.

44. The home health nurse is assessing an older adult patient who refuses to leave the house to see friends or participate in usual activities. She reports taking a bath several times a day and becomes very upset when she has an incontinent episode. What is the priority problem for this patient?
    a. Negative self-image
    b. Stress Urinary Incontinence
    c. Social Isolation
    d. Potential for skin breakdown

45. The nurse is evaluating outcome criteria for a patient being treated for urge incontinence. Which statement indicates the treatment has been successful?
    a. "I'm following the prescribed therapy, but I think surgery is my best choice."
    b. "I still lose a little urine when I sneeze, but I have been wearing a thin pad."
    c. "I had trouble at first, but now I go to the toilet every 3 hours."
    d. "I have been using the bladder compression technique and it works."

46. The nurse is teaching a patient with urge incontinence about dietary modifications. What is the best information the nurse gives to the patient about fluid intake?
    a. Drink at least 2000 mL per day unless contraindicated.
    b. Drink 120 mL every hour or 240 mL every 2 hours and limit fluids after dinner.
    c. Drink fluid freely in the morning hours, but limit intake before going to bed.
    d. Drinking water is especially good for bladder health.

47. A patient has agreed to try a bladder training program. What is the priority nursing intervention in starting this therapy?
    a. Start a schedule for voiding (e.g., every 30 minutes).
    b. Teach the patient to be alert, aware, and able to resist the urge to urinate.
    c. Convince the patient that he or she controls the bladder; the bladder does not control the patient.
    d. Give a thorough explanation of the problem of urge incontinence.

48. An older adult patient with a cognitive impairment is living in an extended-care facility. The patient is incontinent, but as the family points out, "he will urinate in the toilet if somebody helps him." Which type of incontinence does the nurse suspect in this patient?
    a. Urge
    b. Overflow
    c. Functional
    d. Stress

49. The nurse is designing a habit training bladder program for an older adult patient who is alert but mildly confused. What task associated with the training program is delegated to the unlicensed assistive personnel (UAP)?
    a. Tell the patient it is time to go to the toilet and assist him to go on a regular schedule.
    b. Help the patient record the incidents of incontinence in a bladder diary.
    c. Change the patient's incontinence pants (or pad) every 2 hours.
    d. Gradually encourage independence and increase the intervals between voidings.

50. Which patient with incontinence is most likely to benefit from a surgical intervention?
    a. Patient with vaginal atrophy and altered urethral competency
    b. Patient with reflex (overflow) incontinence caused by obstruction
    c. Patient with stress incontinence caused by coughing and sneezing
    d. Patients with urge incontinence or overactive bladder

51. The nurse is teaching a patient a behavioral intervention for bladder compression. In order to correctly perform the Credé method, what does the nurse teach the patient to do?
    a. Insert the fingers into the vagina and gently push against the vaginal wall.
    b. Breathe in deeply and direct the pressure towards the bladder during exhalation.
    c. Empty the bladder, wait a few minutes, and attempt a second bladder emptying.
    d. Apply firm and steady pressure over the bladder area with the palm of the hand.

52. The physician has recommended intermittent self-catheterization for a patient with long-term problems of incomplete bladder emptying. Which information does the nurse give the patient about the procedure?
    a. Perform proper handwashing and cleaning of the catheter to reduce the risk for infection.
    b. Use a large lumen catheter and good lubrication for rapid emptying of the bladder.
    c. Catheterize yourself whenever the bladder gets distended.
    d. Use sterile technique, especially if catheterization is done by a family member.

53. The nurse is reviewing a care plan for a patient who has functional incontinence. There is a note that containment is recommended, especially at night. What is the major concern with this approach?
    a. Skin integrity
    b. Cost of care and materials
    c. Self-esteem of the patient
    d. Fall risk

54. The nurse is caring for a patient with functional incontinence. The UAP reports that "the linens have been changed four times within the past 6 hours, but the patient refuses to wear a diaper." What does the nurse do next?
    a. Thank the UAP for the hard work and advise to continue to change the linens.
    b. Call the health care provider to obtain an order for an indwelling catheter.
    c. Instruct the UAP to stop using the word "diaper" and instead use "incontinence pants."
    d. Assess the patient for any new urinary problems and ask about toileting preferences.

55. Which dietary changes does the nurse suggest to a patient with stress incontinence?
    a. Limit fluid intake to no more than 2 L/day.
    b. Peel all fruit before consuming.
    c. Avoid alcohol and caffeine.
    d. Avoid smoked or salted foods.

56. A patient is considering vaginal cone therapy, but is a little hesitant because she does not understand how it works. What does the nurse tell her about how vaginal cone therapy improves incontinence?
    a. It mechanically obstructs urine loss from the urethra.
    b. It repositions the bladder to reduce compression.
    c. It increases the normal flora of the perineum.
    d. It strengthens pelvic floor muscles.

57. A patient with urinary incontinence is prescribed oxybutynin (Ditropan). What precautions or instructions does the nurse provide related to this therapy?
    a. Avoid aspirin or aspirin-containing products.
    b. Increase fluids and dietary fiber intake.
    c. Report any unusual vaginal bleeding.
    d. Change positions slowly, especially in the morning.

58. Teaching intermittent self-catheterization for incontinence is appropriate for which patient?
    a. 25-year-old male patient with paraplegia
    b. 35-year-old female patient with stress incontinence
    c. 70-year-old patient who wears absorbent briefs
    d. 18-year-old patient with a severe head injury

59. Limiting fluid intake can have what effects on incontinence? *(Select all that apply.)*
    a. Increases the osmolarity and concentration of urine
    b. Makes the urine less irritating
    c. Decreases the risk for incontinence
    d. Makes the urine more irritating
    e. Increases the urge to urinate

60. What role does drug therapy have as an intervention for reflex urinary incontinence?
    a. Medications have no effect.
    b. Sulfa drugs help prevent UTIs with this type of incontinence.
    c. Sodium bicarbonate is used sometimes after surgery.
    d. Cholinergic agents may be used short-term after surgery.

61. A patient is admitted for an elective orthopedic surgical procedure. The patient also has a personal and family history for urolithiasis. Which circumstance creates the greatest risk for recurrent urolithiasis?
    a. Giving the patient milk with every meal tray
    b. Keeping the patient NPO for extended periods
    c. Giving the patient an opioid narcotic for pain
    d. Inserting an indwelling catheter for the procedure

62. A patient reports severe flank pain. The report indicates that urine is turbid, malodorous, and rust-colored; RBCs, WBCs, and bacteria are present; and microscopic analysis shows crystals. What does this data suggest?
    a. Pyuria and cystitis
    b. Staghorn calculus with infection
    c. Urolithiasis and infection
    d. Dysuria and urinary retention

63. A patient reports severe flank pain, bladder distention, and nausea and vomiting with increasingly smaller amounts of urine with frank blood. The patient states, "I have kidney stones and I just need some pain medication." What is the nurse's priority concern?
    a. Controlling the patient's pain
    b. Checking the quantity of blood in the urine
    c. Flushing the kidneys with oral fluids
    d. Determining if there is an obstruction

64. The nurse is caring for a patient with a urolithiasis. Which medication is likely given in the acute phase to relieve the patient's severe pain?
    a. Ketorolac (Toradol)
    b. Oxybutynin chloride (Ditropan)
    c. Propantheline bromide (Pro-Banthine)
    d. Morphine sulfate

65. A patient returns to the medical-surgical unit after having extracorporeal shock wave lithotripsy (ESWL). What is an appropriate nursing intervention for the postprocedural care of this patient?
   a. Strain the urine to monitor the passage of stone fragments.
   b. Report bruising that occurs on the flank of the affected side.
   c. Continuously monitor ECG for dysrhythmias.
   d. Apply a local anesthetic cream to the skin of the affected side.

66. The nurse is teaching self-care measures to a patient who had lithotripsy for kidney stones. What information does the nurse include? *(Select all that apply.)*
   a. Finish the entire prescription of antibiotics to prevent UTIs.
   b. Balance regular exercise with sleep and rest.
   c. Drink at least 3 L of fluid a day.
   d. Watch for and immediately report bruising after lithotripsy.
   e. Urine may be bloody for several days.
   f. Pain in the region of the kidneys or bladder is expected.
   g. Report pain, fever, chills, or difficulty with urination to the health care provider.

67. A patient with a history of kidney stones presents with severe flank pain, nausea, vomiting, pallor, and diaphoresis. He reports freely passing urine, but it is bloody. The priority for nursing care is to monitor for which patient problem?
   a. Possible dehydration
   b. Impaired tissue perfusion
   c. Impaired urinary elimination
   d. Severe Pain

68. Which clinical manifestation indicates to the nurse that the management intervention for a patient with a kidney stone is effective?
   a. Urine is blood-tinged.
   b. Pulse rate is 75 beats/min.
   c. Urine output is 50 mL/min.
   d. Pulse oximeter reading is 94%.

69. The urine output of a patient with a kidney stone has decreased from 40 mL/hr to 5 mL/hr. What is the nurse's priority action?
   a. Ensure IV access and notify the physician.
   b. Perform the Credé maneuver on the patient's bladder.
   c. Test the urine for ketone bodies.
   d. Document the finding and continue monitoring.

Matching. *Indicate which intervention is most appropriate for each type of stone.*

Interventions
a. Captopril
b. Thiazide diuretic
c. Sodium bicarbonate
d. Pyridoxine

Types of Stones
_____ 70. Calcium-containing stone
_____ 71. Uric acid-containing stone
_____ 72. Oxalate-containing stone
_____ 73. Cysteine-containing stone

74. Which patient has the highest risk for bladder cancer?
    a. 60-year-old male patient with chronic alcoholism
    b. 25-year-old male patient with type 1 diabetes mellitus
    c. 60-year-old female patient who smokes two packs of cigarettes per day and works in a chemical factory
    d. 25-year-old female patient who has had three episodes of bacterial *(Escherichia coli)* cystitis in the past year

75. The employee health nurse is conducting a presentation for employees who work in a paint manufacturing plant. In order to protect against bladder cancer, the nurse advises that everyone who works with chemicals should do what?
    a. Shower with mild soap and rinse well before they come to work.
    b. Use personal protective equipment such as gloves and masks.
    c. Limit their exposure to chemicals and fumes at all times.
    d. Avoid hobbies such as furniture refinishing that further expose to chemicals.

76. The nurse is talking to a 68-year-old male patient who is a smoker and has a long history of occupational exposure to toxic chemicals. Because this patient has a high risk for bladder cancer, the nurse is concerned about which urinary complaint?
    a. Frequency
    b. Nocturia
    c. Painless hematuria
    d. Incontinence

77. A patient has had surgery for bladder cancer. To prevent recurrence of superficial bladder cancer, the nurse anticipates that the physician is likely to recommend which treatment?
    a. No treatment is needed for this benign condition.
    b. Intravesical instillation of a single-agent chemotherapy.
    c. Radiation therapy to the bladder, ureters, and urethra.
    d. Intravesical instillation of bacille Calmette-Guérin.

78. Which statement by a patient indicates effective coping with a Kock's pouch?
    a. "I don't have any discomfort, but the pouch frequently overflows."
    b. "My wife has been irrigating the pouch daily. She likes to do it."
    c. "I check the pouch every 2 to 3 hours depending on my fluid and diet."
    d. "I wash the pouch every day, just like they told me to do in the hospital."

79. A patient has had a bladder suspension and a suprapubic catheter is in place. The patient wants to know how long the catheter will remain in place. What is the nurse's best response?
    a. "Typically it remains for 24 hours postoperatively."
    b. "It will be removed at your first clinic visit."
    c. "When you can void on your own, it will be removed."
    d. "When you can void and the residual urine is less than 50 mL."

80. A patient is returning from the postanesthesia care unit after surgery for bladder cancer resulting in a cutaneous ureterostomy. Where does the nurse expect the stoma to be located?
    a. On the perineum
    b. At the beltline
    c. On the posterior flank
    d. In the midabdominal area

CASE STUDY: THE PATIENT WITH URINARY INCONTINENCE

Use a separate sheet of paper to answer the questions in this Case Study, or go to the "Prepare for Class" folder on your Evolve website at http://evolve.elsevier.com/Iggy/ to download and complete as a word processing file. Answer guidelines for this Case Study are also available on your Evolve website.

The patient is a 45-year-old female who has had several full-term pregnancies. She is active and generally healthy, saying, "I take good care of myself." She comes to the clinic for advice about "losing a little urine when I laugh." She reports voiding between 6 and 10 times a day depending on fluid intake. She denies dysuria, back pain, hematuria, fever, or vaginal discharge.

1. What should be included in the assessment of a patient with incontinence?

2. What are the most common types of urinary incontinence? Which type is the patient most likely to have?

3. Why is this patient a good candidate for Kegel exercises? What information should the nurse give about performing the exercises?

4. What topics would the nurse include in the teaching plan for this patient?

5. Document a nursing note for the patient using a systems format.

Care of Patients with Renal Disorders

STUDY/REVIEW QUESTIONS

1. A patient's parent has the autosomal dominant form of polycystic kidney disease (PKD). Which abnormal vital sign is the greatest concern for the nurse to follow up with because of the family history of PKD?
   a. Pulse of 100 beats/min
   b. Temperature of 100.6° F
   c. Blood pressure of 130/84 mm Hg
   d. Respiratory rate of 22/min

2. Which descriptions about the autosomal recessive gene trait of PKD are correct? *(Select all that apply.)*
   a. Both parents must carry a mutated allele; and both mutated alleles must be inherited.
   b. Half of people with this form of PKD develop kidney failure by age 50.
   c. Most people with this form of PKD die in early childhood.
   d. One parent must carry a mutated allele that is inherited.
   e. A child has a 1 in 4 chance of inheriting autosomal PKD.

3. Which descriptions about the autosomal dominant gene trait of PKD are correct? *(Select all that apply.)*
   a. 25% of patients with this form of PKD develop kidney failure by age 30.
   b. This is the most common form of PKD.
   c. Half of people with this form of PKD develop kidney failure by age 50.
   d. Nearly 100% of people who inherit a PKD gene will develop kidney cysts by age 50.
   e. Most people with this form of PKD die in young adulthood.

4. The nurse is interviewing a patient with suspected PKD. What questions does the nurse ask the patient? *(Select all that apply.)*
   a. "Is there any family history of PKD or kidney disease?"
   b. "At what age was your parent diagnosed with PKD?"
   c. "Have you had any constipation or abdominal discomfort?"
   d. "Have you noticed a change in urine color or frequency?"
   e. "Do you have a history of sexually transmitted disease?"
   f. "Is there a family history of sudden death from a myocardial infarction?"
   g. "Have you had any problems with headaches?"

5. A patient has a family history of autosomal dominant form of PKD and has therefore been advised to monitor for and report symptoms. What is an early symptom of PKD?
   a. Headache
   b. Pruritus
   c. Edema
   d. Nocturia

6. A patient reports dull, aching pain and the urinalysis is negative for infection. The nurse identifies that the pain is chronic related to enlarging kidneys compressing abdominal contents. What nursing intervention is best for this patient?
   a. Administer trimethoprim/sulfamethoxazole (Bactrim).
   b. Apply dry heat to the abdomen or flank.
   c. Teach methods of relaxation such as deep-breathing.
   d. Administer around-the-clock NSAIDs.

7. Why may a patient with PKD experience constipation?
   a. Polycystic kidneys enlarge and put pressure on the large intestine.
   b. Patient becomes dehydrated because the kidneys are dysfunctional.
   c. Constipation is a side effect from the medications given to treat PKD.
   d. Patients with PKD have special dietary restrictions that cause constipation.

8. The nurse is developing a teaching plan for a patient with PKD. Which topics does the nurse include? *(Select all that apply.)*
   a. Teach how to measure and record blood pressure.
   b. Assist to develop a schedule for self-administering drugs.
   c. Instruct to take and record weight twice a month.
   d. Teach to keep blood pressure records.
   e. Explain the potential side effects of the drugs.
   f. Review high-protein, low-fat diet plan.

9. A patient with PKD reports sharp flank pain followed by blood in the urine. How does the nurse interpret these signs/symptoms?
   a. Infection
   b. Ruptured cyst
   c. Increased kidney size
   d. Ruptured renal artery aneurysm

10. A patient with PKD reports a severe headache and is at risk for a berry aneurysm. What is the nurse's priority action?
    a. Assess the pain and give a PRN pain medication.
    b. Reassure the patient that this is an expected aspect of the disease.
    c. Assess for neurologic changes and check vital signs.
    d. Monitor for hematuria and decreased urinary output.

11. A patient with PKD reports nocturia. What is the nocturia caused by?
    a. Increased fluid intake in the evening
    b. Increased hypertension
    c. Decreased urine concentrating ability
    d. Detrusor irritability

12. The nurse is reviewing a patient's laboratory results. Which laboratory abnormality in the patient with PKD indicates disease progression?
    a. Hypercalcemia
    b. Hypokalemia
    c. Proteinuria
    d. Homocysteinuria

13. A patient is suspected of having PKD. Which diagnostic study has minimal risks and can reveal PKD?
    a. Kidneys-ureters-bladder (KUB) x-ray
    b. Urography
    c. Renal sonography
    d. MRI with contrast

14. Which pain management strategy does the nurse teach a patient who has pain from infected kidney cysts of PKD?
    a. Take nothing by mouth.
    b. Increase the dose of NSAIDs.
    c. Assume a high-Fowler's position.
    d. Apply dry heat to the abdomen or flank.

15. A patient with PKD usually experiences constipation. What does the nurse recommend?
    a. Stool softeners and increased fluids
    b. Decreased dietary fiber and laxatives
    c. Laxatives and decreased fluids
    d. Daily tap water enemas and fiber supplements

16. A patient with PKD has nocturia. What does the nurse encourage the patient to do?
    a. Drink 2 liters of fluid daily.
    b. Restrict fluid in the evening.
    c. Only drink 1000 mL/24 hr.
    d. Take diuretics as ordered.

17. Which type of medication is the best choice to control hypertension in a patient with PKD?
    a. ACE inhibitors
    b. Beta blockers
    c. Calcium channel blockers
    d. Potassium-sparing diuretics

18. After the nurse instructs a patient with PKD on home care, the patient knows to contact the health care provider immediately when what sign/symptom occurs?
    a. Urine is blood-tinged.
    b. Weight has increased by 3 pounds in 3 days.
    c. Two days have passed since the last bowel movement.
    d. Morning systolic blood pressure has decreased by 5 mm Hg.

19. An older adult male patient calls the clinic because he has "not passed any urine all day long." What is the nurse's best response?
    a. "Try drinking several large glasses of water and waiting a few more hours."
    b. "Are you having any other symptoms such as flank pain or fever?"
    c. "You could have an obstruction, so you should come in to be checked."
    d. "I am sorry, but I really can't comment about your problem over the phone."

20. A patient reports straining to pass very small amounts of urine today, despite a normal fluid intake, and reports having the urge to urinate. The nurse palpates the bladder and finds that it is distended. How does the nurse interpret these findings?
    a. Urethral stricture
    b. Hydroureter
    c. Hydronephrosis
    d. PKD

21. A patient is diagnosed with hydronephrosis. What is a complication that could result from this condition?
    a. Damage to the nephrons
    b. Kidney cancer
    c. Kidney stone
    d. Structural defects

22. Which clinical manifestation in a patient with an obstruction in the urinary system is associated specifically with a hydronephrosis?
    a. Flank asymmetry
    b. Chills and fever
    c. Urge incontinence
    d. Decreased urine volume

23. An older adult male patient reports an acute problem with urine retention. The nurse advises the patient to seek medical attention because permanent kidney damage can occur in what time frame?
    a. In less than 6 hours
    b. In less than 48 hours
    c. Within several weeks
    d. Within several years

24. The nurse is reviewing the laboratory results for a patient being evaluated for trouble with passing urine. The urinalysis shows tubular epithelial cells on microscopic examination. How does the nurse interpret this finding?
    a. The obstruction is resolving.
    b. The obstruction is prolonged.
    c. Glomerular filtration rate (GFR) is reduced.
    d. GFR is adequate.

25. A patient had a nephrostomy and a nephrostomy tube is in place. What is included in the postoperative care of this patient?
    a. Assess the amount of drainage in the collection bag.
    b. Irrigate the tube to ensure patency.
    c. Keep the patient NPO for 6 to 8 hours.
    d. Review the results of the clotting studies.

26. The nurse is caring for a patient with a nephrostomy. The nurse notifies the health care provider about which assessment finding?
    a. Urine drainage is red-tinged 4 hours postsurgery.
    b. Amount of drainage decreases and the patient has back pain.
    c. There is a small steady drainage for the first 4 hours postsurgery.
    d. The nephrostomy site looks dry.

27. Which manifestations are associated with chronic pyelonephritis? *(Select all that apply.)*
    a. Abscess formation
    b. Obstruction with reflex
    c. Acute bacterial infection
    d. Structural deformities
    e. Neurogenic impairment of voiding

Matching. *Match the factors or manifestations to the kidney disorders they are primarily associated with. Answers may be used more than once.*

Kidney Disorders

a. Associated with acute pyelonephritis
b. Common to both acute and chronic pyelonephritis
c. Common to neither acute nor chronic pyelonephritis

Factors and Manifestations

_____ 28. Abscess formation

_____ 29. Alcohol abuse

_____ 30. Active bacterial infection

_____ 31. Decreased urine specific gravity

_____ 32. CVA tenderness/pain

_____ 33. Undergone manipulation of the urinary tract

34. The nurse is assessing a patient who reports chills, high fever, and flank pain with urinary urgency and frequency. On physical examination, the patient has costovertebral angle (CVA) tenderness, pulse is 110 beats/min, and respirations are 28/min. How does the nurse interpret these findings?
    a. Complicated cystitis
    b. Acute pyelonephritis
    c. Chronic pyelonephritis
    d. Acute glomerulonephritis

35. The health care provider informs a patient with acute pyelonephritis that abscess formation is common and recommends diagnostic testing to identify the presence of an abscess. Which test does the nurse prepare the patient for?
    a. Renal arteriography
    b. Cystourethrogram
    c. Radionuclide scintillation
    d. Urodynamic flow studies

36. A patient with chronic pyelonephritis returns to the clinic for follow-up. Which behavior indicates the patient is meeting the expected outcomes to conserve existing kidney function?
    a. Drinks a liter of fluid every day
    b. Considers buying a home blood pressure cuff
    c. Reports self-administration of antibiotics as prescribed
    d. Takes pain medication on a regular basis

37. Which patient is at greatest risk for the development of chronic pyelonephritis?
    a. 80-year-old woman who takes diuretics for mild heart failure
    b. 80-year-old man who drinks four cans of beer per day
    c. 36-year-old woman with diabetes mellitus who is pregnant
    d. 36-year-old man with diabetes insipidus

38. A patient is diagnosed with acute pyelonephritis. What is the priority for nursing care for this patient?
    a. Providing information about the disease process and self-care
    b. Controlling hypertension
    c. Managing pain
    d. Preventing constipation

39. The nurse is giving discharge instructions to a patient who had pyelolithotomy. What topics does the nurse include in the teaching plan? *(Select all that apply.)*
    a. Controlling blood pressure
    b. Restricting fluids
    c. Eating properly to promote healing
    d. Completing oral antibiotics
    e. Monitoring changes in urine output

40. A patient has come to the clinic for follow-up of acute pyelonephritis. Which action does the nurse reinforce to the patient?
    a. Complete all antibiotic regimens.
    b. Report episodes of nocturia.
    c. Stop taking the antibiotic when pain is relieved.
    d. Notify the health care provider of any over-the-counter drug use.

41. A patient with PKD would exhibit which signs/symptoms? *(Select all that apply.)*
    a. Frequent urination
    b. Increased abdominal girth
    c. Hypertension
    d. Kidney stones
    e. Diarrhea

42. In PKD, the effect on the renin-angiotensin system in the kidney ends in which result?
    a. Decreased blood pressure
    b. Increased blood pressure
    c. Increased urine output
    d. Oliguria

43. The common problem of hydronephrosis, hydroureter, and urethral stricture in kidney function is _____.

44. Kidney tissue changes in chronic glomerulonephritis are caused by which factors? *(Select all that apply.)*
    a. Ischemia
    b. Fluid overload
    c. Hypertension
    d. Elevated body temperature
    e. Fluid and electrolyte imbalance

45. A patient diagnosed with renal cell carcinoma that has metastasized to the lungs is considered to be in which stage of cancer?
    a. I
    b. II
    c. III
    d. IV

46. A patient is admitted for acute glomerulonephritis. In reviewing the patient's past medical history, which systemic conditions does the nurse suspect may have caused acute glomerulonephritis and will include in the overall treatment plan?
    a. Systemic lupus erythematosus and diabetic nephropathy
    b. Myocardial infarction and atrial fibrillation
    c. Ischemic stroke and hemiparesis
    d. Blunt trauma to the kidney with hematuria

47. The nurse is assessing a patient with possible acute glomerulonephritis. During the inspection of the hands, face, and eyelids, the nurse is primarily observing for evidence of which factors?
    a. Redness
    b. Edema
    c. Rashes
    d. Dryness

48. The nurse is assessing a patient with glomerulonephritis and notes crackles in the lung fields and neck vein distention. The patient reports mild shortness of breath. Based on these findings, what does the nurse do next?
    a. Check for CVA tenderness or flank pain.
    b. Obtain a urine sample to check for proteinuria.
    c. Assess for additional signs of fluid overload.
    d. Alert the health care provider about the respiratory symptoms.

49. The GFR of a patient with acute glomerulonephritis is 50 mL/min. What is the nurse's interpretation of this finding?
    a. GFR is normal; therapy is effective.
    b. GFR is high; the patient is at risk for dehydration.
    c. GFR is low; the patient is at risk for infection.
    d. GFR is low; the patient is at risk for fluid overload.

50. A patient is very ill and is admitted to the intensive care unit with rapidly progressive glomerulonephritis. The nurse monitors the patient for manifestations of which organ system failure?
    a. Immune system
    b. Cardiac
    c. Liver
    d. Kidney

51. A patient is diagnosed with chronic glomerulonephritis. The patient's spouse reports that the patient is irritable, forgetful, and has trouble concentrating. Which assessment finding does the nurse expect further examination will reveal?
    a. Low oxygen saturation
    b. Elevated blood urea nitrogen
    c. High white count with a left shift
    d. Low blood pressure and bradycardia

52. The nurse is reviewing the laboratory results for a patient with chronic glomerulonephritis. The serum albumin level is low. What else does the nurse expect to see?
    a. Proteinuria
    b. Elevated hematocrit
    c. Very low urine specific gravity
    d. Low white blood cell count

53. A patient has chronic glomerulonephritis. In order to assess for uremic symptoms, what does the nurse do?
    a. Evaluate the blood urea nitrogen (BUN).
    b. Ask the patient to extend the arms and hyperextend the wrists.
    c. Gently palpate the flank for asymmetry and tenderness.
    d. Auscultate for the presence of an S_3 heart sound.

54. The nurse is reviewing the laboratory results for a patient with chronic glomerulonephritis. The phosphorus level is 5.3 mg/dL. What else does the nurse expect to see?
    a. Serum calcium level below the normal range
    b. Serum potassium level below the normal range
    c. Falsely elevated serum sodium level
    d. Elevated serum levels for all other electrolytes

55. The nurse is reviewing arterial blood gas results of a patient with acute glomerulonephritis. The pH of the sample is 7.35. As acidosis is likely to be present because of hydrogen ion retention and loss of bicarbonate, how does the nurse interpret this data?
    a. Normal pH with respiratory compensation
    b. Acidosis with failure of respiratory compensation
    c. Alkalosis with failure of metabolic compensation
    d. Normal pH with metabolic compensation

56. The nurse is taking a history on a patient with chronic glomerulonephritis. What is the patient most likely to report?
    a. History of antibiotic allergy
    b. Intense flank pain
    c. Malnutrition and weight loss
    d. Mild edema and hypertension

57. Which patient history factor is considered a causative factor for acute glomerulonephritis?
    a. Cystitis 6 months ago
    b. Strep throat 3 weeks ago
    c. Kidney stones 2 years ago
    d. Mild hypertension diagnosed 1 year ago

58. A patient with acute glomerulonephritis has edema of the face. The blood pressure is moderately elevated and the patient has gained 2 pounds within the past 24 hours. The patient reports fatigue and refuses to eat. What is the priority for nursing care?
    a. Cluster care to allow rest periods for the patient.
    b. Obtain a dietary consult to plan an adequate nutritional diet.
    c. Monitor urine output with accurate intake and output amounts.
    d. Assess for signs and symptoms of fluid volume overload.

59. A patient with acute glomerulonephritis is required to provide a 24-hour urine specimen. What does the nurse expect to see with the specimen?
    a. Smoky or cola-colored urine
    b. Clear and very dilute urine
    c. Urine that is full of pus and very thick
    d. Bright orange-colored urine

60. Which nursing intervention is applicable for a patient with acute glomerulonephritis?
    a. Restricting visitors to adults only
    b. Using a lift sheet to turn the patient
    c. Inspecting the vascular access
    d. Measuring weight daily

61. Which diagnostic tests and results does the nurse expect to see with acute glomerulonephritis? *(Select all that apply.)*
    a. Urinalysis revealing hematuria
    b. Urinalysis revealing proteinuria
    c. Microscopic red blood cell casts
    d. Normal urine sedimentation assay
    e. 24-hour urine for creatinine clearance decreased
    f. Serum nitrogen level decreased
    g. Serum albumin levels decreased
    h. Antistreptolysin-O titers increased

62. A patient has late-stage chronic glomerulonephritis. Which treatment does the nurse discuss and educate the patient about?
    a. Appropriate anti-infective medications
    b. Dialysis or transplantation
    c. Radiation therapy
    d. Immunosuppressive agents

63. The nurse is caring for a patient with nephrotic syndrome. What interventions are included in the plan of care for this patient? *(Select all that apply.)*
    a. Dietary protein must be increased.
    b. Administer mild diuretics.
    c. Assess for edema.
    d. Administer antihypertensive medications.
    e. Assess the patient's hydration status.

64. The nurse is reviewing laboratory results for a patient with suspected kidney problems. Which manifestation is a hallmark for nephrotic syndrome?
    a. Flank asymmetry
    b. Proteinuria greater than 3.5 g of protein in 24 hours
    c. Serum sodium 148 mmol/L
    d. Serum cholesterol (total) 190 mg/dL

65. A patient is newly admitted with nephrotic syndrome and has proteinuria, edema, hyperlipidemia, and hypertension. What is the priority for nursing care?
    a. Consult the dietitian to provide adequate nutritional intake.
    b. Prevent urinary tract infection.
    c. Monitor fluid volume from intake and output amounts.
    d. Provide instruction on a plan of care related to the disease process.

66. A patient is diagnosed with chronic interstitial nephritis. Which nursing action is relevant and specific for this patient's medical condition?
    a. Avoid analgesic use.
    b. Use disposable gloves.
    c. Monitor for fever.
    d. Place the patient in isolation.

67. Which ethnic groups are mostly likely to develop end-stage kidney disease related to hypertension? *(Select all that apply.)*
    a. Caucasian Americans
    b. Asian Americans
    c. American Indians
    d. African Americans
    e. Hispanic Americans

68. A patient with diabetic nephropathy reports having frequent hypoglycemic episodes "so my doctor reduced my insulin which means my diabetes is improving." What is the nurse's best response?
    a. "Congratulations! You must be following the diet and lifestyle instructions very carefully."
    b. "When kidney function is reduced, the insulin is available for a longer time and thus less of it is needed."
    c. "You should probably talk to your doctor again. You have been diagnosed with nephropathy and that changes the situation."
    d. "Let me get you a brochure about the relationship of diabetes and kidney disease. It is a complex topic and hard to understand."

69. The student nurse is assisting in the postoperative care of a patient who had a recent nephrectomy. The student demonstrates a reluctance to change the linens because "the patient seems so tired." The nurse reminds the student that a priority assessment for this patient is to assess for which factor?
    a. Skin breakdown on the patient's back
    b. Blood on the linens beneath the patient
    c. Urinary incontinence and moisture
    d. The patient's ability to move self in bed

70. After a nephrectomy, a patient has a large urine output because of adrenal insufficiency. What does the nurse anticipate the priority intervention for this patient will be?
    a. ACE inhibitor to control the hypertension and decrease protein loss in urine
    b. Straight catheterization or bedside bladder scan to measure residual urine
    c. IV fluid replacement because of subsequent hypotension and oliguria
    d. IV infusion of Temsirolimus to inhibit cell division and prevent metastasis

71. A patient with a kidney abscess who is receiving antibiotics is ordered an additional treatment by the health care provider. The nurse prepares patient education material for which procedure?
    a. Surgical incision or needle aspiration
    b. Hemodialysis
    c. Insertion of a suprapubic catheter
    d. Cystostomy

72. A 53-year-old patient is newly diagnosed with renal artery stenosis. What clinical manifestation does the nurse observe when the patient first seeks health care?
    a. Sudden onset of hypertension
    b. Urinary frequency and dysuria
    c. Nausea and vomiting
    d. Flank pain and hematuria

73. A patient has been informed by the health care provider that treatment will be needed for renal artery stenosis. The nurse prepares to teach about a variety of treatment options. What treatments will the nurse include in the teaching plan? *(Select all that apply.)*
    a. Kidney transplant
    b. Hypertension control
    c. Balloon angioplasty
    d. Renal artery bypass surgery
    e. Synthetic blood vessel graft
    f. Percutaneous ultrasonic pyelolithotomy

74. What change in diabetic therapy may be needed for a patient who has diabetic nephropathy?
    a. Fluid restriction
    b. Decreased activity level
    c. Decreased insulin dosages
    d. Increased caloric intake

75. A patient has had one kidney removed as a treatment for kidney cancer. The patient's spouse asks, "Does the good kidney take over immediately? I know a person can live with just one kidney." What is the nurse's best response?
    a. "The other kidney will provide adequate function, but this may take days or weeks."
    b. "The other kidney alone isn't able to provide adequate function, so supplemental therapies will be needed."
    c. "That's a good question. Remember to ask your doctor next time he or she comes in."
    d. "It varies a lot, but within a few days we expect everything to normalize."

76. After a nephrectomy, one adrenal gland remains. Based on this knowledge, which type of medication replacement therapy does the nurse expect a patient who had a nephrectomy to receive?
    a. Potassium
    b. Steroid
    c. Calcium
    d. Estrogen

77. The nurse is caring for a patient with kidney cell carcinoma. What symptoms and findings does the nurse expect to see in this patient? *(Select all that apply.)*
    a. Urinary tract infection
    b. Erythrocytosis
    c. Hypercalcemia
    d. Liver dysfunction
    e. Decreased sedimentation rate
    f. Hypertension
    g. Hematuria

78. The nurse is caring for a patient with kidney cell carcinoma. What does the nurse expect to find documented about the patient's initial assessment?
    a. Flank pain, gross hematuria, palpable kidney mass, and renal bruit
    b. Gross hematuria, hypertension, diabetes, and oliguria
    c. Dysuria, polyuria, dehydration, and palpable kidney mass
    d. Nocturia and urinary retention with difficulty starting stream

79. A patient is diagnosed with kidney cancer and the health care provider recommends the best therapy. Which treatment does the nurse anticipate teaching the patient about?
    a. Chemotherapy
    b. Surgical removal
    c. Hormonal therapy
    d. Radiation therapy

80. A patient returning to the unit after a left radical nephrectomy for kidney cell carcinoma is concerned about severe pain on the right side. What does the nurse tell the patient?
    a. "The right kidney was repositioned to take over the function of both kidneys."
    b. "I'll call your doctor for an order to increase your pain medication."
    c. "The pain is likely to be from being positioned on your right side during surgery."
    d. "Would you like to talk with someone who had this surgery last year and now is fully recovered?"

81. The nurse is caring for a postoperative nephrectomy patient. The nurse notes during the first several hours of the shift a marked and steady downward trend in blood pressure. How does the nurse interpret this finding?
    a. Hypertension has been corrected.
    b. Internal hemorrhage is possible.
    c. The other kidney is failing.
    d. This is an expected response to medication.

82. The nurse is caring for a patient after a nephrectomy. The nurse notes that the urine flow was 50 mL/hr at the beginning of the shift, but several hours later has dropped to 30 mL. What is the nurse's priority action?
    a. Notify the health care provider for an order for an IV fluid bolus.
    b. Document the finding and continue to monitor for downward trend.
    c. Troubleshoot the drainage system to make sure there are no obstructions.
    d. Obtain the patient's weight and compare it to baseline.

83. The nurse is caring for a patient who had a nephrectomy yesterday. To manage the patient's pain, what is the best plan for analgesia therapy?
    a. Limit narcotics because of respiratory depression.
    b. Give an oral analgesic when the patient can eat.
    c. Alternate parenteral and oral medications.
    d. Give parenteral medications on a schedule.

84. A patient is brought to the emergency department (ED) after being involved in a fight in which the patient was kicked and punched repeatedly in the back. What does the nurse include in the initial physical assessment? *(Select all that apply.)*
    a. Take complete vital signs.
    b. Check apical and peripheral pulses.
    c. Inspect both flanks for asymmetry or penetrating injuries of the lower chest or back.
    d. Inspect the abdomen for bruising or penetrating wounds.
    e. Deeply palpate the abdomen for signs of rigidity.
    f. Percuss the abdomen for distention.
    g. Inspect the urethra for gross bleeding.

85. The ED nurse is preparing a patient with kidney trauma for emergency surgery. What is the best task to delegate to the unlicensed assistive personnel (UAP)?
   a. Set the automated blood pressure machine to cycle every 30 minutes.
   b. Inform the family about surgery and assist them to the surgery waiting area.
   c. Go to the blood bank and pick up the units of packed red cells.
   d. Insert a Foley catheter if there is no gross bleeding at the urethra.

86. A patient has sustained a kidney injury. In order to assist the patient to undergo the best diagnostic test to determine the extent of injury, what does the nurse do?
   a. Obtain a clean-catch urine specimen for urinalysis.
   b. Give an IV fluid bolus before renal arteriography.
   c. Give an explanation of computed tomography.
   d. Obtain a blood sample for hemoglobin and hematocrit.

CASE STUDY: THE PATIENT WITH PKD

Use a separate sheet of paper to answer the questions in this Case Study, or go to the "Prepare for Class" folder on your Evolve website at http://evolve.elsevier.com/Iggy/ to download and complete as a word processing file. Answer guidelines for this Case Study are also available on your Evolve website.

A 30-year-old white male patient comes to the clinic reporting dull, aching abdominal and flank pain. He reports nocturia and a family history of autosomal dominant PKD. He reports no known personal health problems, although he was instructed to monitor his blood pressure at home and he admits to "not doing so well with that." Today his blood pressure is 130/90 mm Hg; pulse is 72 and regular; respirations 12/min, and temperature is 98.8° F.

1. What additional information should the nurse elicit during the interview?
2. What are the key features of PKD?
3. Describe the causes of pain for patients with PKD.
4. What are typical findings of a urinalysis in a patient with PKD?
5. What are the causes of hypertension and kidney ischemia in a patient with PKD?
6. What is the risk involved with other organs and tissues in the progression of PKD?
7. Patients with PKD often have other tissue involvement. List several of the complications that can be present.
8. Identify priority nursing care needs for the patient with PKD.
9. What would the nurse include in the teaching plan for this patient?
10. Document a nursing note for this patient using a body systems approach.

71 CHAPTER

Care of Patients with Acute Kidney Injury and Chronic Kidney Disease

STUDY/REVIEW QUESTIONS

1. Which problems occur with acute kidney injury? *(Select all that apply.)*
   a. Deficient fluid volume
   b. Acid-base abnormalities
   c. Loss of kidney hormone function
   d. Excess fluid volume
   e. Buildup of nitrogen-based wastes

2. The community health nurse is designing programs to reduce kidney problems and kidney injury among the general public. In order to do so, the nurse targets health promotion and compliance with therapy for people with which conditions?
   a. Diabetes mellitus and hypertension
   b. Frequent episodes of sexually transmitted disease
   c. Osteoporosis and other bone diseases
   d. Gastroenteritis and poor eating habits

3. What are common causes of prerenal azotemia? *(Select all that apply.)*
   a. Urethral cancer
   b. Heart failure
   c. Athletes (such as a marathon runner)
   d. Sepsis
   e. Shock

4. A patient can develop intrarenal kidney injury from which causes? *(Select all that apply.)*
   a. Vasculitis
   b. Renal artery stenosis or thrombosis
   c. Heart failure
   d. Exposure to nephrotoxins
   e. Kidney stones

5. Postrenal azotemia can result from which conditions? *(Select all that apply.)*
   a. Sepsis
   b. Urethral cancer
   c. Kidney stones
   d. Exposure to nephrotoxins
   e. Atony of the bladder

6. When shock or other problems cause an acute reduction in blood flow to the kidneys, how do the kidneys compensate? *(Select all that apply.)*
   a. Constrict blood vessels in the kidneys
   b. Activate the renin-angiotensin-aldosterone pathway
   c. Release beta-blockers
   d. Constrict blood vessels in the kidneys
   e. Release antidiuretic hormones

7. When pressure in the kidney tubules exceeds glomerular pressure, glomerular filtration
   _____.

8. Acute kidney injury may occur with the loss of _____% of nephrons.

9. The nurse is caring for a patient who had hypovolemic shock secondary to trauma in the emergency department (ED) 2 days ago. Based on the pathophysiology of hypovolemia and prerenal azotemia, what does the nurse assess every hour?
   a. Urinary output
   b. Presence of edema
   c. Urine color
   d. Presence of pain

10. The nurse is talking to an older adult male patient who is reasonably healthy for his age, but has benign prostatic hyperplasia (BPH). Which condition does the BPH potentially place him at risk for?
    a. Prerenal azotemia
    b. Postrenal azotemia
    c. Acute tubular necrosis
    d. Acute glomerulonephritis

11. Which combination of drugs is the most nephrotoxic?
    a. Angiotensin-converting enzyme (ACE) inhibitors and aspirin
    b. Angiotensin II receptor blockers and antacids
    c. Aminoglycoside antibiotics and NSAIDs
    d. Calcium channel blockers and antihistamines

12. The nurse is caring for a patient with the nonoliguric form of acute kidney injury (AKI). Which factor contributes to the prognosis for this patient?
    a. The clinical manifestations are more readily and easily observed.
    b. Attentive nursing care has resulted in the patient having the nonoliguric form.
    c. The urine output remains nearly normal and the treatment is less complicated.
    d. The nonoliguric form occurs in younger people who have better baseline health.

13. A patient with AKI secondary to which factor has the worst prognosis and the lowest chance for recovery?
    a. Radiographic contrast dye
    b. Glomerulonephritis
    c. Kidney stone
    d. Dehydration

14. The nurse has obtained a urine specimen from a patient and has used a dipstick to test the urine. Which abnormal finding is the earliest sign of kidney tubular damage?
    a. Presence of blood
    b. Presence of leukocytes
    c. Presence of glucose
    d. Decreased urine specific gravity

15. The nurse is caring for a patient receiving gentamicin. Because this drug has potential for nephrotoxicity, which laboratory results does the nurse monitor? *(Select all that apply.)*
    a. Blood urea nitrogen (BUN)
    b. Creatinine
    c. Drug peak and trough levels
    d. Prothrombin time (PT)
    e. Platelet count
    f. Hemoglobin and hematocrit

16. The nurse is assessing a patient with AKI. The nurse notes bladder distention and the patient reports "feeling the urge to urinate." Urine sodium level is 40 mEq/L; specific gravity of 1.010. How does the nurse interpret these findings?
    a. Prerenal azotemia
    b. Intrarenal AKI
    c. Postrenal azotemia
    d. Oliguric phase

17. A patient has been diagnosed with AKI, but the cause is uncertain. The nurse prepares patient education material about which diagnostic test?
    a. Flat plate of the abdomen
    b. Renal ultrasonography
    c. Computed tomography
    d. Kidney biopsy

18. A patient is in the diuretic phase of AKI. During this phase, what is the nurse mainly concerned about?
    a. Assessing for hypertension and fluid overload
    b. Monitoring for hypovolemia and electrolyte loss
    c. Adjusting the dosage of diuretic medications
    d. Balancing diuretic therapy with intake

19. A patient with prerenal azotemia is administered a fluid challenge. In evaluating response to the therapy, which outcome indicates that the goal was met?
    a. Patient reports feeling better and indicates an eagerness to go home.
    b. Patient produces urine soon after the initial bolus.
    c. The therapy is completed without adverse effects.
    d. The health care provider orders a diuretic when the challenge is completed.

20. The nurse is caring for a patient with AKI and notes a trend of increasing elevated BUN levels. How does the nurse interpret this information?
    a. Breakdown of muscle for protein which leads to an increase in azotemia
    b. Sign of urinary retention and decreased urinary output
    c. Expected trend that can be reversed by increasing dietary protein
    d. Ominous sign of impending irreversible kidney failure

21. The nurse is caring for a patient with prerenal azotemia. What are the primary treatment goals in the initial phase that prevents permanent kidney damage for this patient? *(Select all that apply.)*
    a. Correct blood volume.
    b. Increase blood pressure.
    c. Manage kidney infections.
    d. Relieve the obstruction.
    e. Improve cardiac output.

22. A patient sustained extensive burns and depletion of vascular volume. The nurse expects which changes in vital signs and urinary function?
    a. Decreased urine output, postural hypotension, tachycardia
    b. Increased urine output, bounding pulses, tachycardia
    c. Bradycardia, hypertension, polyuria
    d. Dysrhythmias, hypertension, oliguria

23. The nurse is taking a history of a patient at risk for kidney failure. What does the nurse ask the patient about during the interview? *(Select all that apply.)*
    a. Exposure to nephrotoxic chemicals
    b. Recent weight loss
    c. History of diabetes mellitus, hypertension, systemic lupus erythematosus
    d. Recent surgery, trauma, or transfusions
    e. Leakage of urine when coughing or laughing
    f. Use of antibiotics, NSAIDs, or ACE inhibitors

24. Which disorder may mimic the presentation of prerenal azotemia?
    a. Heart failure
    b. Diabetes mellitus
    c. Pneumonia
    d. Compartment syndrome

25. A patient with AKI is anorexic and refuses to eat. The nurse notifies the health care provider to obtain an order for which intervention?
    a. Normal saline to prevent dehydration
    b. Nutritional consult for a calculated diet
    c. Total parenteral nutrition (TPN) with appropriate laboratory monitoring
    d. Nasogastric tube for enteral feedings

26. Which symptoms does the nurse expect to see in the patient with intrarenal AKI? *(Select all that apply.)*
    a. Oliguria/anuria
    b. Hypotension
    c. Shortness of breath
    d. Jugular vein distention
    e. Decreased central pressure
    f. Weight loss
    g. Crackles
    h. Nausea and anorexia

27. The nurse is caring for a patient with signs and symptoms of prerenal azotemia. A fluid challenge is performed to promote kidney perfusion by doing what?
   a. Administering normal saline 500 to 1000 mL infused over 1 hour
   b. Administering drugs to suppress aldosterone release
   c. Instilling warm, sterile normal saline into the bladder
   d. Having the patient drink several large glasses of water

28. A patient has AKI related to nephrotoxic acute tubular necrosis (ATN). In order to maintain cell integrity, improve glomerular filtration rate (GFR), and improve blood flow to the kidneys, which medication does the nurse anticipate the health care provider will prescribe?
   a. Digoxin
   b. Alpha-adrenergic blockers
   c. Beta blockers
   d. Calcium channel blockers

29. A patient with AKI has a high rate of catabolism. What is this related to?
   a. Increased levels of catecholamines, cortisol, and glucagon
   b. Inability to excrete excess electrolytes
   c. Conversion of body fat into glucose
   d. Presence of retained nitrogenous wastes

30. The nurse is caring for a patient in the ICU who sustained blood loss during a traumatic accident. In order to assess for prerenal azotemia, which signs and symptoms does the nurse observe for? *(Select all that apply.)*
   a. Hypotension
   b. Bradycardia
   c. Decreased urine output
   d. Decreased cardiac output
   e. Increased central venous pressure
   f. Lethargy

31. A patient with AKI is receiving total parenteral nutrition (TPN). What is the goal of TPN?
   a. Preserve lean body mass
   b. Promote tubular reabsorption
   c. Create a negative nitrogen balance
   d. Prevent infection

Matching. *Match each characteristic with its corresponding device. Answers may be used more than once, and there may be more than one answer for a characteristic.*

Devices
a. Continuous arteriovenous hemofiltration (CAVH)
b. Continuous arteriovenous hemodialysis and filtration (CAVHD)
c. Continuous venovenous hemofiltration (CVVH)

Characteristics
_____ 32. Requires placement of arterial and venous catheter

_____ 33. Requires a double-lumen venous catheter

_____ 34. Uses pump

_____ 35. Arterial pressure of at least 60 mm Hg

_____ 36. Removes water and electrolytes

_____ 37. Risk of air embolus

_____ 38. Uses dialysate to remove nitrogenous waste

Matching. *Match each characteristic with its corresponding stage of kidney disease. Answers may be used more than once, and there may be more than one answer for a characteristic.*

Stages

a. Stage 1 chronic kidney disease
b. Mild chronic kidney disease
c. End-stage kidney disease

Characteristics

_____ 39. Excessive waste products

_____ 40. Increased BUN and creatinine

_____ 41. Dialysis

_____ 42. Primary reduction in function

_____ 43. Nephrons compensate

_____ 44. Hypertension

_____ 45. Stress of illness can rapidly compromise this stage

_____ 46. Severe fluid overload

_____ 47. Severe electrolyte and acid-base imbalances

_____ 48. Renal osteodystrophy

49. The nurse is taking a history on a patient with diabetes and hypertension. Because of the patient's high risk for developing kidney problems, which early sign of chronic kidney disease (CKD) does the nurse assess for?
  a. Decreased output with subjective thirst
  b. Urinary frequency of very small amounts
  c. Pink or blood-tinged urine
  d. Increased output of very dilute urine

50. Increased BUN and creatinine, hyperkalemia, and hypernatremia are all characteristics of which stage of kidney disease?
  a. Stage 1 CKD
  b. Mild CKD
  c. Moderate CDK
  d. End-stage kidney disease

51. A patient's laboratory results show an elevated creatinine level. The patient's history reveals no risk factors for kidney disease. Which question does the nurse ask the patient to shed further light on the laboratory result?
  a. "How many hours of sleep did you get the night before the test?"
  b. "How much fluid did you drink before the test?"
  c. "Did you take any type of antibiotics before taking the test?"
  d. "When and how much did you last urinate before having the test?"

52. The nurse is reviewing a patient's laboratory results. In the early phase of CKD, what does the nurse expect to see?
  a. Higher than normal potassium
  b. Lower than normal sodium
  c. Higher than normal calcium
  d. Lower than normal phosphorus

53. A patient with CKD has a potassium level of 8 mEq/L. The nurse notifies the health care provider after assessing for which sign/symptom?
  a. Cardiac dysrhythmias
  b. Respiratory depression
  c. Tremors or seizures
  d. Decreased urine output

54. The nurse is assessing a patient with kidney injury and notes a marked increase in the rate and depth of breathing. The nurse recognizes this as Kussmaul respiration, which is the body's attempt to compensate for which condition?
  a. Hypoxia
  b. Alkalosis
  c. Acidosis
  d. Hypoxemia

55. A patient is diagnosed with renal osteodystrophy. What does the nurse instruct the unlicensed assistive personnel (UAP) to do in relation to this patient's diagnosis?
    a. Assist the patient with toileting every 2 hours.
    b. Gently wash the patient's skin with a mild soap and rinse well.
    c. Handle the patient gently because of risk for fractures.
    d. Assist the patient with eating because of loss of coordination.

56. A patient with CKD develops severe chest pain, an increased pulse, low-grade fever, and a pericardial friction rub with a cardiac dysrhythmia and muffled heart tones. The nurse immediately alerts the health care provider and prepares for which emergency procedure?
    a. Pericardiocentesis
    b. Continuous venovenous hemofiltration
    c. Kidney dialysis
    d. Cardiopulmonary resuscitation

57. All patients with hypertension or diabetes should have yearly screenings for which factor?
    a. Creatinine
    b. BUN
    c. Glycosuria
    d. Microalbuminuria

58. The nurse is assessing a patient with kidney failure. What is an early neurologic manifestation of kidney failure that could potentially be resolved with dialysis?
    a. Lethargy
    b. Unequal pupils
    c. Severe motor impairment
    d. Unilateral weakness

59. The night shift nurse sees a patient with kidney failure sitting up in bed. The patient states, "I feel a little short of breath at night or when I get up to walk to the bathroom." What assessment does the nurse do?
    a. Check for orthostatic hypertension because of potential volume depletion.
    b. Auscultate the lungs for crackles which indicate fluid overload.
    c. Check the pulse and blood pressure for possible decreased cardiac output.
    d. Assess for normal sleep pattern and need for a PRN sedative.

60. What does the breath often smell like in a patient with CKD?
    a. Fruit
    b. Feces
    c. Urine
    d. Blood

61. The patient with CKD reports chronic fatigue and lethargy with weakness and mild shortness of breath with dizziness when rising to a standing position. In addition, the nurse notes pale mucous membranes. Based on the patient's illness and the presenting symptoms, which laboratory result does the nurse expect to see?
    a. Low hemoglobin and hematocrit
    b. Low white cell count
    c. Low blood glucose
    d. Low oxygen saturation

62. The nurse is assessing the skin of a patient with ESKD. Which clinical manifestation is considered a sign of very advanced disease?
    a. Ecchymoses
    b. Sallowness
    c. Pallor
    d. Uremic frost

63. The nurse notes an abnormal laboratory test finding for a patient with CKD and alerts the health care provider. The nurse also consults with the registered dietitian because an excessive dietary protein intake is directly related to which factor?
    a. Elevated serum creatinine level
    b. Protein presence in the urine
    c. Elevated BUN level
    d. Elevated serum potassium level

64. In collaboration with the registered dietitian, the nurse teaches the patient about which diet recommendations for management of CKD? (Select all that apply.)
    a. Controlling protein intake
    b. Limiting fluid intake
    c. Restricting potassium
    d. Increasing sodium
    e. Restricting phosphorus
    f. Eating enough calories to meet metabolic need
    g. Avoiding vitamin supplements

65. A patient receives dialysis therapy and the health care provider has ordered sodium restriction to 3 g daily. What does the nurse teach the patient?
    a. Add only small amounts of salt at the table or during cooking.
    b. Foods high in sodium (e.g., processed foods, fast foods) should be strictly avoided.
    c. Herbs and spices can be used in place of salt to enhance food flavor.
    d. Bland foods with very minimal amounts of spicing are the best choice.

66. In order to assist a patient in the prevention of osteodystrophy, which intervention does the nurse perform?
    a. Administer phosphate binders.
    b. Encourage the patient to eat high-quality protein foods.
    c. Assist the patient to ambulate and exercise several times a day.
    d. Encourage the patient to drink extra milk at mealtimes.

67. The nurse prepares to administer medications to a patient with CKD. The nurse calls the health care provider as a reminder that the patient might need which nutritional supplements? *(Select all that apply.)*
    a. Iron
    b. Magnesium
    c. Phosphorus
    d. Calcium
    e. Vitamin D
    f. Water-soluble vitamins

68. The nurse is caring for a patient with ESKD and dialysis has been initiated. Which drug order does the nurse question?
    a. Erythropoietin
    b. Diuretic
    c. ACE inhibitor
    d. Calcium channel blocker

69. The nurse monitors a CKD patient's daily weights because of the risk for fluid retention. What instructions does the nurse give to the UAP?
    a. Weigh the patient daily at the same time each day, same scale, with the same amount of clothing.
    b. Weigh the patient daily and add 1 kilogram of weight for the intake of each liter of fluid.
    c. Weigh the patient in the morning before breakfast and weigh the patient at night just before bedtime.
    d. Ask the patient what his or her normal weight is and then weigh the patient before and after each voiding.

70. A patient with CKD is taking digoxin. Which signs of digoxin toxicity does the nurse vigilantly monitor for? *(Select all that apply.)*
    a. Nausea and vomiting
    b. Visual changes
    c. Respiratory depression
    d. Restlessness or confusion
    e. Headache or fatigue
    f. Tachycardia

71. The nurse is caring for a patient with CKD. The nurse anticipates that dosage adjustments will be made for which drugs? *(Select all that apply.)*
    a. Antibiotics
    b. Opioids
    c. Insulin
    d. NSAIDs
    e. Oral antidiabetics

72. The nurse is evaluating a patient's treatment response to erythropoietin (Epogen). Which hematocrit reading indicates that the goal is being met?
    a. 10%
    b. 30%
    c. 50%
    d. At baseline

73. A patient has been receiving erythropoietin (Epogen). Which statement by the patient indicates that the therapy is producing the desired effect?
    a. "I can do my housework with less fatigue."
    b. "I have been passing more urine than I was before."
    c. "I have less pain and discomfort now."
    d. "I can swallow and eat much better than before."

74. Which behavior is the strongest indicator that a patient with ESKD is not coping well with the illness and may need a referral for psychological counseling?
    a. Displays irritability when the meal tray arrives
    b. Refuses to take one of the drugs because it causes nausea
    c. Repeatedly misses dialysis appointments
    d. Seems distracted when the health care provider talks about the prognosis

75. A patient with CKD is restless, anxious, and short of breath. The nurse hears crackles that begin at the base of the lungs. The pulse rate is increased and the patient has frothy, blood-tinged sputum. What does the nurse do next?
    a. Facilitate transfer to the ICU for aggressive treatment.
    b. Place the patient in a high-Fowler's position.
    c. Monitor vital signs and assess breath sounds.
    d. Administer a loop diuretic such as furosemide (Lasix).

76. Which patients are candidates for CAVH? *(Select all that apply.)*
    a. Patient with fluid volume overload
    b. Patient who needs long-term management
    c. Hemodynamically unstable patient
    d. Patient who is ready for discharge to home
    e. Patient who is resistant to diuretics

77. As a patient with ESKD experiences isosthenuria, what must the nurse be alert for?
    a. The diuretic stage
    b. Fluid volume overload
    c. Dehydration
    d. Alkalosis

78. The nurse is caring for a patient with CKD. The family asks about when renal replacement therapy will begin. What is the nurse's best response?
    a. "As early as possible to prevent further damage in stage I."
    b. "When there is reduced kidney function and metabolic wastes accumulate."
    c. "When the kidneys are unable to maintain a balance in body functions."
    d. "It will be started with diuretic therapy to enhance the remaining function."

79. Which are the most accurate ways to monitor kidney function in the patient with CKD? *(Select all that apply.)*
    a. Monitoring intake and output
    b. Checking urine specific gravity
    c. Reviewing BUN and serum creatinine levels
    d. Reviewing x-ray reports
    e. Consulting the dietitian's notes

80. As a result of kidney failure, excessive hydrogen ions cannot be excreted. With acid retention, the nurse is most likely to observe what type of respiratory compensation?
    a. Cheyne-Stokes respiratory pattern
    b. Increased depth of breathing
    c. Decreased respiratory rate and depth
    d. Increased arterial carbon dioxide levels

81. The nurse is assessing a patient with uremia. Which gastrointestinal changes does the nurse expect to find? *(Select all that apply.)*
    a. Halitosis
    b. Hiccups
    c. Anorexia
    d. Nausea
    e. Vomiting
    f. Salivation
    g. Stomatitis

82. Which patients with CKD are candidates for hemodialysis? *(Select all that apply.)*
    a. Patient with fluid overload who does not respond to diuretics
    b. Patient with medication-controlled hypertension
    c. Patient with severe neurologic problems
    d. Patient with a decreased attention span and decreased cognition
    e. Patient with worsening anemia and pruritus

83. The home health nurse is evaluating the home setting for a patient who wishes to have in-home hemodialysis. What is important to have in the home setting to support this therapy?
    a. Specialized water treatment system to provide a safe, clean water supply
    b. Large dust-free space to accommodate and store the dialysis equipment
    c. Modified electrical system to provide high voltage to power the equipment
    d. Specialized cooling system to maintain strict temperature control

84. The nursing student is explaining principles of hemodialysis to the nursing instructor. Which statement by the student indicates a need for additional study and research on the topic?
    a. "Dialysis works as molecules from an area of higher concentration move to an area of lower concentration."
    b. "Blood and dialyzing solution flow in opposite directions across an enclosed semipermeable membrane."
    c. "Excess water, waste products, and excess electrolytes are removed from the blood."
    d. "Bacteria and other organisms can also pass through the membrane."

85. A patient and family are trying to plan a schedule that coordinates with the patient's dialysis regimen. The patient asks, "How often will I have to go and how long does it take?" What is the nurse's best response?
    a. "If you are compliant with the diet and fluid restrictions, you spend less time in dialysis; about 12 hours a week."
    b. "Most patients require about 12 hours per week; this is usually divided into three 4-hour treatments."
    c. "It varies from patient to patient. You will have to call your health care provider for specific instructions."
    d. "If you gain a large amount of fluid weight, a longer treatment time may be needed to prevent severe side effects."

86. A patient is undergoing a dialysis treatment and exhibits a progression of symptoms which include headache, nausea, and vomiting; decreased level of consciousness; and seizure activity. How does the nurse interpret these symptoms?
    a. Dialysis disequilibrium syndrome
    b. Expected manifestations in ESKD
    c. Transient symptoms in a new dialysis patient
    d. Adverse reaction to the dialysate

87. The nurse is caring for a patient with an arteriovenous shunt. What instructions are given to the UAP regarding the care of this patient?
    a. Palpate for thrills and auscultate for bruits every 4 hours.
    b. Check for bleeding at needle insertion sites.
    c. Assess the patient's distal pulses and circulation.
    d. Do not take blood pressure readings in the arm with the shunt.

88. The nurse is assessing a patient's extremity with an arteriovenous graft. The nurse notes a thrill and a bruit, and the patient reports numbness and a cool feeling in the fingers. How does the nurse interpret this information in regards to the shunt?
    a. It is functional and symptoms are expected.
    b. It is functional but the patient has "steal syndrome."
    c. It is directing the blood flow in the wrong direction.
    d. It is not functional and therefore causing numbness.

89. The nurse is providing postdialysis care for a patient. In comparing vital signs and weight measurements to the predialysis data, what does the nurse expect to find?
    a. Blood pressure and weight are reduced.
    b. Blood pressure is increased and weight is reduced.
    c. Blood pressure and weight are similar to predialysis measurements.
    d. Blood pressure is low and weight is the same.

90. The nurse is assessing a patient who has just returned from hemodialysis. What is an unexpected finding that warrants notification of the health care provider?
    a. Feeling of malaise
    b. Nausea and anorexia
    c. Muscle cramps in the legs
    d. Bleeding at the access site

91. The nurse is caring for a patient with an arteriovenous fistula. What is included in the nursing care for this patient? *(Select all that apply.)*
    a. Keep small clamps handy by the bedside.
    b. Encourage routine range-of-motion exercises.
    c. Avoid venipuncture or IV administration on the arm with the access device.
    d. Instruct the patient to carry heavy objects to build muscular strength.
    e. Assess for manifestations of infection at needle sites.
    f. Instruct the patient to sleep on the side with the affected arm in the dependent position.

92. A patient has returned to the medical-surgical unit after having a dialysis treatment. The nurse notes that the patient is also scheduled for an invasive procedure on the same day. What is the primary rationale for delaying the procedure for 4 to 6 hours?
    a. The patient was heparinized during dialysis.
    b. The patient will have cardiac dysrhythmias after dialysis.
    c. The patient will be incoherent and unable to give consent.
    d. The patient needs routine medications that were delayed.

93. The nurse alerts the health care provider about changes in a patient's condition and the patient is diagnosed with dialysis disequilibrium syndrome. The nurse prepares to assist in the administration of which treatment?
    a. IV normal saline fluid bolus
    b. Diuretics and antihypertensives
    c. Barbiturates and anticonvulsants
    d. Morphine and anticoagulants

94. Which patient with kidney problems is the best candidate for peritoneal dialysis (PD)?
    a. Patient with peritoneal adhesions
    b. Patient with a history of extensive abdominal surgery
    c. Patient with peritoneal membrane fibrosis
    d. Patient with a history of difficulty with anticoagulants

95. Place the sequence of steps of PD in the correct order using the numbers 1 through 3.

    _____ a. Fluid stays in the cavity for a specified time prescribed by the health care provider.

    _____ b. 1 to 2 L of dialysate is infused by gravity over a 10- to 20-minute period.

    _____ c. Fluid flows out of the body by gravity into a drainage bag.

96. The health care provider has ordered intraperitoneal heparin for a patient with a new
PD catheter to prevent clotting of the catheter.
What does the nurse advise the patient to do?
a. Watch for signs of bleeding such as bruising or bleeding from the gums.
b. Make a follow-up appointment for coagulation studies.
c. Be aware that intraperitoneal heparin does
not affect clotting times.
d. Be aware that heparin will be given with a
small subcutaneous needle.

Matching. *Match the terms with their correct descriptions.*

Terms
a. Continuous ambulatory peritoneal dialysis
(CAPD)
b. Continuous connect system
c. Disconnect system
d. Automated peritoneal dialysis (APD)
e. Intermittent peritoneal dialysis (IPD)
f. Continuous-cycle peritoneal dialysis (CCPD)

Descriptions
_____ 97. Combines osmotic pressure gradients
with true dialysis
_____ 98. Infusion of four 2 L exchanges of dialysate; exchanges occur 7 days a week
_____ 99. The extra opening of the system increases the risk for infection
_____ 100. Empty bag and tubing are folded be-
neath clothing until they are used for
outflow
_____ 101. Permits in-home dialysis during sleep,
allowing dialysis-free waking hours
_____ 102. Uses an automated cycling machine

103. The home health nurse is visiting a patient who
independently performs PD. Which question
does the nurse ask the patient to assess for the
most common problem associated with PD?
a. "Have you noticed any signs or symptoms
of infection?"
b. "Are you having any pain during the dialysis treatments?"
c. "Is the dialysate fluid slow or sluggish?"
d. "Have you noticed any leakage around the
catheter?"

104. The nurse is teaching a patient about performing PD at home. In order to identify the earliest manifestation of infection, what does the
nurse instruct the patient to do?
a. Monitor temperature routinely.
b. Check the effluent for cloudiness.
c. Be aware of feelings of malaise.
d. Monitor for abdominal pain.

105. During PD, the nurse notes slowed dialysate
flow. What does the nurse do to troubleshoot
the system? *(Select all that apply.)*
a. Ensure that the drainage bag is elevated.
b. Inspect the tubing for kinking or twisting.
c. Ensure that clamps are open.
d. Turn the patient to the other side.
e. Make sure the patient is in good body
alignment.
f. Instruct the patient to stand or cough.
g. Milk the tubing for particulate matter.

106. A patient has just started PD therapy and reports some mild pain when the dialysate is flowing in. What does the nurse do next?
    a. Immediately report the pain to the health care provider.
    b. Try warming the dialysate in the microwave oven.
    c. Reassure the patient that some pain is expected for the first week or two.
    d. Assess the connection tubing for kinking or twisting.

107. The nurse is caring for a patient requiring PD. In order to monitor the patient's weight, what does the nurse do?
    a. Check the weight after a drain and before the next fill to monitor the patient's "dry weight."
    b. Calculate the "dry weight" by weighing the patient every day and comparing the measurements to baseline.
    c. Determine "dry weight" by comparing the patient's weight to a standard weight chart based on height and age.
    d. Weigh the patient each day and count fluid intake and dialysate volume to determine the patient's "dry weight."

108. The nurse is monitoring a patient's PD treatment. The total outflow is less than the inflow. What does the nurse do next?
    a. Instruct the patient to ambulate.
    b. Notify the health care provider.
    c. Record the difference as intake.
    d. Put the patient on fluid restriction.

109. Which patients are likely to be excluded from receiving a transplant? *(Select all that apply.)*
    a. Patient who had breast cancer 6 years ago
    b. HIV-positive patient
    c. Patient with a chemical dependency
    d. 70-year-old patient
    e. Patient with diabetes mellitus

110. A daughter is considering donating a kidney to her mother for organ transplant. What information does the nurse give to the daughter about the criteria for donation? *(Select all that apply.)*
    a. Age limit is at least 21 years old.
    b. Systemic disease and infection must be absent.
    c. There must be no history of cancer.
    d. Hypertension or kidney disease must be absent.
    e. There must be adequate kidney function as determined by diagnostic studies.
    f. The donor must understand the surgery and be willing to give up the organ.
    g. There must be no allergies to medications.

111. The nurse is caring for the kidney transplant patient in the immediate postoperative period. During this initial period, for what time frame does the nurse assess the urine output at least hourly?
    a. First 8 hours
    b. First 12 hours
    c. First 24 hours
    d. First 48 hours

112. The intensive care nurse is caring for the kidney transplant patient who was just transferred from the recovery unit. Which finding is the most serious within the first 12 hours after surgery and warrants immediate notification of the transplant surgeon?
    a. Diuresis with increased output
    b. Pink and bloody urine
    c. Abrupt decrease in urine
    d. Low-grade fever

113. The nurse is caring for the kidney transplant patient who is 3 days postsurgery. The nurse notes a sudden and abrupt decrease in urine. The nurse alerts the health care provider because this is a sign of which anomaly?
    a. Rejection
    b. Thrombosis
    c. Stenosis
    d. Infection

CASE STUDY: THE PATIENT ON HEMODIALYSIS

Use a separate sheet of paper to answer the questions in this Case Study, or go to the "Prepare for Class" folder on your Evolve website at http://evolve.elsevier.com/Iggy/ to download and complete as a word processing file. Answer guidelines for this Case Study are also available on your Evolve website.

A 47-year-old man is being sent back to the hospital unit after undergoing hemodialysis in the dialysis unit. The patient was initially admitted for pneumonia but has been receiving hemodialysis Mondays, Wednesdays, and Fridays for the past year for kidney failure. He has a functioning arteriovenous fistula of the left arm. On assessment a positive thrill and bruit are confirmed. The nurse from the dialysis unit informs the unit nurse assigned to the patient that 1 L of fluid was removed. She reports that prior to dialysis the patient's weight was 80 kg, and after dialysis it is 79 kg. At the end of the dialysis treatment the patient's vital signs are: temp 36.7° C (98.0° F); heart rate 87/min; respirations 20/min; blood pressure 90/61 mm Hg. A 2" × 2" gauze dressing covers the accessed site of the AV fistula and it is clean, dry, and intact. The patient is alert and oriented but reports feeling tired after the treatment.

1. Using the SBAR format, outline the conversation the nurse from the dialysis unit will have with the hospital unit nurse in the handoff of this patient.

2. What side effects is the patient experiencing in the post-dialysis stage?

3. What is the reason for the patient's low blood pressure?

CASE STUDY: THE PATIENT WITH CONTINUOUS AMBULATORY PERITONEAL DIALYSIS (CAPD)

Use a separate sheet of paper to answer the questions in this Case Study, or go to the "Prepare for Class" folder on your Evolve website at http://evolve.elsevier.com/Iggy/ to download and complete as a word processing file. Answer guidelines for this Case Study are also available on your Evolve website.

A 36-year-old woman is married and has two adopted children. She is diagnosed with polycystic kidney disease (PKD), and she will soon have to go on dialysis or consent to a kidney transplant.

1. What additional data should the nurse collect to help the patient make the best decision for herself?

2. How would the nurse briefly describe the process of dialysis to the patient? Include information about the following questions:
   a. In peritoneal dialysis, what is the membrane through which the process occurs?
   b. Identify the types of peritoneal dialysis.
   c. What is used to prevent fibrin clot formation in peritoneal dialysis?
   d. How is peritonitis identified and diagnosed in the patient receiving dialysis?
   e. List three advantages of using peritoneal dialysis instead of hemodialysis.

3. Identify the source of possible problems with the flow of dialysate in patients with peritoneal dialysis.

4. What are the protein needs of the patient receiving peritoneal dialysis?

5. Due to the long distance the patient lives from the medical center, she elects to begin CAPD. What would be included in a plan of hospital care for the patient for this procedure?

6. What could the nurse explain and demonstrate about the steps of caring for the dialysis catheter?

7. The patient has been performing PD at home. She calls the nurse to report about outflow from the first peritoneal dialysis. What does the nurse tell the patient about the appearance of the outflow?

Assessment of the Reproductive System

STUDY/REVIEW QUESTIONS

1. When a patient has a rectal exam to evaluate the prostate, it can be palpated through the rectum. How far into the rectal lumen does the prostate normally project?
   a. The prostate does not project into the rectal lumen.
   b. No more than 1 1/2 inches
   c. No more than 3/8 inches
   d. One-half inch

2. What is the site for a Papanicolaou (Pap) test?
   a. Cervix
   b. Walls of the vagina
   c. Cervical canal
   d. Fallopian tubes

3. The epididymis of the internal male reproduction system is the maturation site of

   _____.

4. The nurse is interviewing a 52-year-old woman reporting irregular and decreased flow of menses for several months. Which question does the nurse ask the patient?
   a. "Is there any chance you could be pregnant?"
   b. "Are you having any discomfort during intercourse?"
   c. "Do your breasts feel tender or swollen?"
   d. "Are you having any unusual vaginal discharge?"

5. Which statements about what is included in a hysteroscopy procedure are true? *(Select all that apply.)*
   a. The patient is placed in the lithotomy position.
   b. Removal of an intrauterine device can be done with this procedure.
   c. Tubal ligation can be performed.
   d. The exam can reveal the cause of any abnormal bleeding.
   e. The procedure can correct any infertility problems.

6. A laparoscopy can be used for which purposes? *(Select all that apply.)*
   a. Rule out ectopic pregnancy
   b. Diagnose cervical lesions
   c. Evaluate ovarian disorders
   d. Diagnose infertility problems
   e. Evaluate pelvic masses

7. A laparoscopy is used to perform which procedures? *(Select all that apply.)*
   a. Cervical biopsy
   b. Cyst aspiration
   c. Ovarian biopsy
   d. Tubal sterilization
   e. Retrieval of "lost" intrauterine devices

8. A male patient reports that he has a decreased libido (sex drive). The nurse assesses for which factors related to this condition? *(Select all that apply.)*
   a. Tobacco use
   b. Type and amount of exercise pattern
   c. Alcohol consumption
   d. Type of occupation
   e. Illicit drug use

9. A male patient had mumps as a child which caused orchitis. This patient is likely to have which potential complications? (*Select all that apply.*)
   a. Decreased libido
   b. Early development of secondary sex characteristics
   c. Testicular atrophy
   d. Increased libido
   e. Sterility

10. Which statements about prostate-specific antigen (PSA) testing are true? (*Select all that apply.*)
    a. It is used to screen for prostate cancer.
    b. PSA levels above 25 ng/mL are associated with prostate cancer.
    c. Older men often have a lower normal PSA level.
    d. It is done on patients over 60 years of age.
    e. PSA levels less than 4 ng/mL are normal.

11. Failure of ovulation in women is associated with an increased risk for _____ _____.

12. Most diseases that alter a woman's metabolism or nutrition can result in which condition?
    a. Excessive bleeding
    b. Endometriosis
    c. Amenorrhea
    d. Pelvic inflammatory disease

13. Females who fail to ovulate are associated with a greater risk for what complication?
    a. Tubal pregnancies
    b. Endometrial cancer
    c. Abdominal cramps
    d. Ovarian cancer

14. A 30-year-old female informs the nurse that she has been a diabetic for 10 years. What gynecologic change will the patient likely experience as a result?
    a. White, excessive vaginal drainage
    b. Burning and itching of the vagina
    c. Vaginal bleeding mid-menstrual cycle
    d. Vaginal dryness

Fill in the blanks.

15. The normal pH of the vagina is _____ to _____, which is necessary to decrease the vagina's susceptibility to infection.

16. Men with _____-degree relatives with prostate cancer are at greater risk for the disease than men in the general population.

17. A delayed or early development of secondary sex characteristics can be related to a _____ pattern.

18. Penile erection can result from _____ stimulation and _____ mechanisms.

19. The prostate gland secretes a milky alkaline fluid that enhances sperm _____ and neutralizes acidic _____ secretions.

20. A _____ diet may increase the risk for cancer of the breast, ovary, and prostate gland.

21. A patient taking oral contraceptives will have an increased need for which elements in her diet? (*Select all that apply.*)
    a. Vitamin D
    b. Folic acid
    c. Calcium
    d. Vitamins B_6 and B_{12}
    e. Vitamin C

22. A certain level of body fat and weight is essential to which factors regarding the female reproductive system? (*Select all that apply.*)
    a. Maintenance of secondary sex characteristics
    b. The onset of menses
    c. Prevention of the development of endometriosis
    d. Maintenance of regular menstrual cycles
    e. Maintenance of libido

23. An insufficient estrogen level is related to what condition?
    a. Osteoporosis
    b. Stroke
    c. Coronary artery disease
    d. Decreased immune function

24. A patient with chronic congestive heart failure and chronic obstructive pulmonary disease can have alterations of which factor?
    a. Decreased reproductive function
    b. Decreased sexual response
    c. Increased libido
    d. Decreased susceptibility to sexually-transmitted infections

25. An adult 29-year-old patient has strictures and adhesions in her fallopian tubes. This may be the result of which conditions? *(Select all that apply.)*
    a. Ruptured appendix followed by peritonitis
    b. Frequent bouts of colitis
    c. Gallbladder disease
    d. Frequent urinary tract infections
    e. Pelvic inflammatory disease

26. Young women who have intercourse as teenagers and/or have multiple sex partners are at high risk for which disease?
    a. Endometriosis
    b. Cervical cancer
    c. Amenorrhea
    d. Ovarian cancer

27. A 37-year-old patient reports abnormal vaginal bleeding not related to her menstrual cycle. About what associated symptoms would the nurse ask the patient? *(Select all that apply.)*
    a. Pain
    b. Change in bowel habits
    c. Back pain
    d. Abdominal fullness
    e. Urinary difficulties

28. The nurse is assigned to a patient who reports a discharge from his penis that started 3 days ago. About what associated characteristics does the nurse ask the patient regarding the discharge? *(Select all that apply.)*
    a. Pain
    b. Odor
    c. Amount
    d. Change in bowel habits
    e. Consistency

29. In a patient with a reproductive health problem, what health and lifestyle habits would the nurse assess? *(Select all that apply.)*
    a. Diet
    b. Socioeconomic status
    c. Exercise pattern
    d. Occupation
    e. Sleep pattern

30. Other than determining pregnancy or infertility, a pelvic examination is indicated to assess for which conditions? *(Select all that apply.)*
    a. Rape trauma
    b. Frequent urinary tract infections
    c. Menstrual irregularities
    d. Decreased libido
    e. Vaginal discharge or itching

31. Which imaging is used to differentiate solid tissue masses from cystic or hemorrhagic structures in the abdomen and pelvis?
    a. Hysterosalpingography
    b. Computed tomography
    c. Kidney, ureter, and bladder (KUB) x-ray
    d. Colposcopy

32. What imaging is selected to assess for pelvic masses, calcified tumors or fibroids, metastatic bone changes, and demoid cysts?
    a. Bone scan
    b. Hysterosalpingography
    c. Computed tomography
    d. X-ray of kidneys, ureters, and bladder (KUB)

33. Which test detects cancerous and precancerous cells of the cervix?
    a. Serologic studies
    b. Culture
    c. Pap smear
    d. HPV test

34. A 79-year-old man is being seen for difficulty voiding and some blood in the urine. Which is the first screening test likely to be done?
    a. HIV testing
    b. PSA
    c. Culture
    d. Serologic studies

35. When prostate cancer is suspected in a man, what does the nurse suggest the next step may be?
    a. "You will need to have a needle biopsy of the prostate gland."
    b. "An MRI with contrast will be done of your pelvis and genitals."
    c. "There is no need for further tests or treatments at this time."
    d. "Increase your fluid intake and take your prescribed antibiotics."

36. A 23-year-old female has a decreased level of follicle-stimulating hormone (FSH). What may this finding indicate? *(Select all that apply.)*
    a. Beginning menses
    b. Anorexia nervosa
    c. Fertility
    d. Infertility
    e. Neoplasm

37. What test is used to assess tubal anatomy and patency, and uterine problems?
    a. Computed tomography
    b. X-ray of kidney, ureters, and bladder (KUB)
    c. Colposcopy
    d. Hysterosalpingography

38. A patient is diagnosed with a chlamydial infection but is reluctant to spend the money for treatment because she is asymptomatic and does not have a job or health insurance. The nurse advises her that chlamydial infections can result in which condition?
    a. Female infertility
    b. Male partner infertility
    c. Amenorrhea
    d. Teratogenic effects

39. In recalling dietary intake for a recent 24-hour period, a female patient describes eating eggs, whole milk, and bacon for breakfast; fried chicken and French fries for lunch; three-cheese pizza and ice cream for dinner. This type of diet places her at increased risk for which disorder?
    a. Osteoporosis
    b. Fatigue and low libido
    c. Early menopause
    d. Cancer of the breast and ovaries

40. A 40-year-old woman has heavy vaginal bleeding. Which question is the priority in evaluating the patient's chief complaint?
    a. "Is the bleeding related to the menstrual cycle or intercourse?"
    b. "Are you having any sensations of pain or cramping?"
    c. "Are you sexually active and do you use oral contraceptives?"
    d. "Are you feeling weak, dizzy, or lightheaded?"

41. A young woman reports that she has a genital discharge causing irritation and odor. She feels embarrassed, but insists that she has not had recent sexual relations. What does the nurse assess for? *(Select all that apply.)*
    a. Current use of antibiotic medications
    b. Type of clothing and undergarments
    c. Age of onset of menses
    d. Presence of genital or orifice lesions
    e. Recent change of diet
    f. Chronic presence of the discharge

42. A patient calls to make an appointment for a routine pelvic exam which includes a Pap smear. What type of instructions does the nurse give the patient about preparing for the exam?
    a. Do not douche for at least 24 hours before the exam.
    b. Do not eat or drink anything after midnight to decrease bowel and bladder discomfort.
    c. The genital area must be cleaned with mild soap and water before the exam.
    d. If you are having your period, do not wear a tampon; use a menstrual pad.

43. The nurse is teaching a patient about the contraindications for hysteroscopy. What does the nurse tell the patient?
    a. During the procedure, normal or abnormal cells can be pushed through the fallopian tubes and into your pelvic cavity; therefore pregnancy is contraindicated.
    b. The procedure causes irritation and can be very painful if your vaginal tissue is dry or fragile; therefore, the procedure is not recommended for postmenopausal women.
    c. The procedure can cause a lot of bleeding so a recent prescription of an anticoagulant is contraindicated.
    d. During the procedure, an iodine-based dye is used, so allergies to shellfish or iodine are contraindications.

Matching. Match each dysfunction with its etiology.

Dysfunctions
a. Vaginal dryness, increased yeast infections, impotence
b. Failure of ovulation
c. Ovarian dysfunction
d. Decreased spermatogenesis, libido, or impotence
e. Orchitis
f. Altered sexual response

Etiology
_____ 44. Low levels of body fat or poor nutrition
_____ 45. Mumps
_____ 46. Substance abuse
_____ 47. Endocrine disorders
_____ 48. Chronic disorders of nervous, respiratory, or cardiovascular system
_____ 49. Associated with a greater risk for endometrial cancer

50. A 31-year-old woman is being seen for follow-up of salpingitis. What possible complication can this patient develop?
    a. Infertility
    b. Ovarian dysfunction
    c. Abdominal cramps
    d. Pelvic scarring

51. The nurse explains to a patient that the American Cancer Society (ACS) advises to begin annual Pap testing for women who meet which criteria? *(Select all that apply.)*
    a. Within 1 year of becoming sexually active
    b. No later than 21 years of age if not sexually active
    c. By age 18 years of age if not sexually active
    d. Within 3 years of becoming sexually active
    e. By 16 years of age whether or not sexually active

52. The nurse is caring for a patient who had a laparoscopy. What does postoperative care for this patient include? *(Select all that apply.)*
    a. Administer oral analgesics for incisional pain.
    b. Notify the physician of postoperative shoulder pain.
    c. Reassure the patient that most painful sensations disappear within 4 to 6 weeks.
    d. Instruct the patient to change the small adhesive bandage as needed.
    e. Teach the patient to observe the incision for signs of infection or hematoma.
    f. Remind the patient to avoid strenuous activity for 4 to 6 weeks after the procedure.

53. The nurse is helping a patient schedule an appointment for a hysteroscopy. When does the nurse advise the patient that the procedure should be done?
    a. 5 days after menses have ceased
    b. 5 days before the beginning of menses
    c. During the menstrual period
    d. Whenever she can take 3 to 4 days off of work

54. In which patients is a hysteroscopy contraindicated? *(Select all that apply.)*
    a. Patient with suspected cervical cancer
    b. Infertile patient
    c. Patient with an infection of the reproductive tract
    d. Menopausal patient
    e. Pregnant patient
    f. Patient with suspected endometrial cancer

55. What serum levels are typically obtained to help diagnose male or female reproductive tract disorder? *(Select all that apply.)*
    a. Follicle-stimulating hormone (FSH)
    b. Total iron-binding capacity (TIBC)
    c. Prolactin
    d. Luteinizing hormone (LH)
    e. Thyroid-stimulating hormone (TSH)

56. A _____ allows for three-dimensional magnification and intense illumination of epithelium that has suspected disease of cervical, vaginal, and vulvular epithelium.

CASE STUDY: THE PATIENT WITH ABNORMAL VAGINAL BLEEDING

Use a separate sheet of paper to answer the questions in this Case Study, or go to the "Prepare for Class" folder on your Evolve website at http://evolve.elsevier.com/Iggy/ to download and complete as a word processing file. Answer guidelines for this Case Study are also available on your Evolve website.

A 32-year-old woman comes to the clinic for a routine gynecologic exam. She reports noticing heavy bleeding with periods and pelvic pain. She reports that her form of birth control is the intrauterine device. She is married with no children. Her weight is 179 lbs, and her height is 5'4".

1. Document a nursing note for this patient using a free text format.

2. What exam might be ordered for this patient besides the routine pelvic and PAP exam?

3. What information will be needed in the patient history? Review of systems? What components of the physical assessment will be used to assess this patient?

Care of Patients with Breast Disorders

STUDY/REVIEW QUESTIONS

Matching. *Match the terms with their correct definitions.*

Terms
a. Macrocysts
b. Ductal ectasia
c. Gynecomastia
d. Lymphedema of the affected limb
e. Breast augmentation
f. Papilloma
g. Ductal carcinoma in situ (DCIS)
h. Peau d'orange

Definitions

_____ 1. Dimpling, orange-peel appearance of the skin

_____ 2. Surgery to enhance the size, shape, or symmetry of breasts

_____ 3. Fluid-filled and painful, enlarging in response to monthly hormonal changes

_____ 4. Benign breast problem usually seen in women approaching menopause

_____ 5. Pedunculated outgrowth of tissue

_____ 6. Early noninvasive form of breast cancer

_____ 7. Usually a benign condition of breast enlargement in men

_____ 8. Abnormal accumulation of protein fluid in the subcutaneous tissue

9. Danazol (Danocrine) is used in patients with type of fibrocystic breast condition (FBC)? *(Select all that apply.)*
   a. Mild
   b. Moderate
   c. Severe
   d. New onset
   e. Recurrent

10. A 29-year-old woman is being seen for a self-detected mass in her right breast. Clinical examination reveals an oval-shaped, freely mobile, and rubbery lesion measuring 1 cm x 2.5 cm. What type of tumor is this most likely to be?
    a. Ductal ectasia
    b. Papilloma
    c. Fibroadenoma
    d. Macrocyst

11. A 33-year-old woman reports that the skin over her left breast is reddened, warm, and has swelling. These characteristics are typically found in which type of breast disorder?
    a. Intraductal papilloma
    b. Fibroadenoma
    c. Inflammatory breast cancer
    d. Infiltrating ductal carcinoma

12. The nurse reads a history of a patient with small, nonpalpable cysts inside the breast glands that were discovered 3 months ago. What likely breast disorder is this?
    a. Papilloma
    b. Microcysts
    c. Ductal ectasia
    d. Fibroadenoma

13. The nurse is preparing an information packet about reconstructive breast surgery. What information does the nurse include about health risks for large-breasted women?
    a. Increased risk for fungal infections and backaches
    b. Decreased difficulty in nursing a baby
    c. Likelihood of foul discharge from the nipples
    d. Increased risk for fibrocystic disease

14. For which associated serious side effects does the nurse instruct a patient when taking danazol (Danocrine) for fibrocystic breast condition? *(Select all that apply.)*
    a. Irritable bowel syndrome
    b. Sudden numbness
    c. Hypotension
    d. Chest pain
    e. Severe headache

15. A patient with fibrocystic breast condition (FBC) has just undergone fine needle aspiration to drain the cyst fluid and reduce pressure and pain. At what points does the nurse prepare patient education material about breast biopsy? *(Select all that apply.)*
    a. If hormonal replacement therapy is prescribed
    b. If fluid is not aspirated
    c. If the mammogram shows suspicious findings
    d. If fluid buildup recurs
    e. If the mass remains palpable after aspiration
    f. If aspirated fluid reveals cancer cells

16. A patient with FBC is prescribed drug therapy to manage symptoms. The nurse prepares teaching materials for which group of medications?
    a. Anti-androgen agents, calcium supplements, opioids
    b. Monoclonal antibody agents, corticosteroids
    c. Aromatase inhibitors, potassium supplements, NSAIDs
    d. Oral contraceptives, vitamin therapy, diuretics

17. The nurse recommends which self-care measures to help a patient reduce pain and manage symptoms associated with FBC? *(Select all that apply.)*
    a. Temporarily discontinue drug therapy just before menses.
    b. Take mild analgesics as needed.
    c. Limit salt intake before menses to help decrease swelling.
    d. Wear a supportive bra.
    e. Locally apply ice or heat to provide temporary relief of pain.
    f. Massage breasts frequently during peak episodes of pain.

18. A 54-year-old woman has identified a hard breast mass with irregular borders, redness, and edema. She reports a greenish-brown nipple discharge and enlarged axillary nodes. Based on the patient's age and description of the symptoms, what does the nurse suspect?
    a. Fibroadenoma
    b. Fibrocystic breast condition
    c. Ductal ectasia
    d. Intraductal papilloma

19. The nurse notes in the electronic medical record that the patient has a round, firm, non-tender, mobile breast mass not attached to breast tissue or the chest wall. What does this describe?
    a. Fibroadenoma
    b. Fibrocystic disease
    c. Breast cysts
    d. Ductal ectasia

20. The nurse is reviewing discharge instructions for a patient who had breast augmentation surgery. What does the nurse include in these instructions? *(Select all that apply.)*
    a. Expect soreness in chest and arms for several months.
    b. Breasts will feel tight and sensitive; the breast skin may feel warm or itchy.
    c. Anticipate having difficulty raising the arms over the head.
    d. Perform lifting, pushing, and pulling exercises several times a day.
    e. Walk every few hours to prevent deep vein thrombi.
    f. Expect some swelling for 3 to 4 weeks after surgery.

21. What is the most common breast dysfunction found in the male breast?
    a. Nipple discharge
    b. Nipple retraction
    c. Gynecomastia
    d. Disseminated breast cancer

Fill in the blank.

22. The two main features of FBC are _____ and _____.

23. The 5-year survival rate for women with localized breast cancer is 98%, whereas the rate drops to 81% when the breast cancer has spread to the _____ _____ nodes.

24. The most common sites of metastatic disease from breast cancer are _____, _____, _____, and _____.

25. _____ are the most common benign tumor in women during the reproductive years.

26. FBC is thought to be caused by an imbalance in the normal _____ to progesterone ratio.

27. What does the nurse instruct the patient who is scheduled to have a breast augmentation surgery to do before the surgery? *(Select all that apply.)*
    a. Take an aspirin.
    b. Stop smoking.
    c. Avoid taking NSAIDs.
    d. Avoid taking Ginkgo biloba.
    e. Take garlic supplements.

28. After surgery, a female patient has been told her breast tumor contains estrogen receptors (ER positive). How will this type of cancer be treated?
    a. Surgery alone
    b. Hormonal therapy
    c. Radiation therapy
    d. Targeted therapy with trastuzumab

29. According to the latest studies, which woman has the greatest risk of developing breast cancer?
    a. Physician, age 56, who had her first child at age 38
    b. Ballet dancer, age 20, who has a 5-year-old son
    c. Radiation technician, age 24, who had her menarche at age 13
    d. Postmenopausal woman, age 52, who had breast reduction surgery at age 26

30. The nurse is counseling a woman recently diagnosed with breast cancer. Which factor has the most influence on the patient's choice for treatment?
    a. Age at the time of diagnosis
    b. Overall health status
    c. Personal choice and type of insurance
    d. Extent and location of metastasis of the breast mass

31. A young patient is suspected of having invasive breast cancer. Based on the types and frequencies of breast cancer, what is the patient most likely to be diagnosed with?
    a. FBC
    b. Infiltrating ductal carcinoma
    c. Lobular carcinoma in situ
    d. DCIS

32. Which factor is the incidence of breast disease most closely related to?
    a. Weight
    b. Aging
    c. Ethnic background
    d. Socioeconomic status

33. Cancer surveillance in high-risk women involves breast self-examination (BSE), clinical breast examination (CBE), and mammography. Cancer surveillance is used to detect cancer in its early stages and is referred to as what kind of prevention?
    a. Primary
    b. Secondary
    c. Tertiary
    d. Prophylactic

34. The American Cancer Society recommends early detection by screening for breast masses with a mammogram for women aged _____ years and older.

35. Which factor makes the mammogram a more sensitive screening tool than other tests?
    a. Higher compliance rate than BSE because it is less painful
    b. Less expensive than other tests that identify tumor markers
    c. Able to reveal masses too small to be palpated manually
    d. Able to differentiate between fluid and solid masses

36. The nurse is teaching a 24-year-old patient about BSE. When does the nurse tell her to perform BSE?
    a. The day before her menstrual flow is due
    b. On the third day after her menstrual flow starts
    c. When ovulation occurs
    d. One week after her menstrual flow starts

37. The nurse is teaching a thin, small-breasted woman how to perform BSE. The patient keeps palpating her ribs and reporting lumps. What technique does the nurse use to help her identify the ribs?
    a. Have her stand in front of a mirror and look at the rib contour.
    b. Reassure her that because she is thin, she is feeling her ribs.
    c. Demonstrate how to follow the rib to the sternum.
    d. Put her in a supine position so that breast tissue falls to the sides.

38. A patient stopped having menses about a year ago. When does the nurse advise the patient to perform BSE?
    a. The first day of every other month
    b. Continue on schedule even though menses have ceased
    c. The last day of each month
    d. Any day as long as the schedule is consistent

39. The student nurse is preparing to teach a Navajo patient about breast cancer and BSE. After reading culturally relevant material, which teaching methods does the student decide are best for this patient? *(Select all that apply.)*
    a. Show the patient a video.
    b. Have the patient attend a lecture.
    c. Supply reading material for the patient.
    d. Practice on a manikin.
    e. Provide helpful Internet sites that the patient can view.

40. The nurse is teaching a young patient about BSE. Which statement by the patient indicates a need for further instruction?
    a. "I should perform BSE on a monthly basis from now on."
    b. "I see my health care provider annually, but I should perform BSE."
    c. "BSE is a self-care measure that I can use to prevent breast cancer."
    d. "The best time to perform BSE is 1 week after my menstrual period."

41. What type of teaching increases the likelihood that a woman will be more compliant with the performance of regular monthly BSE?
    a. Learning from a pamphlet at home
    b. Learning at a clinic or office
    c. Seeing a television program about the risks for developing breast cancer
    d. Reading magazine articles

42. The advanced-practice nurse is performing a CBE. The practitioner places the patient in which position to begin the examination?
    a. Supine position with a pillow under the shoulder and the arm raised above the head
    b. The arms raised over the head to expose the surface underneath the breast for inspection
    c. Standing position with the hands on the hips
    d. Sitting or standing with the arms down at the sides

43. During a CBE, the examiner observes a discharge from the nipple. What is most important to include in the documentation of this finding?
    a. Area of "the clock" that was compressed when the discharge was released
    b. Amount of pressure required for the discharge to be released
    c. Frequency and technique the patient uses for BSE
    d. History of difficulty or pain when attempting to breast-feed

44. Upon performing a CBE, the patient with which symptom suggests advanced disease?
    a. Gynecomastia
    b. Oval-shaped, mobile, rubbery mass
    c. Thin, milky discharge from the nipple
    d. Skin change of peau d'orange

45. Which screening techniques are best for early detection of breast cancer? *(Select all that apply.)*
    a. Mammogram
    b. Clinical breast exam
    c. Needle aspiration of breast tissue
    d. Breast self-awareness
    e. Computed tomography

46. Fibroadenomas are the most common benign tumor in women during the _____ years.

47. Many symptoms of breast cancer are similar to those seen in _____ disorders.

48. Women who have a personal history of breast cancer are at high risk for developing a reoccurrence or new breast cancer with the presence of which factors? *(Select all that apply.)*
    a. BRCA 3 genetic mutation
    b. Strong family history
    c. BRCA 2 genetic mutation
    d. BRCA 1 genetic mutation
    e. Occupation

49. The nurse is instructing a patient with ductal ectasia about her risk for breast cancer. What does the nurse tell the patient?
    a. It increases the risk of breast cancer by 25%.
    b. It has no effect to the risk of developing breast cancer.
    c. It increases the risk of breast cancer by 75%.
    d. It doubles the risk of developing breast cancer.

50. Which are characteristics of patients with a high risk for breast cancer? *(Select all that apply.)*
   a. Early menarche
   b. Multiple births
   c. Late menopause
   d. Nullipara
   e. First pregnancy after 30 years of age

51. Most men who present with nipple discharge are diagnosed with _____ _____.

52. A patient has returned from breast reconstruction surgery with a Jackson-Pratt drain in place that is patent and draining serosanguineous fluid. The nurse notices that at 8:00 AM, the drainage container is full. It was last emptied at 6:00 AM. The total drainage for the last 2 hours is measured at 145 mL. What is the priority nursing intervention?
   a. Notify the health care provider about the amount and type of drainage for last 2 hours.
   b. Empty the drain every 2 hours so the suction will be more effective.
   c. Chart the type and amount of drainage and continue to monitor.
   d. Reinforce the drain site with a sterile bulky dressing.

53. A patient had a partial mastectomy yesterday and the nurse writes on the nursing care plan "Anxiety related to removal of breast tissue." What is the nurse's priority intervention?
   a. Use distraction until the patient improves and is able to think more clearly.
   b. Encourage the patient to have a positive attitude so she will heal faster.
   c. Ensure that the patient takes PRN anxiolytic medication every 4 to 6 hours.
   d. Encourage the patient to discuss her fears and ask questions about her concerns.

54. A patient had a partial mastectomy. When teaching about care of the arm on the affected side, what does the nurse tell the patient?
   a. Start arm exercises as soon as the drains are removed from the incision.
   b. Keep the arm elevated so the elbow is above the shoulder and the wrist is above the elbow.
   c. Do not take blood pressure in the arm on the affected side for the first 6 months after surgery.
   d. Do push-ups and arm circles on a routine basis for a full recovery.

55. A patient has recently been diagnosed with breast cancer. What is the most likely priority preoperative nursing care for this patient?
   a. Providing patient education
   b. Assisting the patient to make independent decisions
   c. Providing reassurance
   d. Providing a safe environment so the patient can talk openly about his or her feelings

56. Which intervention is priority in the nursing care plan for a patient after a modified radical mastectomy?
   a. Position the patient on the affected side to aid with gravity flow of drainage from the incision site.
   b. Immobilize the arm on the affected side for the first 24 hours postoperatively.
   c. Assess the patient for anxiety because it can impede the healing process.
   d. Teach the patient signs and symptoms of infection and how to monitor for altered wound healing.

57. A patient who had surgery for breast cancer appears in need of continued community support. The nurse refers the patient to which organization?
   a. Reach to Recovery
   b. Empty Arms
   c. Resolve
   d. NAMI

58. The nurse is counseling a woman who has had several discussions with the health care provider about her risk for breast cancer. The nurse reinforces that prophylactic mastectomy would have what effect on her risk for developing breast cancer?
    a. Increases the risk
    b. Eliminates the risk
    c. Decreases the risk
    d. Doubles the risk

59. Which woman has the highest risk for developing breast cancer?
    a. 68-year-old who has taken hormone replacement therapy
    b. 35-year-old with three children
    c. 23-year-old who started menstruating at age 12
    d. 40-year-old who has two cousins who have had breast cancer

60. Which interventions incorporate research findings related to higher breast cancer mortality rates among African-American women? *(Select all that apply.)*
    a. Ask high-end retail stores to do promotional campaigns encouraging mammograms.
    b. Make a list of facilities that do diagnostic screenings in low-income neighborhoods.
    c. Identify bus routes that serve hospitals and clinics and advocate for increased service.
    d. Encourage women to have breast cancer screening because insurance pays for it.
    e. Take all opportunities to teach patients to do BSE.

61. A patient found a mass in her breast 6 months ago. What question does the nurse ask related to possible metastases of a potential cancer?
    a. "Why did you wait 6 months before seeking medical attention?"
    b. "Have you noticed any joint or bone pain or other changes in your body?"
    c. "Have you ever had any exposure to radiation or toxic chemicals?"
    d. "Has your sister or mother ever been diagnosed with breast cancer?"

62. A patient has just been diagnosed with advanced breast cancer. Which behavior by the patient is the strongest indicator of readiness for additional patient teaching and information?
    a. Cheerfully talking about her family and the vacation they will take to Europe
    b. Being active and angrily throwing her belongings into her suitcase
    c. Crying and being upset, asking the nurse to call a spiritual counselor
    d. Being quiet and thoughtfully fingering the lace on her new bra

63. A patient in the medical-surgical unit says to the nursing student, "My doctor told me I have advanced breast cancer and I want to give you this bracelet, because you have been so sweet to me today." What does the student nurse do next?
    a. Contact the charge nurse because the patient may be signaling intentions of suicide.
    b. Sit with the patient and allow her to take the lead in the conversation.
    c. Contact the nursing instructor because the news is overwhelming.
    d. Explain to the patient that it is unethical for students to accept expensive gifts.

64. The nurse is reviewing the laboratory results from a postmenopausal woman being evaluated for a breast mass. What type of metastases does the increased serum calcium and alkaline phosphatase levels suggest?
    a. Brain
    b. Bone
    c. Lung
    d. Liver

65. The nurse is talking to a woman recently diagnosed with breast cancer who confides, "I am going to use nutritional and herbal therapy instead of taking drugs and radiation that would make my hair fall out." What is the nurse's best response?
    a. "Some research shows benefits when complementary therapy is combined with conventional medicine."
    b. "What did your physician tell you about all of your possible treatment options?"
    c. "You really shouldn't use alternative nutritional therapies as a replacement for conventional therapies."
    d. "Where did you hear about this nutritional and herbal treatment?"

66. The nurse is caring for a patient who had a right-sided modified radical mastectomy. Which task does the nurse delegate to the UAP?
    a. Observe the drainage in the Jackson-Pratt drain.
    b. Take blood pressure on the right arm only.
    c. Assist the patient to ambulate the day after surgery.
    d. Instruct the patient about arm positioning.

67. A patient is lying in bed after a mastectomy. How does the nurse position the patient?
    a. Head of the bed up at least 30 degrees with the affected arm elevated on a pillow
    b. Supine body position with the affected arm positioned straight by the side
    c. Any position that is the most comfortable to the patient
    d. Side-lying position with the unaffected side down towards mattress

68. A patient is one day postsurgery after a mastectomy and is anxious to begin the prescribed exercises. Which exercise is appropriate for the patient's first efforts?
    a. Flex the fingers so that the hands slowly "walk" up the wall.
    b. Squeeze the affected hand around a soft, round object.
    c. Swing the rope in small circles and gradually increase to larger circles.
    d. Grab the ends of the rope, and extend the arms until they are straight.

69. A patient is being discharged with a prescription for tamoxifen to decrease the chance of breast cancer recurrence. Because of the common side effect, what does the nurse suggest to the patient in taking this drug?
    a. Have soda crackers and ginger ale on hand.
    b. Install a handrail around the bathtub.
    c. Purchase a scale to monitor body weight.
    d. Buy a soft-bristle toothbrush.

70. A patient is prescribed trastuzumab (Herceptin) for breast cancer. What is the priority nursing intervention for this patient?
    a. Obtain an order for baseline ECG.
    b. Assess for signs of bleeding.
    c. Premedicate with an antiemetic.
    d. Rotate injection sites.

71. The nurse is designing a teaching plan for a patient who had surgery for breast cancer. What information does the nurse include in the plan? *(Select all that apply.)*
    a. Do not use lotions or ointments on the area.
    b. Delay using deodorant under the affected arm until healing is complete.
    c. Swelling and redness of the scar itself are considered normal and permanent.
    d. Report any increased heat and tenderness of the area to the surgeon.
    e. Wear loose pajamas at home for 6 to 8 weeks.
    f. Begin active range-of-motion exercises 1 week after surgery.

CASE STUDY: THE PATIENT WITH FIBROCYSTIC BREAST DISEASE

Use a separate sheet of paper to answer the questions in this Case Study, or go to the "Prepare for Class" folder on your Evolve website at http://evolve.elsevier.com/Iggy/ to download and complete as a word processing file. Answer guidelines for this Case Study are also available on your Evolve website.

A 26-year-old woman reports during her annual gynecologic examination that she has been feeling fullness and soreness before her menstrual period and that she has felt some "marbles" in her breast. She is using contraceptive gel for prevention of pregnancy. The nurse palpates numerous nodules in both breasts and tells the patient that this is most likely fibrocystic changes in the breast tissue.

1. What should the nurse tell the patient about diagnostic testing that will be done?

2. What kinds of treatments might the nurse instruct the patient about after the diagnosis of fibrocystic breast disease (FBD) is confirmed?

3. What teaching should the nurse do to prepare the patient to care for her symptoms?

4. Identify six instructions necessary for the nurse to teach a woman before having her demonstrate a BSE.

5. Document a nursing note for the patient using the following format:
   - Problem:
   - Note:
   - Exam:

74
CHAPTER

Care of Patients with Gynecologic Problems

STUDY/REVIEW QUESTIONS

Matching. Match each term to its corresponding definition.

Terms

a. Uterine prolapse
b. Myometrium
c. Cystocele
d. Dyspareunia
e. Vulvovaginitis
f. Fibroid
g. Rectocele
h. Polyp
i. Bartholin cyst

Descriptions

_____ 1. Protrusion of the bladder through the vaginal wall

_____ 2. Painful sexual intercourse

_____ 3. Protrusion of the rectum through the vaginal wall

_____ 4. Inflammation of the lower genital tract

_____ 5. A common disorder of the vulva

_____ 6. Weakened pelvic floor muscles and a full feeling in the vagina

_____ 7. Uterine muscle

_____ 8. Slow-growing solid tumor of the uterus

_____ 9. Most common benign neoplastic growth of the cervix

Fill in the blank.

10. _____ is the most common symptom of endometriosis.

11. Teach the patient who is receiving _____ therapy for menopausal symptoms that fibroids may continue to grow because of estrogen stimulation.

12. In endometriosis, the monthly cyclic bleeding occurs at an _____ site of implantation, which irritates and scars the surrounding tissue.

13. Without _____, prolonged estrogen stimulation causes the endometrium to grow, causing disordered shedding of the uterine lining.

14. Management of symptoms for endometriosis include which medications or supplements? *(Select all that apply.)*
    a. Oral progestins
    b. Goserelin (Zoladex)
    c. Injectable progestins
    d. Calcium
    e. Magnesium

15. A 20-year-old woman is being seen for possible toxic shock syndrome. Which conditions could be the cause? *(Select all that apply.)*
    a. Surgical wound infection
    b. Nonsurgical wound infection
    c. Multiple sexual partners
    d. Internal contraceptives
    e. Tampon use for prolonged times

16. A patient with endometriosis is likely to have what manifestation from this disorder?
    a. Bartholin cyst
    b. Chocolate cyst
    c. Fibroid
    d. Leiomyomas

17. A 22-year-old patient reports pain associated with her menstrual periods. What questions does the nurse ask when taking the patient's history? *(Select all that apply.)*
    a. "How old were you when you started menstruation?"
    b. "When did you first start having pain?"
    c. "What is a typical menstrual period for you?"
    d. "Have you ever been pregnant?"
    e. "What kind of contraceptives do you use?"
    f. "Do you have a history of frequent urinary tract infections?"

18. What nonpharmacologic therapy may be recommended to a patient to prevent vulvovaginitis?
    a. Wear nylon underwear.
    b. Douche daily until symptoms are gone.
    c. Wear a cold pack on the lower abdomen.
    d. Avoid wearing tight-fitting clothing.

19. A current treatment of nonemergent dysfunctional uterine bleeding includes which medication?
    a. Oral or patch contraceptives
    b. Tamoxifen (Nolvadex)
    c. Nonsteroidal anti-inflammatory drugs (NSAIDs)
    d. Prostaglandin stimulators

20. The nurse is taking care of a 39-year-old woman who is 2 days postoperative for an abdominal hysterectomy. What complications may occur after the surgery? *(Select all that apply.)*
    a. Urinary incontinence
    b. Pneumonia
    c. Atelectasis
    d. Intestinal obstruction (paralytic ileus)
    e. Hemorrhage

21. What types of examinations are done to reveal the presence of uterine enlargement related to fibroids? *(Select all that apply.)*
    a. Abdominal examination
    b. Vaginal examination
    c. Rectal examination
    d. Magnetic resonance-guided focused ultrasound
    e. Transvaginal ultrasound with saline infusion

22. Which woman is at greatest risk for developing pelvic organ prolapse?
    a. 16-year-old caring for her first child
    b. 25-year-old who became sexually active at age 15
    c. 34-year-old who just gave birth to her first child
    d. 48-year-old mother of four who is recently divorced

23. Which woman is at risk for dysfunctional uterine bleeding?
    a. 20-year-old who has one child
    b. 45-year-old attorney with a stressful life
    c. 30-year-old who has smoked for 10 years
    d. 25-year-old who rarely exercises

24. Following a uterine embolization using a vascular closure device, the nurse must provide what patient care? *(Select all that apply.)*
    a. Assist the patient to ambulate 2 hours after the procedure.
    b. Keep the patient on bedrest with the leg immobilized for 4 hours before ambulating.
    c. Keep the head of the bed flat.
    d. Assess the patient's pain level and administer analgesics as needed.
    e. Raise the head of the bed.

25. An obese 54-year-old patient describes excessive menstrual bleeding that occurs approximately every 10 days. The nurse prepares the patient for which diagnostic test that is used to evaluate for endometrial cancer?
    a. Bimanual pelvic examination
    b. Transvaginal ultrasound
    c. Sonohysterography
    d. Endometrial biopsy

26. A 25-year-old patient is diagnosed with dysfunctional uterine bleeding. During the pelvic exam, the health care provider determines that the bleeding is acute and heavy. What is the nurse's priority action?
    a. Prepare the patient for immediate transport to the operating room.
    b. Prepare to administer combination hormonal therapy.
    c. Anticipate an order for a hormonal contraceptive patch.
    d. Prepare to administer injectable medroxyprogesterone acetate (Depo-Provera).

27. A patient who is very upset asks the nurse, "My doctor says I have endometriosis. That sounds so horrible. What does it mean?" What is the nurse's best response?
    a. "It is an early warning sign of endometrial cancer, but you still need more testing."
    b. "A special type of tissue, called *endometrial tissue*, is outside of your uterus."
    c. "It's the growth of a special tissue which grows rapidly, but it is not dangerous."
    d. "It is a type of infection and inflammation of the endometrial tissue."

28. Dysfunctional uterine bleeding is classified into which types? *(Select all that apply.)*
    a. Occasional
    b. Excessive
    c. Anovulatory
    d. Frequent
    e. Ovulatory

29. What signs/symptoms does the nurse assess in a patient with dysfunctional uterine bleeding? *(Select all that apply.)*
    a. Male hair pattern
    b. Gastric ulcers
    c. Thyroid enlargement
    d. Abdominal pain
    e. Abdominal masses

30. What is the primary treatment for dysfunctional uterine bleeding in perimenopausal women?
    a. Hysterectomy
    b. Progestins
    c. Radiation
    d. Chemotherapy

31. A patient has excessive bleeding from uterine fibroids. Which therapy stops the blood flow to the fibroids?
    a. An infusion of conjugated estrogens
    b. Dilation and curettage (D&C)
    c. Vaginal estrogen therapy (ET) as a ring, tablet, or cream
    d. Endometrial ablation

32. What is the major reason for the onset of menopause and resulting atrophy of the vulvar organs?
    a. Decrease in levels of follicle-stimulating hormone
    b. Increase in levels of prostaglandin
    c. Decrease in levels of estrogen
    d. Increase in levels of luteinizing hormone

33. A patient has undergone a total hysterectomy with vaginal repair. The nurse advises her to use which over-the-counter product to decrease sexual discomfort related to intercourse?
    a. Hydrocortisone cream
    b. Water-soluble gel
    c. Petroleum jelly
    d. Vitamin A and D ointment

34. Potential complications following hysteroscopic surgery can include which conditions? *(Select all that apply.)*
    a. Hemorrhage
    b. Embolism
    c. Severe headache
    d. Perforation of uterus
    e. Severe low back pain

35. Which is a common cause of vulvovaginitis?
    a. Taking antibiotics
    b. Swimming in lakes
    c. Wiping from front to back
    d. Wearing inappropriate clothing

36. The nurse is advising a patient about self-care for vulvovaginitis, which is caused by a nonpathologic condition. What information does the nurse provide? *(Select all that apply.)*
    a. Wash the area daily with hydrogen peroxide.
    b. Take a sitz bath for 30 minutes several times a day.
    c. Apply prescribed topical drugs, such as estrogens or lidocaine.
    d. Remove any irritants or allergens (e.g., change detergents).
    e. Apply a topical lindane cream or lotion.
    f. Apply wet compresses.

37. A patient with a high fever, headache, flu-like symptoms, and fainting is admitted with the diagnosis of toxic shock syndrome. What additional clinical manifestations does the nurse assess for?
    a. Sunburn-like rash with peeling of palms
    b. Sore throat and swollen lymph nodes
    c. Severe hypertension and confusion
    d. Polyuria and diaphoresis

38. The nurse is teaching a group of women about prevention of toxic shock syndrome. What preventive measures does the nurse include? *(Select all that apply.)*
    a. "Avoid the use of tampons."
    b. "Use sanitary napkins at night."
    c. "Avoid using internal contraceptives."
    d. "Have your partner avoid using condoms."
    e. "Change your tampon every 8 hours."

39. A patient is admitted with toxic shock syndrome. What organism is frequently associated with this syndrome when it occurs as a menstrually related infection?
    a. *Escherichia coli*
    b. *Staphylococcus aureus*
    c. *Haemophilus influenzae*
    d. Beta-hemolytic streptococcus

40. A patient reports the sensation of feeling as if "something is falling out" along with painful intercourse, backache, and a feeling of heaviness or pressure in the pelvis. Which question does the nurse ask to assess for a cystocele?
    a. "Are you having urinary frequency or urgency?"
    b. "Do you feel constipated?"
    c. "Have you had problems with hemorrhoids?"
    d. "Have you had any heavy vaginal bleeding?"

41. A patient is recovering from repair of a cystocele. What postprocedure intervention does the nurse teach the patient?
    a. Perform perineal floor exercises.
    b. Take sitz baths three times a day.
    c. Perform povidone-iodine douches every other day.
    d. Maintain bedrest for the first 6 weeks.

42. A patient has had a posterior colporrhaphy. What is included in the nursing care of this patient? *(Select all that apply.)*
    a. Administer pain medication before having a bowel movement.
    b. Instruct to avoid straining during a bowel movement.
    c. Resume regular activities after discharge from the hospital.
    d. Provide sitz baths.
    e. Promote a low-residue (low-fiber) diet.

43. A patient reports a feeling of "heaviness" in her vagina. Upon examination, the nurse observes that the uterus is bulging into the vagina, and the cervix is protruding through the entrance to the vagina. This assessment finding would be graded as which type of uterine prolapse?
    a. Grade I
    b. Grade II
    c. Grade III
    d. Grade IV

Matching. Match the terms with their correct definitions.

Terms
a. Intramural leiomyomas
b. Submucosal leiomyomas
c. Subserosal leiomyomas
d. Pedunculated leiomyomas
e. Parasitic fibroid

Definitions
_____ 44. May extend to the broad ligament, pressing other organs

_____ 45. Contained in the uterine wall within the myometrium

_____ 46. Occasionally breaks off and attaches to other tissues

_____ 47. Can cause bleeding and disrupt pregnancy

_____ 48. Attached by a stalk to the outside of the uterus

49. A patient is diagnosed with uterine leiomyomas. What does the nurse expect to see in the documentation for this patient as the chief presenting complaint?
    a. Vaginal pressure and fullness
    b. Heavy vaginal bleeding
    c. Intermittent pain
    d. Urinary dysfunction

50. A patient with uterine leiomyomas reports a feeling of pelvic pressure, constipation, urinary frequency, and says "I can't button my pants anymore." What does the nurse assess for to further evaluate the patient's symptoms?
    a. Fluid imbalance
    b. Abdominal distention or enlargement
    c. Bowel and bladder incontinence
    d. Vaginal bleeding or discharge

51. A patient has had a pelvic examination and needs an additional diagnostic test for possible uterine leiomyomas. The nurse prepares the patient for which first-choice diagnostic test?
    a. Transvaginal ultrasound
    b. Laparoscopy
    c. Hysteroscopy
    d. Magnetic resonance imaging (MRI)

52. What is the priority nursing care most commonly seen preoperatively and postoperatively in a patient with leiomyomas?
    a. Preventing infection
    b. Managing severe pain
    c. Monitoring for adequate tissue perfusion
    d. Assessing for and managing anxiety

53. What disease is strongly associated with prolonged exposure to estrogen without the protective effects of progesterone?
    a. Endometriosis
    b. Uterine cancer
    c. Leiomyomas
    d. Endometrial cancer

54. The main symptom of endometrial cancer is _____ bleeding.

55. _____ women most often get endometrial cancer in the United States.

56. A patient with cancer has also been diagnosed with uterine leiomyomas. Which procedure does the nurse prepare the patient for?
    a. Myomectomy
    b. Hysterectomy
    c. HRT
    d. Magnetic resonance-guided focused ultrasound

57. A patient who had a total abdominal hysterectomy is anxious to resume her activities because she has young children at home. What postprocedure information does the nurse provide to the patient? *(Select all that apply.)*
    a. Climb stairs to build strength and endurance.
    b. Avoid sitting for prolonged periods.
    c. Do not lift anything heavier than 5 to 10 lbs.
    d. Walk 2 to 3 miles per day.
    e. When sitting, do not cross the legs.

58. A patient who had a total abdominal hysterectomy comes to the clinic for a 6-week follow-up appointment. Which patient demeanor is the strongest indicator that there is a need for psychological referral?
    a. Quiet and withdrawn but able to correctly answer questions
    b. Tense and impatient but answers questions correctly
    c. Disheveled and lackluster but answers correctly with repeated prompting
    d. Cheerful and distractible but answers correctly with excessive detail

59. What does discharge teaching for a woman who had a local cervical ablation include? *(Select all that apply.)*
    a. Sexual activity may be resumed usually in 1 week.
    b. Refrain from sexual intercourse for 3 weeks.
    c. Daily exercise such as walking is encouraged after the first 6 weeks.
    d. Showering is permitted, but no tub baths.
    e. Avoid lifting heavy objects for 3 weeks.

60. A patient reporting swelling in the perineal area is diagnosed with a Bartholin cyst. Nonsurgical management is recommended. What does the nurse instruct the patient to do?
    a. Apply moist heat (e.g., sitz baths or hot wet packs) to the vulva.
    b. Return immediately to the clinic if the cyst ruptures.
    c. Contact all sexual partners about the need for treatment.
    d. Change the dressing at least three times a day.

61. What gold standard tests are done to determine the presence of endometrial thickening and cancer? *(Select all that apply.)*
    a. Transvaginal ultrasound
    b. Abdominal ultrasound
    c. Magnetic resonance imaging (MRI)
    d. Computed tomography (CT) of the pelvis
    e. Endometrial biopsy

62. The surgical procedure for stage I disease of endometrial cancer involves removal of which components? *(Select all that apply.)*
    a. Uterus
    b. Vagina
    c. Fallopian tubes
    d. Peritoneum
    e. Ovaries

63. The nurse is caring for a patient with a radio-active implant. Which task can be delegated to unlicensed assistive personnel (UAP)?
    a. Save linens until radioactive source is removed, then dispose of linens as usual.
    b. Wear a dosimeter film badge while caring for the patient for protection.
    c. Use a long-handled forceps to dispose of the radioactive source in the toilet.
    d. Arrange beds so that two patients undergoing the treatment can share the room.

64. A patient is receiving external radiation therapy for treatment of endometrial cancer. What task does the nurse delegate to the UAP?
    a. Gently wash the markings outlining the treatment site.
    b. Monitor for signs of skin breakdown, especially in the perineal area.
    c. Assist the patient to ambulate if she feels fatigue or tiredness.
    d. Clean the Foley catheter and meatus with mild soap and water.

65. A patient receiving chemotherapy treatments reports fatigue, loss of energy, and experiencing an "emotional crisis every day and my hair is falling out." What does the nurse do first to help the patient adapt to body changes?
    a. Suggest participation in self-management.
    b. Encourage the patient to ventilate feelings.
    c. Help the patient to select a wig or scarf.
    d. Encourage the patient to talk to her family.

66. The nurse encourages a teenage patient to receive the human papillomavirus (HPV) vaccine (Gardasil) because it protects against which type of cancer?
    a. Endometrial cancer
    b. Cervical cancer
    c. Ovarian cancer
    d. Uterine cancer

67. Which statement about pelvic examinations and Pap smears is correct?
    a. Begin screening precautions within 3 years after having sexual intercourse or by the age of 21.
    b. Sexually active women should have annual screening regardless of underlying health problems or history.
    c. Postmenopausal women should have a final pelvic examination 1 to 2 years after the onset of menopause.
    d. Screening precautions every 2 to 3 years are sufficient for adult women who are sexually active.

68. Which classic symptom is indicative of invasive gynecologic cancer in an older patient?
    a. Swelling of one leg
    b. Dark and foul-smelling discharge
    c. Painless vaginal bleeding
    d. Flank pain

69. The nurse is taking a history on a patient with probable gynecologic cancer. Which clinical manifestation is a sign of metastasis?
    a. Watery, blood-tinged vaginal discharge
    b. Painless vaginal bleeding
    c. Dark and foul-smelling discharge
    d. Dysuria and hematuria

70. A patient had loop electrosurgical excision procedure (LEEP) for treatment and diagnosis of cervical cancer. In the discharge instructions, what does the nurse tell the patient to expect after the procedure?
    a. Spotting
    b. Vaginal bleeding similar to menses
    c. Clotting and cramps lasting 24 hours
    d. Heavy watery discharge

71. The nurse is teaching several patients being discharged after having a total abdominal hysterectomy. Which conditions does the nurse tell each patient to report to the surgeon immediately? *(Select all that apply.)*
    a. Vaginal drainage that becomes thicker or foul-smelling
    b. Hot flushes and night sweats
    c. Temperature of 100.5° F
    d. Burning during urination
    e. Feeling more tired and sleeping longer

72. A patient had a total abdominal hysterectomy. Which patient behavior is the best indicator that she is coping and adapting successfully?
    a. Refusing to look at the wound site, but encouraging the nursing students to look
    b. Withdrawn and quiet, sitting passively when the nurse performs wound care
    c. Asking questions about the wound care, but reluctant to do self-care
    d. Frequently staring at the wound site, but appearing afraid to touch the area

73. A patient has undergone surgery for ovarian cancer and will be receiving chemotherapy. Which drugs may be part of the patient's therapy? *(Select all that apply.)*
    a. Cisplatin (Platinol)
    b. Carboplatin (Paraplatin)
    c. Methotrexate (MTX)
    d. Taxanes
    e. Tamoxifen (Nolvadex)

74. The nurse is giving instructions to a patient who is undergoing brachytherapy for cervical cancer. What information does the nurse include? *(Select all that apply.)*
    a. "Limit interactions with others between treatments for their protection."
    b. "You are not radioactive between treatments."
    c. "Report any blood in the urine or severe diarrhea immediately."
    d. "Expect heavy vaginal bleeding during this time."
    e. "You will be on bedrest during the treatment session."

75. A patient undergoing which procedure has the greatest need for referral to sexual counseling because of the nature of the surgery?
    a. Vulvectomy
    b. Myomectomy
    c. Vaginectomy
    d. Hysterectomy

CASE STUDY: THE PATIENT WITH ENDOMETRIOSIS

Use a separate sheet of paper to answer the questions in this Case Study, or go to the "Prepare for Class" folder on your Evolve website at http://evolve.elsevier.com/Iggy/ to download and complete as a word processing file. Answer guidelines for this Case Study are also available on your Evolve website.

A 28-year-old woman comes to the gynecologist's office reporting persistent lower abdominal pain that peaks just before menstrual flow, and she has had difficulty getting pregnant. She is very frustrated and wants to know "what's wrong" with her. The patient is scheduled to have a laparoscopy tomorrow. Vital signs are: temp 36.9° C (98.4° F); heart rate 79/min; respirations 22/min; blood pressure 128/67 mm Hg. The patient states that she has no known allergies. She has no other medical history. The patient reports that she had an appendectomy 10 years ago without complications. She takes a daily multivitamin and is on no prescribed medications.

1. What will the nurse focus on during the history-taking?
2. What will the nurse tell the patient about usual testing procedures for endometriosis?
3. What interventions will the nurse describe to the patient as usual treatment for endometriosis?
4. What type of complementary and alternative therapies could the nurse discuss with the patient?
5. What are the goals of nursing management for the patient with endometriosis?
6. Document a nursing note for the patient using the SBAR format directed to the nurse scheduling the patient for the laparoscopy.

75 CHAPTER

Care of Male Patients with Reproductive Problems

STUDY/REVIEW QUESTIONS

Fill in the blanks.

1. Of all malignancies, prostate cancer is one of the _____ growing, and it metastasizes in a _____ pattern.

2. Starting at the age of _____, men should discuss having a prostate-specific antigen testing with their health care provider.

3. Men are at a higher risk for testicular cancer if they have a _____ history of the disease.

4. Which groups of men are at a higher risk for prostate cancer? *(Select all that apply.)*
   a. Asian Americans
   b. Men with a first-degree relative with prostate cancer
   c. Hispanic Americans
   d. African Americans
   e. Men with a second-degree relative with prostate cancer

5. Prostate-specific antigen (PSA) is a glycoprotein produced solely by the prostate. After treatment for prostate cancer, what does an elevated PSA level indicate?
   a. Recurrence of the prostate cancer
   b. Intolerance of cancer therapy
   c. Presence of a malignancy elsewhere in the body
   d. Reduction of the prostate gland tissue

6. A 49-year-old man is admitted with penile cancer. The nurse would expect to find which manifestations related to this condition? *(Select all that apply.)*
   a. Painful lesion on the penis
   b. Wartlike growth on the penis
   c. Reddened lesion with plaques
   d. Drainage from the urethra
   e. Ulcer on the glans under the prepuce (foreskin)

7. What are common serum tumor markers that confirm a diagnosis of testicular cancer? *(Select all that apply.)*
   a. Lactate dehydrogenase (LDH)
   b. Early testicular cancer antigen (EPCA-2)
   c. Glutathione S-transferase (GST P1)
   d. Alpha-fetoprotein (AFP)
   e. Beta human chorionic gonadotropin (hCG)

8. The nurse is reviewing the laboratory results for a patient with metastasis of prostate cancer to the bone. Which elevated level does the nurse expect to see?
   a. Alpha fetoprotein
   b. Blood urea nitrogen
   c. Serum alkaline phosphatase
   d. Serum creatinine

9. Which assessment tool is commonly used to ask patients about the effect of urinary symptoms on their quality of life?
   a. American Urological Assessment Tool
   b. International Urological Assessment Tool
   c. American Prostate Symptom and Assessment Tool
   d. International Prostate Symptom Score

10. A patient reports scrotal pain, edema, a heavy feeling in the testicle, dysuria, and discharge from the penis. These clinical manifestations are common to which two disorders?
    a. Orchitis and epididymitis
    b. Priapism and scrotal torsion
    c. Benign prostatic hyperplasia (BPH) and prostate cancer
    d. Hydrocele and varicocele

11. An adult patient who had a prostatectomy earlier this morning has a Foley catheter. What type of urinary drainage does the nurse expect to see in this patient?
    a. Light pink with small clots
    b. Bright red with small clots
    c. Dark burgundy with no clots
    d. Minimal for the first 12 hours

12. The nurse is teaching a patient diagnosed with erectile dysfunction about the common treatments and therapies. Which topics does the nurse include? *(Select all that apply.)*
    a. Phosphodiesterace-5 (PDE-5) inhibitors
    b. Intraurethral applications
    c. Vacuum devices
    d. Anticholinergics
    e. Penile injections
    f. Penectomy

13. Which statement about testicular cancer is true?
    a. Testicular cancer typically occurs bilaterally.
    b. Testicular cancer occurs most often in older African-American men.
    c. Elevated alpha-fetoprotein level is used as a tumor marker for testicular cancer.
    d. Elevated alpha-fetoprotein level indicates metastasis of testicular cancer.

14. During the first 24 hours after prostatectomy, what is the priority assessment in the nursing care plan?
    a. Hemorrhage
    b. Infection
    c. Hydronephrosis
    d. Confusion

15. Which type of surgery is used to treat BPH while leaving no incision?
    a. Suprapubic prostatectomy
    b. Perineal prostatectomy
    c. Retropubic prostatectomy
    d. Transurethral resection

16. A patient is diagnosed with prostatitis. Which intervention does the nurse use to alleviate the discomfort associated with this condition?
    a. Stool softeners to prevent straining
    b. Nonsteroidal anti-inflammatory drugs (NSAIDs) to prevent pain
    c. Comfort measures such as sitz baths for pain
    d. Antispasmodics to relieve bladder pain

Matching. *Match each term with its corresponding fact.*

Terms

a. Spermatocele
b. Organic erectile dysfunction
c. Varicocele
d. Cryptorchidism
e. Penectomy
f. Circumcision
g. Phimosis
h. Scrotal support
i. Priapism
j. Orchitis

Facts

_____ 17. Uncontrolled, long-maintained penile erection without sexual desire

_____ 18. Gradual deterioration of function

_____ 19. Increased risk of suicide after this procedure

_____ 20. Acute testicular inflammation

_____ 21. If not done at birth, requires strict personal hygiene to clean the prepuce

_____ 22. Constricted prepuce that cannot be contracted over the glans

_____ 23. Palpation reveals a "wormlike" mass

_____ 24. Usually requires no intervention unless the patient reports discomfort

_____ 25. Promotes drainage and comfort after surgery

_____ 26. Undescended testis with increased risk for testicular cancer

27. Inflammation of the prostate (prostatitis) can be the result of which conditions? *(Select all that apply.)*
    a. Psychosexual problem
    b. Tissue hyperplasia
    c. Sexually transmitted disease (STD)
    d. Viral or bacterial infection
    e. Retrograde ejaculation

28. A patient who has testicular cancer is likely to have which common problem?
    a. Priapism
    b. Erectile dysfunction
    c. Azoospermia
    d. Cryptorchidism

29. Which condition is a result from a disorder in the lymphatic drainage of the scrotum, causing a mass around the testis?
    a. Varicocele
    b. Hydrocele
    c. Cryptorchidism
    d. Tumescence

30. A patient has BPH. Based on this medical diagnosis, with what does the nurse prepare to assist the patient?
    a. PRN pain medications
    b. Urinary stasis or retention
    c. Erectile dysfunction
    d. Constipation

31. The nurse is interviewing a patient to determine the presence of lower urinary tract symptoms (LUTS) associated with BPH. What does the nurse question the patient about? *(Select all that apply.)*
    a. Difficulty in starting and continuing urination
    b. Urinary urgency
    c. Reduced force and size of the urinary stream
    d. Postvoid dribbling
    e. Nocturia
    f. Pain with urination
    g. Sensation of incomplete bladder emptying

32. The nurse is preparing to assess an obese patient who reports subjective symptoms and urinary patterns associated with BPH. Which technique does the nurse use to perform the physical assessment?
    a. Instruct the patient to undress from the waist down, then inspect and palpate the bladder.
    b. Have the patient drink several large glasses of water and percuss the bladder.
    c. Apply gentle pressure to the bladder to elicit urgency; then instruct the patient to void.
    d. Instruct the patient to void and then use the bedside ultrasound bladder scanner.

33. The advanced-practice nurse is preparing to examine a patient's prostate gland. Before the exam, what does the nurse tell the patient?
    a. He may feel the urge to defecate or faint as the prostate is palpated.
    b. He should lie supine with knees bent in a fully flexed position.
    c. The examination is very painful, but it lasts just a few seconds.
    d. The gland will be massaged to obtain a fluid sample for possible prostatitis.

34. The nurse is reviewing the laboratory results from a patient being evaluated for LUTS. What does an elevated PSA level and serum acid phosphatase level in this patient indicate?
    a. Infection
    b. Prostate cancer
    c. Renal involvement
    d. Infertility

35. A patient has an enlarged prostate. Which procedure is used to test for bladder obstruction?
    a. Urodynamic pressure-flow study
    b. Bladder scan
    c. Transrectal ultrasound
    d. Cystoscopy

36. A patient is being treated for both BPH and hypertension. Which alpha blocker does the nurse anticipate will be prescribed for the patient?
    a. Doxazosin (Cardura)
    b. Finasteride (Proscar)
    c. Dutasteride (Avodart)
    d. Sildenafil (Viagra)

37. The nurse is designing a teaching plan for a patient with an enlarged prostate and obstructive symptoms. What does the nurse teach the patient to avoid?
    a. Sexual intercourse
    b. Diuretics
    c. Straining to urinate
    d. Citrus fruits

Matching. *Match the definitions of treatment options for BPH with the correct terminology.*

Terms
a. Thermotherapy
b. Transurethral needle ablation (TUNA)
c. Transurethral microwave therapy (TUMT)
d. Interstitial laser coagulation (ILC)
e. Electrovaporization

Definitions
_____ 38. Low radiofrequency energy shrinks the prostate.

_____ 39. Several noninvasive techniques to destroy excess prostate tissue using heat methods.

_____ 40. High-frequency electrical current cuts and vaporizes excess tissue.

_____ 41. Laser energy coagulates excess tissue.

_____ 42. High temperatures heat and destroy excess tissue.

43. Patients with which condition meet the criteria for a having a transurethral resection of the prostate (TURP)? *(Select all that apply.)*
    a. Acute urinary retention and hematuria
    b. Hydronephrosis
    c. Acute urinary tract infection
    d. Kidney stone
    e. Chronic urinary tract infections

44. A patient is undergoing large volume bladder irrigation. During and after the procedure, the nurse observes the patient for confusion, muscle weakness, and increased gastrointestinal motility related to which potentially adverse effect of large volume irrigation?
    a. Hyponatremia
    b. Hypovolemia
    c. Hypoactivity
    d. Hypotension

45. A patient has had a TURP with a three-way urinary catheter taped to the left thigh. Which position does the nurse instruct the patient to maintain for the left leg?
    a. Abducted
    b. Hip slightly flexed
    c. Elevated
    d. Straight

46. An older adult patient had a TURP at 8:00 AM. At 3:00 PM the nurse assesses the patient. Which finding does the nurse report to the physician?
    a. Patient reports a continuous urge to void.
    b. Patient has painful spasms after trying to void around catheter.
    c. Patient is restless and picks at tubes.
    d. Patient keeps moving and burgundy-colored output is noted.

47. The nurse notes bright red blood with numerous clots on a patient who has had a TURP. After notifying the surgeon, what does the nurse do next?
    a. Irrigate the catheter with normal saline.
    b. Remove the Foley catheter.
    c. Start an IV infusion and draw blood for type and cross.
    d. Give oxygen via nasal cannula and stay with the patient.

48. The nurse is giving discharge instructions to a patient who had a TURP. What does the nurse include in the instructions?
    a. Reassurance that loss of control of urination or dribbling of urine is temporary
    b. Instructions about how to apply a condom catheter and monitor for skin breakdown
    c. Advice about how to control bleeding and passage of blood clots
    d. Information about the side effects related to aminocaproic acid (Amicar)

49. Based on American Cancer Society (ACS) recommendations, what does the nurse teach a patient about screening for prostate cancer?
    a. Beginning at age 30, all men should have an annual digital rectal examination.
    b. All African-American men should start screening at 45 years of age.
    c. Men with multiple first-degree young relatives with prostate cancer at an early age should begin screening at age 40.
    d. Asian-American men should start screening at 55 years of age.

50. The nurse is teaching a patient at risk for prostate cancer about food sources of omega-3 fatty acids. Which food does the nurse suggest?
    a. Red meat
    b. Fish
    c. Watermelon
    d. Oatmeal

51. Which sign or symptom is considered a late sign of prostate cancer?
    a. Difficulty starting urination
    b. Hematuria
    c. Frequent bladder infections
    d. Urinary retention

52. An older patient is scheduled for an annual physical including a PSA and a digital rectal examination (DRE). How are these two tests scheduled for the patient?
    a. PSA is drawn before the DRE.
    b. DRE is done several weeks before the PSA.
    c. PSA is reviewed first because DRE may be unnecessary.
    d. Both tests can be done at the convenience of the patient.

53. The nurse is reviewing PSA results for a patient who had a prostatectomy for prostate cancer several weeks ago. The PSA level is 40 ng/mL. How does the nurse interpret this data?
    a. This is an expected PSA level during this stage of the treatment.
    b. The cancer was completely removed during the surgery.
    c. The cancer is most likely recurring.
    d. There is prostate irritation and infection occurring.

54. A patient had a transrectal ultrasound with biopsy. After this procedure, what does the nurse instruct the patient to do? *(Select all that apply.)*
    a. Report fever, chills, bloody urine, and any difficulty voiding.
    b. Avoid strenuous physical activity.
    c. Limit fluid intake, especially in the first 24 hours after the procedure.
    d. Expect a small amount of bleeding that makes the urine turn pink.
    e. Expect some mild perineal and abdominal pain.

55. An older adult patient's wife is very upset because "my husband was just told that he had prostate cancer. He feels fine now, but the doctor told him to watch and wait. Why are we just watching? What are we watching for?" What is the nurse's best response?
    a. "Prostate cancer is very slow-growing. Your husband will be scheduled for regular DRE and PSA testing and I will make you a list of symptoms to watch for."
    b. "This is very upsetting news. Let's sit down and talk about how you feel and then I will have the doctor talk to you again."
    c. "It's okay, don't be upset. This is a very common way to handle prostate cancer for men who are your husband's age."
    d. "I can get you some information about prostate cancer. This will help you to understand why the doctor said this to your husband."

56. The nurse is caring for a patient who had an open radical prostatectomy. During the assessment, the nurse notes that the penis and scrotum are swollen. What does the nurse do next?
    a. Notify the physician and monitor for an inability to void or increasing pain.
    b. Elevate the scrotum and penis; apply ice to the area, 20 minutes on and 20 minutes off.
    c. Assist the patient to increase mobility, especially early ambulation.
    d. Observe the urethral meatus for redness and discharge and monitor urine output.

57. The nurse is teaching a patient who had an open radical prostatectomy about how to manage the common potential long-term complications. What does the nurse teach the patient?
    a. How to perform testicular self-examination
    b. How to manage a permanent suprapubic catheter
    c. How to perform Kegel perineal exercises
    d. Dietary modifications to acidify the urine

58. A patient has undergone external beam radiation therapy (EBRT) for palliative treatment of prostate cancer. What suggestions does the nurse make to help the patient manage acute radiation cystitis secondary to EBRT?
    a. Limit intake of water and other fluids.
    b. Avoid intake of coffee, colas, and teas.
    c. Increase consumption of dairy products.
    d. Wash genitals with mild soap and water.

59. A patient is receiving internal radiation therapy (brachytherapy) and has had a low-dose radiation seed implanted directly into the prostate gland. What nursing implication is related to this therapy?
    a. Ensure that any staff member or visitor who is pregnant is not exposed to the patient.
    b. Organize the nursing care so that exposure to the patient is limited to a few minutes.
    c. Instruct UAP that all urine specimens should be immediately discarded.
    d. Teach the patient that fatigue is common, but should pass after several months.

60. A patient is prescribed the LHRH agonist leuprolide (Lupron) for treatment of a prostate tumor. What possible side effect of this medication does the nurse advise the patient about?
    a. Nipple discharge
    b. Scrotal enlargement
    c. Fragility of the skin
    d. Erectile dysfunction

61. A patient reports having uncomfortable and unsettling episodes of "hot flashes" after receiving hormonal therapy for a prostate tumor. To alleviate this symptom, which prescription medication does the nurse assist the patient in obtaining?
    a. Biphosphonate drug such as pamidronate (Aredia)
    b. Anti-androgen drug such as bicalutamide (Casodex)
    c. Hormonal inhibitor drug such as megestrol acetate (Megace)
    d. Antimuscarinic agents such as tolterodine (Detrol)

62. The nurse is teaching a patient about self-care following a radical prostatectomy. What does the nurse include in the health teaching? *(Select all that apply.)*
    a. Teach how to care for the indwelling catheter and manifestations of infection.
    b. Walk short distances.
    c. Restrict lifting to no more than 25 lbs. for up to 3 weeks.
    d. Maintain an upright position and do not walk bent or flexed.
    e. Avoid vigorous exercise for at least 4 weeks.
    f. Shower rather than soak in a bathtub for the first 2 to 3 weeks.
    g. PSA blood tests are taken 12 weeks after surgery and then once a year.

63. A patient reports having erectile dysfunction and is seeking a prescription for sildenafil (Viagra). Because of the potential for dangerous drug-drug interactions, the nurse asks the patient specifically if he takes which type of drug?
    a. NSAIDs
    b. Nitrates
    c. Opioids
    d. Antilipemics

64. The advanced-practice nurse is performing a testicular exam on a young Caucasian patient. The practitioner finds a lump, which the patient reports is painless. This finding is considered the most common manifestation of which disease or disorder?
    a. Testicular cancer
    b. Erectile dysfunction
    c. Prostate cancer
    d. Epididymitis

65. The nurse is performing an assessment on a patient with organic erectile dysfunction (ED). What are possible causes of this condition? *(Select all that apply.)*
    a. Hypertension
    b. Gastroesophageal reflux disease (GERD)
    c. Thyroid disorders
    d. Diabetes mellitus
    e. Tibia/fibula injuries

66. A young patient has been diagnosed with testicular cancer. He and his wife had been trying to conceive a child for several months. What information does the nurse give the couple about sperm storage?
    a. Arrangements for sperm storage should be made as soon as possible after diagnosis.
    b. Sperm collection should be completed after radiation therapy or chemotherapy.
    c. Two or three samples should be collected 6 days apart.
    d. Saving sperm prevents fears related to erectile dysfunction.

67. The nurse is caring for a patient who had minimally invasive surgery (MIS) for testicular cancer. The nurse is also caring for the patient who had an open radical retroperitoneal lymph node dissection for testicular cancer. The nurse anticipates that the second patient has more of a risk for which condition?
    a. Paralytic ileus
    b. Urinary incontinence
    c. Metastatic disease
    d. Fluid overload

68. The nurse is teaching a patient who had an open retroperitoneal lymph node dissection. What instructions does the nurse give to the patient? *(Select all that apply.)*
    a. Do not lift anything over 5 lbs.
    b. Limit intake of fluids to 1000 mL per day.
    c. Do not drive a car for several weeks.
    d. Notify the surgeon if chills, fever, or increasing tenderness or pain around the incision site occur.
    e. Resume usual activities within 1 week after discharge, except for lifting.
    f. Perform monthly testicular self-examination on the remaining testis.
    g. Have follow-up diagnostic testing for at least 3 years after the surgery.

69. Yesterday a patient underwent the surgical removal of a hydrocele with a drain inserted. He calls the clinic for advice because he is unable to remember the discharge instructions. The nurse advises him to come into the clinic if he experiences which sign/symptom?
    a. Some serosanguineous drainage
    b. Malodorous and purulent drainage
    c. Moderate incision pain
    d. Scrotal swelling and edema

70. The nurse teaches patients with benign prostatic hyperplasia (BPH) to follow which instructions? *(Select all that apply.)*
    a. Avoid diuretics.
    b. Void only when the bladder feels full.
    c. Avoid antihistamines.
    d. Avoid caffeine.
    e. Avoid drinking large amounts of fluid in a short time.

71. The nurse is caring for a middle-aged patient who had a total penectomy. Which behavior by the patient is the strongest indicator that he needs referral for psychological assistance?
    a. Looking at pictures of his wife and children
    b. Being embarrassed because he has to sit down to urinate
    c. Getting angry at the nurse for leaving the door open
    d. Starting to plan a hunting trip in a remote area

72. The nurse is giving instructions to the UAP about hygienic care for an older adult patient who is uncircumcised. What does the nurse instruct the UAP to do?
    a. Defer cleaning the penis because of patient embarrassment.
    b. Replace the foreskin over the penis after bathing.
    c. Observe the penis and the foreskin for redness or odor.
    d. Avoid touching the foreskin because of hypersensitivity.

73. Which medical conditions can be associated with priapism? *(Select all that apply.)*
    a. Leukemia
    b. Sickle cell disease
    c. Diabetes mellitus
    d. Myocardial infarction
    e. Kidney injury
    f. Malignancies

74. A patient comes to the emergency department reporting fever, chills, dysuria, urethral discharge, and a boggy, tender prostate. On exam there is a urethral discharge which shows WBCs. What does the nurse suspect in this patient?
    a. Acute bacterial prostatitis
    b. Chronic bacterial prostatitis
    c. Chronic pelvic pain syndrome
    d. Asymptomatic inflammatory prostatitis

75. The nurse is teaching a patient who is taking finasteride (Proscar), an 5-alpha reductase inhibitor (5-ARI). Which side effects does the nurse tell the patient may be experienced? *(Select all that apply.)*
    a. Increased libido
    b. Erectile dysfunction
    c. Dizziness
    d. Headaches
    e. Decreased libido

76. What are common sites of metastasis for prostate cancer? *(Select all that apply.)*
    a. Pancreas
    b. Bones of the pelvis
    c. Liver
    d. Bones of the lower extremities
    e. Lungs

CASE STUDY: THE PATIENT WITH ERECTILE DYSFUNCTION

Use a separate sheet of paper to answer the questions in this Case Study, or go to the "Prepare for Class" folder on your Evolve website at http://evolve.elsevier.com/Iggy/ to download and complete as a word processing file. Answer guidelines for this Case Study are also available on your Evolve website.

A 42-year-old man comes to the clinic reporting erectile dysfunction. He states that he has noticed a diminished erection. The patient has no history of pelvic fractures, lumbosacral injuries, and has not had a prostatectomy. He currently is on the ACE inhibitor lisinopril, 5 mg orally daily, for treatment of hypertension. In addition, he is on metformin, 500 mg orally twice daily, for management of his type II diabetes. Further assessment reveals that the patient is not a current smoker and has no history of smoking. He denies any difficulty urinating. The patient reports that he consumes 1 to 2 alcoholic drinks 5 times a week. Vital signs are: temp 37.1° C (98.7° F); pulse 86/min; respirations 18/min; blood pressure 132/81 mm Hg.

1. What may be attributable causes for this patient's case of ED?
2. What recommendations can the nurse make to the patient?
3. What diagnostic tests would likely be ordered for this patient?
4. Document a nursing note for this patient using a body systems approach.

CASE STUDY: THE PATIENT WITH URINARY RETENTION SECONDARY TO PROSTATE ENLARGEMENT

Use a separate sheet of paper to answer the questions in this Case Study, or go to the "Prepare for Class" folder on your Evolve website at http://evolve.elsevier.com/Iggy/ to download and complete as a word processing file. Answer guidelines for this Case Study are also available on your Evolve website.

A 73-year-old man comes to the ambulatory urgent care center reporting burning on urination, urgency, dribbling of urine, and a feeling of bladder fullness. He states that he has noticed a gradual change in his urinary pattern over the past few months but attributes it to "old age." He adds that he would not have come in at all except that he noticed some burning when he urinated today. He also says his back has been hurting, but he attributes that to yard work and gardening.

1. When interviewing this patient, what questions should the nurse ask?
2. What are the symptoms of LUTS?
3. What symptoms differentiate an obstructive problem from a nonobstructive problem?
4. What laboratory tests and/or procedures can be expected for this patient?
5. The patient is diagnosed with BPH. State four effects of BPH on urinary elimination.

Care of Patients with Sexually Transmitted Disease

STUDY/REVIEW QUESTIONS

1. Which is the first symptom of primary syphilis?
   a. Small painless, indurated, smooth, weeping lesion
   b. There are no symptoms, so a history of potential exposure is essential
   c. Malaise, low-grade fever, and general muscular aches and pains
   d. Rash that tends to change from papules to squamous papules to pustules

2. A patient calls the nurse suspecting a one-time exposure to syphilis that occurred about 4 weeks ago. The patient reports being asymptomatic and abstinent since the incident. What is the nurse's best response?
   a. "The first sign is a chancre which will usually develop by the third week."
   b. "Continue abstinence for up to 90 days and observe the genitalia for painless sores."
   c. "Use a latex or polyurethane condom for genital and anal intercourse."
   d. "The chancre can appear anywhere and then disappear, so you must come in for testing."

3. A patient is admitted for emergency surgery after an accident. In addition, the patient has a pustular rash related to secondary syphilis. What instructions does the nurse give to the unlicensed assistive personnel (UAP)?
   a. Gloves should be worn at all times when touching the patient.
   b. The lesions are highly contagious, so the patient should do his or her own hygienic care.
   c. No instructions are given to the UAP because patient confidentiality is essential.
   d. If the skin is open and draining pus or fluid, use gloves during patient care.

4. A patient who has no reaction to a penicillin skin test is given benzathine penicillin G intramuscularly. What does the nurse ensure happens immediately after the injection?
   a. Instruct the patient to contact any sexual partners for treatment.
   b. Instruct the patient to go home to rest for 2 to 4 hours.
   c. Observe the patient for 2 hours to detect any allergic reaction.
   d. Observe the patient for at least 30 minutes to detect any allergic reaction.

5. A patient is diagnosed with primary syphilis. The nurse prepares to administer and educate the patient about which treatment regimen?
   a. Benzathine penicillin G given intramuscularly as a single 2.4 million unit dose, and follow-up evaluation at 6, 12, and 24 months
   b. Benzathine penicillin G given intramuscularly for 7 days, and follow-up evaluation at 6, 12, and 24 months
   c. Ceftriaxone (Rocephin) 125 mg intramuscularly in a single dose, plus azithromycin (Zithromax) 1 g orally in a single dose, and follow-up evaluation at 6, 12, and 24 months
   d. Metronidazole (Flagyl) 500 mg orally twice daily for 14 days, and follow-up evaluation at 6, 12, and 24 months

6. How is a Jarisch-Herxheimer reaction treated?
   a. Oxygen, epinephrine, and antihistamines
   b. Emergency IV fluid resuscitation
   c. Analgesics and antipyretics
   d. Monitoring for symptom resolution

7. A patient is diagnosed with late tertiary syphilis. In addition to central nervous system involvement, what findings does the nurse see documented in the patient's record?
   a. Chancres on the genitalia, lips, or nipples
   b. Rash on the palms and soles of the feet
   c. Benign lesions of the skin, mucous membranes, and bone
   d. Contagious wart-like lesions and mucous patches

8. A patient is diagnosed with early latent syphilis. Which medication is prescribed for the patient?
   a. Penicillin-G
   b. Doxycycline
   c. Amoxicillin
   d. Tetracycline

9. A patient reports a possible exposure to syphilis. The nurse informs the patient about which screening test?
   a. ELISA serum
   b. VDRL serum
   c. FTA antibody
   d. MHA assay

10. Which sexually transmitted diseases (STDs) are reportable to the local health authorities in every state? *(Select all that apply.)*
    a. Chlamydia
    b. Pelvic inflammatory disease (PID)
    c. Gonorrhea
    d. Syphilis
    e. Chancroid

11. What is the causative organism of syphilis?
    a. *N. gonorrhoeae*
    b. *C. trachomatis*
    c. *T. pallidum*
    d. Cytomegalovirus

12. _____ _____ _____ is one of the leading causes of infertility and is related to the increase in the number of ectopic pregnancies reported in the United States.

13. Nurses in which setting(s) are responsible for identifying people at risk for STDs? *(Select all that apply.)*
    a. Secondary and tertiary
    b. Tertiary only
    c. Secondary only
    d. Nurses do not have this responsibility.

14. What are the less common diseases in the United States that are transmitted by sexual contact? *(Select all that apply.)*
    a. Human immunodeficiency virus
    b. Lymphogranuloma venereum
    c. Herpes simplex virus
    d. Chancroid
    e. Granuloma inguinale

15. What is the number-one causative agent associated with PID?
    a. *N. gonorrhoeae*
    b. Herpes simplex virus
    c. Cytomegalovirus
    d. *T. pallidum*

16. Standards of care and treatment for STDs are developed by which government organization?

17. What are the goals of medication in treating genital herpes? *(Select all that apply.)*
    a. Reduce symptoms
    b. Reduce the risk of transmission
    c. Reduce discomfort
    d. Prevent recurrence
    e. Cure

18. The spermicide nonoxynol-9 may _____ the risk for transmission of HIV during vaginal intercourse and anal intercourse.

19. A patient has had genital herpes–HSV-2 for several years. She is at the clinic for her annual Papanicolaou (Pap) smear and asks about long-term problems. What is the nurse's best response?
    a. "There is an increased risk for PID."
    b. "You are likely to have frequent episodes of vaginitis."
    c. "You have a greater risk for developing cervical cancer."
    d. "When you are pregnant, the risk of neonatal transmission will be monitored."

20. The nurse is teaching a patient being discharged after treatment for genital herpes. Which patient statement indicates a need for further teaching?
    a. "I can be contagious even when I do not have any lesions."
    b. "If I get pregnant, I need to tell my nurse midwife that I have genital herpes."
    c. "After taking all of my acyclovir, I will not have genital herpes anymore."
    d. "I need to have an annual Pap smear because of my increased risk for cervical cancer."

21. A patient is prescribed a single dose of doxycycline for the treatment of *Chlamydia trachomatis*. What additional information does the nurse give the patient about treatment issues?
    a. Abstinence from sex is required until 7 days from the date of treatment.
    b. Even with treatment, expect long-term complications of carditis and arthritis.
    c. The treatment will cure the infection, but lymph nodes will drain chronically.
    d. Watch for and report headache, malaise, arthralgia, and anorexia.

22. Why do women develop complications more often than men when being treated for gonorrhea?
    a. Treatment for the disease can leave women infertile.
    b. The disease is asymptomatic in the early stages.
    c. Estrogen leaves the woman more resistant to antibiotic therapy.
    d. The disease is much more difficult to cure in women.

23. How long is the usual incubation period for gonorrhea?
    a. 3 to 10 days
    b. 10 to 14 days
    c. 2 to 3 weeks
    d. 2 to 3 months

24. The nurse is performing a history and physical on the male patient who reports an STD. Which symptom is the most common in the male with Chlamydia?
    a. Painful intercourse
    b. Urethritis
    c. Dark yellow urine
    d. Thick, green discharge

25. When obtaining a complete obstetric-gynecologic history, the nurse also takes a sexual history from the patient. Which approach is the most therapeutic to elicit information from the patient?
    a. Use a checklist to ask "yes" and "no" questions.
    b. Ask the patient to explain his or her sexual history.
    c. Ask directly if the patient has ever had an STD.
    d. Ask open-ended questions.

26. For the nurse to be an effective clinician when working with patients concerning sexuality, STDs, or other sexual concerns, what must the nurse do first?
    a. Take a course on sexual relations and counseling.
    b. Know all about his or her patient's concerns, problems, or needs.
    c. Be aware of his or her own sexual values, attitudes, and sexuality.
    d. Set up a meeting with the patient's sexual partner.

27. A female patient reporting a troublesome vaginal discharge is diagnosed with trichomoniasis and is given medication to treat the infection. What does the nurse teach the patient about the diagnosis?
    a. *Trichomonas vaginalis* is self-limiting, but medicine is needed to treat the vaginal itching.
    b. The patient's sexual partner must be treated if the problem is to be resolved.
    c. The medication should be applied liberally to the external genitalia once a day.
    d. The vaginal infection can cause infertility in childbearing women.

28. Women with PID are at an increased risk for which condition?
    a. Ovarian rupture
    b. Appendicitis
    c. Infertility
    d. STDs

29. What is the most common chief complaint that leads a patient with PID to seek medical health care?
    a. Vaginal itching
    b. Lower abdominal pain
    c. Malaise with fever
    d. Abnormal menstrual flow

30. A patient with PID is on bedrest with bathroom privileges. What position is best for the patient while on bedrest?
    a. Prone
    b. Supine
    c. Side-lying
    d. Semi-Fowler's

31. A patient with PID is discharged home on oral antibiotics. What are the important measures for the nurse to include in patient teaching? *(Select all that apply.)*
    a. "Douche 3 times a week to aid in healing."
    b. "Report an increase in temperature right away."
    c. "Continue taking the antibiotics until the medication is gone."
    d. "Do not have intercourse until you and your partner have completed the antibiotic therapy."
    e. "Take antacids if the antibiotics upset your stomach."

32. When performing discharge teaching about resuming sexual relations to a female patient diagnosed with an STD, what does the nurse teach the patient?
    a. Douche within 24 hours after vaginal intercourse.
    b. Sexual relations are prohibited for 3 months.
    c. Intercourse should be postponed until the treatment regimen is completed.
    d. Intercourse is permitted unless there is an increase in abdominal pain.

33. What does the nurse tell a patient with PID about the practice of vaginal douching?
    a. It increases a woman's risk for developing PID.
    b. It should be done daily during the course of the illness.
    c. Vinegar is the only safe solution to use.
    d. Use only disposable equipment.

34. Which infection describes an STD that is limited to the vagina, is very irritating, but has no long-term sequelae?
    a. Chlamydia
    b. Herpes simplex type 2
    c. Candida
    d. Granuloma inguinale

35. Which STD carried by a pregnant woman can be transmitted by direct sexual contact and can be transmitted to the fetus during a vaginal delivery?
    a. Chancroid
    b. Candida
    c. Human papillomavirus
    d. Gonorrhea

36. A patient with human papillomavirus will commonly develop which disease?
    a. Herpes genitalis
    b. Genital warts
    c. Granuloma inguinale
    d. Chancroid

Matching. *Match each STD with its corresponding definition. Not all options will be used.*

Sexually Transmitted Diseases

a. Herpes simplex type 2
b. Secondary syphilis
c. Lymphogranuloma venereum
d. Genital herpes
e. Pediculosis pubis
f. Primary syphilis
g. Granuloma inguinale
h. Gonorrhea
i. Bacterial vaginosis
j. Chlamydia
k. Human papillomavirus (HPV)
l. Candida

Definitions

_____ 37. Highly infectious state with the presence of a chancre

_____ 38. Viral cause of an STD

_____ 39. STD that is seen less often in affluent countries

_____ 40. In 2006, the U.S. Food and Drug Administration approved a vaccine which provides almost 100% immunity

_____ 41. Flu-like symptoms and a generalized rash

_____ 42. Women tend to have a "silent" infection more often than men

_____ 43. Men experience dysuria but women often have no symptoms

_____ 44. Normal flora on the skin that is easily relocated to the vagina

_____ 45. Initial infection that causes blisters which rupture and cause painful lesions

46. The nurse is preparing an information packet about women's health considerations for STDs. What information does the nurse include? *(Select all that apply.)*
   a. Young women generally have excellent knowledge about the risk of STDs.
   b. Young women frequently believe that they are vulnerable to STDs.
   c. Young women mistakenly believe that contraceptives protect them from STDs.
   d. Mucosal tears in postmenopausal women may also place them at greater risk for STDs.
   e. Women have more asymptomatic infections that may delay diagnosis and treatment.

47. A young female patient requires hospitalization for a severe case of genital herpes. What information is given to the patient regarding the long-term consequences?
   a. There is an increased risk of recurrence with an increased susceptibility to reinfection.
   b. There is a risk of neonatal transmission and an increased risk for acquiring HIV infection.
   c. There is an increased risk of recurrence with greater severity of symptoms with each episode.
   d. There is an increased risk for multiple types of reproductive cancers at a young age.

48. The nurse is counseling a patient experiencing recurrent outbreaks of genital herpes. What suggestions for symptomatic treatment does the nurse include?
    a. Oral analgesics, sitz baths, and increased oral fluid intake
    b. Topical anesthetics, nutritional therapy, and warm compresses
    c. Abstinence, frequent bathing, and fluid restriction
    d. Bedrest and application of podofilox (Condylox) 0.5% solution

49. A patient is diagnosed with *Condylomata acuminata*. What are the desired outcomes of management for this patient?
    a. Reduce pain and prevent recurrence
    b. Prevent long-term complications to the cardiac system
    c. Remove the warts and treat the symptoms
    d. Prevent infertility and systemic infection

50. A patient requires treatment for genital warts. Which treatment is done by the patient at home if given the proper instructions?
    a. Imiquimod (Aldara) 5% cream
    b. Cryotherapy with liquid nitrogen
    c. Podophyllin resin 10% in a compound of tincture of benzoin
    d. Trichloroacetic acid (TCA) or bichloroacetic acid (BCA)

51. What is the incubation period for genital warts?
    a. 3 to 7 days
    b. 2 to 20 days
    c. 10 to 90 days
    d. 2 to 3 months

52. A patient has had podophyllin treatment for *Condylomata acuminata*. For which sign/symptom does the nurse tell the patient to return for further treatment?
    a. Discomfort at the site
    b. Bleeding from the site
    c. Infection at the site
    d. Sloughing of parts of warts

53. A male patient reports that a female sexual partner just told him that she was treated for gonorrhea. What symptoms does the nurse ask him about, because they are the most likely to occur with gonorrhea in a male?
    a. Small, painless lump that occurred on the penis, but spontaneously disappeared
    b. Numerous small, painless papillary growths in the genital area
    c. Painful intercourse because of scrotal swelling and epididymitis
    d. Dysuria and a profuse yellowish green or scant clear penile discharge

54. A patient is being treated for gonorrhea. Which single-dose medication order does the nurse question?
    a. Ceftriaxone (Rocephin) 125 mg
    b. Cefixime (Suprax) 400 mg
    c. Azithromycin (Zithromax) 1 g orally
    d. Ciprofloxacin (Cipro) 250 mg

55. A patient is tested for and diagnosed with gonorrhea. The nurse advocates that the choice of drug therapy include medications that concurrently treat which condition?
    a. Genital herpes
    b. Chlamydia
    c. Syphilis
    d. Genital warts

56. A young woman discovers she has Chlamydia after going to her doctor for a routine Pap smear and pelvic exam. She is reluctant to accept the diagnosis, because she is asymptomatic and "does not have any money for unnecessary treatment right now." What is the nurse's best response?
    a. Explain that there is a single-dose of medication which has a one-time cost.
    b. Talk to the woman about her financial situation and help her find resources.
    c. Encourage the patient to express her reluctance and disbelief.
    d. Tell her that it is possible to have Chlamydia without having any symptoms.

57. A patient with an STD freely admits to being a commercial sex worker. In talking to this patient, the nurse recognizes that she has not disclosed a true name, address, or partner contact information. What is the best treatment strategy to use with this patient?
    a. Reassure her that all health data is confidential and will be handled with discretion.
    b. Spend extra time with the patient to enlist trust so that she will give correct information.
    c. Administer a one-dose course of treatment and dispense a box of condoms.
    d. Give her all the medications for a 7-day treatment and convey a nonjudgmental attitude.

58. Which factors increase the risk for PID? *(Select all that apply.)*
    a. Age younger than 26 years
    b. Multiple sexual partners
    c. Intrauterine device (IUD) in place
    d. Caffeine use
    e. History of Chlamydia or gonococcal infection
    f. History of gastrointestinal infections

59. A young female patient with a history of previous STDs has a hunched-over gait and has difficulty getting on the examination table. On observing this behavior, what does the nurse first assess for?
    a. Lower abdominal pain
    b. Lower back pain
    c. Musculoskeletal weakness
    d. Vaginal bleeding

60. The nurse is reviewing laboratory results for a patient with PID. Which lab results does the nurse expect to see? *(Select all that apply.)*
    a. Elevation in white blood cell (WBC) count
    b. Elevation in erythrocyte sedimentation rate (ESR)
    c. Decreased level of C-reactive protein
    d. Presence of human chorionic gonadotropin (hCG) in urine
    e. Presence of more than 10 WBCs per high-power field for vaginal discharge

61. In the ED, a patient is diagnosed with PID and there is an order to discharge the patient home with a prescription for antibiotics. What circumstance causes the nurse to question the order for discharge to home?
    a. The patient is several months postpartum, but had very mild symptoms.
    b. The patient is nauseated, but able to tolerate small amounts of oral fluids.
    c. The patient is pregnant, but willing to attempt self-care if properly instructed.
    d. The patient is afraid to go home, but the sister and husband are available to help.

62. The nurse is caring for a patient admitted for PID. Which task does the nurse delegate to the UAP?
    a. Apply a heating pad to the lower abdomen or back.
    b. Place the patient in semi-Fowler's position.
    c. Ask the patient if the pain is a 2 to 3 on a pain scale of 0 to 10.
    d. Report to the nurse if the patient is anxious about infertility.

63. A patient reports an itching or tingling sensation felt in the skin 1 to 2 days followed by a blister on the penis which ruptured spontaneously with painful erosion. What are these symptoms consistent with?
    a. Syphilis
    b. Genital warts
    c. Genital herpes
    d. Gonorrhea

64. The nurse is teaching a group of high-school students about the use of condoms. What information does the nurse include? *(Select all that apply.)*
    a. Condoms are primarily effective for vaginal intercourse.
    b. Female condoms are too difficult to use for inexperienced partners.
    c. Keep condoms (especially latex) in a cool, dry place out of direct sunlight.
    d. Do not use condoms that are in damaged packages or that are brittle or discolored.
    e. Avoid damaging the condom with fingernails, teeth, or other sharp objects.
    f. Put condoms on the penis before foreplay or arousal.
    g. If you use a lubricant, make sure that the lubricant is water-based.

65. Which STD is associated with an increased risk for cervical cancer?
    a. Syphilis
    b. *Condylomata acuminata*: HPV type 16
    c. *Condylomata acuminata*: HPV type 6
    d. PID

66. In performing a genital exam on a teenage patient, the examiner sees multiple large cauliflower-like growths in the perineal area. The patient reports these appeared about 3 months after her first sexual experience. What does the examiner suspect?
    a. *Condylomata acuminata*
    b. Genital herpes
    c. Salpingitis
    d. Gonorrhea

CASE STUDY: THE PATIENT WITH A SEXUALLY TRANSMITTED DISEASE

Use a separate sheet of paper to answer the questions in this Case Study, or go to the "Prepare for Class" folder on your Evolve website at http://evolve.elsevier.com/Iggy/ to download and complete as a word processing file. Answer guidelines for this Case Study are also available on your Evolve website.

A young woman comes to the STD clinic. She is defensive and seems disgusted as she explains to the nurse that she believes she was exposed to an STD. She bases her belief on something a friend told her, but she is reluctant to be more forthcoming about the details. She currently denies symptoms. She is also very angry about "false accusations" that people are making. The nurse validates her decision to come in for examination and diagnosis.

1. The nurse explains that women have more health problems associated with STDs than men. What should the nurse tell the patient?

2. Explain why the patient could present with this angry and defensive behavior. What can the nurse do?

3. What should be included in a nursing assessment of the patient with symptoms of an STD?

4. What are six nursing responsibilities associated with the management of a patient who is newly diagnosed with an STD?

5. The patient is reluctant to disclose the names of sexual partners or talk about partners. What could the nurse do?

6. The patient is diagnosed with Chlamydia. What should be included in the patient education material?

7. What should the nurse include in the patient teaching for a patient who was prescribed oral antibiotics?

8. Document a nursing note for this patient using the following format:
   • Problem:
   • Note:

Answer Key for Study/Review Questions

CHAPTER 1

1. d
2. b
3. a, b, c, f
4. a, b, c, e
5. b
6. d
7. b
8. b
9. a, b, d, e
10. c

CHAPTER 2

1. a, d, e
2. a, b, c, e
3. c
4. b
5. d
6. a
7. e
8. a, b, c, e
9. a, c, d
10. c
11. a, b, e, f
12. a, b, c
13. a
14. d
15. b
16. a, b, c, e

CHAPTER 3

1. a, b, c, d
2. a, b, d, e
3. a, c, d, e, g
4. c
5. a, d, e, f
6. b, c, e
7. a, c, d, e
8. a, d
9. a
10. a, b, c, d, e
11. b, c, d
12. a, e
13. a, b, e
14. c

15. a, c, d
16. c
17. d
18. b
19. a
20. a, b, c, e
21. d
22. c
23. a
24. b

CHAPTER 4

1. c
2. d
3. a
4. i
5. h
6. f
7. g
8. b
9. e
10. d
11. T
12. T
13. T
14. F; have varied health care needs
15. T
16. F; is displayed differently among cultures
17. a
18. d
19. b, d
20. a, c, e
21. a, b, c, e

CHAPTER 5

1. b, c, d
2. a, b, c, d, e
3. b
4. c
5. a, b, c, d
6. c
7. a, e, g, j
8. c, d, f
9. b, d, h, i

10. a, e
11. b
12. c
13. a
14. d
15. a
16. CP
17. B
18. AP
19. CP
20. CP
21. B
22. AP
23. a, b
24. b
25. a, b, c, d, e
26. a, c
27. a, b, e
28. a, b, c, d
29. c, e
30. b, c, e
31. b, c, e, g
32. b
33. c
34. a, c
35. b
36. b
37. c
38. b
39. c
40. c
41. b
42. Precipitating or palliative
    Quality or quantity
    Region or radiation
    Severity scale
    Timing
43. a, c, d, f
44. a, c, d, e
45. b
46. d
47. d
48. e
49. c
50. b
51. a

52. a
53. a
54. b
55. d
56. d
57. a
58. c
59. a
60. c
61. b

CHAPTER 6

1. **Across**
   3. RNA
   4. Centromere
   6. Autosomes
   8. Genome
   9. Dizygotic
   10. Transcription
   11. Diploid
   Down
   1. Chromosome
   2. Phenotype
   5. Haploid
   7. Monozygotic
2. Application of known genetic variation to enhance health care to individuals and their families
3. 46; 23
4. a
5. same
6. different
7. same
8. a. AR
   b. AD
   c. B
   d. AD
   e. AR
   f. AD
   g. AR
   h. AR
9. Looking at a specific trait expressed through several generations of a family, one can determine how that gene is passed from genera-

tion to generation. These patterns indicate whether a gene is dominant or recessive, and is located on an autosomal or sex chromosome. This can predict the risk for any one person to transmit a trait to his or her children.
10. d
11. a, c, d
12. a, c, e, f
13. a. SLR
    b. FC
    c. FC
    d. SLR
    e. SLR
    f. FC

CHAPTER 7

1. Nurses using available research and evidence found in policies, procedures, and guidelines in the agency to guide clinical practice
2. c
3. b
4. d
5. f
6. e
7. a
8. a, b, c, d
9. a, b, c, d, e
10. Population, Intervention, Comparison, Outcome, Time
11. a, b, c, d, e
12. a, b, e

CHAPTER 8

1. e
2. j
3. b, c, d
4. d
5. a
6. h, i
7. h
8. b
9. c
10. k
11. g
12. f
13. b
14. e
15. b
16. b, h
17. l
18. c
19. d
20. c
21. a, b, c, d, e

22. a, b, c, d, e
23. a
24. d
25. a
26. a, b, c, d, e
27. a, c, d, e, f
28. a
29. b
30. a
31. a
32. b
33. b
34. a
35. b
36. a
37. b
38. d
39. a, b, c, e
40. a
41. a, b, c, e
42. c
43. c
44. c
45. b
46. b
47. c
48. a, b, c
49. c
50. d
51. a, b, c
52. c
53. a
54. c
55. d
56. c
57. a
58. e
59. c
60. e
61. b

CHAPTER 9

1. c
2. a
3. d
4. b
5. d
6. c
7. c
8. a, c, d, e
9. a. 2
   b. 3
   c. 1
10. c, e, f
11. d
12. b, c, d, e
13. b
14. d
15. a
16. c

17. b
18. a
19. c
20. c
21. a, c, e
22. a, c
23. a, b, d, e
24. Discontinuing one or more therapies that might prolong the life of a person who cannot be cured by the therapy; death occurs by doing nothing and letting a condition or disease process take its course
25. Taking action that purposefully and directly causes a patient's death; death occurs by direct action

CHAPTER 10

1. d
2. b
3. c
4. a
5. e
6. a, b, d, f, g
7. d
8. c
9. b
10. d
11. b
12. c
13. b, d, e
14. a, b, c, d
15. d
16. b
17. c
18. a
19. d
20. b, c, e
21. d
22. a. U
    b. E
    c. E
    d. U
    e. N
    f. U
    g. E
    h. N
23. a, c, e, f
24. c, e, b, a, d
25. a, c
26. c
27. b, c, e
28. c
29. a
30. d
31. c
32. b

33. a
34. e
35. c
36. c
37. a
38. a
39. a
40. a
41. c
42. b, c
43. b
44. d
45. a, b, e
46. a. 2
    b. 1
    c. 3
    d. 4
47. b
48. c
49. b
50. a, d
51. F; the nurse may search the patient for protection of the patient, staff, and others
52. T
53. b, e
54. b, d, e
55. c, b, a, d, e

CHAPTER 11

1. a, c, e, f, g
2. b, d, e
3. c
4. c, d, e
5. b
6. a, c, d
7. c
8. c
9. a
10. d
11. b, c, e
12. a
13. a, c, e
14. a, c, d, e
15. c
16. d
17. c
18. a
19. a, c, d
20. a
21. d
22. b
23. a
24. b, c
25. a
26. b
27. a
28. a, b, d, g
29. c
30. b

31. a
32. a
33. b
34. c
35. a
36. b
37. a
38. c
39. **Across**
   1. Urticating
   3. Brown recluse
   4. Honeybee
   6. Black widow
   Down
   2. Tarantula
   5. Bark
40. a, b
41. a
42. b
43. b
44. a
45. b
46. b
47. b
48. a
49. c
50. c
51. c
52. a
53. a, c, d, e
54. b
55. b, c, d, a
56. c
57. d
58. a, b, e
59. c
60. b
61. b
62. c
63. a
64. c, e
65. c
66. b
67. a
68. b, d, e
69. c
70. b
71. b
72. a, c, d
73. b
74. c
75. b
76. c
77. d
78. c
79. d
80. a, c, d, e, f
81. c
82. c
83. b, c, d

84. b
85. a, b, d, e
86. a
87. a
88. c
89. a, b, e
90. b
91. b, e, g, h
92. a
93. b
94. d
95. b
96. b
97. a
98. a, b, e
99. b, d, e
100. b
101. c
102. d
103. c, e
104. b, e, c, a, d

CHAPTER 12

1. weapons of mass destruction (or WMDs)
2. hazardous materials
3. disaster mortuary operational response (or DMORTs)
4. hospital incident command
5. HAZMAT
6. emergency operations or command
7. d
8. a, c, d, g
9. b
10. d
11. a, c, d
12. a
13. b
14. c
15. d
16. c
17. b
18. b
19. c
20. c
21. a
22. a
23. a, c, d, e
24. c
25. triage officer
26. d
27. c
28. a
29. d, b, e, c, a
30. a
31. a, c, d, f
32. d
33. b, d, e

34. d
35. a, c, d
36. a, c, e
37. a
38. c
39. b
40. c, e

CHAPTER 13

1. diffusion
2. osmosis
3. filtration
4. hydrostatic pressure
5. osmolarity
6. osmolality
7. a, b, d, f, h
8. b
9. b
10. a, c, d, e
11. b
12. b
13. a, d, e
14. b
15. aldosterone
16. a, b, c, e, f
17. a
18. d
19. 2
20. b, c, e
21. c
22. a
23. a
24. b
25. b, d, e
26. c
27. excess
28. d
29. c
30. c
31. b
32. a
33. c
34. b
35. b
36. f
37. f
38. a
39. d
40. a
41. e
42. b
43. b
44. c
45. d
46. d
47. c
48. e
49. b, d, e
50. b, c, d
51. a, d, e

52. a, d, e
53. b, c, e
54. Potassium
55. c
56. a
57. a, d, e
58. b, d, e
59. a, c, d, f
60. d
61. c, a, b, d
62. c, d, e
63. a
64. a
65. d
66. a
67. hyponatremia
68. b
69. a, e
70. d
71. b, e
72. a, c, d, e
73. hypernatremia
74. c
75. a
76. a, b, d
77. a, d, e, g
78. b
79. b
80. b
81. a
82. a
83. a
84. b
85. b
86. a
87. a
88. b
89. b
90. a
91. b
92. b
93. b, c, d
94. d
95. b, c, e
96. a
97. c, e
98. a, b, c, d
99. d
100. a, c, e
101. b
102. a
103. b
104. b
105. d
106. b, c, d
107. a, c, d
108. b
109. b, c, d
110. a
111. c

112. b
113. b, d, e
114. c
115. b
116. b
117. b
118. a
119. b, c, e
120. a, e, f, g, h
121. a, c, e
122. b
123. a
124. a, b, c, d
125. c
126. d
127. b
128. c
129. a
130. a
131. a
132. a, c, d
133. d
134. b
135. b, e
136. a
137. b, c, d
138. b, c, d
139. c
140. a
141. Hypocalcemia
142. b
143. a, d, e
144. a, c, d
145. hypophosphatemia
146. b, d, e
147. d
148. d
149. a
150. c, a, b, d
151. d
152. a
153. c
154. a, b, c

CHAPTER 14

1. a, b, d
2. c, b, a, d
3. a
4. a, d, e
5. b, c, d
6. b, c, d
7. a, b, e
8. acidic
9. 1:20
10. bicarbonate; CO_2
11. b
12. a
13. a
14. c
15. d
16. a
17. d
18. b
19. c
20. $CO_2 + H_2O \rightarrow H_2CO_3 \rightarrow H^+ + HCO_3^-$
21. a. D
   b. D
   c. D
   d. I
   e. I
22. b
23. c
24. c
25. a
26. d
27. b
28. b
29. a, b, e
30. b
31. c
32. a
33. b
34. d
35. c
36. a, c, d, e
37. a
38. b, d
39. d
40. a
41. d
42. c
43. c
44. b
45. a
46. d
47. c
48. b
49. a
50. b
51. b
52. b
53. d
54. a
55. c
56. b
57. b, c
58. c
59. b, d, f
60. b
61. a
62. c
63. a
64. b
65. a
66. b
67. b
68. a
69. a, b, c, e, f
70. c
71. b
72. c
73. d
74. d
75. d
76. b
77. c
78. b
79. c
80. a
81. b, d, e
82. a, c
83. b, d, e
84. a
85. d
86. c
87. b
88. c
89. d
90. a
91. a
92. c
93. e
94. b
95. b
96. c
97. c
98. a. Acid
   b. Acid
   c. Alkaline
   d. Acid

CHAPTER 15

1. a
2. b, d, e
3. b, c, a, d
4. a, b, c, e, g
5. a, b, c
6. c
7. b, d, e, g
8. d, c, b, a
9. a, c, e
10. d
11. b
12. a
13. d
14. a
15. d
16. b
17. c
18. b
19. c
20. c
21. a, d, e
22. b
23. b, c, e
24. c
25. c
26. a
27. b, e, f
28. c
29. a
30. c, d, e
31. d
32. d
33. b
34. d
35. b, c, d
36. b
37. a. P
   b. CID
   c. P
   d. P
   e. CID
38. a, b, c, e
39. c
40. d
41. a, c, e
42. d
43. a, b, e
44. d
45. a
46. a, b, c, d
47. a
48. a. 5
   b. 4
   c. 6
   d. 3
   e. 1
   f. 7
   g. 2
49. c
50. b
51. b, c, e
52. c
53. b, c, f
54. c
55. a
56. a, b, c, e
57. d
58. c
59. d
60. c
61. a
62. d
63. a
64. **Across**
   1. Infection
   3. Infiltration
   4. Vesicant
   8. Thrombosis
   Down
   2. Extravasation
   5. Phlebitis
   6. Ecchymosis
   7. Allergic
   9. Speed shock

CHAPTER 16

1. b, d, e

2. d
3. b
4. a
5. c
6. a
7. b
8. c
9. d
10. b, c, e
11. b
12. a, b, c, d, e
13. a, b, c
14. a, c, e
15. b, d, e
16. a
17. c
18. c, a, d, b
19. a, d, e

CHAPTER 17

1. a
2. a, b, e
3. b, c
4. a, b, c, d, e
5. a
6. d
7. a
8. b
9. f
10. e
11. c
12. a, b, c, d
13. d
14. b
15. a
16. c
17. b
18. a, b, c, e, g
19. d
20. b, c, e
21. d, a, c, b, e
22. a, d, e
23. b
24. e
25. d
26. a
27. c
28. b, d, e
29. h
30. d
31. e
32. g
33. f
34. a
35. c
36. b
37. c
38. c
39. e
40. c

41. a
42. b
43. d
44. a, c, d, g
45. b
46. d

CHAPTER 18

1. d
2. b
3. d
4. c, d, e
5. c
6. b, c, e
7. b, c, a, d
8. a. Situation: Nurse transfers a patient to the PACU who had an incision and drainage for an abscess in the right groin with general anesthesia.
   b. Background: Patient had an abscess in the right groin. History of vulvar cancer, had a needle biopsy of right groin 1 week ago, and hypertension treated with lisinopril 5 mg PO daily. No known drug allergies. Is a full code.
   c. Assessment: Blood pressure is 80/47 mm Hg, HR 117/min in sinus tachycardia, respiratory rate 28/min, pulse oximeter reading 93% on oxygen at 3 L nasal cannula, temp 38.5° C. Jackson-Pratt drain has cream-colored output, 70 mL.
   d. Recommendation: Surgeon sending orders to bolus patient with 500 mL IV over 1 hour of normal saline, draw two sets of blood cultures, and culture drainage from Jackson-Pratt drain.
9. a, b, e
10. a, b, e
11. c, b, d, e
12. d
13. a
14. c, e
15. b
16. a
17. g
18. b

19. c
20. d
21. f
22. a
23. b, c
24. g
25. c
26. c, d, f
27. d
28. a
29. f
30. g
31. e
32. c, g
33. b, c
34. g
35. f
36. a, b, c
37. d
38. b
39. g
40. a
41. a
42. a. 7
    b. 3
    c. 4
    d. 5
    e. 6
    f. 2
    g. 1
43. b
44. a. 2
    b. 3
    c. 4
    d. 5
    e. 1
45. An evisceration is a surgical emergency. First, call for help and stay with the patient. The person who responds should notify the surgeon immediately and ensure that supplies are brought to the room. Immediately cover the wound with nonadherent dressing premoistened in warm sterile normal saline. If premoistened dressings are not available, moisten the sterile gauze or sterile towels in a sterile irrigation tray with sterile saline, then cover the wound. Do not allow the dressings to dry. Do not attempt to reinsert the protruding organ or viscera. While one nurse is dressing the wound, another should be taking the patient's vital signs, and ensuring that the patient

is in a supine position with the hips and knees bent. (See Figure 18-2 in the text for more details.)
46. d
47. b
48. a, c, e

CHAPTER 19

1. a, b, c, e
2. a, b, c, d, e
3. a, c, e
4. d
5. b
6. a, b, e
7. a, b, d, e
8. d
9. b
10. a, b, c, d, e
11. b
12. c
13. a
14. d
15. c
16. b
17. a
18. a
19. b
20. c
21. d
22. a, b, c
23. a, b, c, d, e
24. a
25. b
26. c, d, e
27. b
28. a
29. b
30. a, c, d
31. c
32. c
33. a, b, d
34. a
35. b
36. b
37. c
38. a
39. e
40. d
41. a
42. d
43. c
44. b
45. e
46. a
47. a, b, c
48. c
49. a
50. d
51. c

52. b
53. c
54. a
55. c, d
56. c
57. c
58. a
59. a
60. b
61. a
62. b
63. c
64. b
65. c
66. a
67. c
68. c
69. a
70. a, c, e
71. b, d, e
72. a
73. d
74. b
75. a
76. c
77. a, b, d, e
78. a
79. c, e
80. a, b
81. b, c, d, e

CHAPTER 20

1. a. Connective tissue disease
   b. Degenerative joint disease
   c. Osteoarthritis
   d. Erythrocyte sedimentation rate
   e. Total joint replacement
   f. Total joint arthroplasty
   g. Deep vein (venous) thrombosis
   h. Continuous passive motion
   i. Rheumatoid arthritis
   j. Temporomandibular joint
   k. Systemic lupus erythematosus
2. d
3. a, c, d
4. a, b, c, e
5. b, e, f
6. c
7. a, e
8. b, c, e
9. a, b, d, e

10. c
11. b
12. d, e
13. b, c, d
14. c, e
15. a, b, c, d, e
16. c
17. a, b, c, d
18. a, c, d
19. a, b, d, e
20. a. increased pain
    b. shortening of affected leg
    c. leg rotation
21. a, b, c, d, e
22. T
23. T
24. T
25. a, b, c, e
26. b
27. a, b, d, e
28. b
29. a
30. b, c, e
31. a
32. a, c d
33. b, d, e
34. d
35. c, e
36. b, c, d
37. b, c, e, f
38. a, e
39. c
40. b
41. b
42. a, b, c
43. b
44. d
45. a
46. a. L
    b. E
    c. L
    d. L
    e. L
    f. E
    g. E
    h. L
47. a, c, d, e
48. a
49. c
50. a, b, c
51. c
52. a, b
53. a
54. a, b, e
55. a, b, c, d
56. d
57. a, c
58. a. Low
    b. Low

c. Low
d. High
e. High
59. b, e
60. c
61. f
62. b
63. a
64. d
65. h
66. g
67. c
68. e
69. i
70. b
71. a, c
72. a
73. b
74. c
75. c
76. b
77. d
78. d
79. d
80. a, c, e
81. a, b, c, d
82. b, d
83. c
84. T
85. T
86. a
87. a, b, c
88. a
89. a, c, e
90. d, e
91. a, b
92. T
93. F; is a disease that mimics the clinical manifestations of gout, but the crystals deposited in the joints are calcium pyrophosphate, not sodium urate
94. a, c, d
95. c
96. g
97. e
98. b
99. d
100. a
101. c
102. f

CHAPTER 21

1. b, c, e
2. d
3. a
4. c
5. b
6. e

7. Retrovirus: The family of viruses to which the HIV virus belongs.
8. HIV protease: "Chemical scissors" which clip the new virus particle in the form of one long protein strand made within the HIV-infected CD4+ T cell. The clipped strand is a smaller functional piece which forms the new-finished viral particle.
9. HIV: Human immunodeficiency virus; a virus which attacks the immune system
10. AIDS: Acquired immunodeficiency syndrome; the end result of HIV altering the patient's immune system. A person with AIDS is HIV-positive and has either a CD4+ T cell count of < 200 cells/mm^3 or an opportunistic infection.
11. b, e
12. a, b, c, d, e
13. a, b, d
14. b, c
15. a, c, d
16. d, e
17. b
18. b, c, e
19. b
20. a
21. a, e
22. Pathogenic infections are caused by virulent organisms and occur even among people whose immune systems are functioning normally. Opportunistic infections are those caused by organisms that are present as part of the normal environment and are kept in check by normal immune function. Only when immune function is depressed are such organisms capable of causing infection.
23. a, b, c, d
24. a, e
25. a, c, d, e
26. d
27. a, b, c
28. T
29. F; Histoplasmosis progresses to a widespread infection.
30. T
31. a, c, d
32. b, c, d

33. c
34. a, b, c, d, e
35. b, c, d, e
36. a, b, c
37. a, b, d
38. a, b, d
39. a, b, d, e
40. a, c, d
41. T
42. F; lesions resulting from Kaposi's sarcoma are small, purplish-brown, raised, and usually not painful or itchy
43. T
44. F; patients with HIV should know that as CD4+ counts lower, clinical manifestations increase, not decrease
45. T
46. F; antiretroviral therapy only inhibits viral replication and does not kill the virus.
47. F; HIV is more easily transmitted from infected male to uninfected female than infected female to uninfected male
48. a, c
49. b
50. a. D
    b. NC
    c. D
    d. D
51. d

CHAPTER 22

1. b
2. a, b, c
3. a
4. b
5. d
6. a
7. e
8. c
9. a
10. b
11. d
12. a
13. c
14. d
15. An antigen that provokes allergic sensitization
16. Stimulates further inflammatory response
17. A short-acting biochemical agent that causes capillary leak, nasal and conjunctival mucus secretion, and itching and erythema

18. Runny nose, clear drainage, and pink mucosa
19. a, b, e
20. b, d
21. b
22. a
23. c
24. d
25. e
26. b, d
27. a, b, e
28. a, b, e, f
29. b
30. T
31. F; after the proper dose of epinephrine is administered to a patient having an anaphylactic reaction, the same dose may be repeated every 15 to 20 minutes if needed
32. F; latex allergens may enter the body through inhalation, direct contact with blood vessels during surgery, or via direct contact with the skin
33. T
34. F; patients with bee sting allergies should carry a kit that contains injectable epinephrine for immediate treatment as needed
35. a
36. a, e
37. a
38. a, d, e
39. b
40. c, e
41. a, b, d, e
42. c
43. b
44. a, b, c, d
45. a, b
46. a, b, c, e
47. Glomerular basement membrane and neutrophils
48. a, d, f
49. c, e
50. a, b
51. c
52. a
53. d
54. a
55. a

CHAPTER 23

1. b, c
2. b
3. a, c, e, f
4. a, b, c, f
5. b, d, e

6. e
7. b
8. a
9. c
10. d
11. f
12. g
13. c
14. a, b, c, d, f
15. b, c, d, f
16. a, b, c, d
17. a, b, e
18. T
19. T
20. T
21. F; if promotion occurs and the cancer cell is able to divide
22. T
23. a, b, e
24. a, b, c, e
25. c
26. a
27. a, b, c, d, e
28. a, c, e
29. c, e
30. a, b, c, d
31. a, c, d, e
32. Exposure to carcinogens, genetic predisposition, immune function
33. a, b, c, d
34. a, b, c, e
35. a, b, e
36. a, b, c, d
37. a, b, d, e
38. a, b, c, d, e
39. a, b, c, e
40. a, b, c
41. c, e
42. a
43. b, c
44. a, b, c, d, e
45. a, b, c, e
46. a, c, f

CHAPTER 24

1. b
2. b, c, e
3. b, d
4. b, d
5. F; pain does not always accompany cancer
6. T
7. F; the purpose of cancer treatment is to prolong survival time or improve quality of life
8. T
9. a, c, e

10. a, b, c, d
11. a, b
12. b
13. a, b
14. a, b, c
15. T
16. F; the total dose of radiation needed depends on the size and location of the tumor and on the radiation sensitivity of the tumor and surrounding normal tissues
17. F; some damage to normal tissues cannot be avoided during radiation therapy
18. T
19. F; the optimum dose of radiation is one that can kill the cancer cells with an acceptable level of damage to normal tissues
20. T
21. T
22. F; with needles and seed implants, the patient emits radiation while the implant is in place, but the excreta are not radioactive
23. T
24. a
25. a, b, c
26. b, c, d
27. b
28. a
29. a, b, e
30. a, b, c, e
31. c
32. a, c
33. c
34. b
35. d
36. a
37. b
38. b
39. b
40. b, c
41. b, c
42. d
43. a, c
44. a. V
    b. V
    c. I
    d. V
    e. I
45. a, b
46. a, b
47. d
48. c
49. a, c, f
50. a, c, d

51. b, c, f
52. T
53. T
54. a, e
55. Interleukins are a group of substances the body makes to help regulate inflammation and immune protection, and help different immune system cells recognize and destroy abnormal body cells. They appear to "charge up" the immune system and enhance attacks on cancer cells by macrophages, natural killer (NK) cells, and tumor-infiltrating lymphocytes.
56. Interferons are cell-produced proteins that have been effective to some degree in the treatment of melanoma, hairy cell leukemia, renal cell carcinoma, ovarian cancer, and cutaneous T cell lymphoma. They assist in cancer therapy by slowing tumor cell division, stimulating the growth and activation of NK cells, inducing cancer cells to resume a more normal appearance and function, and inhibiting the expression of oncogenes.
57. a, d
58. a, b, c, e
59. b
60. a
61. a, b, c, e
62. b
63. c
64. d
65. a
66. c
67. b, e
68. c
69. d
70. c

CHAPTER 25

1. c
2. f
3. d
4. g
5. h
6. e
7. b
8. a
9. a
10. b
11. c

12. a
13. a, b, c, d, g
14. a
15. e
16. d
17. a
18. a
19. c
20. b
21. d
22. e
23. a, b, e
24. e
25. c
26. a, b
27. 167
28. b
29. d
30. a, b, d
31. b
32. b
33. d
34. c
35. d
36. b
37. a
38. a, b, c, d, e
39. d, e, f, g
40. g
41. h
42. f
43. e
44. d
45. c
46. b
47. a
48. d
49. T
50. F; a fever, generally a temperature greater than 101° F, is one of the indicators of a systemic infection
51. T
52. F; a superinfection is either a reinfection or a second infection with the same kind of microorganism
53. a, b, c, d
54. a. Erythromycin, tetracycline, gentamicin
    b. Antifungal agents
    c. Actinomycin
    d. Penicillins and cephalosporins
55. b
56. g
57. i
58. f
59. h
60. b

61. a
62. c
63. d
64. e
65. b
66. c
67. a
68. c
69. b
70. d

CHAPTER 26

1. b
2. a
3. b
4. b
5. c
6. a
7. a
8. b
9. c
10. c
11. b
12. c
13. a
14. c
15. a
16. c
17. d
18. e
19. h
20. c
21. b
22. i
23. j
24. f
25. g
26. a
27. a
28. b
29. b, c, e, f, g
30. d
31. b
32. a
33. a, b, c, e
34. c
35. d
36. b
37. a
38. b
39. d
40. d
41. a, b, d, f
42. a
43. c
44. c
45. b
46. c
47. d
48. d

49. a
50. b
51. e
52. c
53. a
54. c
55. a
56. b
57. c
58. d
59. a
60. b
61. c
62. a
63. a, b, c, d, f, g
64. d
65. b
66. a
67. i
68. h
69. e
70. d
71. f
72. g
73. c
74. b
75. c
76. d
77. c
78. a, c, e, f
79. a
80. j
81. a
82. c
83. e
84. h
85. i
86. b
87. d
88. f
89. g

CHAPTER 27

1. m
2. k
3. i
4. d
5. b
6. f
7. l
8. j
9. c
10. a
11. e
12. h
13. g
14. a
15. b, c, d, f
16. d
17. b

18. b
19. c
20. c
21. b
22. d
23. a
24. a, b, e
25. c
26. a
27. b
28. b
29. a, c, d, e
30. c
31. b
32. a, b, d, e
33. a
34. a
35. d
36. a
37. a, b, c, e
38. b
39. a, d, e, g
40. d
41. b
42. c
43. a
44. e
45. a, b, c, e
46. b
47. b
48. c
49. c
50. a
51. a
52. a, c, d
53. a
54. a
55. c
56. c
57. e
58. b
59. h
60. g
61. a
62. d
63. e
64. f
65. i
66. j
67. k
68. l
69. c
70. d
71. c
72. b
73. b
74. a
75. a. 1
    b. 8
    c. 7

d. 4
e. 6
f. 5
g. 3
h. 2
76. c
77. a, c, d
78. b
79. c
80. a
81. c
82. c
83. d
84. b
85. b
86. b
87. c
88. a, b, c, e, f
89. b
90. d
91. a
92. c
93. d
94. a
95. a
96. b
97. d
98. c
99. a
100. c

CHAPTER 28

1. i
2. e
3. g
4. a
5. d
6. h
7. c
8. f
9. b
10. k
11. j
12. a
13. c
14. b, c, d, e
15. d
16. a
17. c
18. d
19. c
20. b
21. b
22. b
23. b
24. a, c, d, e
25. b
26. a
27. b
28. c

29. b
30. b, c, d
31. a, b, c
32. b
33. b
34. d
35. c
36. d
37. c
38. d
39. b
40. d
41. b
42. b
43. a, b, c, e
44. c
45. b
46. a
47. c
48. b
49. a
50. c
51. a
52. 40 mL/hr
53. c
54. b
55. c
56. b
57. a
58. c
59. b
60. a, c, e
61. c
62. c, d, e
63. d
64. a, c, e
65. a
66. b
67. a, b, c, e
68. a
69. b
70. c
71. d
72. a, b, d, e
73. b
74. a, d
75. b
76. a, b, d, f
77. c
78. a
79. a
80. a
81. b, c, d
82. T
83. T
84. F
85. F
86. T
87. a
88. a

89. a
90. a
91. a
92. c
93. c
94. c
95. b
96. f
97. e
98. a
99. d
100. g
101. b
102. b
103. b, c, d
104. c
105. c
106. d
107. b, d, f
108. a
109. a
110. d
111. **Across**
     2. Desquamation
     3. Eschar
     5. Shock
     7. Superficial
     8. Partial
     9. Blanch
     11. Emergent
     13. Third-spacing
     Down
     1. Pigskin
     4. Remobilization
     6. Full
     10. Contact
     12. Moist
     14. Dry

CHAPTER 29

1. a
2. a
3. b
4. b
5. b
6. a
7. b
8. a
9. a
10. a
11. b
12. b
13. a
14. diffuses
15. b
16. c
17. a
18. c
19. e
20. b

21. a
22. d
23. b
24. a, b, c, e
25. c
26. a
27. b
28. d
29. c
30. b
31. b, c, e
32. b
33. b
34. c
35. b
36. c
37. a
38. (Refer to Fig. 29-11 in the text)
39. a, b, e
40. a, b, c, d, f
41. d
42. c
43. a
44. c
45. c
46. c
47. a
48. a, e
49. c
50. pneumothorax
51. a, b, e
52. a
53. e
54. a
55. c
56. b
57. d
58. b
59. c
60. a
61. a
62. c
63. b, d
64. d
65. d
66. b
67. b
68. increased
69. alkalosis
70. d
71. d
72. b
73. a

CHAPTER 30

1. a, c, e
2. b, c, d, e
3. b, c, e
4. Tracheomalacia

5. a, d, e
6. b, c, e
7. b, d, e
8. b
9. b
10. c
11. c
12. c
13. d
14. c
15. a, b, c, d, e
16. b
17. c
18. c
19. a, c, d, e
20. a
21. d
22. d
23. c
24. c
25. c
26. a
27. c
28. a
29. a
30. c
31. d
32. c
33. c
34. b
35. a, c, d, e
36. a
37. a
38. b
39. a, b, c, e
40. a, c, d, e, f, g
41. a
42. b
43. a. 1
    b. 2
    c. 6
    d. 9
    e. 3
    f. 4
    g. 8
    h. 7
    i. 5
44. a. 2
    b. 10
    c. 1
    d. 4
    e. 7
    f. 3
    g. 8
    h. 6
    i. 5
    j. 9
45. d
46. a
47. d

48. d
49. d
50. a, b, e
51. b, e
52. h
53. c
54. d
55. a
56. g
57. f
58. b
59. e
60. d
61. a, d, e
62. c
63. b
64. c
65. b
66. c
67. c

CHAPTER 31

1. c
2. a, b, e
3. c
4. a
5. a
6. c, e
7. a, c, e
8. d
9. c
10. c
11. b
12. b, a, d, c, e
13. c
14. a
15. b
16. b
17. c
18. c
19. a
20. b, d, e
21. a
22. a
23. c
24. a, c, d, e
25. b
26. d
27. a
28. a
29. c
30. b
31. c
32. d
33. d
34. T
35. T
36. T
37. F; erythroplakia; white lesions are leukoplakia

38. T
39. F; partial laryngectomy
40. T
41. T
42. a, c, d, e
43. d
44. d
45. a, c, e, f
46. a
47. c
48. b
49. a
50. a
51. d
52. c
53. c
54. a
55. d
56. a
57. a
58. b
59. c
60. d
61. d
62. b, e
63. c
64. a
65. c
66. a
67. b
68. d
69. a, d, e, f
70. c
71. a, c, e

CHAPTER 32

1. a, b
2. b
3. c
4. c
5. b, c
6. b
7. b, c
8. a
9. b
10. a, b, c
11. a
12. a
13. a
14. c
15. a
16. c
17. a
18. b, c
19. a
20. a
21. a
22. a, c, d, f
23. c
24. b

25. a, b, d, e
26. food; weight
27. a
28. d
29. b
30. a, d
31. d
32. Improve air flow
    Relieve symptoms
    Prevent asthma episodes
33. c
34. b
35. b
36. b
37. a, d, e
38. c
39. c
40. b
41. d
42. c
43. d
44. b
45. b
46. c
47. d
48. b
49. a
50. b
51. b
52. c
53. a
54. a
55. b
56. c
57. d
58. b
59. c
60. c
61. c
62. a. 2
    b. 6
    c. 5
    d. 3
    e. 4
    f. 7
    g. 1
63. a
64. b
65. c
66. a
67. b, c, e
68. a, c, d, f
69. d
70. b
71. c
72. a
73. brain; bone
74. b, c, e
75. T
76. T

77. T
78. T
79. F; symptoms are a late sign
80. F; a CT scan can detect early cancer; x-rays may indicate advanced disease
81. T
82. T
83. a, c, e
84. c
85. d
86. a
87. d
88. c
89. c
90. b
91. b
92. c
93. c
94. d
95. b
96. b
97. a
98. T
99. T
100. a
101. a, c, e
102. a
103. c
104. a

CHAPTER 33

1. c
2. d
3. a, c, d, e
4. d
5. b
6. c
7. b
8. b
9. a, c, d, e
10. c
11. c
12. a
13. a, c, e
14. c, d
15. c
16. a
17. b
18. b
19. b, c, d
20. c
21. a
22. b
23. c
24. a, b, c, e
25. a. 8
    b. 6
    c. 7

d. 11
e. 3
f. 12
g. 2
h. 5
i. 10
j. 4
k. 9
l. 1
26. b
27. b
28. a, d, e
29. a, e
30. d
31. a
32. c
33. c
34. b
35. a
36. d
37. a
38. c
39. a
40. c
41. c
42. d
43. d
44. a
45. b
46. b
47. c
48. a
49. c, a, d, b, e
50. b
51. a
52. a, b, d, e
53. a, b, d, e
54. b
55. c
56. b, c, d, f
57. c
58. b
59. b, c, d
60. airborne
61. a, c, e
62. a, c, e
63. a
64. d
65. c
66. 6 months
67. d
68. d
69. b
70. a
71. b
72. b
73. b
74. d
75. a
76. a, b, c, d

77. a
78. a
79. a, b, c
80. c
81. d
82. b
83. c
84. c
85. b
86. b, c, e
87. a, b, d, e, f
88. b

CHAPTER 34

1. a, c, e
2. b
3. amniotic fluid
4. blood clots
5. a, c, e
6. c, a, b, d, e
7. c
8. a, b, c, g
9. a
10. b
11. d
12. b
13. b, c, e
14. d
15. a, d, e
16. a, b, e
17. b
18. c
19. d
20. b
21. d
22. b, c, d, f
23. c
24. c
25. b
26. a
27. c
28. ventilatory failure
29. b, c, d, e
30. oxygenation failure
31. asthma
32. a, b, d, e
33. Transfusion-related acute lung injury, or TRALI
34. b
35. a, c, d, f
36. c
37. a
38. b
39. d
40. b, c, e, g
41. a
42. c
43. b
44. d
45. b

46. b
47. a, c, d, e
48. b, c, e
49. b
50. c
51. a
52. c
53. a
54. b
55. b
56. c
57. a
58. a
59. b
60. a
61. a
62. c
63. b
64. a
65. a
66. a, b, c, e, g
67. b
68. c
69. a, c, e
70. c
71. c
72. c
73. a
74. b
75. d
76. a
77. c
78. b, c, d, e, f
79. c
80. c
81. a
82. a
83. b
84. b
85. a
86. a
87. a, b, c, e, g
88. b, c, e
89. a, b, d
90. b, c, d
91. f
92. c
93. b
94. h
95. a
96. g
97. e
98. d
99. i
100. j
101. a, d, e
102. c
103. d
104. c
105. b

106. a
107. d
108. d
109. a. 3
     b. 5
     c. 7
     d. 4
     e. 8
     f. 1
     g. 2
     h. 6
110. a, b, d
111. b, d, e, f
112. c
113. d
114. b
115. a
116. a
117. b
118. a
119. a, d

CHAPTER 35

1. g
2. b
3. i
4. h
5. f
6. e
7. c
8. d
9. a
10. a. SA node rate is 60 to 100 beats/min
    b. AV node rate is 40 to 60 beats/min
    c. Purkinje fibers rate is 20 to 40 beats/min
11. c
12. e
13. a
14. d
15. b
16. a, c, d
17. a, d, e, f
18. a
19. oxygenation, perfusion
20. a
21. a, b, d, f
22. a, b, e
23. b
24. parasympathetic, sympathetic
25. c
26. a
27. b, d, e
28. a, c, d
29. Uncontrollable: diabetes, ethnic background, age, postmenopause

Controllable: smoking, obesity, sedentary lifestyle
30. F; the left ventricle
31. T
32. a. 3
    b. 1
    c. 2
    d. 5
    e. 4
33. c
34. b
35. b
36. d
37. c
38. a
39. c
40. d
41. One-half pack/day × 2 years = 1 pack-year
42. a
43. a
44. a
45. b
46. a
47. a
48. c
49. d
50. b, d
51. c
52. a
53. (Refer to Fig. 35-7 in the text.)
54. F; begins with inspection
55. T
56. T
57. F; detected by auscultation
58. T
59. F; best heard at the lower left sternal border or the apex
60. F; to listen for high-frequency sounds
61. T
62. a, b, c
63. f
64. d
65. c
66. a, b, c
67. a
68. f
69. b
70. e
71. b
72. e
73. c
74. d
75. b
76. a, c, d, e, f
77. a, c, d
78. c

79. c
80. b, c, e
81. hypersensitivity
82. T
83. F
84. F
85. T
86. a
87. b
88. a
89. c
90. d
91. b
92. a
93. d
94. b
95. a
96. e
97. c
98. a
99. a
100. a, b, d
101. c
102. a, b, d
103. a
104. b
105. a
106. c
107. d
108. b, e
109. F; do not require informed consent
110. T
111. F; effective for detecting an acute MI and define its location and size
112. F; is not placed in isolation
113. T
114. T
115. T
116. T
117. T
118. F; multigated blood pool scanning is a noninvasive test that evaluates cardiac motion and calculates ejection fraction
119. T
120. T
121. F; is useful
122. d
123. a
124. a
125. b, d, e
126. c, d, e, f, g
127. b
128. b, d
129. a, d, e

CHAPTER 36

1. sinoatrial (SA) node
2. Bundle of His; Purkinje fibers
3. delay
4. automaticity
5. Contractility
6. conductivity
7. excitability
8. Atrial kick
9. b
10. b
11. c
12. c
13. d
14. a
15. c
16. f
17. e
18. b
19. (Refer to Fig. 36-5 in the text.)
20. a
21. c
22. a
23. a
24. d
25. a
26. c
27. c
28. d
29. c
30. a
31. c
32. d
33. a. 6
    b. 3
    c. 1
    d. 5
    e. 4
    f. 2
34. a
35. b
36. a, b, e, f
37. d
38. b, c, e
39. a
40. b
41. QRS complex
42. S-T segment
43. d
44. electrical activity
45. T
46. T
47. T
48. F; of ventricles to occur
49. b
50. a
51. d
52. 60 (1500 divided by 25)

53. 50; bradycardia
54. b
55. b
56. a, c, e
57. g
58. d
59. e
60. f
61. h
62. c
63. a
64. b
65. f
66. b
67. c
68. a, b, c, d
69. d
70. c
71. d
72. a
73. b, d, e
74. a
75. b
76. b
77. a
78. d
79. a
80. b
81. a, c, d, e
82. a
83. a
84. a, c, d, e
85. decrease
86. b, c, e
87. syncope; diaphoresis
88. T
89. F; there is a delay in the AV node conduction, but all impulses reach the ventricles
90. T
91. T
92. c
93. b
94. c
95. d
96. a
97. b
98. b
99. b
100. d
101. b
102. c
103. b
104. c
105. a
106. a, b, c, d
107. a, b, d, f
108. c
109. b
110. d

111. c
112. d
113. e
114. a
115. b
116. f
117. c
118. a, c
119. c
120. a. 1
     b. 3
     c. 6
     d. 4
     e. 5
     f. 7
     g. 2
121. c
122. a
123. a, b, d
124. b, c, e
125. ventricular
126. a, d, e
127. F; treats spontaneous sustained ventricular tachycardia (VT) or ventricular fibrillation (VF) unrelated to a myocardial infarction or other causes amenable to correction
128. T
129. a
130. b, d, e
131. a
132. c
133. b, c, d, f
134. a. 4
     b. 1
     c. 3
     d. 5
     e. 2
135. b, c, e
136. c
137. a, c, d, f
138. *Rate:* Atrial rate: Approx. 300 beats/min
Ventricular rate: 75 beats/min
Rhythm: Irregular (due to PACs)
P waves: 2 flutter waves per QRS complex; no P waves present
PR interval: None
QRS duration: 0.08 seconds
Interpretation: 2:1 atrial flutter with occasional PACs
139. *Rate:* About 50 beats/min
Rhythm: Regular
P waves: Regular; 1 per QRS
PR interval: 0.20 seconds
QRS duration: 0.08 seconds

110. d
Interpretation: Sinus bradycardia with PAC
140. *Rate:* 150 beats/min
Rhythm: Regular
P waves: Regular; notched 1 per QRS
PR interval: 0.12 seconds
QRS duration: 0.08 seconds
Interpretation: Atrial tachycardia
141. *Rate:* Beat-to-beat variability approx. 130 beats/min
Rhythm: Irregular, irregular
P waves: Fibrillation waves
PR interval: None
QRS duration: 0.08 seconds
Interpretation: Atrial fibrillation with rapid ventricular response
142. *Rate:* 83 beats/min
Rhythm: Regular
P waves: 1 per QRS
PR interval: 0.16 seconds
QRS duration: 0.08 seconds
Interpretation: Sinus rhythm with 2.3-second pause/sinus arrest
143. *Rate:* 150 beats/min
Rhythm: Regular
P waves: Regular; 1 per QRS
PR interval: 0.12 seconds
QRS duration: 0.04 seconds
Interpretation: Sinus tachycardia
144. *Rate:* Cannot be determined
Rhythm: Chaotic
P waves: None
PR interval: None
QRS duration: None
Interpretation: Ventricular fibrillation
145. *Rate:* 78 beats/min
Rhythm: Regular
P waves: Regular; 1 per QRS
PR interval: 0.20 seconds
QRS duration: 0.04 seconds
Interpretation: Sinus rhythm with PVC
146. *Rate:* Cannot be determined
Rhythm: Chaotic
P waves: None
PR interval: None
QRS duration: None
Interpretation: Ventricular fibrillation
147. *Rate:* Approx. 200 beats/min

Rhythm: Regular with wide-complex QRS
P waves: None
PR interval: None
QRS duration: Wide—0.28 seconds
Interpretation: Monomorphic ventricular tachycardia
148. *Rate:* None
Rhythm: None
P waves: None
PR interval: None
QRS duration: None
Interpretation: Asystole
149. *Rate:* 107 beats/min
Rhythm: Irregular, irregular
P waves: Fibrillation waves
PR interval: None
QRS duration: 0.08 seconds
Interpretation: Atrial fibrillation
150. *Rate:* Ventricular rate: Varies—starts at 42 beats/min, speeds up to 83 beats/min
Atrial rate: Approx. 350 beats/min
Rhythm: Regular
P waves: Flutter waves present
PR interval: None—not measured in this rhythm
QRS duration: 0.08 seconds
Interpretation: Atrial flutter (latter half looks like 3:1 flutter)
151. *Rate:* 75 beats/min
Rhythm: Regular
P waves: Regular; 1 per QRS
PR interval: 0.20 seconds
QRS duration: 0.08 seconds
Interpretation: Sinus rhythm with PJC
152. *Rate:* Ventricular: 35 beats/min
Atrial: 100 beats/min
Rhythm: Regular wide complex
P waves: Do not correspond with QRS complex
PR interval: None
QRS duration: 0.20 seconds
Interpretation: Third-degree AV block with underlying ventricular escape rhythm

CHAPTER 37

1. b
2. e
3. c
4. d
5. f
6. a
7. left ventricle
8. diminishes; pulmonary
9. fluid overload
10. increase
11. sympathetic stimulation
12. c
13. c
14. a, c, e
15. a, b, c, e, f
16. d
17. d
18. d
19. b
20. a. Medications
    b. Activity
    c. Weight
    d. Diet
    e. Symptoms
21. a. Medications: Take as prescribed; keep prescriptions filled; know purpose and side effects for each drug
    b. Activity: Stay active but avoid overexertion; know your limits; make it a goal to be able to converse while exercising
    c. Weight: Weigh daily at the same time using the same scale and amount of clothing; monitor for fluid retention
    d. Diet: Limit daily sodium to 2-3 g; limit daily fluid intake to 2 L
    e. Symptoms: Notify health care provider immediately of any new or worsening symptoms
22. c
23. d
24. d
25. b
26. b
27. a
28. a
29. a, b, c, e
30. a, d, e
31. a
32. d
33. c
34. b
35. c
36. a
37. d
38. c
39. a
40. d
41. a
42. b
43. a
44. c
45. b
46. a, b, c, e
47. b
48. c, d, e, f
49. b
50. a
51. b
52. d
53. a
54. e
55. a, b
56. c
57. a
58. e
59. b
60. a
61. a, b
62. c
63. c
64. d
65. d
66. b
67. a, b, c
68. b
69. a
70. a
71. c
72. c
73. a
74. a
75. b
76. b
77. c
78. b
79. a
80. c
81. a
82. b, c, e, f, g, h
83. d
84. c
85. b
86. e
87. a
88. f
89. g
90. b
91. a
92. a
93. c
94. a
95. b
96. a
97. c
98. a, d, e, f
99. b
100. c
101. a
102. b
103. b
104. b
105. a, c, e
106. d
107. a, c, e
108. cardiac tamponade
109. b
110. c
111. b
112. a
113. c
114. b
115. a
116. b
117. a, b, c, e
118. c
119. b
120. d
121. a, c, d, e
122. a, b, e
123. a
124. b
125. a, e, f, g

CHAPTER 38

1. T
2. T
3. T
4. F; taken at bedtime
5. a, b, c, e
6. African American; diabetes mellitus; obese; sedentary lifestyle; genetic predisposition
7. b, c, d
8. a, b, d
9. a, d
10. d
11. b
12. a
13. d
14. b
15. d
16. b
17. a
18. b, c, d
19. b, c, d
20. a
21. b
22. b
23. b, c, d, e, g
24. b
25. a
26. d
27. a
28. b, c, d, e
29. c

30. a
31. b
32. d
33. a
34. c
35. a
36. b
37. a, b, c, f
38. b
39. a, c, d, e
40. b
41. b
42. b
43. d
44. b
45. a, b, c, f
46. a
47. b
48. c
49. d
50. b
51. b
52. a
53. c
54. a, b, d, f
55. c
56. c
57. a, c, d, e
58. a, c, d
59. a, c, e
60. b, c, d
61. b
62. a, b, c, e
63. b
64. a
65. d
66. a
67. b
68. d
69. a
70. a
71. b
72. c
73. b
74. a
75. a
76. c
77. a
78. b, c
79. a, b, e
80. a
81. b, d, e, f, g, h
82. a
83. c
84. b
85. b
86. d
87. b
88. a
89. b

90. a, b, c, e, f
91. a
92. c
93. c
94. d
95. a
96. a
97. c
98. a, b, c, d
99. b
100. a
101. d
102. b
103. a. BD
    b. RD
    c. RD
    d. BD
    e. BD
    f. RD
104. b
105. a
106. c
107. a
108. d
109. a
110. c
111. a
112. c
113. d
114. a
115. T
116. T
117. F; within 5 days
118. T
119. F; associated with stasis of blood flow, endothelial injury, and/or hypercoagulability, known as *Virchow's triad*
120. T
121. T
122. T
123. F; UFH inhibits fibrin formation; the drug does nothing to the existing clot
124. d
125. b
126. c, d, e
127. c
128. c
129. a, b, c
130. a
131. a, b, c, d, f, g
132. b
133. c
134. d
135. a
136. a, b, c, e
137. a
138. c
139. c

140. a, c, e
141. b, c, e
142. Healing of the ulcer; preventing infection; preventing stasis with reoccurrence of ulcer formation
143. b
144. a
145. a, b, d, e
146. a
147. a, b, c, d, e, f
148. a
149. c
150. a, b, d, e
151. c
152. c
153. b
154. b
155. a. 6
    b. 3
    c. 2
    d. 5
    e. 4
    f. 1
156. c

CHAPTER 39

1. e
2. a
3. f
4. b
5. h
6. c
7. d
8. i
9. g
10. j
11. a, b, d
12. b, c, d, e
13. a, e
14. d
15. b, c, d, f
16. a, b, d, e
17. d
18. b, e
19. c
20. d
21. d
22. a, b, c, d
23. c
24. d
25. c
26. a
27. b
28. a, b
29. b
30. a
31. a
32. b
33. a

34. a. Cry
    b. Col
    c. Col
    d. Cry
    e. Col
35. c, e
36. a
37. c
38. d, e
39. c
40. a, b, e, f, g
41. b
42. a
43. c
44. a
45. a, b, c
46. b
47. a, b, c, d
48. b
49. d
50. c
51. a
52. b
53. b
54. b
55. c
56. c
57. a
58. c
59. d
60. d
61. c
62. d
63. b
64. c
65. a
66. a
67. d
68. c
69. c
70. a, c, d, f
71. d
72. a, b, c, e, f
73. b
74. d
75. b
76. a
77. T
78. F; shock progresses in a predictable, orderly fashion, but death is not inevitable
79. F; in the early stages of shock, the blood pressure is within normal limits or slightly increased because of adequate compensatory mechanisms
80. T
81. T
82. T

83. T
84. T
85. F; cause an increase in cardiac output
86. T
87. d
88. f
89. e
90. b
91. a
92. d
93. e
94. a
95. f
96. d
97. a
98. c
99. a
100. a
101. f
102. a
103. f
104. a

CHAPTER 40

1. f
2. b
3. g
4. d
5. c
6. h
7. k
8. i
9. e
10. j
11. a
12. b, e
13. c, d, e
14. b
15. d
16. b, c, f
17. c
18. a
19. c
20. a
21. a. 4
  b. 5
  c. 1
  d. 2
  e. 3
22. a. A
  b. MI
  c. MI
  d. A
  e. MI
  f. A
  g. A
  h. MI
  i. MI
23. T

24. T
25. F; have an incidence of MI that equals that of men
26. T
27. a, c
28. b
29. b, c, d, e
30. b
31. d, e
32. c
33. a
34. a
35. d
36. a, b, d, e
37. a
38. c
39. F; accounts for over one-third of deaths
40. T
41. F; does not reduce the risk of CAD
42. T
43. F; does not increase
44. b
45. a, b, c, e, g
46. a, c, d, f, g
47. a
48. b
49. a, f, g
50. b
51. c
52. b, e
53. a, b, c, d
54. c
55. b
56. b
57. a, b, c, e, g
58. b
59. a, b, d
60. b
61. a, b, c, e, f
62. a, b, d, e, f
63. b, c, d
64. a
65. b
66. a
67. b
68. b
69. a
70. b
71. c
72. a
73. a
74. c
75. a
76. a, b, d, e, f
77. c
78. b
79. a
80. c

81. a
82. c
83. a
84. b
85. a
86. a, c, d, f
87. a, b, e
88. b
89. b, c, d, e
90. a, b, d, e, f
91. b
92. b
93. d
94. a
95. b
96. d
97. b
98. a
99. c
100. a, b, c, e
101. b
102. b, c, d
103. c
104. a
105. b
106. a
107. a, b, c, d, e, f
108. b
109. c
110. e
111. b
112. a
113. c
114. d

CHAPTER 41

1. T
2. T
3. T
4. F; globulins transport substances and protect the body against infection
5. F; 120 days
6. T
7. T
8. T
9. F; the kidney produces
10. T
11. F; the smallest
12. T
13. F; the liver
14. F; Vitamin K
15. T
16. T
17. F; provide the first step in the clotting process
18. T
19. T
20. T
21. T

22. T
23. F; an enzyme
24. T
25. a, b, c, d
26. d
27. a, b, c, d, e
28. b
29. F; anticoagulants prevent new clots from forming
30. T
31. T
32. T
33. F; fibrinolytic agents can break down clots older than 6 hours, but tissue that has been anoxic for greater than 6 hours will not benefit from fibrinolytic drugs
34. F; thrombotic strokes
35. a
36. a, b, d, e
37. a, c, d
38. d
39. T
40. T
41. F; the iliac crest
42. F; an aspirin-free mild analgesic
43. T

CHAPTER 42

1. a, b, c, d, e, f
2. a, b, c, d, e
3. b, d, e
4. a
5. a, d, f
6. c
7. a, e
8. c
9. b
10. b
11. a
12. a, b, c, d, e
13. d
14. a, b, c, d, e
15. a, b, c, d, e
16. a
17. a
18. c
19. a, b, d, e, f
20. a
21. a, b
22. a, b, c, d, e
23. a
24. c
25. b
26. c
27. a, b, c, e, f
28. a
29. c

30. b
31. a, b, c, d, e
32. c
33. a, c, d, e
34. a
35. a
36. a
37. a
38. b
39. a
40. a
41. b
42. a
43. ATP
44. TTP
45. ATP
46. TTP
47. ATP
48. ATP
49. TTP
50. ATP
51. ATP
52. b
53. c, e
54. b
55. b
56. a
57. a
58. b
59. c
60. a, c, d

CHAPTER 43

1. b
2. c
3. a
4. f
5. d
6. g
7. e
8. a
9. a
10. d
11. b
12. a. P
    b. B
    c. B
    d. P
    e. P
    f. P
    g. B
    h. P
13. b
14. d
15. a
16. c
17. PNS
18. SNS
19. PNS
20. PNS

21. SNS
22. SNS
23. d
24. a, b, d
25. a
26. d
27. c
28. a
29. a
30. c
31. d
32. c
33. a
34. a
35. d
36. c
37. e
38. b
39. a
40. f
41. a
42. a
43. d
44. e
45. a
46. c
47. b
48. b
49. b
50. a
51. b
52. b
53. c
54. d
55. b
56. c
57. d
58. a
59. d
60. c
61. a
62. d
63. a, b, c, d, f
64. a

CHAPTER 44

1. a
2. b
3. b
4. a
5. a
6. a
7. b
8. a
9. a
10. a
11. b
12. b
13. b
14. a

15. b
16. a
17. b
18. b
19. a
20. a, b, e, f
21. d
22. d
23. a
24. b
25. a
26. c
27. c
28. b
29. a
30. d
31. c
32. a
33. b
34. d
35. b
36. d
37. b
38. c
39. a
40. b
41. a
42. c
43. b
44. c
45. b
46. c
47. d
48. b
49. a, b, e, f
50. c
51. b
52. c
53. a
54. b
55. a, b, c, e
56. a
57. c
58. d
59. b
60. b
61. c
62. b
63. b

CHAPTER 45

1. b
2. b
3. a
4. d
5. b
6. a, b, c, e
7. b
8. c, e
9. a

10. a
11. d
12. b
13. a, b, d
14. 125 mL/hr
15. b
16. a
17. a
18. b
19. b
20. a
21. a
22. b
23. a
24. b
25. b
26. c, e
27. b
28. a
29. b, c, e
30. c
31. a
32. b
33. b
34. d
35. a, e, f
36. c
37. e
38. b
39. a
40. d
41. a, b, c, e, f
42. c
43. b, e
44. d
45. a
46. b, c, e
47. c
48. d
49. a, b, e
50. b

CHAPTER 46

1. j
2. d
3. a
4. c
5. m
6. h
7. g
8. f
9. i
10. b
11. k
12. l
13. e
14. b, e, f
15. c
16. c, e
17. d

18. c, e
19. a
20. c
21. a
22. a, b, d, e
23. c
24. a
25. b
26. b, d, e, f
27. a
28. b
29. a
30. a
31. a, b, d
32. a, c, e, f
33. b
34. b
35. c
36. a, b, c, f
37. a
38. d
39. c
40. b
41. a
42. c
43. a
44. c
45. b
46. c
47. b
48. d, e, f
49. b
50. b
51. d
52. b
53. c
54. a
55. b
56. d
57. d
58. b
59. a, c, e
60. a
61. c, e
62. c
63. d
64. b, c, e
65. a, b, e, f
66. d
67. c
68. c
69. c
70. c
71. b
72. b
73. d
74. a
75. a, b, c, f
76. c
77. a

78. a
79. b
80. a
81. b
82. b
83. b
84. a
85. b
86. b
87. a
88. b
89. a
90. b, c, d, f
91. d
92. c

CHAPTER 47

1. b
2. a
3. b
4. b
5. b
6. a
7. b
8. a
9. b
10. b
11. a, b, d, e
12. d
13. c
14. a
15. b
16. b
17. b
18. b
19. d
20. g
21. e
22. b
23. c
24. f
25. a
26. c
27. b
28. a
29. a
30. a, c, d, e
31. d
32. b
33. b
34. c
35. a, b, d, e, f
36. a, b, c, e
37. a, b, d, f
38. a
39. a
40. b
41. a
42. b
43. a

44. b
45. a
46. b
47. a
48. a
49. c
50. b
51. a
52. c
53. a
54. b
55. a
56. d
57. b
58. a
59. h
60. d
61. a
62. b
63. g
64. e
65. i
66. f
67. c
68. c
69. c
70. a
71. b
72. c
73. a
74. d
75. c
76. a
77. c
78. c
79. c
80. b
81. a, c, d, e
82. a
83. b
84. a
85. a
86. a
87. b
88. b
89. a
90. a
91. b
92. a
93. b
94. b
95. a
96. b
97. c
98. d
99. a, c, d, f
100. b
101. a
102. d
103. c

104. b
105. d
106. c
107. d
108. d
109. b
110. a
111. c

CHAPTER 48

1. c
2. a. 4
   b. 2
   c. 3
   d. 1
   e. 5
3. b, d
4. d
5. c
6. a
7. d
8. b
9. d
10. d
11. e
12. a
13. c
14. b
15. a, b, c
16. a, b, c, d
17. d
18. b, c
19. c
20. a
21. d
22. b
23. c
24. e
25. a, e, f
26. a, c, d
27. b
28. b, d, f
29. d, e
30. c
31. a
32. d
33. b
34. e
35. c
36. d, e
37. c
38. a, d, e
39. c
40. 20, 70
41. T
42. F; located in the upper outer part of the orbit
43. a, c, d, f, g
44. a, c, d
45. b

46. e
47. a
48. d
49. c
50. a, c, e
51. b, c, e
52. a, c, d
53. blindness, retinopathy

CHAPTER 49

1. b
2. c
3. d
4. lashes
5. b, d, e
6. a, b, c
7. a, b, c, d, e
8. c
9. c
10. a, b, e
11. b, c, d, e
12. a, b, c
13. c
14. a, c, d
15. c, e
16. c
17. a
18. (Refer to Table 49-1 in the text.)
19. a, b, c, d, e,
20. a. Physically constrict-ing the pupil so that the ciliary muscle is contracted, which allows better circulation of the aqueous humor to the site of absorption
    b. Reducing the produc-tion of aqueous humor
21. a, b, e
22. d
23. a, b, e
24. c
25. a, b, c, e
26. a
27. b
28. c
29. c
30. b, c, e
31. c
32. reading, writing, close work, activities which increase IOP
33. b
34. d
35. b
36. c
37. c, e
38. c
39. c

40. d
41. Melanoma
42. d
43. a, b, c, d
44. d
45. b
46. c

CHAPTER 50

1. 1. Incus
   2. Malleus
   3. Semicircular canals
   4. Eighth cranial (ves-tibulocochlear) nerve
   5. Cochlea
   6. Eustachian tube
   7. Vestibule
   8. Stapes
   9. Tympanic membrane
   10. External canal
2. a
3. c
4. b, d
5. b, c, d, e
6. a
7. b
8. b
9. c
10. a
11. c
12. b
13. a. 2
    b. 3
    c. 4
    d. 5
    e. 1
    f. 6
14. a, c
15. Hyperacusis
16. a
17. b
18. c
19. d
20. a, c, e, f
21. b
22. d, e
23. c
24. Air conduction
25. b, d, e
26. d
27. d
28. e
29. f
30. b
31. c
32. a
33. b
34. a, b, c
35. b
36. c

37. a
38. d
39. b
40. a
41. a
42. c
43. c
44. a
45. b

CHAPTER 51

1. a, b, c, e
2. b, c, d, e
3. d
4. b, c, d, e
5. c
6. a, c, d, e
7. b
8. a
9. a
10. b
11. b, c, e, f
12. a
13. a
14. a, b, e
15. b
16. a, b, c, d, e
17. b, c, d, e
18. vertigo
19. a, b, e
20. a, b, c, e
21. c
22. a, c, d
23. a, b, e
24. b, c, e
25. c, e
26. sensorineural
27. b, c, d, e
28. b
29. a, b, c, d, e
30. a, b, e
31. a, c, e
32. a, b, c, e
33. c, d
34. c
35. e
36. d
37. i
38. h
39. f
40. b
41. g
42. a
43. b, d, e
44. d, e
45. a, c, e
46. c

CHAPTER 52

1. a
2. b, c
3. h
4. c
5. b
6. e
7. d
8. a
9. k
10. f
11. j
12. i
13. g
14. b
15. c
16. a
17. b
18. a, c, e
19. a
20. d
21. b
22. d
23. c
24. g
25. a
26. b
27. i
28. e
29. h
30. f
31. d
32. c
33. b
34. b, c, e
35. d
36. increases
37. a, c, d, e
38. c
39. d
40. a
41. b
42. a, c, d, e
43. d
44. b, d, e
45. b, c, e
46. a
47. b
48. c
49. d
50. a
51. a, b, d, e
52. a, b
53. a
54. growth
55. c
56. a, b, d
57. c
58. b

59. F; African-American men have denser bones than African-American women
60. T
61. F; such as dark green leafy vegetables
62. **Across**
    1. Varum
    3. Gait
    4. Mobility
    Down
    1. Valgum
    2. Scoliosis
63. k
64. e
65. a
66. f
67. b
68. c
69. g
70. i
71. j
72. l
73. d
74. h
75. a, c, e

CHAPTER 53

1. b
2. c
3. a
4. b
5. c
6. c
7. a
8. b
9. a
10. b, c
11. a
12. c
13. b, c, d
14. a, c, e
15. b, c
16. b
17. a
18. a, c, f
19. b
20. a
21. c
22. a
23. c
24. b, c, d
25. d
26. b, d, e
27. raloxifene (Evista) or estrogen agonist/antagonist
28. a, c, e
29. hypercalcemia
30. testosterone

31. hip
32. b
33. T-score
34. b
35. a
36. b
37. a
38. b
39. d
40. a
41. b
42. d
43. a
44. c
45. a
46. b
47. a, c, d
48. d
49. a, b, d
50. b
51. c
52. b, d, e
53. a, c, d
54. Primary
55. d
56. c
57. a, b, f
58. a
59. a
60. c
61. c
62. e
63. a
64. b
65. d
66. a
67. c
68. b
69. c
70. d
71. a
72. b
73. b
74. a
75. c
76. b
77. a
78. b
79. b
80. a
81. b
82. b
83. a
84. b
85. b
86. a
87. b
88. c
89. a
90. c

91. d
92. e
93. a
94. b
95. b
96. d
97. e
98. e
99. a
100. a, b, d, e
101. d
102. a, b, d, e

CHAPTER 54

1. c
2. d
3. b
4. a
5. a, b, d, f
6. d
7. b
8. a
9. b
10. c
11. a
12. c
13. a. 4
    b. 5
    c. 1
    d. 3
    e. 2
14. d
15. b, c, d
16. c
17. a
18. b
19. b
20. d
21. c
22. b
23. b
24. d
25. a
26. Ilizarov
27. electrical
28. pulsed ultrasound
29. a
30. c
31. a
32. b, c
33. a, b, d, e
34. d
35. c
36. a
37. b, d
38. a, d, e
39. b
40. e
41. b
42. a

43. f
44. d
45. c
46. a
47. ischemia-edema
48. d
49. d
50. a
51. d
52. b
53. a. 6
    b. 4
    c. 1
    d. 2
    e. 5
    f. 3
54. b
55. b
56. c
57. a
58. c
59. b
60. b, e
61. d
62. b
63. d
64. b
65. c
66. a
67. c
68. d
69. c
70. a
71. c
72. c
73. a, b, c, e
74. b
75. a, b, e
76. a, b, c
77. b, c, d
78. F; medial meniscus is more likely to tear
79. T
80. F; 6 to 9 months or longer
81. F; athletes who participate in strenuous sports
82. F; a strain is excessive stretching of a muscle or tendon
83. T
84. F; cannot maintain abduction
85. a, b, c, d
86. b
87. c
88. a, c, d, e
89. c
90. d
91. d

92. b
93. a
94. c
95. d
96. a. 5
     b. 1
     c. 2
     d. 4
     e. 3
     f. 6
97. b, c, e, g
98. b
99. a
100. a, b, e

CHAPTER 55

1.   i
2.   q
3.   m
4.   b
5.   o
6.   n
7.   p
8.   d
9.   h
10. l
11. e
12. c
13. a
14. j
15. f
16. k
17. b, d, e
18. a, c, e
19. b, e
20. a, b, c
21. d
22. a, c
23. a, b, c, d, e
24. a. 4
     b. 3
     c. 2
     d. 1
25. a. 1
     b. 3
     c. 4
     d. 2
26. d
27. d
28. c
29. b
30. a
31. a, b, e
32. c, e
33. c
34. i
35. h
36. d
37. f
38. g

39. j
40. computed tomography
     (or CT) colonography
41. b
42. d
43. c
44. a
45. c
46. e
47. b
48. a

CHAPTER 56

1.   d
2.   a
3.   a
4.   b
5.   c
6.   a
7.   a
8.   c
9.   a, d, e
10. a
11. d
12. b
13. c
14. d
15. d
16. b
17. c
18. a
19. c
20. b, d, e
21. c
22. b, d, e
23. fatigue
24. saliva
25. a
26. c
27. c
28. a

CHAPTER 57

1.   b
2.   a
3.   a, e
4.   a
5.   d
6.   b
7.   e
8.   c
9.   f
10. h
11. g
12. i
13. b
14. d
15. a
16. a

17. d
18. d
19. b
20. a, b, c, d, e
21. diaphragmatic
22. d
23. premalignant
24. b
25. a
26. a, c, e
27. a
28. a, b, c, d
29. d
30. b
31. c
32. a, b, c, d, e

CHAPTER 58

1.   a, c, d
2.   a, c, d, e
3.   F; is made with lab tests
     for *H. pylori*, physical assess-
     ment, EGD
4.   T
5.   F; long-term use of
     NSAIDs
6.   T
7.   a, c, d
8.   a
9.   b
10. d
11. a
12. b
13. d
14. a
15. d
16. T
17. T
18. F; Curling's ulcer
19. T
20. F; at or above
21. T
22. a, c, d, e
23. c
24. a
25. d
26. b
27. d
28. a, b, c, d, e
29. b
30. c
31. a, b, c, e
32. a, b, c, d, e
33. a
34. a
35. c
36. a, b, c
37. a, c
38. b, c, d, e
39. c

40. T
41. T
42. T
43. F; high in protein, high
     in fat, low in carbohydrate
44. T
45. a
46. a

CHAPTER 59

1.   T
2.   T
3.   F; in young adulthood
4.   T
5.   F; left lower quadrant
6.   T
7.   T
8.   a
9.   b, c
10. d
11. a
12. f
13. c
14. b
15. e
16. g
17. c
18. c, e
19. c
20. b
21. a
22. T
23. T
24. T
25. F; usually decreased
26. F; positive test result
27. T
28. T
29. b
30. a
31. a
32. d
33. a
34. c
35. d
36. b
37. a
38. T
39. T
40. T
41. F; metabolic alkalosis
42. F; volvulus is
43. F; intussusception is
44. T
45. T
46. a
47. a, b, c, d, e
48. b
49. a, b
50. d

51. c
52. a
53. T
54. T
55. T
56. T
57. a
58. b, c, d, e
59. c
60. a, c, d
61. a
62. b
63. T
64. T
65. T
66. F; of diarrhea
67. T
68. d

CHAPTER 60

1. T
2. T
3. T
4. F; in the epigastric or periumbilical area
5. F; in the right lower quadrant
6. T
7. a, b
8. b
9. b, c
10. a, b, d
11. c
12. a
13. b
14. c
15. c
16. T
17. T
18. F; without penetrating it
19. T
20. d
21. b
22. c, d
23. c
24. a. UC
     b. CD
     c. UC
     d. CD
     e. UC
     f. UC
     g. CD
25. a
26. a
27. b
28. a, b, e
29. c
30. e
31. d
32. f

33. a
34. b
35. c
36. d
37. a, b, c, d
38. T
39. T
40. F; low in cereal fiber
41. T
42. T
43. F; usually does not undergo
44. d
45. a
46. c
47. c
48. c
49. a
50. b
51. b
52. c
53. a
54. b
55. a, b, c, d
56. F; is not communicable
57. T
58. T
59. T
60. T
61. T

CHAPTER 61

1. T
2. T
3. F; by alcohol abuse
4. T
5. F; sodium and water retention
6. T
7. T
8. T
9. T
10. F; a slow onset with a prolonged, destructive course
11. a, b, c, d, e
12. d
13. b
14. j
15. a
16. f
17. i
18. c
19. g
20. e
21. h
22. d
23. b
24. a, b, c, d, e, f
25. b
26. c

27. b
28. a, c, d, e, f
29. a
30. a
31. d
32. T
33. T
34. T
35. T
36. T
37. a
38. d
39. F; Hepatitis C
40. T
41. T
42. F; have no signs
43. F; not transmitted
44. T
45. T
46. a, b, c, d, e
47. a, b, c, d, e
48. T
49. F; three injections
50. F; only prevents hepatitis B
51. T
52. T
53. T
54. F; can continue to transmit
55. T
56. T
57. a
58. a, b, c, d
59. b, c, d, e
60. a, b, c
61. T
62. T
63. T
64. F; Selective internal radiation
65. T
66. T
67. T
68. T
69. T

CHAPTER 62

1. a
2. c
3. c
4. a
5. c
6. a
7. d
8. b
9. e
10. f
11. g
12. b

13. d
14. a
15. b
16. a
17. a, c, d, e
18. d
19. e
20. c
21. a
22. d
23. b
24. b
25. c
26. a
27. d
28. b
29. T
30. T
31. T
32. T
33. T
34. F; a side-lying position
35. T
36. T
37. b
38. c
39. d
40. c
41. c
42. T
43. T
44. F; is fatigue
45. T
46. F; combination chemotherapy and radiation
47. T

CHAPTER 63

1. a, c, e
2. a, b, c, e
3. b
4. a
5. c
6. a, b, c, d, e
7. a, c, d, e
8. a
9. b
10. a, b, c, d, e
11. b
12. f
13. g
14. b
15. a
16. d
17. e
18. b or c
19. h
20. i
21. b
22. b, c

23. d
24. b, c, d
25. c, d, e
26. a, b, e
27. a
28. b, c, e
29. a, c, d, e
30. e
31. f
32. c
33. d
34. a
35. b
36. b
37. d
38. b
39. c
40. a
41. b
42. a, b, c, e
43. b
44. a
45. a, c, d, e
46. b
47. a
48. d
49. d
50. a, b, c, d
51. b
52. c
53. a
54. b
55. b, e
56. b, c, d, e
57. a, c, d, e
58. d
59. d
60. d

CHAPTER 64

1. a, c, d, e
2. c
3. b
4. h
5. e
6. c
7. d
8. l
9. a
10. f
11. i
12. c
13. e
14. j
15. g
16. k
17. b
18. b
19. e
20. a

21. a
22. d
23. a, b, e
24. a
25. c
26. a
27. b
28. a, b, e
29. a
30. b
31. d
32. a, e
33. b
34. b, c, e
35. a, b, c, e
36. b, c, d
37. a
38. d
39. a, b, c, e
40. b, c, d
41. d
42. d
43. a, c, e
44. b
45. d
46. b
47. b, c, d, e
48. b
49. c
50. b
51. d
52. a
53. a
54. b
55. b
56. a, b, c, d
57. b
58. c, d, e, f
59. a, b, d, e
60. b
61. d
62. b

CHAPTER 65

1. d
2. a, b, c, e
3. c, e
4. a, b, d, e
5. c
6. a
7. a, e
8. d
9. b
10. a
11. a, b, c, d, e
12. d, e
13. a, b, c, d
14. c
15. d
16. c

17. c, d, e
18. a, b, c, d
19. b, c, d, e, f
20. b
21. b
22. a
23. c
24. b
25. a, c, d
26. b, c, e
27. a, b
28. a
29. a, b, d
30. c
31. b
32. b
33. c
34. a, c, d
35. a
36. c
37. a. Decreases
    b. Increases
    c. Increases
38. a, d
39. b
40. b
41. d
42. b
43. b
44. d
45. d
46. d
47. d
48. a, d, f, h
49. c
50. b, c, e
51. a
52. a
53. c
54. b
55. b
56. d
57. b
58. a, b, c, d, e
59. a
60. a
61. a, c, d
62. b
63. d
64. d
65. a, b, c

CHAPTER 66

1. d
2. a
3. b
4. a
5. a
6. a
7. b

8. a
9. a
10. b
11. a
12. a
13. b
14. a
15. b
16. a
17. b
18. a
19. a
20. b
21. b
22. a
23. a
24. c
25. b
26. b
27. d
28. b
29. a
30. b
31. d
32. b
33. c
34. c
35. a, b, e
36. c
37. b
38. b
39. a, b, c, d
40. a, b, d, e
41. a, b
42. d
43. c
44. a
45. b
46. d
47. e
48. a
49. b
50. c
51. a, c, d
52. a
53. b
54. a, c, d, e
55. a, b, c, e
56. b, c, d, e, g, h
57. a, b, c, d, e
58. d
59. c, d
60. b
61. a, b, d, e
62. a, b, e
63. d
64. a
65. b
66. a
67. c

68. b
69. d
70. c
71. b
72. b
73. a
74. b
75. b
76. a
77. a
78. a, b, c
79. a, b, c, d, e
80. a, c
81. b
82. a, c, d

CHAPTER 67

1. c
2. b
3. a
4. c
5. b
6. a
7. c
8. b
9. b
10. a, b, d
11. c
12. d
13. d
14. c
15. c
16. a, b, d
17. b, c, d, e
18. a, b
19. a
20. c
21. d
22. c
23. c
24. b
25. a, c, d
26. a, b, d, e
27. d, e
28. a
29. b, c, e
30. b
31. a
32. b
33. d
34. c
35. c
36. b
37. c
38. b
39. d
40. c
41. d
42. 40 mL/hr
43. b, d, e

44. a
45. d
46. c
47. a
48. b
49. a
50. c
51. b
52. c
53. c
54. c, d, e
55. a, b, c, d, e
56. b
57. c
58. a
59. a, b, d, e
60. d
61. b
62. c
63. a
64. a
65. c, e, f
66. d
67. a, c, d, e, f
68. c
69. b
70. c
71. c
72. c
73. b
74. b, c, d, e
75. a, b, d
76. d
77. a. 2
    b. 1
    c. 3
    d. 4
    e. 6
    f. 7
    g. 5
78. b
79. d
80. d
81. a. 4
    b. 1
    c. 2
    d. 3
82. a
83. a
84. b
85. b
86. a

CHAPTER 68

1. e
2. b
3. f
4. i
5. g
6. b

7. glomerulus
8. a, c, e
9. b
10. erythropoietin
11. b
12. a, b, c
13. b
14. b
15. b
16. a
17. a
18. b
19. a
20. a
21. volume; composition; waste
22. acid-base
23. 20; 25
24. 125
25. pressure; flow
26. Antidiuretic hormone (ADH)
27. water
28. antidiuretic hormone (ADH)
29. reabsorption
30. b
31. c
32. c
33. a, b, e
34. c
35. d
36. c
37. b
38. b
39. d
40. b
41. b
42. d
43. b
44. a
45. a
46. d
47. b
48. d
49. a, d
50. e
51. h
52. k
53. m
54. a
55. d
56. g
57. i
58. l
59. j
60. f
61. c
62. b
63. b

64. a
65. a
66. a
67. c
68. c
69. b
70. c
71. a
72. c
73. b
74. c
75. a. 2
    b. 5
    c. 4
    d. 1
    e. 7
    f. 3
    g. 6
    h. 8
76. a
77. c
78. b
79. c
80. a
81. b
82. d
83. b
84. a
85. c
86. b
87. a, d, e, f

CHAPTER 69

1. b
2. f
3. a
4. h
5. c
6. k
7. d
8. j
9. g
10. i
11. l
12. e
13. a, e, g
14. b
15. cystitis
16. 50%
17. a
18. a
19. a, b, d
20. d
21. c
22. a
23. c
24. a
25. b
26. b
27. d

28. c
29. b, c, d, e
30. a
31. b
32. a
33. b
34. c
35. a
36. d
37. c
38. a
39. c
40. d
41. a
42. a, b, c, d, f
43. b
44. a
45. c
46. b
47. d
48. c
49. a
50. b
51. d
52. a
53. a
54. d
55. c
56. d
57. b
58. a
59. a, d, e
60. d
61. b
62. c
63. d
64. d
65. a
66. a, b, c, e, g
67. d
68. b
69. a
70. b
71. c
72. d
73. a
74. c
75. b
76. c
77. d
78. c
79. d
80. d

CHAPTER 70

1. b
2. a, c, e
3. b, c, d
4. a, b, c, d, g
5. d

6. c
7. a
8. a, b, d, e
9. b
10. c
11. c
12. c
13. c
14. d
15. a
16. a
17. a
18. b
19. c
20. a
21. a
22. a
23. b
24. b
25. a
26. b
27. b, d, e
28. a
29. c
30. a
31. c
32. b
33. b
34. b
35. c
36. c
37. c
38. c
39. a, c, d, e
40. a
41. b, c, d
42. b
43. obstruction
44. a, c, e
45. d
46. a
47. b
48. c
49. d
50. d
51. b
52. a
53. b
54. a
55. a
56. d
57. b
58. d
59. a
60. d
61. a, b, c, e, g, h
62. b
63. b, c, d, e
64. b
65. c

66. c
67. c, e
68. b
69. b
70. c
71. a
72. a
73. b, c, d, e
74. c
75. a
76. b
77. b, c, f, g
78. a
79. b
80. c
81. b
82. c
83. d
84. a, b, c, d, f, g
85. c
86. c

CHAPTER 71

1. b, c, d, e
2. a
3. b, d, e
4. a, b, d
5. b, c, e
6. b, d, e
7. stops
8. 50%
9. a
10. b
11. c
12. c
13. a
14. d
15. a, b, c
16. c
17. d
18. b
19. b
20. a
21. a, b, e
22. a
23. a, c, d, f
24. a
25. c
26. a, c, d, g, h
27. a
28. d
29. a
30. a, c, d, f
31. a
32. a
33. b, c
34. c
35. a
36. a
37. c

38. b
39. c
40. b, c
41. c
42. a
43. a
44. a, b, c
45. a
46. c
47. c
48. c
49. d
50. d
51. c
52. b
53. a
54. c
55. c
56. a
57. d
58. a
59. b
60. c
61. a
62. d
63. c
64. a, b, c, e, f
65. c
66. a
67. a, d, e, f
68. b
69. a
70. a, b, d, e, f
71. a, c, e
72. b
73. a
74. c
75. b
76. a, c, e
77. b
78. c
79. a, b, c
80. b
81. a, b, c, d, e, g
82. a, c, d, e
83. a
84. d
85. b
86. a
87. d
88. b
89. a
90. d
91. b, c, e
92. a
93. c
94. d
95. a. 2
    b. 1
    c. 3

96. c
97. e
98. a
99. c
100. b
101. d
102. f
103. a
104. b
105. b, c, d, e, g
106. c
107. a
108. c
109. b, c
110. b, c, d, e, f
111. d
112. c
113. b

CHAPTER 72

1. c
2. a
3. sperm
4. b
5. a, b, d
6. a, c, d, e
7. b, c, d, e
8. a, c, e
9. c, e
10. a, e
11. endometrial cancer
12. c
13. b
14. d
15. 3.5; 5
16. first
17. familial
18. tactile; psychogenic
19. movement; vaginal
20. high-fat
21. b, d, e
22. b, d
23. a
24. b
25. a, e
26. b
27. a, b, d, e
28. a, b, c, e
29. a, c, e
30. a, c, e
31. b
32. d
33. c
34. b
35. a
36. b, d, e
37. d
38. a
39. d
40. d

41. a, b, d, f
42. a
43. a
44. c
45. e
46. d
47. a
48. f
49. b
50. a
51. b, d
52. a, d, e
53. a
54. a, c, e, f
55. a, c, d
56. colposcopy

CHAPTER 73

1. h
2. e
3. a
4. b
5. f
6. g
7. c
8. d
9. c, e
10. c
11. c
12. b
13. a
14. b, e
15. b, c, e, f
16. d
17. b, c, d, e
18. c
19. a
20. b, c, e, f
21. c
22. fibrosis; cysts
23. regional lymph
24. bone; lungs; brain; liver
25. Fibroadenomas
26. estrogen
27. b, c, d
28. b
29. a
30. d
31. b
32. b
33. b
34. 40
35. c
36. d
37. c
38. d
39. a, c, d
40. c
41. b
42. d

43. a
44. d
45. a, b, d
46. reproductive
47. benign
48. b, c, d
49. b
50. a, c, d, e
51. breast cancer
52. a
53. d
54. b
55. d
56. d
57. a
58. c
59. a
60. b, c, e
61. b
62. d
63. b
64. b
65. b
66. c
67. a
68. b
69. c
70. a
71. a, b, d, f

CHAPTER 74

1. c
2. d
3. g
4. e
5. i
6. a
7. b
8. f
9. h
10. Pain
11. hormone
12. ectopic
13. progesterone
14. a, c, d, e
15. a, b, d, e
16. b
17. a, b, c, d, e
18. d
19. a
20. b, c, d, e
21. a, b, c, e
22. d
23. b
24. a, d, e
25. d
26. b
27. b
28. c, e
29. a, c, d, e

30. b
31. d
32. c
33. b
34. a, b, d
35. a
36. b, c, d, f
37. a
38. a, b, c
39. b
40. a
41. a
42. a, b, d, e
43. b
44. c
45. a
46. e
47. b
48. d
49. b
50. b
51. a
52. c
53. d
54. postmenopausal
55. White or Caucasian
56. b
57. b, c, e
58. c
59. b, d, e
60. a
61. a, e
62. a, c, e
63. a
64. c
65. b
66. b
67. a
68. c
69. d
70. a
71. a, c, d
72. c
73. a, b, d
74. b, c, e
75. c

CHAPTER 75

1. slowest; predictable
2. 50
3. family
4. b, d
5. a
6. b, c, e
7. a, d, e
8. c
9. d
10. a
11. a
12. a, b, c, e

13.	c	47.	a	3.	a	35.	d
14.	a	48.	a	4.	d	36.	b
15.	d	49.	c	5.	a	37.	f
16.	c	50.	c	6.	c	38.	a
17.	i	51.	b	7.	c	39.	c
18.	b	52.	a	8.	a	40.	k
19.	e	53.	c	9.	b	41.	b
20.	j	54.	a, b, d	10.	a, c, d, e	42.	h
21.	f	55.	a	11.	c	43.	j
22.	g	56.	b	12.	pelvic inflammatory dis-	44.	i
23.	c	57.	c		ease	45.	d
24.	a	58.	b	13.	a	46.	c, d, e
25.	h	59.	d	14.	b, e	47.	b
26.	d	60.	d	15.	a	48.	a
27.	a, c, d	61.	c	16.	Centers for Disease Con-	49.	c
28.	c	62.	a, b, d, f		trol and Prevention (CDC)	50.	a
29.	b	63.	b	17.	a, b, c	51.	d
30.	b	64.	a	18.	increase	52.	c
31.	a, c, d, e, g	65.	a, c, d	19.	d	53.	d
32.	d	66.	a	20.	c	54.	d
33.	d	67.	a	21.	a	55.	b
34.	b	68.	c, d, e, f, g	22.	b	56.	b
35.	a	69.	b	23.	a	57.	c
36.	a	70.	a, c, d, e	24.	b	58.	a, b, c, e
37.	b	71.	d	25.	d	59.	a
38.	b	72.	b	26.	c	60.	a, b, e
39.	a	73.	a, b, c, f	27.	b	61.	c
40.	e	74.	a	28.	c	62.	b
41.	d	75.	b, c, e	29.	b	63.	c
42.	c	76.	b, c, e	30.	d	64.	c, d, e, g
43.	a, b, e			31.	b, c, d	65.	b
44.	a			32.	c	66.	a
45.	d	**CHAPTER 76**		33.	a		
46.	d	1.	a	34.	c		
		2.	d				